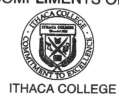

P9-CEJ-288

Cardiopulmonary Rehabilitation: Basic Theory and Application

Third Edition

Contemporary Perspectives in Rehabilitation

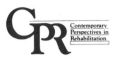

Steven L. Wolf, PhD, FAPTA
Editor-in-Chief

PUBLISHED VOLUMES

Pharmacology in Rehabilitation, 2nd Edition

Charles D. Ciccone, PhD, PT

Dynamics of Human Biologic Tissues

Dean P. Currier, PhD, PT, and Roger M. Nelson, PhD, PT

The Biomechanics of the Foot and Ankle, 2nd Edition

Robert A. Donatelli, PhD, PT, OCS

Electrotherapy in Rehabilitation

Meryl Roth Gersh, MMSc, PT

Rehabilitation of the Knee: A Problem-Solving Approach

Bruce H. Greenfield, MMSc, PT

Vestibular Rehabilitation

Susan J. Herdman, PhD, PT

Wound Healing: Alternatives in Management, 2nd Edition

Joseph M. McCulloch, PhD, PT, Luther C. Kloth, MS, PT, and Jeffrey A. Feedar, PT

Fundamentals of Orthopedic Radiology

Lynn N. McKinnis, PT, OCS

Thermal Agents in Rehabilitation, 3rd Edition

Susan L. Michlovitz, MS, PT, CHT

Burn Care and Rehabilitation: Principles and Practice

Reginald L. Richard, MS, PT, and Marlys J. Staley, MS, PT

Concepts in Hand Rehabilitation

Barbara G. Stanley, PT, CHT, and Susan M. Tribuzi, OTR, CHT

Cardiopulmonary Rehabilitation: Basic Theory and Application

Third Edition

Frances J. Brannon, PhD
Professor and Coordinator of
Exercise Science
Department of Physical Education
Slippery Rock University
Slippery Rock, Pennsylvania

Margaret Wiley Foley, RN, MN
Previously Affiliated:
St. Joseph's Hospital
Atlanta, Georgia

Julie Ann Starr, MS, PT, CCS
Clinical Assistant Professor
Department of Physical Therapy
Sargent College of Health and Rehabilitation Sciences
Boston University
Boston, Massachusetts

Physical Therapist II
Beth Israel Deaconess Medical Center
Boston, Massachusetts

Lauren M. Saul, RN, MSN
Cardiovascular Clinical Nurse Specialist
Shadyside Hospital
Pittsburgh, Pennsylvania

 F. A. DAVIS COMPANY • Philadelphia

F. A. Davis Company
1915 Arch Street
Philadelphia, PA 19103

Printed in the United States of America

Last digit indicates print number: 10 9 8 7 6

Publisher, Health Professions: Jean-François Vilain
Developmental Editor: Marianne Fithian
Production Editor: Michael Schnee
Cover Designer: Louis J. Forgione

As new scientific information becomes available through basic and clinical research, recommended treatments and drug therapies undergo changes. The authors and publisher have done everything possible to make this book accurate, up to date, and in accord with accepted standards at the time of publication. The authors, editors, and publisher are not responsible for errors or omissions or for consequences from application of the book, and make no warranty, expressed or implied, in regard to the contents of the book. Any practice described in this book should be applied by the reader in accordance with professional standards of care used in regard to the unique circumstances that may apply in each situation. The reader is advised always to check product information (package inserts) for changes and new information regarding dose and contraindications before administering any drug. Caution is especially urged when using new or infrequently ordered drugs.

Library of Congress Cataloging-in-Publication Data

Cardiopulmonary rehabilitation : basic theory and application /
    Frances J. Brannon . . . [et al.].—3rd ed.
        p.   cm.—(Contemporary perspectives in rehabilitation.)
    Previous ed. cataloged under Brannon.
    Includes bibliographical references and index.
    ISBN 0-8036-0318-5 (hc)
        1. Cardiopulmonary system—Diseases—Patients—Rehabilitation.
    2. Cardiopulmonary system—Diseases—Exercise therapy.   I. Brannon,
    Frances J., 1935–   . II. Series.
    RC702.C383   1997
    616.1′206—dc21   97-24298
                                                            CIP

To the memory of my nephew, Charlie Stephens, Jr., to his wife, Sue, to his daughter Savanna, and to his daughter and my pal, Miika, who struggles to recover from surgery to remove a benign brain tumor.
Frances J. Brannon

To my family—Terry, Allison, and Sean—with love and appreciation. And to Chuck Kesler—in his memory.
Margaret W. Foley

To my family—George, Jillian, Jana, and Adam—for their support, assistance, and patience, and to my Mom and Dad, who taught me to finish what I start.
Julie Ann Starr

To the Lord—who is the great Author of Life.
Lauren M. Saul

Foreword

When a text has successfully fulfilled its intent, one is hard-pressed to justify modest changes, let alone profound ones. The first two editions of *Cardiac Rehabilitation: Basic Theory and Application* have been well received by practitioners and students. The notoriety achieved with the first edition favorably impacted on the second edition. At the time, it was felt that inclusion of sections addressing pulmonary function and rehabilitation would strengthen the text even further. The popular sections of ECG interpretation and case histories were expanded and all references were updated.

Then what could possibly be added? Fortunately, the collective wisdom of Frances Brannon, Margaret Foley, Julie Starr, and Lauren Saul saw changes in cultural attitudes in health and changing patterns of treatment. Consequently, they have taken these issues into consideration and, as a result, have provided a Preface that succinctly defines the refinements in this edition and the rationale underlying their inclusion. Teachers, students, and clinicians should note the emphasis placed on functional outcomes and their measurement. This consideration is essential to justify reimbursement for treating even the most obvious of diagnoses. Complementing this emphasis is the presentation of new material on imaging techniques, surgical interventions, and new pharmacological management strategies.

As Editor-in-Chief of this series on *Contemporary Perspectives in Rehabilitation,* and as a firm believer in the role of behavioral management and monitoring as an essential adjunct to all forms of physiotherapeutic interventions, I am particularly impressed with the sensitivity shown toward involvement of patients in planning outcomes and in assuming responsibility for aspects of health care (dietary intake, smoking cessation, hypertension). Clearly, more responsibility for all aspects of physiological homeostasis, particularly that affecting the cardiac and pulmonary systems, continues to be relegated toward the patient. In this regard, this new text emphasizes this point and serves as a model by which students can become indoctrinated into assisting their patients to become active participants in choices that can profoundly affect their lives.

If ever we can stress the "contemporary" aspect of this series, the third edition of *Cardiopulmonary Rehabilitation: Basic Theory and Application* is a blueprint for so doing. I daresay that few texts on this subject can more adequately provoke thought processes or can better challenge critical analytic skills of a readership committed to the study of optimizing cardiac and pulmonary capabilities.

Steven L. Wolf, Ph.D., FAPTA
Series Editor

Preface to the Third Edition

Although extensive revisions have been made to the third edition of *Cardiopulmonary Rehabilitation: Basic Theory and Application,* a major goal of the text remains. It continues to provide students and practicing clinicians with information necessary to develop their decision-making skills to provide comprehensive and quality rehabilitation programs for cardiac and pulmonary patients. A major strength of the text continues to be the presentation of case studies that reinforce and illustrate problem-solving techniques and provide guidance for the clinician in the practical application of current theoretical concepts vital to quality cardiopulmonary rehabilitation programs. References in all chapters have been updated and extensive revisions have been made to incorporate the current theories, practices, and procedures used in formulating patient goals, evaluations, and measurement of outcomes.

Chapter 1 presents an overview of cardiac and pulmonary rehabilitation programs and redefines the recovery phases of cardiac rehabilitation from the traditional three phases (inpatient, outpatient, and community) to include four phases: inpatient, immediate outpatient, intermediate outpatient, and maintenance outpatient. Progression of the patient through each of the four phases is presented in terms of patient goals, patient evaluations, and measurement of patient outcomes. An overview of pulmonary rehabilitation programs includes a discussion of inpatient acute and outpatient chronic phases of pulmonary rehabilitation. As with cardiac rehabilitation, the primary goal of pulmonary rehabilitation is to increase the functional capacity of patients and to assist them in attaining normal function, insofar as possible, in their daily lives.

Extensive revisions in Chapter 5, "Pathophysiology of Coronary Artery Disease," include current information of the pathogenesis of atherosclerosis, and a new section on the lipid-insudation hypothesis has been added. The discussion of angina has been expanded to include new information on asymptomatic (silent) angina, and more detailed presentations of history and current symptoms of myocardial infarction and thrombolytic therapy have been included.

The information in Chapter 7, "The Medical and Surgical Management of Cardiopulmonary Disease," has been extensively updated and new medications and their uses have been included. The discussion on drug therapy has been expanded to include anisoylated plasminogen streptokinase activator, aspirin, ticlopidine, heparin, abciximab, and warfarin. New sections on surgical interventions in coronary artery disease include discussions of directional coronary atherectomy, laser angioplasty, coronary stents, coronary artery bypass graft surgery without cardiopulmonary bypass, and dynamic cardiac myoplasty. Surgical interventions in pulmonary disease include tumor resection, bullae resection, pneumectomy, and lung transplantation.

Chapter 9, "Assessment of the Cardiac Patient," has been revised, and information on body mass index, waist-to-hip ratio, ramping tests, and assessment of functional outcomes has been added. The addition of a new section on advances in cardio-vascular testing technology include radionuclide imaging as it relates to myocardial perfusion imaging, assessment of ventricular function, and pharmacologic stress perfusion imaging. Discussions on echocardiography and coronary angiography are also new additions to the third edition.

In Chapters 11 and 12, current information and guidelines for the exercise prescription and the exercise therapy sessions have been included. Additions to Chapter 12 include guidelines to assist the clinician in exercise prescription and programming for the patient with chronic heart failure (CHF) and for patients with cardiac transplantation. Psychosocial variables, quality-of-life issues, and outcomes are also discussed.

Revisions to Chapter 13, "Risk Factor Modification," present new approaches to assist the patient in smoking cessation, and include pharmacologic intervention, behavioral instruction, techniques for behavioral modification, and measurement of smoking outcomes. The pharmacologic treatment of hypertension has been revised, and treatment algorithms are presented in accordance with the *Fifth Report of the Joint National Committee on Detection, Evaluation, and Treatment of High Blood Pressure (1995)*. Dietary recommendations for treatment of high blood cholesterol have been revised and pharmacologic therapy presented according to the recommendations of the *Second Report of the Expert Panel on Detection, Evaluation, and Treatment of High Blood Cholesterol in Adults (1993)*. Measurement of outcomes in management of hypertension and lipid levels is also discussed.

A new addition to Chapter 14 is a section on self-administered secretion removal techniques. This section discusses the VRP1, positive expiratory pressure (PEP) masks, and autogenic drainage.

We hope that the practical nature of this edition will continue to serve those educators responsible for disseminating information to future clinicians. We also hope that this text will assist practicing clinicians in their decisions so that they may provide comprehensive and quality rehabilitation programs for the cardiopulmonary patient.

FJB
MWF
JAS
LMS

Acknowledgments

For the variety of ways in which they made the writing of this edition easier, we would like to thank the following:

My family, who have always encouraged and supported me, and with whom I have had countless good times—a special thanks to Marjorie B. Stephens and Dee; Elise, Clovis, Joan, John, and Kaye Faltot; Patricia and Leonard Pike; Emma, Alan, Diane, and Ann Armstrong; Robert and Linda Fox; and Jean and Pete Sawchuck. My friends, who help whenever needed—especially those at the "Round Table" at Slippery Rock University. I also express my appreciation to Slippery Rock University for awarding me a sabbatical leave, which gave me precious time to write. My gratitude also extends to my co-authors, Peggy Foley, Julie Starr, and Lauren Saul, not only for their cooperation with this edition but also for their concern and compassion for me and my family. Acknowledgments would be incomplete without thanking Jean-François Vilain for his continued support and encouragement in the writing of this text.

FJB

To my husband, Terry—thank you for encouraging me to stay with this edition and for your unending enthusiasm and many, many hours of work as it came together. To Allison and Sean—thank you for your patience and thousands of smiles. To my family and friends, whose encouragement for my completing "the book" never faltered and to my computer-literate neighbors—Jon Barton and Judy Abraham, I couldn't have gotten there without you. Thanks! To Lauren Saul, a co-author and friend—thanks for joining us and adding your expertise to this project. And many, thanks to Dr. Frances Brannon, my co-author and friend, for sparking my interest in cardiac rehabilitation so many years ago and for all her help through the three editions of this text!

MWF

I would like to thank George B. Coggeshall, Jr., for his support, expertise, and enthusiasm for this project. I also want to acknowledge the patience of my ever-delightful trio: Jillian, Jana, and Adam. Although they lost a Mom and a playmate for a while—I'm back! A special thanks to Rick and Joyce for providing technical support when I really needed it. And a final thanks to Jean-François Vilain and Frances Brannon for their faith that we could get this job done.

JAS

Many thanks to my parents, siblings, and friends, who were a great support to me throughout this new and, sometimes, rigorous adventure. To John Schlicht, PharmD, who generously offered his expertise and wisdom in the myriad of cardiac drugs. To the gracious gentlemen in the MIS Department at Shadyside Hospital, who lent me a laptop, allowing me to "keyboard away" on weekends. To the Librarians at Shadyside Hospital and to Ray Tate, who cajoled me with political banter as we journal-searched and photocopied. To Peggy Wiley Foley, my first graduate student, who remembered me, encouraged me, and empathized with me during late-night phone calls. And finally, to Fran Brannon, who displayed much grace under pressure and gentle encouragement throughout.

LMS

Preface to the Second Edition

The first edition of this text, *Cardiac Rehabilitation: Basic Theory and Application*, was an attempt to give students and practicing clinicians information necessary to develop their decision-making skills so as to provide comprehensive and quality rehabilitation programs for cardiac patients. Practical application of theoretical concepts based on current research was emphasized, with a particular strength of the text being the presentation of case studies to reinforce and illustrate problem-solving techniques.

The second edition follows the practical approach of the first, but the scope of the second edition has been broadened to include knowledges, and applications of those knowledges, necessary to provide quality rehabilitation programs for the pulmonary patient. The title of the text has, therefore, been changed to *Cardiopulmonary Rehabilitation: Basic Theory and Application.*

All chapters have been updated, and four new chapters have been added that specifically address the rehabilitation of the pulmonary patient. Chapter 3 presents the anatomy and physiology of respiration; Chapter 6 discusses the pathophysiology of COPD; Chapter 10 addresses the assessment of the pulmonary patient; and Chapter 14, "Additional Components of Pulmonary Rehabilitation," presents skills and techniques of pulmonary rehabilitation that are not commonly encountered in programs designed primarily for the cardiac patient.

Extensive revisions have been made in Chapters 11, 12, and 13 to reflect the current theories, practices, and procedures used in exercise prescription and programming for cardiopulmonary patients.

We hope that the practical nature of this text will continue to serve those educators responsible for disseminating information to future clinicians. The text was also written to assist practicing clinicians who are responsible for providing quality care in the rehabilitation of the cardiopulmonary patient.

FJB
MWF
JAS

Contents

CHAPTER 1

Cardiopulmonary Rehabilitation: Overview

HISTORICAL PERSPECTIVE OF CORONARY HEART DISEASE

During the early part of the twentieth century, standard treatment for patients with diagnosed myocardial infarction included 2 months of bed rest.[1] By the late 1940s and early 1950s, ambulation was begun within 14 days of an acute episode and by the 1960s, a 3-week hospitalization was the standard practice following an acute myocardial infarction (AMI).[2,3] As more health professionals became interested in early ambulation and its beneficial effects, early ambulation was transformed into what we currently know as inpatient cardiac rehabilitation,[4,5] and outpatient cardiac rehabilitation programs soon followed.[6–8] Despite the recent advances in technology and new treatment regimens for coronary heart disease (CHD) and the fact that the rate of deaths from CHD has decreased during the past 30 years, CHD remains the leading cause of premature death and disability in the United States and coronary artery disease (CAD) is the major factor in deaths caused by CHD.[9,10]

The decline in mortality caused by CHD during the past 3 decades has been attributed to the American public's lifestyle changes and awareness of primary and secondary prevention procedures. Primary prevention is based on adoption of lifestyle changes to prevent the onset of cardiovascular disease. Secondary prevention uses current techniques to restore, maintain, or improve a patient's status after a diagnosis of cardiovascular disease has been made.[11,12] High-technology care has increased the survival rate of patients with acute cardiac disease, but it has also increased the costs of medical care.[11] In an effort to reduce health care costs, emphasis is being placed not only on primary and secondary prevention but also on managed health care.[11,12] The length of time a patient spends in the acute-care setting (hospital) has decreased and secondary prevention services have been shown to be cost-effective and to reduce the rate of death and disability.[11,12] Cardiac rehabilitation programs have a history of providing secondary preventive care and outpatient cardiac rehabilitation has been shown to be cost-effective and to reduce hospital readmissions by 62 percent. In addition to cost-effectiveness, positive outcomes of cardiac rehabilitation programs include increased functional capacity and quality of life, improved coronary risk profile, and decreased cardiac symptoms.[13,14]

Primary and secondary prevention programs for CHD emphasize modification of cardiovascular disease risk factors through positive lifestyle changes. Elevated blood pressure, increased plasma lipids and blood sugar, cigarette smoking, physical inactivity, obesity, and psychosocial factors have all been shown to increase the risk for CHD.[15-29] Current research indicates that positive lifestyle changes that modify the risk of CHD have reduced the rates of mortality and morbidity and are important behavioral approaches to the primary and secondary prevention of CHD.[9,11,16–18,22,28,30–33] Increasing evidence supports the concept that regular physical activity, decreases in plasma lipids, maintenance of appropriate body weight, cessation of smoking, and controlling blood pressure not only are important factors in primary and secondary prevention, but are also useful interventions that may promote the regression of CHD and prolong life.[18,24,27,31,33–43] Therefore quality primary and secondary prevention programs must provide not only exercise training but also guidance in the multifaceted area of risk-factor modification.[44,45]

Comprehensive cardiac rehabilitation programs require personnel who can provide interventions for restoring functional capacity, reducing risk factors, and promoting positive psychosocial behavioral changes that lead to maintenance of health and social independence.[44] The specialized skills of several professionals working as a team may be required to provide effective rehabilitation services to the cardiac patient. These professionals include nurses, exercise physiologists, nutritionists, mental health professionals, physical and occupational therapists, health educators, vocational rehabilitation counselors, and other health and education specialists. Under the supervision of a physician, these health care specialists provide primary care to cardiac rehabilitation patients and offer the broad range of services that characterize a comprehensive program, including supervised exercise training, patient education, counseling, and instruction in nutrition.[44–48]

The delivery of health care services through systems of managed care is rapidly becoming the standard for health care in this country. Managed care plans (e.g., health maintenance and preferred provider organizations) organize services for their members and emphasize cost-effective prevention and care of disease. Although providers of managed care and other third-party payers (e.g., Blue Cross, Medicare) have no control over the way in which services such as cardiac rehabilitation are provided, they influence health care delivery by specifying the health care services for which insurance reimbursement will be made. It is important for the survival of cardiac rehabilitation that program personnel evaluate and measure the outcomes of intervention strategies so that information is obtained on mortality, morbidity, quality of life, and the impact of rehabilitation on health, clinical status, and patient behavioral changes.[49,50] Outcomes for evaluation following cardiac rehabilitation programs include information on survival, return to work, risk-factor changes, improvement in exercise capacity, improved quality-of-life issues, education, and psychosocial adjustment. Data must be collected and the outcomes in these areas measured for all cardiac rehabilitation programs to evaluate their efficacy, not only to provide information for their improvement but for accreditation purposes and reimbursement considerations.[5,13,47,49–53]

Issues affecting cardiac rehabilitation programs include not only managed care, cost containment, evaluation of outcomes, efficacy, personnel, and the like, but also changes in the structure of cardiac rehabilitation programs. The recovery phases of rehabilitation have been redefined from the traditional three phases (inpatient, outpatient, and community-based) to include four phases: inpatient, immediate outpatient, intermediate outpatient, and maintenance outpatient.[54] After a brief discussion of the inpatient phase, the major focus of this text will be to provide the basic theory of outpatient cardiac rehabilitation and the practical application of that theory so that health care professionals who care for patients in Phases II and III outpatient rehabilitation may gain sufficient information to function optimally.

INPATIENT CARDIAC REHABILITATION

Phase I, the inpatient phase of cardiac rehabilitation, begins in the hospital, as soon after an acute cardiac event as possible. Candidates for inpatient rehabilitation include those having had myocardial infarctions (MI), coronary artery bypass grafts (CABG), percutaneous transluminal coronary angioplasty (PTCA), compensated heart failure, dilated cardiomyopathy, controlled arrhythmias, organ transplantation, postvalve repair, peripheral artery disease (PAD), and patients with other chronic diseases.[54] The inpatient program, like all rehabilitation programs, should be individualized, and there is no specific length of time for inpatient rehabilitation because cost-containment issues dictate that patients be progressed through intervention, recovery, and discharge in as little time as possible.[50,54]

The goals of inpatient cardiac rehabilitation include:

1. Providing appropriate medical care
2. Preventing the deleterious effects of bed rest through physical activity
3. Assessing the hemodynamic response to exercise
4. Managing the psychosocial issues of cardiac disease
5. Educating the patient and family[54–57]

Phase I rehabilitation begins with the physician referral and initial consultation, which includes information regarding age, diagnosis, laboratory and other test results, medical and/or surgical history, patient interview, physical examination, and overall assessment of the patient. Once the assessment of the patient has been completed and the patient is deemed medically stable, the inpatient program may commence. Components of Phase I, which may begin as early as day 1 of hospitalization, include low-level exercise, patient and family education, group and individual counseling, and group discussions. The length of the inpatient rehabilitation depends on patient progress and risk for further cardiovascular events, but the current emphasis on early discharge has resulted in hospital dismissal in as few as 3 days after uncomplicated cardiovascular conditions.[58] Many patients are hospitalized for 5 to 7 days and Phase I cardiac rehabilitation is therefore limited to only a few days.[59,60]

Inpatient exercise is usually begun at a low intensity, that is, 1 to 2 metabolic equivalents (METs). (One MET is the amount of oxygen consumed at rest and is equal to approximately 3.5 milliliters of oxygen per kilogram of body weight per minute.) The types of exercise prescribed include active assisted or active range-of-motion activities, ambulation, and self-care. These are usually performed at least twice a day under the supervision of a health professional trained in assessing the patient's response, and may also be monitored by ECG. Exercise intensity is gradually increased to 2 to 3 METs. The major exercise in inpatient rehabilitation is walking. According to patient response, gradual increases in pace and distance are encouraged and should be performed several times a day under supervision.[55,56]

Exercise intensity during Phase I cardiac rehabilitation is usually prescribed according to heart rate and by using the Borg rating of perceived exertion. The training heart rate prescribed is either (1) a low-level fixed heart rate at approximately 120 beats per minute (not appropriate for all patients) or (2) the patient's standing heart rate plus 10 to 20 beats per minute (usually appropriate for most patients). Patients should try to achieve levels that are classified as "light" in intensity on the Borg scale.[55,56] Blood pressures should also be measured before and after exercise. Systolic blood pressure should not usually rise more than 20 mm Hg or fall more than 10 to 15 mm Hg. Systolic blood pressures in excess of 180 mm Hg and diastolic pressures above 110 mm Hg with low-intensity activity usually warrant antihypertensive therapy.[5,55,56] Table 1-1 illustrates activities and progressions that have been used in inpatient rehabilitation programs to help patients achieve functional capacities that permit self-care.

TABLE 1-1 Mayo Clinic Inpatient Cardiac Rehabilitation Physical Activity Protocol

| Stage | Days of Program | | | Activity Schedule |
	6-day plan	9-day plan	12-day plan	
I	1	1	1	Use bedside commode. Begin physical therapy range-of-motion exercises to each extremity. Sit at side of bed 5-10 min.
		2	2	Sit in chair 5-15 min twice daily. Begin education program at bedside. Continue physical therapy as above.
	2	3	3	Sit in chair up to 30 min twice daily. Continue physical therapy as above.
II	3	4	5	Move to step-down area. Bathe above waist, shave, and comb hair. Begin self-exercise program with appropriate supervision. Sit in chair 60-120 min twice daily.
		5	7	Continue self-exercise program with appropriate supervision. Begin ambulation with exercise therapist. Sit in chair 90-150 min twice daily. Begin attending education classes and discussion groups.
		6	8	Take wheelchair shower and use bathroom ad lib. Continue physical activity as above.
III	4	7	9	Move to general cardiovascular ward. Dress in street clothes if desired. Be up and around room as tolerated. Begin climbing stairs with therapist.
	5	8	11	Take predismissal graded-exercise test. Continue physical activity as above. Take standing shower.
	6	9	12	Receive final going-home instructions.

Source: Adapted from Squires, RW, et al. Cardiovascular rehabilitation. Status, 1990. Mayo Clin Proc 65: 731-755, 1990. Used by permission.

Before discharge from the hospital, a low-level exercise test should be administered. The exercise test begins at a low intensity and is often terminated:

1. At a heart rate of 120 to 130 beats per minute
2. At 70 percent of age-predicted maximum heart rate
3. To a termination point of 5 to 6 METs
4. To a symptom-limited end point[56,58]

The benefits of a predischarge exercise test include identification of patients at high risk (risk stratification, see Chapter 11), those in need of further intervention and definition of safely tolerated activity levels, which is important for further rehabilitation.[5,56,60] Discharge instructions to the patient should include guidelines for daily physical activity, information regarding medications, signs and symptoms of heart-related problems, and a discussion of the patient's emotional feelings. As part of the discharge plan, patients should be referred to an appropriate outpatient rehabilitation program, which should begin within 2 weeks after hospital discharge.[54] A major outcome to be achieved during inpatient cardiac rehabilitation is that patients will improve in functional capacity and become fully ambulatory.[51]

OUTPATIENT CARDIAC REHABILITATION PROGRAMS

Immediate Outpatient Program

The immediate outpatient cardiac rehabilitation program (Phase II) begins immediately after hospitalization and usually lasts from 2 to 12 weeks.[58] The length of this stage of rehabilitation is partly determined by risk stratification (see Chapter 11), individual patient need for supervision and intensive monitoring, and managed-care or other insurance-reimbursement policies. During Phase II cardiac rehabilitation, there is a greater degree of supervision and more ECG monitoring (by either telemetry or hard wire), and greater attention is given to risk-factor modification. Supervision during Phase II includes education of the patient in self-assessment as to symptoms and compliance with medications. Frequent measurements of blood pressures, body weights, heart rates, and perceived exertions are obtained and recorded.[54]

The major goals of Phase II are:

1. To increase the patient's functional capacity through an individualized exercise program and to teach safe activity guidelines
2. To educate the patient as to risk-factor modification, including smoking cessation, stress reduction, weight control, reduction in plasma cholesterol, and instruction in dietary guidelines
3. To educate the patient regarding medications, signs and symptoms of heart disease and its progression, and sexual activities
4. To promote psychological, behavioral, and educational improvement[31,60]

Each patient entering into Phase II cardiac programs must have physician approval and an initial assessment. The initial assessment should include a medical history, a patient-family interview, a physical examination, an exercise stress test, a blood chemistry panel, a description of current symptoms, nutritional and body composition analyses, a stratification of risk, and notations of physical limitations and disabilities.[54,60] Because of the individualized nature of Phase II cardiac rehabilitation and the amount of supervision required, a minimum staff-to-patient ratio of 1:5 is necessary. A second person should be immediately available in case of emergency.[61]

Frequency of visits for patients in Phase II cardiac rehabilitation is usually 2 or 3 times a week and length of stay in the program varies. A recent national survey indicated that, in the programs that stratify their patients according to risk, low-risk patients attended outpatient programs an average of 5.6 weeks, moderate-risk patients averaged 7.8 weeks, and high-risk patients were in the program for an average of 10 weeks. For those programs that did not stratify their patients, the length of the outpatient program was 8 to 12 weeks.[62] Although it is difficult to say exactly how long a patient will remain in Phase II cardiac rehabilitation, patients are progressed to Phase III cardiac rehabilitation programs only when they are determined to be clinically stable, can demonstrate independence in performing self-monitoring techniques (especially during their physical activities), and no longer require intensive ECG monitoring.[54,60]

Intermediate Outpatient Cardiac Rehabilitation

Intermediate outpatient cardiac rehabilitation (Phase III) is a continuation of the Phase II program and usually lasts 6 to 8 weeks beyond Phase II.[60] It begins when the patient is stabilized and no longer needs frequent ECG monitoring. Exercise training and risk-factor modification continue to be the major focus of Phase III cardiac rehabilitation.[54] Interventions are designed to prevent or delay the progression of the disease and to restore optimal physical, psychological, emotional, social, and vocational function. A comprehensive, individualized approach to Phase III cardiac rehabilitation that includes physical activity; patient and family education; and psychosocial, nutritional, and vocational counseling is important.[63]

Most Phase III patients meet once a week in a formal program and continue progression in their exercise training, which usually includes light weight training. Patients and their families attend weekly education classes on risk-factor modification and various topics about heart disease.[60] The staff-to-patient ratio is a minimum of 1:15, and at least one person who is certified in advanced cardiac life support (ACLS) and has the medical and legal authority to provide such care must be present if the supervised program is provided for high- and intermediate-risk patients. The staff members continue to monitor heart rates, blood pressures, weight, and symptoms.[61] When the staff and the patient feel it is prudent, the patient advances to Phase IV cardiac rehabilitation.

Maintenance Outpatient Cardiac Rehabilitation

Maintenance outpatient cardiac rehabilitation (Phase IV) begins when the patient can maintain the outcomes achieved during Phases II and III. These outcomes include survival, attainment of optimal functional capacity, return to work, smoking cessation and other risk-factor changes, and attainment of positive psychosocial and quality-of-life issues.[64] A goal of maintenance cardiac rehabilitation is that patients continue indefinitely with their exercise and educational programs, either in a formal setting or on their own. Phase IV cardiac rehabilitation can occur in the hospital, in a community-based organization, or at home. The patient in Phase IV can self-monitor at rest and during exercise, and blood pressures and heart rates are noted and recorded. Follow-up exercise tests are recommended every 6 to 12 months so that the patient and the physician can note the progress of functional capacity and reduction of risk factors.[60]

As patients move through the various stages of outpatient rehabilitation (from Phase II to III to IV), at each stage they should go through a discharge procedure, which includes:

1. A summary of accomplishments in physical activity, management of risk factors, emotional issues, and return to work
2. A summary of goals that need to be achieved
3. Guidelines for daily exercise and other activities
4. Information on all medications
5. Information on signs and symptoms of heart-related problems
6. Recommendations for check-ups and visits with their primary physicians[54]

MEASUREMENT OF PATIENT OUTCOMES

As patients progress through the four phases of recovery, assessments are made for entry into each phase and each patient is stratified according to risk (see Chapter 11). On the basis of the results of these assessments, an individualized program is prescribed for each patient, including exercise and educational and behavioral modification.[54] Program plans with expected goals and outcomes should be developed for each patient at each stage of cardiac rehabilitation. Documentation of patients' progress will enable the rehabilitation staff to continually evaluate exercise and educational and behavioral changes and establish new patient goals in a timely manner. Table 1–2 illustrates the parameters that might be addressed in the evaluation of the patient, the program from which a patient may benefit, and the expected outcomes from the individualized program plan.[64]

Evaluation of patient outcomes by the rehabilitation staff will provide information for program evaluation, which is required for accreditation of rehabilitation programs by the Joint Commission on Accreditation of Healthcare Organizations (JCAHO) and Medicare.[64] The best method of showing the effectiveness of cardiac rehabilitation is through outcome results that show patient improvement in behavior, functional capacity, and psychosocial status.[64] An example of the data to be collected for assessment of patient outcomes can be found in Table 1–3. The rapidly changing health care delivery system should prove challenging for cardiac rehabilitation professionals. It has been estimated that, by the year 2000, 55 percent of all cardiovascular procedures will be performed on an outpatient basis and cardiac rehabilitation programs are likely to increase in number and in availability to patients.[64] The cardiac rehabilitation staff must be competent in the ability to prescribe appropriate exercise and provide education that is successful in risk-factor modification and psychosocial interventions. These competencies are essential in the primary and secondary prevention of CHD.

TABLE 1–2 Design for Patient Assessment, Recommended Program,
and Expected Outcome Measures

Patient Assessment and Profile	Educational Needs	Expected Outcomes
Recent open chest or heart surgery (CABG, valve, AICD)	Disease process, treatment, recovery, activity guidelines, risk factors, sexual activity, medications, and return to work	Return to self-care activities; knowledge of medications; activity progression; risk factor modification
Recent diagnosis of CAD/MI or its treatment or sequelae, e.g., cath, PTCA, atherectomy, stent, CHF, dysrhythmia	Disease process, signs and symptoms, treatment options, risk factors, activity guidelines, sexual activity, medications, and return to work	Return to self-care activities; knowledge of activity progression, recognition and treatment of angina, risk factor modification
Reduced activity level, decreased functional capacity, or sedentary lifestyle	Individualized exercise program based on risk stratification: • monitored • unmonitored, supervised • home exercise program and education	Increase in activity level and functional capacity; attainment of an improved level of fitness and regular exercise participation
Tobacco use or abuse	Smoking cessation program	Reduction or smoking cessation
Blood lipid and/or lipoprotein abnormality (confirmed by repeat measurement)	Dietary lipid/modification and medical intervention program in accordance with NCEP (2nd report) guidelines. Weight-reduction and exercise program when appropriate	Progress toward or attainment of appropriate blood lipid and lipoprotein levels as set forth in the NCEP guidelines
High blood pressure (confirmed by repeat measurement)	Blood-pressure management program including medical intervention and education in accordance with the NHBPEP guidelines: weight reduction, dietary modification, stress management, and/or exercise programs when appropriate	Decreased blood pressure or attainment of appropriate blood pressure as set forth in the NHBPEP guidelines and reduction or elimination of blood-pressure medication
Excess body weight or relative fatness as determined by scale, body mass index, skinfold calipers, or hydrostatic weighting	Dietary weight reduction program and/or exercise program in accordance with the American Dietetic Association (ADA) guidelines	Reduction in body weight and fat stores; attainment of desirable body weight
High stress levels and/or inappropriate response to stress as determined by patient/family report, stress assessment tools, or psychological evaluation	Stress-management program. Coping and relaxation techniques	Reduction in stress and/or increase of appropriate responses to stress

Source: Reprinted by permission from American Association of Cardiovascular Pulmonary Rehabilitation, 1995, Guidelines for Cardiac Rehabilitation Programs, ed 2. Human Kinetics, Champaign, 1995, p 61.

TABLE 1–3 Data Required for the Assessment of Patient Outcomes

Data	Minimal Expectations	Other Options
Demographic and clinical information	Age, gender, race, and marital status Diagnosis (ICD-9 code)	
Functional status	Change in distance walked in 6 min Change in METs from graded exercise tests	
Return to vocation/avocation	Timing Work modification	
Smoking cessation	Self-reported number of cigarettes smoked per day in past week	Carbon monoxide level Serum thiocyanate levels Salivary, urine, or plasma cotinine levels
Weight control	Height, weight, and body mass index (BMI)	Percent body fat by multiple techniques
Lipids	Lipid profile	Dietary assessments Fat intake diet diary
Managed blood pressure	Regular, averaged BP	Ambulatory BP monitor
Stress management	Self-perceived report of stress—Likert scale	Self-report through diary of relaxation tape use frequency mm Hg change in SBP or DBP
Quality of life (QOL)	Measure multiple domains of QOL	Standardized QOL tools

Source: Reprinted by permission from American Association of Cardiovascular and Pulmonary Rehabilitation, 1995, Guidelines for Cardiac Rehabilitation Programs, ed 2. Human Kinetics, Champaign, 1995, p. 79.

HISTORICAL PERSPECTIVE OF PULMONARY DISEASE

A few decades ago, patients with pulmonary disease were given a standard prescription for rest and avoidance of exercise.[65] Well into the 1960s, the stress imposed by exercise was considered deleterious to such people.[66] Patients with pulmonary disease were treated as invalids and sometimes referred to as respiratory cripples.[67] An impetus to change direction in the treatment of pulmonary dysfunction came in 1964 as a result of a study by Pierce and his co-workers.[66] Patients with severe chronic obstructive pulmonary disease (COPD) were pretested for their exercise abilities and trained via treadmill walking programs. With post-test data, decreases in exercising heart rate, respiratory rate, minute ventilation, oxygen consumption, and carbon dioxide production at similar exercise intensities were noted. An increase in exercise tolerance was also reported. In 1966, the Eighth Aspen Emphysema Conference, chaired by Dr. Thomas Petty, reviewed current therapies for patients with advanced COPD. Out of this conference came the directives to define and examine pulmonary rehabilitation.[68]

The American College of Chest Physicians' Committee on Pulmonary Rehabilitation adopted the following definition of Pulmonary Rehabilitation at its 1974 annual meeting:

> Pulmonary rehabilitation may be defined as an art of medical practice wherein an individually tailored, multidisciplinary program is formulated which through accurate diagnosis, therapy, emotional support, and education, stabilizes or reverses both the physio- and psychopathology of pulmonary diseases and attempts to return the patient to the highest possible functional capacity allowed by his pulmonary handicap and overall life situation.[69]

Exercise training is a major component of the rehabilitation of the patient with chronic pulmonary disease. The exercise portion of the pulmonary rehabilitation program is prescribed by mode, intensity, duration, and frequency of exercise. Each exercise program is individualized according to the patient's abilities, the severity of the disease, and the patient's goals. There is no standard exercise regimen, but certain characteristics prevail. A circuit program often includes upper-body, lower-extremity, and respiratory-muscle training to increase functional abilities as well as to decrease boredom. Activity periods are frequently interspersed with rest periods so that patients may accumulate a greater amount of total exercise time. Symptoms of overexertion, and shortness of breath, along with heart rate, are monitored often and are instrumental in gauging exercise intensity. Much research has shown the positive effects of exercise training on patients with COPD.[70–80] Other types of chronic pulmonary diseases, termed nonobstructive pulmonary disease, are also debilitating, and their rehabilitation potential has been investigated. In one study, the results of a pretraining and post-training 6-minute walk test revealed that patients with pulmonary diseases other than COPD (primarily restrictive pulmonary diseases) could significantly increase their walking distances.[81] The authors concluded that patients with both COPD and nonobstructive pulmonary disease appear to benefit from monitored exercise programs. These results have been supported by other authors.[82]

Another major emphasis in pulmonary rehabilitation is education. The education sessions are best provided by a variety of health care professionals. Topics such as the pulmonary disease process, available treatment modalities, smoking cessation, and energy-saving techniques give patients the information they need to be better participants and managers in their own care.

Chronic pulmonary disease has been steadily increasing in incidence and is now estimated to afflict as many as 14 to 16 million Americans.[83] Because it is a leading cause of chronic disability, pulmonary rehabilitation programs are more necessary now than ever before. Therefore, a major purpose of this text is to provide the basic theory of pulmonary rehabilitation and the practical application of the theory so that allied health professionals at all educational levels might gain sufficient information to function optimally in their roles as pulmonary rehabilitation specialists.

ACUTE PULMONARY CARE

Acute respiratory-tract infections are the most frequently occurring infections; they range in severity from the common cold to pneumonia.[84] The effects of these infections range from minimal discomfort to respiratory failure. The goals of acute pulmonary care are to improve ventilation, improve gas exchange, promote secretion clearance, and maintain functional capacity.[85] The role of the clinician involved in acute pulmonary care is to:

1. Instruct patients in breathing exercises in order to promote greater lung volumes, a more evenly distributed ventilation, and more efficient breathing patterns.
2. Perform secretion removal techniques to enhance gas exchange and decrease airflow obstruction.
3. Prescribe general conditioning exercises to maintain and improve present levels of function.

It is not within the scope of this text to provide detailed information on acute pulmonary care, although some aspects of breathing exercises and secretion-removal techniques are briefly explained in Chapter 14. General activity provided to maintain baseline functional abilities in the acute care setting should be carried out while monitoring heart rate, blood pressure, rate of perceived exertion, and arterial saturation of oxygen (SaO_2). Activity should be of an intensity such that heart rate does not rise more than 20 to 30 beats above the resting heart rate. (Resting heart rate may be relatively high because of the side effects of some pulmonary medications.) The patient, when rating his or her activity, should report it as "light" and the report on breathing should not be more than "mildly short of breath." The measurement of SaO_2 should remain above 88 percent and supplemental oxygen should be used as needed for patients with hypoxemia at rest and/or during exercise. Because of the limitations on length of hospital stay, there is insufficient time to gain the physiologic adaptations of exercise training. Achievement of premorbid activity level is more compatible within the time frame of an acute and subacute care hospitalization.

CHRONIC PULMONARY CARE

Chronic pulmonary disease and its associated dysfunction have a slow and insidious onset. Persons with pulmonary dysfunction generally avoid activities that result in the uncomfortable sensation of dyspnea. Family and friends often discourage these persons from exerting themselves for fear of untoward effects.[86] A slow but steady decrease in activity level soon follows. It is not uncommon for these people to lose many functional abilities before seeking medical help. One goal of pulmonary rehabilitation is to interrupt this downward spiraling of physical ability.[87]

A rehabilitation program can be initiated on an inpatient admission or on an outpatient basis. Because of the confines of hospital admission, however, most increases in functional capacity occur during outpatient rehabilitation. Candidates for outpatient pulmonary rehabilitation come from a variety of sources. In some cases, the outpatient program begins after hospitalization for an acute exacerbation of the disease. Other patients receive a diagnosis of chronic pulmonary disease as outpatients and are then referred for pulmonary rehabilitation. Finally, patients who have lived with the diagnosis of lung disease for some time can be referred to pulmonary rehabilitation when their dyspnea interferes with their ability to maintain acceptable levels of physical activity. Enrollment in an outpatient pulmonary rehabilitation program is usually by physician referral.

An exercise test is often performed before admission to a pulmonary rehabilitation program. The results of this exercise test help the rehabilitation staff to quantify patient symptoms, assess functional abilities, determine the need for supplemental oxygen and bronchodilators during exercise, predict the potential for return to work, and prescribe appropriate exercise programs.[88–90] Clinicians monitor patients by using rates of perceived exertion and perceived shortness of breath, heart rates, blood pressures, respiratory rates, and oxygen saturation.

Generally, conditioning exercises are conducted three times per week for 6 to 8 weeks. During the course of the exercise therapy program, patients should gradually be weaned to self-monitoring and a home program of exercise. They can be assigned a home exercise program when, on the basis of exercise performance and laboratory data, the rehabilitation staff deems it feasible. The patients perform their home programs during an "off day" and return to the rehabilitation program with exercise logs including exercise heart rates, perceived exertion rates, exercise parameters, and any problems that may have occurred during the home program. The staff members analyze the data, adjust the home program if necessary, and suggest methods for self-monitoring the changes in the home program. Progression of patients to home programs is an ultimate goal of both the cardiac and pulmonary rehabilitation programs. Once the patient reaches an increased funtional capacity, demonstrates an ability to exercise safely without supervision, and has met educational goals, he or she is discharged from the program. At the end of the rehabilitation program, an exercise retest may be performed to document the efficacy of the program and to reassess the exercise prescription for continuation of care.

An unfortunate reality is that pulmonary patients often have respiratory setbacks. Continued contact and encouragement in the form of periodic rechecks is essential to attain and maintain new levels of physical activity. However, insurance reimbursement for such care (maintenance) is difficult to obtain.[91] Many pulmonary rehabilitation programs have low-cost maintenance sessions to help patients maintain the gains made during the program. Patients are also advised to join community-based groups that encourage compliance with their medical care. The Better Breathing Club, which is sponsored by the American Lung Association and Emphysema Anonymous, are groups patients can join for encouragement and support.

BENEFITS OF PULMONARY REHABILITATION

The benefits of a pulmonary rehabilitation program include increased exercise tolerance, increased ability for self-care, decreased sensation of dyspnea and exertion during activities, improved quality of life, decreased utilization of health care, decreased anxiety and depression, and perhaps increased survival.[92–95]

With exercise training, most patients show an impressive increase in exercise tolerance. If this increase in exercise ability has been specifically designed toward improving a patient's functional abilities, the patient will be better able to perform activities of daily living independently and do so with a decreased sensation of exertion and dyspnea.[96,97]

Pulmonary rehabilitation programs also offer education and counseling. The benefit of improved functional abilities becomes intertwined with many of the other stated benefits. Patients report a decrease in pulmonary symptoms, more control over their disease, and an increase in their self-esteem, along with decreased depression and anxiety.[94]

Cost-effectiveness is a necessity in any program in today's health care environment. Pulmonary rehabilitation programs have been shown to reduce the number of in-hospital days for years following participation in a pulmonary rehabilitation program.[94,98]

Finally, although some articles have described an increase in survival rate in patients who have participated in pulmonary rehabilitation programs, this issue has not been definitively resolved in the research literature. Prospective randomized controlled studies are needed to prove or disprove this potential benefit of pulmonary rehabilitation.[94]

MULTISPECIALTY APPROACH TO CARDIAC AND PULMONARY REHABILITATION

The primary goals of cardiac and pulmonary rehabilitation programs should be to increase the functional capacity of patients and to assist them in attaining normal function, insofar as possible, in their daily lives. Throughout the many aspects of cardiopulmonary care, input from a diversity of health professionals is essential to provide the knowledge required to meet the medical, physical, social, and psychologic needs of the patient with cardiac and pulmonary disease. The rehabilitation team may include nurses, physicians, exercise physiologists, physical therapists, occupational therapists, respiratory therapists, vocational counselors, sex therapists, dietitians, psychiatrists, psychologists, social workers, recreational therapists, clergy, and, most important, the patient and the patient's family. It appears that hospitals and geographic regions differ in the extent of participation by the various allied health professionals in the rehabilitative process. A comprehensive program dedicated to fulfilling the various needs of the patients that it serves should avail itself of these disciplines.[99]

SUMMARY

This chapter has presented a basic overview of cardiac and pulmonary rehabilitation programs. The recovery phases of cardiac rehabilitation have been redefined from the traditional three phases (inpatient, outpatient, and community-based) to include four phases: inpatient, immediate outpatient, intermediate outpatient, and maintenance outpatient. Phase I (the inpatient phase) of cardiac rehabilitation should be individualized, and there is no specific length of time for inpatient rehabilitation because cost-containment issues dictate that patients be progressed through intervention, recovery, and discharge in as little time as possible. The current trend toward early hospital discharge has resulted in hospital dismissal in as few as 3 days. Many patients, however, are hospitalized for 5 to 7 days, and Phase I cardiac rehabilitation is therefore limited to only a few days. Phase II (immediate outpatient) cardiac rehabilitation begins following hospital discharge and usually lasts from 2 to 12 weeks. The length of this stage is usually determined by risk stratification, individual patient need for supervision and intensive monitoring, and managed-care or other insurance reimbursement policies. Patients are progressed to Phase III (intermediate outpatient) cardiac rehabilitation programs when they are determined to be clinically stable, that is, when they demonstrate independence in self-monitoring, and no longer require intensive ECG monitoring. Phase III is a continuation of the Phase II program and usually lasts 6 to 8 weeks beyond Phase II. Phase IV (maintenance outpatient cardiac rehabilitation) begins when the patient can maintain the outcomes achieved during Phases II and III. A goal of maintenance cardiac rehabilitation is that patients continue their exercise and educational programs either in a formal setting or on their own. Phase IV cardiac rehabilitation can occur in the hospital, in a community-based organization, or at home. Follow-up evaluations are recommended every 6 to 12 months. Program plans with expected goals and outcomes should be developed and documented for each patient at each stage of cardiac rehabilitation. Guidelines for patient assessment, recommended programs, and measurement of expected outcomes in cardiac rehabilitation were also presented.

Pulmonary rehabilitation programs are divided into inpatient acute and outpatient chronic phases. Inpatient care is directed toward improvement in ventilation, airflow obstruction, and gas exchange. It is usually of insufficient duration to allow any physiologic training effects. Outpatient programs are usually conducted three times per week for a period of 6 to 8 weeks. As in cardiac rehabilitation, patients are gradually weaned from the structured programs and encouraged to begin home exercise programs. Follow-up evaluations by the outpatient pulmonary rehabilitation staff are important to ensure the highest level of patient compliance.

REFERENCES

1. Froelicher, V: Cardiac Rehabilitation. In: Parmley, W and Chatterjee, K (eds): Cardiology. JB Lippincott, Philadelphia, 1988, pp 1–17.
2. Levine, S and Lown, B: Armchair treatment of acute coronary thrombosis. JAMA 148:1365–1369, 1952.
3. Cain, HD, Frasher, WG, and Stivelman, R: Graded activity program for safe return to self-care after myocardial infarction. JAMA 177:111–115, 1961.
4. Abraham, A, et al: Value of early ambulation in patients with and without complications after acute myocardial infarction. N Engl J Med 292:719–722, 1975.
5. Pashkow, F: Issues in contemporary cardiac rehabilitation: A historical perspective. J Am Coll Cardiol 21(3):822–834, 1993.
6. Zohman, L: Early ambulation of post-myocardial infarction patients. In: Naughton J, Hellerstein H, and Mohler I (eds): Exercise Testing and Exercise Training in Coronary Heart Disease. Academic Press, New York, 1973, pp 330–331.
7. Miller, H and Ribisl, P: Cardiac rehabilitation program at Wake Forest University. J Cardiac Rehabil 2:503–505, 1982.
8. Pashkow, F, Schafer, M, and Pashkow, P: HeartWatchers—low cost, community centered cardiac rehabilitation in Loveland, Colorado. J Cardpulm Rehabil 6:469–473, 1986.
9. Leon, AS: Scientific rational for preventive practices in atherosclerotic and hypertensive cardiovascular disease. In: Pollock, ML and Schmidt, DH (eds): Heart Disease and Rehabilitation, ed 3. Human Kinetics, Champaign, 1995, p 115.
10. Agency for Health Care Policy and Research: Ischemic heart disease PORT publishes latest findings. Research Activities No. 183:1, March/April, 1995.
11. American Association of Cardiovascular and Pulmonary Rehabilitation: Secondary prevention of cardiovascular and pulmonary diseases under health care reform. In: News & Views 9:3, summer, 1995.
12. American Association of Cardiovascular and Pulmonary Rehabilitation: Health care reform in the 1990. J Cardpulm Rehabil 14(1):11–12, 1994.
13. Hall, LK: The future of health care: Implications for cardiac and pulmonary rehabilitation. J Cardpulm Rehabil 14:(4)228–231, 1994.
14. Ades, PA, Huang, D, and Weaver, SO: Cardiac rehabilitation participation predicts lower hospitalization costs. Am Heart J 123:916–921, 1992.
15. American Association of Cardiovascular and Pulmonary Rehabilitation: Guidelines for Cardiac Rehabilitation Programs, ed 2. Human Kinetics, Champaign, 1995, p 75.
16. Burnett, RE and Blumenthal, JA: Biobehavioral aspects of coronary artery disease: Considerations for prognosis and treatment. In: Pollock, ML and Schmidt, DH (eds): Heart Disease and Rehabilitation, ed 3. Human Kinetics, Champaign, 1995, pp 41–55.
17. Eaton, CB, et al: Physical activity and coronary heart disease risk factors. Med Sci Sports Exerc 27(3):340–346, 1995.
18. Foster, C, Schrager, M, and Cohen, J: The value of cardiac rehabilitation: Secondary prevention. In: Pollock, ML and Schmidt, DH (eds): Heart Disease and Rehabilitation, ed 3. Human Kinetics, Champaign, 1995, pp 177–183.
19. Frasure-Smith, N: The Montreal heart attack readjustment trial. J Cardpulm Rehabil 15(2):103–106, 1995.
20. Frasure-Smith, N, Lesperance, F, and Talajic, M: Depression after myocardial infarction. Circulation 91:999–1005, 1995.
21. Hare, DL, et al: Cardiac rehabilitation based on group light exercise and discussion. J Cardpulm Rehabil 15(3):186–192, 1995.
22. Kannel, WB: Epidemiologic insights into atherosclerotic cardiovascular disease—from the Framingham study. In: Pollock, ML and Schmidt, DH (eds): Heart Disease and Rehabilitation, ed 3. Human Kinetics, Champaign, 1995, pp 3–16.
23. Leon, AS: Scientific rationale for preventive practices in atherosclerotic and hypertensive cardiovascular

disease. In: Pollock, ML and Schmidt, DH (eds): Heart Disease and Rehabilitation, ed 3. Human Kinetics, Champaign, 1995, pp 115–146.

24. LaFontaine, T: The role of lipid management by diet and exercise in the progression, stabilization, and regression of coronary artery atherosclerosis. J Cardpulm Rehabil 15:(4):262–268, 1995.

25. DeBusk, RF, et al: A case-management system for coronary risk factor modification after acute myocardial infarction. Ann Intern Med 120:721–729, 1994.

26. Nelson, DV, et al: Six-month follow-up of stress management training versus cardiac education during hospitalization for acute myocardial infarction. J Cardpulm Rehabil 14(6):384–390, 1994.

27. Niebauer, J, et al: Five years of physical exercise and low fat diet: Effects on progression of coronary artery disease. J Cardpulm Rehabil 15(1):47–64, 1995.

28. Powell, KE and Blair, SN: The public health burdens of sedentary living habits: Theoretical but realistic estimates. Med Sci Sports Exerc 26(7):851–856, 1994.

29. Taylor, CB and Berra, K: Assessing depression. J Cardpulm Rehabil 14(6):376–377, 1994.

30. Joreteg, T, et al: Evaluation of outcomes in patients post cardiac event following participation in cardiac rehabilitation or conventional medical management. J Cardpulm Rehabil 15(5):366, 1995.

31. Rosenson, RS: Reversing coronary artery disease.The Physician and Sportsmedicine 22(11):59–64, 1994.

32. American Association of Cardiovascular and Pulmonary Rehabilitation: Round Table: The primary prevention of coronary artery disease. J Cardpulm Rehabil 14(2):79–86, 1994.

33. Friedman, DB: Exercise and the Heart. University of Texas, Southwestern Medical Center, Dec 9, 1993.

34. American Heart Association: Position Statement: Cardiac rehabilitation programs. Circulation 90(3):1602–1610, 1994.

35. Froelicher, VF, et al: Exercise and the Heart. Mosby, St. Louis, 1993, pp 347–377.

36. Hambrecht, R, et al: Various intensities of leisure time physical activity in patients with coronary artery disease: effects of cardiorespiratory fitness and progression of coronary atherosclerotic lesions. J Am Coll Cardiol 22:468–477, 1993.

37. Ornish, D, et al: Can lifestyle changes reverse coronary heart disease? Lancet 336(8708):129–133, 1990.

38. Paffenbarger, RS and Blair, SN: Exercise in the primary prevention of coronary artery disease. In: Pollock, ML and Schmidt, DH (eds): Heart Disease and Rehabilitation, ed 3. Human Kinetics, Champaign, 1995, pp 169–176.

39. Paffenbarger, RS, et al: Changes in physical activity and other lifeway patterns influencing longevity. Med Sci Sports Exerc 26(7):857–865, 1994.

40. Paffenbarger, RS, et al: The association of changes in physical-activity level and other lifestyle characteristics with mortality among men. N Engl J Med 328:538–545, 1993.

41. Sherman, C: Reversing heart disease: Are lifestyle changes enough? The Physician and Sportsmedicine 22(1).91–95, 1994.

42. Schuler, G, et al: Regular physical exercise and low-fat diet: Effects on progression of coronary artery disease. Circulation 86:1–11, 1992.

43. Hurst, JW: Coronary heart disease: The overview of a clinician. In: Wenger, NK and Hellerstein, HK (eds): Rehabilitation of the Coronary Patient, ed 3. Churchill Livingstone, New York, 1992, p 14.

44. American Association of Cardiovascular and Pulmonary Rehabilitation: Guidelines for Cardiac Rehabilitation Programs, ed 2. Human Kinetics, Champaign, 1995, pp 87–95.

45. Balady, GJ, et al: Cardiac rehabilitation programs: A statement for healthcare professionals from the American Heart Association. Circulation 90(3):1602–1610, 1994.

46. Irwin, S: Philosophy and structure of a cardiac rehabilitation program. In: Irwin, S and Tecklin, JS (eds): Cardiopulmonary Physical Therapy, ed 3. Mosby, St. Louis, 1995, p 4.

47. Southard, DR, et al: Core competencies for cardiac rehabilitation professionals: Position statement of the American Association of Cardiovascular and Pulmonary Rehabilitation. J Cardpulm Rehabil 14(2): 87–92, 1994.

48. Paris, W, et al: A comparison of role expectations and conflict resolution style between patients and cardiac rehabilitation staff. J Cardpulm Rehabil 14(6):418–419, 1994.

49. American Association of Cardiovascular and Pulmonary Rehabilitation: Guidelines for Cardiac Rehabilitation Programs, ed 2. Human Kinetics, Champaign, 1995, pp 73–79.

50. Comoss, PA: Standards for cardiac rehabilitation programs and practice. In: Pollock, ML and Schmidt, DH (eds): Heart Disease and Rehabilitation, ed 3. Human Kinetics, Champaign, 1995, pp 287–306.

51. Hall, LK and Gettman, LR: Policies and procedures in P&R programs. In: ACSM's Resource Manual for Guidelines for Exercise Testing and Prescription, ed 2. Lea & Febiger, Philadelphia, 1993, pp 562–569.

52. Oldridge, NB: Universal access and insurance coverage: Missing pieces. J Cardpulm Rehabil 15(1):9–13, 1995.

53. Sallis, RE and Massimino, F: Sports medicine and managed care. The Physician and Sportsmedicine 23(4):33–35, 1995.

54. American Association of Cardiovascular and Pulmonary Rehabilitation: Guidelines for Cardiac Rehabilitation Programs, ed 2. Human Kinetics, Champaign, 1995, pp 1–25.

55. Pollock, ML, Welsch, MA, and Graves, JE: Exercise prescription for cardiac rehabilitation. In: Pollock ML

and Schmidt, DH (eds): Heart Disease and Rehabilitation, ed 3. Human Kinetics, Champaign, 1995, pp 243–276.

56. Wenger, NK: In-hospital exercise rehabilitation after myocardial infarction and myocardial revascularization: Physiologic basis, methodology, and results. In: Wenger, NK and Hellerstein, HK (eds): Rehabilitation of the Coronary Patient, ed 3. Churchill Livingstone, New York, 1992, pp 351–363.

57. Fletcher, GF, et al: Exercise standards: A statement for health professionals from the American Heart Association. Circulation 82(6):2286–2322, 1990.

58. Squires, RW, et al: Cardiovascular rehabilitation: Status, 1990. Mayo Clin Proc 65:731–755, 1990.

59. American College of Sports Medicine: ACSM's Guidelines for Exercise Testing and Prescription, ed 5. Williams & Wilkins, Baltimore, 1995, p 178.

60. Temes, WC: Cardiac rehabilitation. In: Hillegass, EA and Sadowsky, HS (eds): Essentials of Cardiopulmonary Physical Therapy. Saunders, Philadelphia, 1994, pp 633–675.

61. American Association of Cardiovascular and Pulmonary Rehabilitation: Guidelines for Cardiac Rehabilitation Programs, ed 2. Human Kinetics, Champaign, 1995, p 94.

62. Winslow, A, et al: Exercise prescription for cardiac patients: A national survey of outpatient cardiac rehabilitation programs (CRPs). J Cardpulm Rehabil 15(5):358, 1995.

63. Franklin, BA, Bonzheim, K, Berg, T, and Bonzheim, S: Hospital and home-based cardiac rehabilitation outpatient programs. In: Pollock, ML and Schmidt, DH (eds): Heart Disease and Rehabilitation, ed 3. Human Kinetics, Champaign, 1995, pp 209–227.

64. American Association of Cardiovascular and Pulmonary Rehabilitation: Guidelines for Cardiac Rehabilitation Programs, ed 2. Human Kinetics, Champaign, 1995, pp 57–86.

65. Hughes, R and Davison, R: Limitation of exercise reconditioning in COLD. Chest 83(2):241–249, 1983.

66. Pierce, A, et al: Responses to exercise training in patients with emphysema. Arch Intern Med 114:28–36, 1964.

67. Hale, T, Cumming, G, and Spriggs, J: The effects of physical training in chronic obstructive pulmonary disease. Bulletin of European Physiopathology of Respiration 14:593–608, 1978.

68. Petty, T: Pulmonary rehabilitation: A personal historical perspective. In: Casaburi, R and Petty, T (eds): Principles and Practice of Pulmonary Rehabilitation. W B Saunders, Philadelphia, 1993.

69. American Thoracic Society: Pulmonary Rehabilitation. Am Rev Respir Dis 124:663–666, 1981.

70. Miller, W: Rehabilitation of patients with chronic obstructive pulmonary disease. Med Clin North Am 51:349–361, 1967.

71. Paez, P, et al: The physiological basis of training patients with emphysema. Am Rev Respir Dis 95:944–953, 1967.

72. Bass, H, Whitcomb, J, and Forman, R: Exercise training: Therapy for patients with chronic obstructive pulmonary disease. Chest 57:116–121, 1970.

73. Vyas, M, et al: Response to exercise in patients with chronic airway obstruction. I. Effects of exercise training. Am Rev Respir Dis 103:390–400, 1971.

74. Woolf, C: A rehabilitation program for improving exercise tolerance in patients with chronic lung disease. Can Med Assoc J 106:1289–1292, 1972.

75. Bedout, D, et al: Clinical and physiological outcomes of a university hospital pulmonary rehabilitation program. Respiratory Care 28(11):1468–1471, 1983.

76. Carter, R, et al: Exercise conditioning in the rehabilitation of patients with chronic obstructive pulmonary disease. Arch Phys Med Rehabil 69:118–121, 1988.

77. Casaburi, R: Exercise training in Chronic Obstructive Pulmonary Disease. In: Casaburi, R and Petty, T, (eds): Principles and Practice of Pulmonary Rehabilitation. Saunders, Philadelphia, 1993.

78. Reis, A: The importance of exercise in pulmonary rehabilitation. Clin Chest Med 15(2):327–337, 1994.

79. Punzal, P, et al: Maximum intensity exercise training in patients with chronic obstructive pulmonary disease. Chest 100:618–623, 1991.

80. Barach, A, Bickerman, H, and Beck, G: Advances in the treatment of nontuberculous pulmonary disease. Bull NY Acad Med 28:353–384, 1952.

81. Foster, S and Thomas, H: Pulmonary rehabilitation in lung disease other than chronic obstructive pulmonary disease. Am Rev Respir Dis 141:601–604, 1990.

82. Novitch, R and Thomas, H: Rehabilitation of patients with chronic ventilatory limitation from nonobstructive lung disease. In: Casaburi, R and Petty, T (eds): Principles and Practice of Pulmonary Rehabilitation. Saunders, Philadelphia, 1993.

83. Petty, T: The worldwide epidemiology of chronic obstructive pulmonary disease. Curr Opin Pulm Med 2:84–89, 1996.

84. Price, S and Wilson, L: Pathophysiology: Clinical Concepts of Disease Processes, ed 2. McGraw-Hill, New York, 1982, p 393.

85. Humberstone, N: Respiratory assessment and treatment. In: Irwin, S and Tecklin, J: Cardiopulmonary Physical Therapy, ed 2. Mosby, St. Louis, 1990, p 303.

86. Moser, K, Archibald, C, and Hansen, P: Better Living and Breathing: A Manual for Patients, ed 2. Mosby, St. Louis, 1980, p 46.

87. Frownfelter, D: Pulmonary rehabilitation. In: Frownfelter, D: Chest Physical Therapy and Rehabilitation. Year Book Medical Publishers, Chicago, 1987, p 295.

88. Zadai, C: Rehabilitation of the patient with chronic obstructive pulmonary disease. In Irwin, S and Tecklin, J: Cardiopulmonary Physical Therapy, ed 2. Mosby, St. Louis, 1990, p 496.
89. Hodgkin, J: Exercise testing and training. In Hodgkin, J and Petty, T: Chronic Obstructive Pulmonary Disease: Current Concepts, Saunders, Philadelphia, 1987, p 121.
90. American Thoracic Society Position Statement: Evaluation of impairment/disability secondary to respiratory disease. Am Rev Respir Dis 126:945–951, 1982.
91. Elkousy, N, et al: Outpatient pulmonary rehabilitation: A Medicare fiscal intermediary's viewpoint. J Cardiopulmonary Rehabil 11:492–497, 1988.
92. Belman, M and Wasserman, K: Exercise training and testing in patients with chronic obstructive pulmonary disease. Basics Respir Dis 10:1–6, 1981.
93. Sneider, R, O'Malley, J, and Kahn, M: Trends in pulmonary rehabilitation at Eisenhower Medical Center: An 11-year's experience (1976–1987). J Cardpulm Rehabil 11:453–461, 1988.
94. American Thoracic Society: Standards for the diagnosis and care of patients with chronic obstructive pulmonary disease. Am J Respir Crit Care Med 152(5):S78–S121, 1995.
95. Reis, A: Position Paper for the American Association of Cardiovascular and Pulmonary Rehabilitation: Scientific basis of pulmonary rehabilitation. J Cardpulm Rehabil 10:418–441, 1990.
96. Sinclair, D and Ingram, C: Controlled trial of supervised exercise training in chronic bronchitis. BMJ 280(1):519–521, 1980.
97. O'Donnell, D, et al: The impact of exercise reconditioning on breathlessness in severe chronic airflow limitation. Am J Respir Crit Care Med 152:2005–2013, 1995.
98. Hudson, L, Tyler, M, and Petty, T: Hospitalization needs during an outpatient rehabilitation program for severe chronic airway obstruction. Chest 70:606–610, 1976.
99. Miller, NH, et al: Position paper of the American Association of Cardiovascular and Pulmonary Rehabilitation. J Cardpulm Rehabil 10(6):198–209, 1990.

CHAPTER 2

The Heart and Circulation

THE HEART

The heart is a hollow, cone-shaped organ that in an adult, weighs approximately 300 g. It is not positioned in the center of the chest cavity; most of it lies to the left of center. The base of the heart is broad and is located superiorly, and the apex is at the inferior end and points anteriorly and approximately 45° to the left. The heart is enclosed in a fibrous protective sac called the pericardium, which confines the heart to its position in the chest and allows it to contract freely and vigorously.[1]

Three layers of tissue form the cardiac wall. The outer, external surface is covered with a fibrous membrane, the epicardium (external layer), which merges at the base of the heart with the pericardium. The major portion of the heart itself is the middle layer, which is composed of muscle tissue referred to as the myocardium. The muscular tissue of the myocardium is arranged in layers that run in indefinite, circular, and oblique directions. The inner layer of the myocardium is lined with smooth epithelial tissue called the endocardium, which allows the blood to pass through the chambers of the heart without damage to the blood cells.[1]

The interior of the heart is divided into four chambers: the right and left atria, which are located superiorly; and the right and left ventricles, which are located inferiorly. The apex of the heart is formed by the tip of the left ventricle.[1,2]

The surfaces of the heart are the sternocostal, the diaphragmatic, and the posterior. The sternocostal surface (anterior) is formed primarily by the right atrium and the right ventricle. The diaphragmatic (inferior) surface of the heart is formed by the right and left ventricles. The posterior (base) of the heart is formed primarily by the left atrium, although the right atrium forms a small part of the posterior surface.[2]

The four borders of the heart are the right, left, superior, and inferior. The right border is formed by the right atrium. The left border is formed mainly by the left ventricle, but a small part of it is formed by the left atrium. The superior border is formed by both atria and is located in the area where the great vessels unite with the heart. The inferior border is formed primarily by the right ventricle and, to a lesser extent, by the left ventricle (Fig. 2–1).[2]

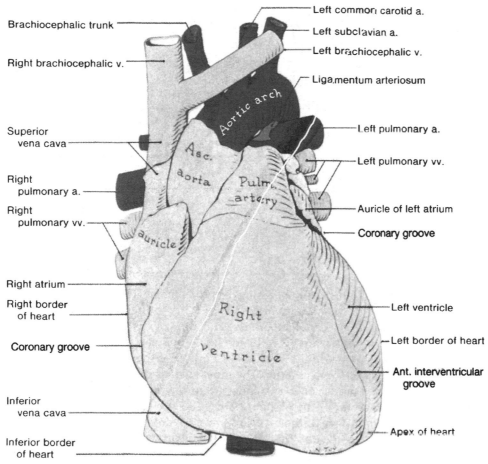

FIGURE 2–1. The sternocostal aspect of the heart. (From Moore, KL,[2] p. 83, with permission.)

Heart Chambers

The four chambers of the heart are arranged in pairs. The two atria are thin-walled cavities designed to receive blood into the heart. The right atrium receives blood from the systemic circulation through two openings: the superior and inferior venae cavae. During systole of the atria, blood from the right atrium is sent through the right atrioventricular orifice to the right ventricle. This orifice contains the tricuspid valve, which opens to allow the blood to pass into the ventricle during atrial systole. During ventricular systole, the tricuspid valve closes so that blood will not be pumped back into the atrium (Fig. 2–2).[2,3]

The left atrium is also thin-walled and has four openings at its superior and posterior walls (Fig. 2–3). These openings accommodate the four pulmonary veins that carry oxygenated blood from the lungs to the left atrium. Blood passes from the left atrium through the left atrioventricular orifice, which is controlled by the bicuspid or

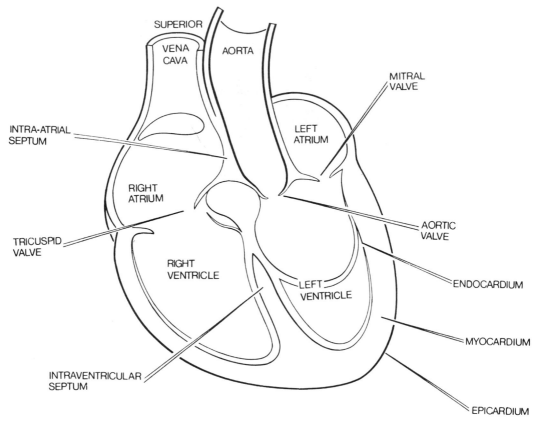

FIGURE 2–2. The heart and its chambers. (From Phillips, RE and Feeney, MK,[7] p. 13, with permission.)

mitral valve. During ventricular contraction, the mitral valve is tightly closed to prevent blood from surging back into the atrium.[2,4]

The walls of the ventricles are much thicker and stronger than those of the atria and are well suited to pumping blood farther. The right ventricle forms most of the front of the heart; it pumps the blood through the pulmonary orifice into the pulmonary artery (Fig. 2–4). The blood flow to the pulmonary artery is controlled by the semilunar or pulmonary valve, which prevents the flow of blood back to the right ventricle during systole. The right ventricle contracts to send the blood via the pulmonary artery through the pulmonary circulation to be oxygenated; hence, the right ventricle is referred to as the pulmonary pump.[4,5]

The walls of the left ventricle are thicker and stronger than those of the right ventricle. The left ventricle forms most of the left margin and the apex of the heart, and it is responsible for pumping blood throughout the entire systemic circulation: it is the systemic pump. Blood enters the systemic circulation from the left ventricle through the aortic orifice, guarded by the aortic valve, and into the aorta. The aorta is the largest artery in the body.[1,2,4]

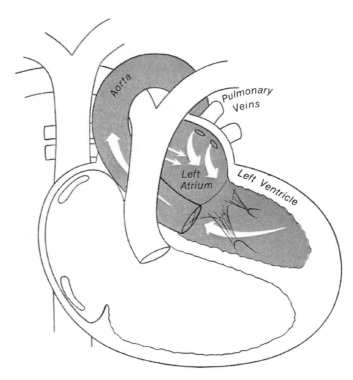

FIGURE 2–3. The left atrium and the pulmonary veins. (From Phillips, RE and Feeney, MK,[7] p. 8, with permission.)

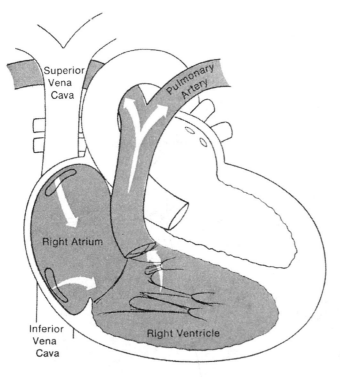

FIGURE 2–4. Blood flow from the right ventricle to the lungs. (From Phillips, RE and Feeney, MK,[7] p. 8, with permission.)

THE CORONARY ARTERIES

The two major arteries that supply the heart with blood arise directly from the aorta at a point near the aortic valve (Fig. 2–5). These major arteries are the right and left coronary arteries, each of which is approximately the size of a soda straw.[2,5–7] Although there is considerable variation among individuals, the right coronary artery branches to send blood to the right atrium, the right ventricle and, in most persons, the inferior wall of the left ventricle, the atrioventricular (AV) node, and the bundle of His. The sinoatrial (SA) node receives its blood supply from the right coronary artery in about 55 percent of human beings.[2]

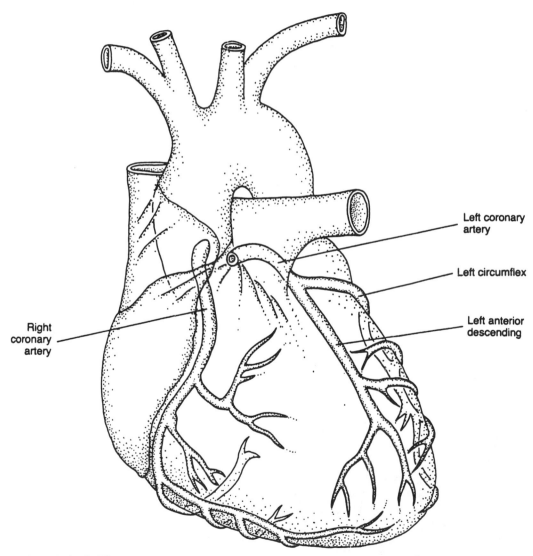

FIGURE 2–5. The coronary arteries. (From Phillips, RE and Feeney, MK,[7] p. 10, with permission.)

The left coronary artery branches into two main divisions within approximately 2 cm from its point of origin. The left anterior descending (LAD) artery supplies the left ventricle, the interventricular septum, the right ventricle, and, in most persons, the inferior areas of the apex and both ventricles.[2,4]

The second main division of the left coronary artery, the left circumflex, supplies blood to the inferior walls of the left ventricle and to the left atrium. In about 45 percent of humans, the left circumflex supplies the SA node with blood.[2,4,6–8]

Circulation to the Heart

Blood circulating to the heart muscle itself via the coronary arteries must do so while the muscle fibers are relaxed, during diastole of the heart. To prevent the occurrence of an ischemic state, this is an important fact to remember when considering whether the heart muscle has adequate blood flow during exercise. Although blood is forced into the coronary arteries from the heart during systole, that blood cannot enter the cardiac muscle fibers to supply oxygen to the tissue until the heart is in diastole and the fibers are relaxed.[5,8,9] Perhaps this is the greatest single reason for keeping the exercising heart rate relatively low in a coronary patient.

METABOLISM OF CARDIAC TISSUE

Cardiac tissue contains large amounts of myoglobin, the enzymes of the Krebs cycle, and the electron transport system, and is thus well suited for aerobic metabolism. To function properly, the heart must receive a constant supply of oxygen to support its almost exclusively aerobic metabolism. The principal source of energy production for cardiac muscle is the oxidation of free fatty acids. Although acetoacetic acid and lactic acid can be metabolized to produce energy, the energy of preference of the heart is supplied by fatty acid metabolism.[8,10–12] Examples of the anaerobic and aerobic pathways for adenosine 5'-triphosphate (ATP) production are given in Table 2–1.

TABLE 2–1 Anaerobic and Aerobic Metabolic Pathways for
Production of ATP

Anaerobic Metabolism

1. Coronary circulation delivers glucose to cardiac tissue
2. Glucose via glycolysis (in cytoplasm) $\longrightarrow$ Pyruvate + 2 ATP
or
3. Lactate delivered by coronary circulation to cardiac tissue
4. Lactate (in cytoplasm) $\longrightarrow$ Pyruvate + 2 ATP

Aerobic Metabolism

1. Coronary circulation delivers free fatty acids to cardiac tissue
2. Free fatty acids undergo β-oxidation $\longrightarrow$ ~4 ATP + Acetyl Co A (Mitochondria)
3. Acetyl Co A enters Krebs cycle + O_2 $\longrightarrow$ ~12 ATP (approximately 6 total ATP with *each* 2-carbon + H_2O + CO_2
or
4. Pyruvate (free cytoplasm) $\longrightarrow$ Acetyl Co A (Mitochondria)
5. Acetyl Co A $\longrightarrow$ Krebs cycle + O_2 $\longrightarrow$ 36 ATP + H_2O + CO_2

The most common fatty acids have chains of 16 and 18 carbons. Through β-oxidation (oxidizing 2 carbons at one time), a 16-carbon-chain fatty acid could produce approximately 128 ATP when completely metabolized (16 ATP × 16 carbon β-oxidation) = 16 ATP × 8 = 128 ATP.[10]

The importance of continuous O_2 delivery to the cardiac muscle can be seen in the relative contributions of anaerobic and aerobic metabolism to the production of ATP. During rest, cardiac tissue extracts approximately 70 percent of the O_2 that is delivered to it via the coronary arteries. This leaves a very limited reserve for increasing oxygen extraction during increased myocardial work. The increased demand for more oxygen during work is met by increasing the blood flow to the cardiac tissue. Consequently, the rate and force of cardiac contraction, and therefore cardiac output, increase in response to increased activity. Increased coronary blood flow is also achieved through a reduction in the resistance (dilation) of the coronary vessels.[12-14]

CONDUCTION

Although there are structural and functional similarities between cardiac and skeletal muscle, there are also major differences. Cardiac muscle has two major types of tissue in addition to ordinary muscle tissue: nodal and Purkinje. The nodal tissue is located at the junction of the superior vena cava and the right atrium (sinoatrial node) and at the junction of the right atrium and the right ventricle (atrioventricular node). The Purkinje fibers are the specialized conducting tissues of both ventricles.[7,9,15]

Sinoatrial Node

The sinoatrial (SA) node (Fig. 2–6) is composed of small, slender, spindle-shaped cells that contain very few myofibrils but large amounts of thick connective tissue. The SA node, called the pacemaker of the heart, has sympathetic and parasympathetic innervation, although, at rest, the SA node is under continuous parasympathetic control via the vagus nerve. Small strands of fibers extend out from the main region of the SA node and are continuous with the ordinary muscle fibers of the atrium. Through this arrangement, once the SA node initiates an impulse (sinus rhythm), that impulse can spread from muscle fiber to muscle fiber throughout both atria (functional syncytium).[7,9,15]

Atrioventricular Node

The atrioventricular (AV) node is a band of fibers located at the lower end of the interatrial septum of the right atrium (Fig. 2–7). The AV nodal tissue merges with the atrioventricular bundle of His near the origin of the ventricles. The AV node normally functions to receive the impulse that originates from the SA node and conducts it to the bundle of His. In cases of impaired SA node function, the AV node can become the pacemaker of the heart and send out its own impulses to keep the heart beating (nodal rhythms). The AV node is also supplied with nerves from the sympathetic and parasympathetic systems.[7,9,15]

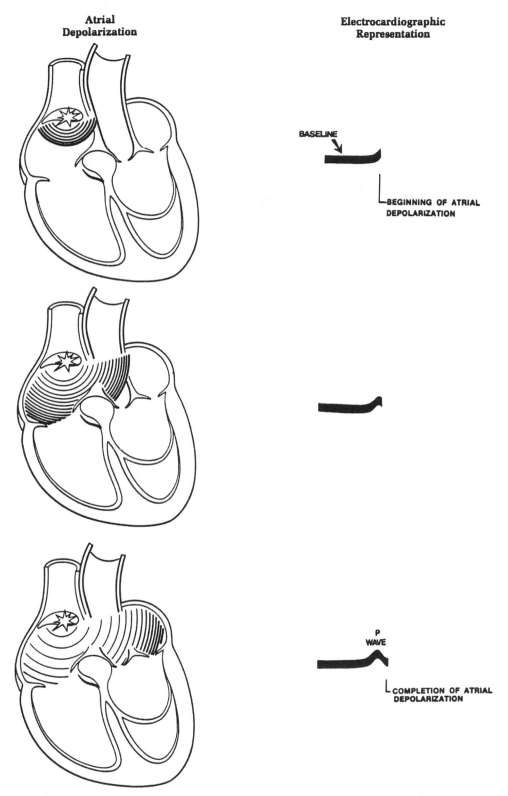

FIGURE 2–6. Atrial impulse conduction. (From Phillips, RE and Feeney, MK,[7] p. 27, with permission.)

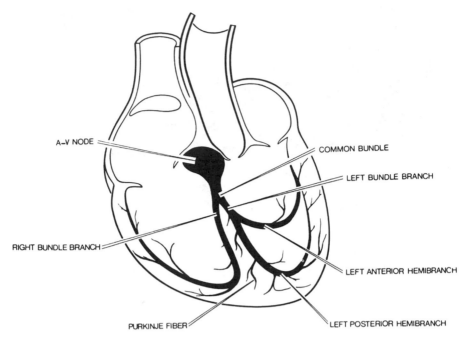

FIGURE 2–7. Ventricular conduction. (From Phillips, RE and Feeney, MK,[7] p. 29, with permission.)

Purkinje Tissue

The AV bundle of His has two branches, the right and the left, located along either side of the intraventricular septum (see Fig. 2–7). These branches terminate in the Purkinje fibers, which are the specialized conducting tissues for both ventricles. The fibers that comprise the Purkinje system have sarcoplasm that contains large amounts of glycogen but few myofibrils. The fibers of the Purkinje system terminate in twigs that penetrate the ventricles and are intimately associated with the contractile fibers of the ventricles.[7,9,15]

Origin and Conduction of Heartbeat

The origin of the electrical impulse that precedes the contraction of the heart is in the SA node (myogenic). This impulse spreads quickly through both atria, which then contract simultaneously. This wave of electrical activity next stimulates the AV node, which transmits the impulse down the bundle of His to the Purkinje fibers. Because the Purkinje fibers merge with the walls of the ventricles, the impulse spreads through the Purkinje system to the cells of the ventricles, and the ventricles contract together (Fig. 2–8). This rhythmic sequence of events occurs an average of 72 times per minute.[7,9,15]

Myocardial Fibers

The microscopic appearance of cardiac muscle fibers is similar to that of skeletal muscle fibers. Both types of muscle appear to be striated; their myofibrils have well-

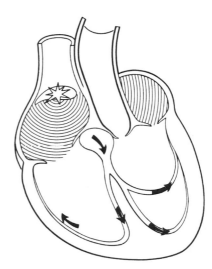

FIGURE 2–8. Schematic illustration of the conduction system of cardiac muscle. (From Phillips, RE and Feeney, MK,[7] p. 29, with permission.)

identified A, I, and Z bands. Compared with skeletal muscle, cardiac tissue has numerous mitochondria and its T-tubules are larger, but the sarcoplasmic reticulum (SR) is not well developed.[16] A major functional difference between skeletal and cardiac muscle is that cardiac muscle exhibits a rhythmicity (myogenicity) of contraction, whereas skeletal muscle contracts in response to direct neural stimulation. This inherent rhythmicity of cardiac tissue originates in the SA node.

GENERAL MYOLOGY

Muscle Tissue

The protoplasm of muscle cells has the ability to contract, and because most muscle cells are elongated, individual cells are called fibers. There are three types of muscle tissue in the body: smooth, skeletal, and cardiac. (Skeletal or striated muscle is sometimes further divided into skeletal and cardiac.[16])

Smooth muscle is closely associated with connective tissue structures and is found in the walls of the digestive tract, urinary tract, and blood vessels. Contraction of smooth muscle in these areas causes the structures to change in size and volume. Smooth muscle is also called involuntary or visceral, and the terms are used interchangeably. Each individual muscle fiber (cell) of smooth muscle tissue has a single oval nucleus. Unlike cardiac and skeletal muscle, smooth muscle can regenerate quite well after injury.[17]

The basic cellular structure of skeletal muscle can be described as a multinucleated cylinder that varies in length and may be longer than 30 cm. Skeletal muscle cells are striped and have light (isotropic) and dark (anisotropic) bands throughout. Synonymous terms for skeletal muscle are somatic, voluntary, and striated muscle. Skeletal muscles are responsible for moving the various parts of the skeleton.[16,17]

The individual cells of cardiac muscle are irregular in shape, contain a single oval nucleus, and seem to have incomplete cell membranes. Like skeletal muscle, cardiac muscle is striated. Unlike skeletal muscle, individual cardiac cells are joined through intercalated discs. Because cardiac cells have branches that appear to connect with adjacent fibers, the cells contract as a unit to act as a syncytium (a functional rather than an anatomic syncytium). The heart has two such functional syncytia: the atria and the ventricles.[16,17]

Although the muscles of the body are composed of three different types of contractile tissues, they are similar in that all are affected by the same kinds of stimuli: they atrophy in response to inadequate activity, and they hypertrophy as a result of increased work. Current theory regarding muscle contraction indicates that skeletal and cardiac muscle contractions are similar physiologic processes.[16,17]

THE MUSCLE FIBER

The sarcolemma is the membrane of a muscle cell. Each muscle cell has at least one nucleus. It is surrounded by the cytoplasm, which, in muscle cells, is called the sarcoplasm. The myofibrils are the structures in the sarcoplasm of muscle cells that provide stability, and they are directly responsible for muscle contraction. The function of the mitochondria found in muscle cells is the same as that for other cells of the body: energy production. There are abundantly more mitochondria in cardiac fibers than there are in skeletal muscle fibers. Skeletal muscle fibers respond to aerobic training by increasing the number and size of mitochondria in their cells, a response that apparently does not occur in cardiac tissue.[18-20]

The two important tubular systems found in muscle fibers are the transverse tubules (T-tubules) and the sarcoplasmic reticulum (Fig. 2–9). The T-tubules occur at regular intervals along the fibers; their function is to conduct waves of depolarization from the sarcolemma to deeper regions of the fiber. The numerous saclike structures that comprise the sarcoplasmic reticulum (SR) are located next to the T-tubules. The SR seems to be a storage place for the calcium (Ca^{2+}) that is necessary for muscle contraction. The T-tubules in cardiac tissue are significantly larger than those in skeletal muscle. Conversely, SRs are not as abundant in cardiac muscle as in skeletal muscle. The amount of Ca^{2+} released into the fiber during the contractile process seems to relate to the force of contraction that is generated by that fiber.[16,21]

The Myofibril

Muscle fibers contain numerous myofibrils, the filaments directly responsible for the contractile process. The smallest functional unit of the myofibril is the sarcomere, which is characterized by alternating light (I-band) and dark (A-band) bands. The A-band contains mainly the myosin protein, which is a thick, dark filament. The I-band is composed primarily of the protein actin, a much thinner filament than myosin (Fig. 2–9). During muscle contraction, cross-bridges located on myosin connect to the actin filaments. The thin actin filaments slide inward toward the center of the sarcomere, and the sarcomere shortens.[16,17,20–24]

Myosin. Chemical studies of myosin indicate that there are several forms and several large components. The fundamental unit of myosin is a protein with an average molecular weight of 465,000.[23] The ATPase (ability to split ATP) activity of the myofibril is confined to myosin; it is activated by Ca^{2+} and inhibited by Mg^{2+}.[16,21–24]

Actin. Actin has been found to exist as G-actin (globular) and as F-actin (fibrous). It has a molecular weight of approximately 43,000.[23] The conversion of F-actin to G-actin, and vice versa, involves a process of polymerization, which is necessary for muscle contraction to occur. ATP has been found to bind to actin, and this binding is stronger to F-actin than to G-actin.[16,21-23]

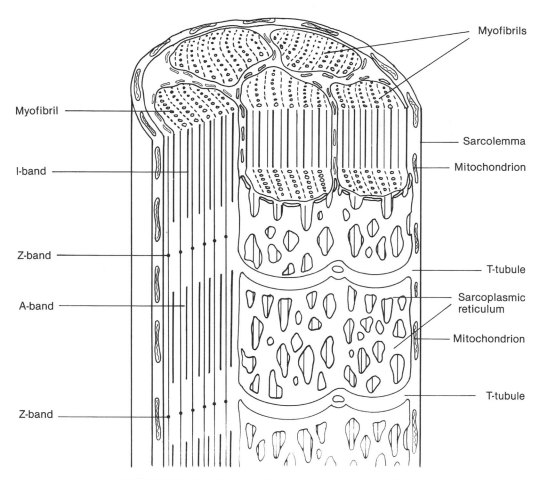

FIGURE 2-9. Schematic illustration of the myocardium.

The Regulatory Proteins. The two major proteins in the myofibril that exert a regulatory effect on contraction are tropomyosin and troponin. In the resting state, tropomyosin seems to prevent actin and myosin from interacting. Once calcium enters the cell, it binds with troponin to remove the inhibiting effect of tropomyosin. At this point, actin and myosin can interact and muscle contraction occurs.[16,21-23]

Calcium plays a role in the contraction of skeletal and cardiac muscle. In the rest-

TABLE 2-2 Energy Formation in Muscle Cells

1. ATP-F-actomyosin $\xrightarrow[\text{Ca}^{2+}]{\text{nerve impulse}}$ G-actomyosin + ATP
2. ATP $\rightleftharpoons$ ADP + Pi (H_3PO_4) + E (energy used for contraction)
3. Phosphocreatine $\rightleftharpoons$ creatine + Pi (H_3PO_4) + E (energy used for resynthesis of ATP)
4. Glycogen (Glycolysis) $\rightleftharpoons$ Lactic acid + E (energy used for resynthesis of phosphocreatine)
5. 1/5 Lactic acid + O_2 (Krebs cycle) $\longrightarrow$ CO_2 + H_2O + E (energy drives reaction 6)
6. 4/5 Lactic acid + E $\longrightarrow$ Glycogen

ing state, the regulatory protein tropomyosin prevents actin and myosin from interacting. When muscle cells are stimulated, Ca^{2+} is released from the SR and binds to the regulatory protein troponin, which removes the inhibiting effect of tropomyosin. Actin and myosin are now free to interact and contraction occurs.[16,21–23]

Contraction Theory

Once a nerve impulse enters the muscle fiber, Ca^{2+} is released by the SR. Some of the Ca^{2+} combines with myosin to form an "activated myosin," which now has the property of an ATPase enzyme. This activated ATPase is able to react with ATP to remove part of its energy. This energy, in turn, is used to "pull" the actin filaments in among the myosin filaments. This process is referred to as the sliding-filament theory of muscle contraction.[16,21–23]

In the resting muscle cell, the myofibril is composed of F-actomyosin with ATP strongly attached to form an ATP-F-actomyosin complex. As a result of the ionic events that occur in response to nerve impulses, the ATP-F-actomyosin linkage is broken and G-actomyosin if formed. Table 2–2 summarizes the energy-forming events that occur during muscle contraction.

NEURAL CONTROL OF HEART RATE AND BLOOD VESSELS

The heart is regulated by the autonomic nervous system, which has two major divisions: the parasympathetic and the sympathetic (Fig. 2–10).

Parasympathetic Center

The parasympathetic system innervates the heart via the vagus nerve (X cranial). The center for this system, located in the medulla oblongata, is considered a cardioinhibitory center. Stimulation of the parasympathetic nerves (Fig. 2–11) causes a release of acetylcholine (cholinergic), which in turn slows the normal intrinsic rate of the heart and also decreases the force of its contraction. Vagal stimulation also causes the coronary arteries to dilate, enhancing coronary blood flow. At rest, the normal heart is under continual vagal control.[16,25,26]

Sympathetic Center

The sympathetic center (adrenergic) is located in the medulla oblongata. Stimulation of this center causes an increase in the rate and the force of contraction of the cardiac muscle. The chemical mediator for sympathetic stimulation is primarily norepinephrine, although epinephrine is also released (see Fig. 2–11). The sympathetic system has two types of receptors that respond to stimulation: the alpha and beta receptors. Both alpha and beta receptors are classified into subtypes: alpha$_1$, (α_1), alpha$_2$ (α_2), beta$_1$ (β_1), and beta$_2$ (β_2). Generally, the alpha receptors are excitatory, whereas some beta receptors are excitatory and others are inhibitory. Norepinephrine excites

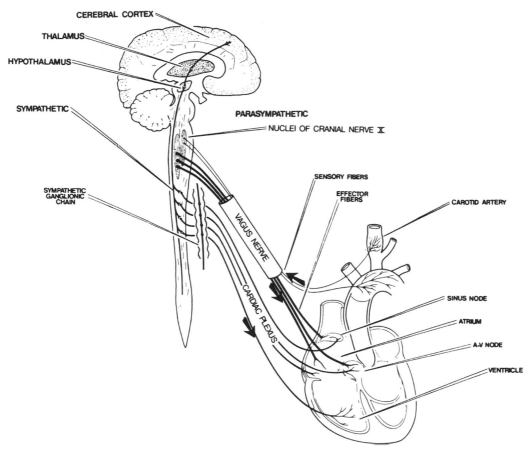

FIGURE 2–10. The autonomic nervous system innervation of cardiac muscle. (From Phillips, RE and Feeney, MK,[7] p. 92, with permission.)

mainly the alpha receptors, whereas epinephrine excites both the alpha and beta receptors. Before the norepinephrine or epinephrine transmitter secreted at the autonomic nerve endings can stimulate the effector organ, it must bind with specific receptors of the effector cells. The effects of norepinephrine and epinephrine on different effector organs are, therefore, dependent on the types of receptors in the organ stimulated. When stimulated, most alpha receptors cause coronary arteriolar vasoconstriction. In contrast, beta receptors, when stimulated, cause coronary arteriolar vasodilation. In cardiac tissue, however, norepinephrine binding to the beta receptors has a stimulating effect that causes the rate and force of contraction to increase. A balance between the alpha and beta receptors is necessary for the heart to function properly.[7,26–28]

Additional Mechanisms That Control the Heart

Although neural regulation seems to be the heart's main mode of control, other factors influence heart action. The baroreceptors (pressoreceptors) located in the aorta

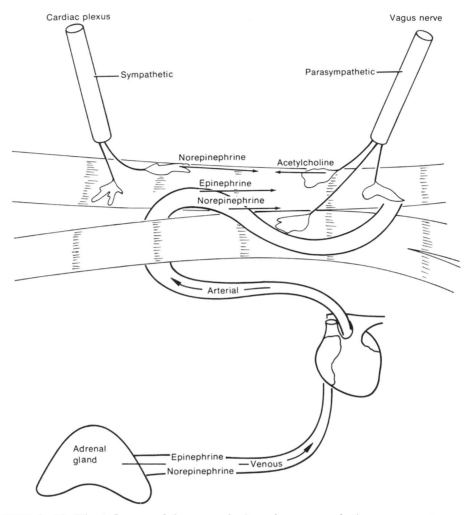

FIGURE 2–11. The influence of the sympathetic and parasympathetic nervous systems on the heart. (From Phillips, RE and Feeney, MK,[7] p. 95, with permission.)

and carotid sinus are sensitive to changes in blood pressure. When blood pressure is increased, the baroreceptors send this information to the medulla oblongata and stimulate the parasympathetic system to decrease the rate and force of the cardiac contraction.[29]

The chemoreceptors located in the carotid body are sensitive to changes in such blood chemicals as O_2, CO_2, and lactic acid. For instance, either an increase in CO_2 (and a decrease in O_2) or lactic acid concentration (causing decreased pH) will cause the heart rate to increase. Increased levels of O_2 will cause the heart action to decrease.[29]

Body temperature plays an important role in controlling the rate of heart action. Increased body temperature causes the heart rate to increase, whereas a decrease in body temperature causes the heart rate to decrease.[16]

The concentration of ions in the blood is important in proper heart action. Increased concentration of potassium (hyperkalemia) widens the PR interval and the QRS complex, produces tall T waves, and decreases the rate and force of contraction.

Hypokalemia (decreased concentration of potassium), if not treated, may cause ST-segment depression, cardiac irritability, and arrhythmias that may progress to ventricular fibrillation.[16,30]

Excessive calcium concentration (hypercalcemia) causes the heart to produce prolonged, spastic contractions. Hypocalcemia depresses heart action and causes the heart to become flaccid. All these factors govern heart action, and proper balance among them is necessary for normal cardiac function.[16]

PERIPHERAL CIRCULATION

Blood circulates when the pressure in one area or structure of the body is higher than in another. Blood flows from an area of higher pressure to one of lower pressure. Blood pressure can be defined as the pressure exerted by the blood against the walls of the vessels.[31] During systole (contraction) of the ventricles, the pressure exerted against the walls of the vessels is greater than during diastole (relaxation) of the ventricles. Systolic and diastolic arterial blood pressures are usually determined indirectly by the auscultatory method with the bell of the stethoscope applied to the brachial artery. Average systolic arterial blood pressures usually range from 90 to 120 mm Hg and the average diastolic arterial pressure range is from 60 to 90 mm Hg. Resting arterial systolic blood pressures consistently above 140 mm Hg and resting diastolic arterial blood pressures in excess of 90 mm Hg are considered to be abnormal.[31,32] Although blood pressures vary with such factors as age, emotional state, and exercise, a primary determinant of blood is the volume of blood in the arteries. Thus, an increase in the blood volume in the arteries tends to cause an increase in arterial pressure; conversely, a decrease in volume tends to cause a decrease in arterial pressure. Two important factors that affect blood volume, and therefore blood pressure, are cardiac output and peripheral resistance.[4,33]

Cardiac Output

An increase in cardiac output (amount of blood ejected from the heart per minute) tends to increase arterial blood volume and therefore increase blood pressure. The volume of blood pumped per minute depends on the number of contractions (heartbeats) per minute and the amount of blood pumped with each contraction. The amount of blood pumped per beat (stroke volume) depends on the force of ventricular contraction. The greater the force of contraction, the greater the stroke volume and the systolic pressure tend to be.[4,33]

Stroke volume is determined by the difference between ventricular filling and ventricular emptying. The volume of blood in the ventricle at the peak of ventricular filling or end of diastole (end diastolic volume) is also referred to as preload. Preload is determined by the contractility of the heart muscle, which is regulated by the Frank-Starling mechanism (ventricles become stretched when they receive more blood, which causes them to contract more forcefully). Afterload is the load against which the muscle exerts its contractile force and is the pressure in the artery leading from the ventricle. Afterload is often described as resistance to ventricular emptying and represents the systolic pressure. The percentage of the end-diastolic volume that is ejected or pumped from the ventricles is called the ejection fraction (usually about 60 percent).[5,16]

Increases in heart rate result in increased cardiac output. This causes arterial blood volume and therefore arterial blood pressure to increase. Conversely, when the heart beats more slowly and/or with less force, there are decreases in cardiac output, arterial volume, and arterial blood pressure.[4,33]

REGULATION OF CARDIAC OUTPUT

Stroke volume is directly related to contractility (preload) and to the strength of the heartbeat. The main regulator for stroke volume is the ratio of sympathetic to parasympathetic impulses innervating the heart. An increase in sympathetic impulses causes a more forceful contraction of the heart, which increases the stroke volume. Blood concentrations of epinephrine also affect stroke volume because increases in blood epinephrine increase stroke volume.[4,33]

The baroreceptors (pressoreceptors) in the aortic arch and carotid sinus are the main mechanisms responsible for controlling heart rate. If the blood pressure within those areas increases, impulses are sent to the cardioinhibitory center in the medulla oblongata, which causes the heart rate to slow. A decrease in the blood pressures in the aortic arch or carotid sinus causes a reflex acceleration of the heart.[4,29,33]

Baroreceptors in the right atrium of the heart also affect heart rate. Increases in the right atrial blood pressure cause a reflex acceleration, and decreases in right atrial pressure cause a reflex slowing of the beat.[4,19,33]

Other factors affecting heart rate, and therefore cardiac output, include emotions, exercise, blood temperature, and hormones. Anxiety, fear, and anger tend to increase heart rate and cardiac output, whereas grief tends to decrease heart rate and cardiac output. Increases in heart rate are observed during exercise, along with increases in the temperature of the blood and levels of epinephrine.[4,33]

Peripheral Resistance

A change in peripheral resistance (resistance to blood flow) tends to cause the volume of blood within the arteries to change and thus, change blood pressure. An increase in peripheral resistance tends to increase arterial blood volume and to increase arterial blood pressure. A decrease in peripheral resistance tends to cause decreased blood volume and decreased arterial blood pressure. Peripheral resistance is influenced by the viscosity of the blood and the diameter of the arterioles and capillaries. When the amount of blood flowing from the arteries to the arterioles decreases, more blood is left in the arteries. This increases blood volume and tends to cause an increase in arterial blood pressure.[4,33]

REGULATION OF PERIPHERAL RESISTANCE

The amount of resistance encountered by the peripheral circulation depends primarily on the viscosity of the blood and the diameter of the arterioles. To a large extent, the viscosity (thickness) of the blood determines the ease with which the blood flows. The hematocrit, or the ratio of the formed elements (red blood cells, white blood cells, and platelets) to the plasma content of whole blood, exerts a great influence on viscosity, as does the number of plasma proteins circulating in the blood. If the formed elements (mainly red blood cells) increase, then viscosity increases and so does peripheral resistance. Normally, blood viscosity changes very little. In conditions such as hemorrhage, viscosity decreases (as does total blood volume) and thereby lowers peripheral resistance and arterial blood pressure. When the hematocrit rises above 50 percent (as in polycythemia), the corresponding increase in blood viscosity causes decreased blood flow and also increases the work of the heart.[33]

Arteriole diameter (vasoconstriction and vasodilation) is influenced by many factors, among which are arterial blood pressure, oxygen and carbon dioxide content of the blood, pH of the blood, and substances such as hormones (epinephrine, norepinephrine), histamines, and lactic acid. Decreases in arteriole diameters (vasoconstriction) increase the peripheral resistance and therefore increase blood pressure. Increases in arterial blood pressure stimulate the aortic and carotid baroreceptors and thereby cause parasympathetic impulses to be sent to the cardioinhibitory system in the medulla oblongata, which inhibits the vasoconstriction center. As a result, impulses are sent to the heart and blood vessels, thereby causing the heart rate to decrease and the arterioles to dilate and reduce arterial blood pressure. Decreases in arterial blood pressure have the opposite effect.[4,33]

SUMMARY

This chapter has dealt with the basic structure and function of the heart, cardiac contraction, and similarities between skeletal muscle and cardiac tissue. A discussion of muscle fiber structure included the comments that more mitochondria are found in cardiac fibers than in skeletal fibers and that aerobic training does not appear to increase the number and size of mitochondria in cardiac muscle cells. The T-tubules in cardiac tissue are larger than those in skeletal muscle, but the sarcoplasmic reticulum is not as abundant in cardiac tissue.

The ultrastructure of the myofibril and the A-bands and I-bands and their relation to actin and myosin were presented. Muscle contraction theory, including the roles of tropomyosin and troponin as regulatory proteins, was discussed.

In presenting the function of the heart, particular attention was given to the fact that the heart has three kinds of tissue: nodal, Purkinje, and ordinary muscle. The origin and conduction of the heartbeat are functions of the coordination of these three tissues.

A discussion of the anatomy of the heart included the four chambers (two atria and two ventricles), the three surfaces (sternocostal, diaphragmatic, and posterior), and the four borders (right, left, superior, and inferior). Circulation to the heart is provided by two major arteries: the right and left coronary arteries.

Metabolism of the heart was described as primarily aerobic, with the preferred substrate being fatty acids. The importance of continuous O_2 delivery to cardiac muscle was emphasized.

Factors controlling the rate and force of cardiac contraction were shown to be primarily neural (cholinergic or adrenergic). Other factors influencing heart action are the baroreceptors, chemoreceptors, body temperature, and concentration of ions (potassium and calcium) in the blood.

A primary determinant of peripheral blood pressure is the volume of blood in the arteries. Increases in arterial blood volume tend to increase blood pressure. Factors affecting blood volume and thus blood pressure are cardiac output and peripheral resistance. Increases in heart rate and stroke volume increase cardiac output, which tends to increase arterial blood pressure. Increases in peripheral resistance tend to increase arterial blood volume and therefore to increase arterial blood pressure. Peripheral resistance is influenced by the viscosity of the blood and the diameter of the arterioles and capillaries. Blood viscosity is determined largely by the hematocrit, and arteriole diameter is influenced by blood pressure; pH; and blood concentrations of oxygen, carbon dioxide, hormones, lactic acid, and histamines.

REFERENCES

1. Tortora, GJ: Principles of Human Anatomy, ed 7. HarperCollins College Publishers, New York, 1995, pp 323–410.
2. Moore, KL: Clinical Oriented Anatomy, ed 3. Williams & Wilkins, Baltimore, 1992, pp 33–125.
3. McArdle, WD, Katch, FI, and Katch, VL: Essentials of Exercise Physiology, Lea & Febiger, Philadelphia, 1994, pp 237–277.
4. Anthony, CP and Thibodeau, GA: Textbook of Anatomy and Physiology, ed 12. Mosby, St. Louis, 1987, pp 416–477.
5. Brooks, GA, Fahey, TD, and White, TP: Exercise Physiology: Human Bioenergetics and Its Applications, ed 2. Mayfield Publishing, Mountain View, Calif, 1996, pp 243–280.
6. DeVries, HA and Housh, TJ: Physiology of Exercise, ed 5. Brown & Benchmark, Dubuque, Iowa, 1994, pp 312–333.
7. Phillips, RE and Feeney, MK: The Cardiac Rhythms, ed 3. Saunders, Philadelphia, 1990, pp 1–131.
8. Guyton, AC: Textbook of Medical Physiology, ed 8. Saunders, Philadelphia, 1991, pp 234–244.
9. Hole, JW: Human Anatomy & Physiology, ed 6. William C. Brown, Dubuque, Iowa, 1993, pp 650–713.
10. Guyton, AC: op cit, pp 744–770.
11. Starnes, JW: Introduction to respiratory control in skeletal muscle. Med Sci Sports Exerc 26(1):27–29, 1994.
12. Wasserman, K, et al: Principles of Exercise Testing and Interpretation, ed. 2. Lea & Febiger, Philadelphia, 1994, pp 9–49.
13. Protas, EJ: Normal cardiovascular anatomy, physiology, and responses at rest and during exercise. In: Hasson, SM (ed): Clinical Exercise Physiology, Mosby, St. Louis, 1994, pp 101–120.
14. Johnson, AT: Biomechanics of Exercise Physiology. John Wiley & Sons, New York, 1991, pp 1–30.
15. Memmler, RL, Cohen, BJ, and Wood, DL: Structure and Function of the Human Body, ed 5. JB Lippincott, Philadelphia, 1992, pp 151–177.
16. Guyton, AC: op cit, pp 67–117.
17. Tortora, GJ: op cit, pp 205–227.
18. Brooks, GA, Fahey, TD, and White, TP: op cit, pp 81–99.
19. McArdle, WD, Katch, FI, and Katch, VL: op cit, pp 343–369.
20. Cahalin, LP: Exercise tolerance and training for healthy persons and patients with cardiovascular disease. In: Hasson, SM (ed): Clinical Exercise Physiology, Mosby, St. Louis, 1994, pp 121–156.
21. Williams, JH: Normal musculoskeletal and neuromuscular anatomy, physiology, and responses to training. In: Hasson, SM (ed): Clinical Exercise Physiology, Mosby, St. Louis, 1994, pp 159–177.
22. Guyton, AC: Basic Neuroscience: Anatomy & Physiology, ed 2. Saunders, Philadelphia, 1992, pp 295–297.
23. Southerland, WM: Biochemistry. Churchill Livingstone, New York, 1990, pp 491–504.
24. Montgomery, R, Conway, TW, and Spector, MC: Biochemistry: A Case-Oriented Approach, ed 5. Mosby, St. Louis, 1990, pp 497–549.
25. Guyton, AC: Basic Neuroscience: Anatomy & Physiology, ed 2. Saunders, Philadelphia, 1992, pp 320–329.
26. Tortora, GT: op cit. pp 579–591.
27. Guyton, AC: Textbook of Medical Physiology, ed 8. Saunders, Philadelphia, 1991, pp 589–678.
28. Smith, JJ and Kampine, JP: Circulatory Physiology, ed 3. Williams & Wilkins, Baltimore, 1990, pp 25–172.
29. Guyton, AC: Textbook of Medical Physiology, ed 8. Saunders, Philadelphia, 1992, pp 194–220.
30. Lowenthal, DT, Guillen, GJ, and Kendrick, ZV: Drug effects. In: Pollock, ML and Schmidt, DH (eds): Heart Disease and Rehabilitation, ed 3. Human Kinetics, Champaign, 1995, pp 379–392.
31. Thomas, CL (ed): Taber's Cyclopedic Medical Dictionary, ed 17. FA Davis, Philadelphia, 1993, p 243.
32. US Department of Health and Human Services. The Fifth Report of the Joint National Committee on Detection, Evaluation, and Treatment of High Blood Pressure. National Institutes of Health, Bethesda, NIH Publication No. 95–1008, 1995.
33. West, JB (ed): Best and Taylor's Physiological Basis of Medical Practice, ed 12. Williams & Wilkins, Baltimore, 1991, pp 276–330.

CHAPTER 3

Anatomy and Physiology of Respiration

This chapter presents a brief review of respiratory anatomy and physiology. Respiratory anatomy includes the bony structure of the thorax; the musculature of ventilation; and the composition of the lungs, the conducting airways, and the distal respiratory unit. Respiratory physiology includes an overview of lung volumes and capacities, flow rates, external and internal respiration, the regulation of respiration, the respiratory system's contribution to the acid-base balance within the body, and arterial oxygenation.

BONY STRUCTURES

The bony thorax has three major functions: It protects the vital organs of the cardiopulmonary system and upper abdominal viscera; it supports the shoulder girdle; and it provides skeletal attachment for the muscles of the upper limbs, chest, neck, and back.[1] The bony structures of the thorax include the sternum anteriorly, the ribs laterally, the thoracic vertebrae posteriorly, and the shoulder girdle including the clavicle, humerus, and scapula (Figs. 3–1 and 3–2).

The sternum is the anterior border of the thorax, which comprises the manubrium, the body, and the xiphoid process. A palpable landmark of the sternum is the sternal angle, which is the bony ridge of fibrocartilage at the union of the manubrium and the body. The sternum provides articulating surfaces for the ribs and the clavicle.

Twelve pairs of ribs form the lateral borders of the thorax. The first seven pairs are called true ribs because they attach by a single costocartilage to the sternal body. Ribs 8 to 12 are called false ribs because they lack direct anterior attachment to the sternum. Ribs 8 to 10 attach anteriorly to the cartilage of the rib above them, and not directly to the sternum. The last two pairs of ribs, 11 and 12, are called floating ribs because they have no anterior attachment.

The thoracic vertebrae (T-1 through T-12) constitute the posterior aspect of the thorax. A synovial gliding joint is present between the head of a rib and the facets of

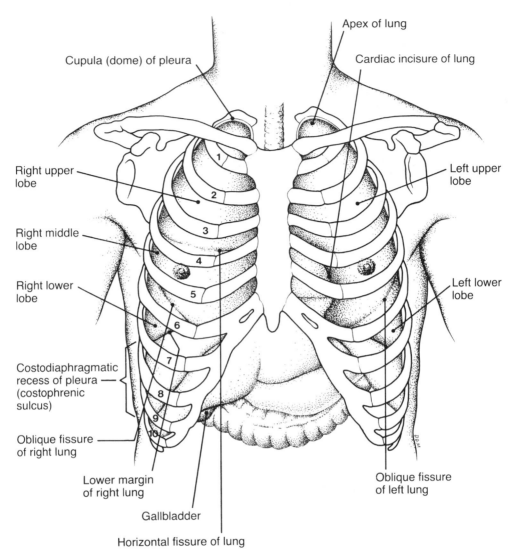

FIGURE 3–1. The bony thorax, anterior view. (From Rothstein, JM, Roy, SH, and Wolf, SL: The Rehabilitation Specialist's Handbook, ed 2. FA Davis, Philadelphia, 1998, p. 494, with permission.)

the vertebral bodies, superiorly and inferiorly to each rib. (Ribs 1, 10, 11, and 12 articulate with only one vertebral body.) Additional articulations exist between the neck and tubercle of the rib and the adjacent transverse process of the vertebrae.

The shoulder girdle can affect the motion of the thorax. The sternal end of the clavicle articulates with the superior border of the manubrium. The acromion of the scapula attaches to the distal end of the clavicle. The glenoid fossa of the scapula articulates with the head of the humerus. The muscular attachments from the shoulder girdle to the thorax, head, and cervical spine can potentially be used to assist ventilation.

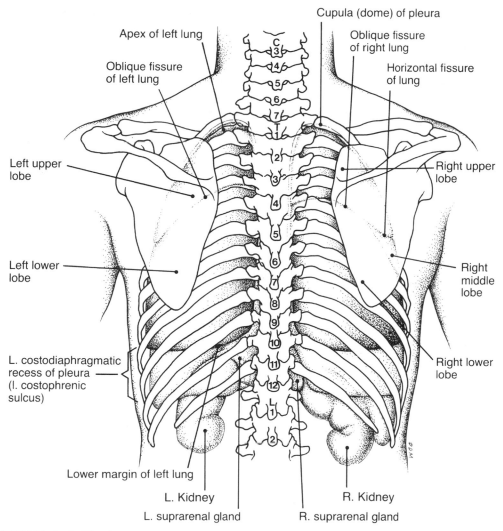

FIGURE 3–2. The bony thorax, posterior view. (From Rothstein, JM, Roy, SH, and Wolf, SL: The Rehabilitation Specialist's Handbook, ed. 2. FA Davis, Philadelphia, 1998, p. 495, with permission.)

MUSCULATURE

The musculature about the thorax can be divided into muscles of inspiration and those of expiration.

Inspiration

The principal inspiratory muscle is the diaphragm.[2] This dome-shaped muscle originates from the sternum, ribs, lumbar vertebrae, and lumbocostal arches; it forms the inferior border of the thorax. The muscle fibers insert into a central tendon. A right leaf (or right hemidiaphragm) is innervated by the right phrenic nerve, and a left leaf is innervated by the left phrenic nerve (Fig. 3–3).

When stimulated, the muscle fibers of the diaphragm contract; in doing so, they pull the central tendon and therefore the dome caudally. Thus, the descending diaphragm increases the volume of the thorax. Boyle's law states that at a constant temperature, the volume to which a given quantity of gas is compressed is inversely proportional to the pressure ($V \propto 1/P$).[3] Therefore, according to Boyle's law, increasing the volume within the thorax reduces the pressure within the thorax. The pressure inside the thorax (intrathoracic) during a diaphragmatic contraction becomes less than the pressure outside the thorax (atmospheric). Air then enters the lungs to equalize the two pressures.

During quiet inspiration, muscles of ventilation other than the diaphragm also are active.[4-6] Both the internal and external intercostals contract to keep the ribs aligned rather than to actually raise the rib cage.[7,8] The scaleni muscles are used to stabilize and may help to elevate the rib cage.[9,10]

Deep inspiration requires that the accessory muscles of inspiration contract more fully and thereby further increase the volume (by decreasing the pressure) within the thorax. The external intercostals contract to lift the ribs; the sternocleidomastoids elevate the sternum; and the levatores costarum and serratus posterior superior raise the ribs. The trapezius, rhomboid major, rhomboid minor, and levator scapulae elevate

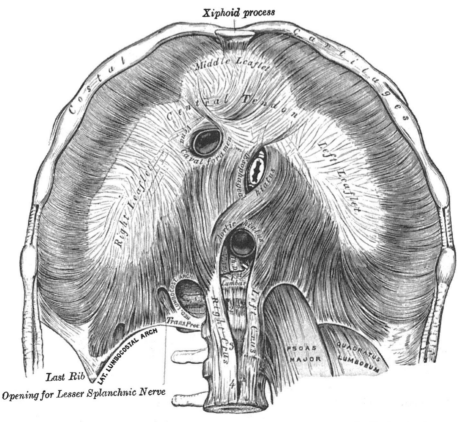

FIGURE 3–3. The diaphragm, abdominal surface. (From Clemente, C [ed]: Gray's Anatomy, ed 30. Lea & Febiger, Philadelphia, 1985, with permission.)

and fix the scapulae when the head and neck are fixed. With stabilization of the shoulder girdle, the pectoralis minor, pectoralis major, and serratus anterior also elevate the ribs. The sacrospinalis can further assist in raising the ribs and increasing the volume within the thorax by extending the vertebral column.[4]

Expiration

Quiet expiration is mainly a passive process involving relaxation of the inspiratory muscles. With relaxation of the muscles of inspiration, the elastic properties of lung tissue recoil and pull the chest wall inward, which returns the thorax to its resting position.[11] By Boyle's law, as the thorax decreases in volume, there is an increase in the intrathoracic pressure. Air is passively exhaled to preserve a pressure equilibrium between intrathoracic and atmospheric pressures. In the standing position, the abdominal muscles have been shown to actively generate some tension during quiet expiration.[12]

The elastic properties of the lung parenchyma, with its inward recoiling force, are opposed by the tendency of the force within the thoracic cage to spring outward and upward. These two forces are at equilibrium at the end of a quiet exhalation. This state of equilibrium is referred to as resting end-expiratory pressure (REEP).

Forced expiration is an active process. The abdominal muscles (rectus abdominis, external and internal obliques, and transverse abdominis) contract to compress the abdominal viscera. Because the viscera are prevented from moving posteriorly by the vertebral column and caudally by the pelvis, the abdominal contents are forced cephally, which pushes the diaphragm upward. The ribs are pulled downward by the action of the quadratus lumborum, internal intercostals, and the serratus posterior inferiores.[4] Flexing the vertebral column[13] and exerting pressure with the arms on the chest wall[14] can enhance forced expiration. As the thorax decreases in volume, intrathoracic pressure is increased and air is forced out of the lungs.

LUNGS

The lungs are the primary organs of external respiration. Each lung has an apex, a base, a costal surface, and a mediastinal surface. The apex may reach as high as 1.5 to 2.5 cm above the clavicle.[11] The base of the lung is concave, and it rests on the diaphragm. The dome of the right hemidiaphragm is higher than that of the left because of the size of the underlying liver. The costal surface is large and convex; it conforms to the inner contour of the rib cage. The mediastinal surface is concave, which enables it to accommodate the heart. Because the heart is situated more within the left hemithorax than the right, the cardiac impression is larger and deeper on the left lung than on the right lung (Figs. 3–4 and 3–5). As a result, the left lung is narrower and longer and the right lung is larger, shorter, and wider.[11]

The inner surfaces of the thorax, sternum, ribs, vertebrae, and diaphragm are covered by a thin serous membrane called the parietal pleurae. Each lung is enveloped by a thin membrane called the visceral pleura. Both the visceral and the parietal pleurae are actually continuous with each other around the root of the lung; in the healthy individual, they are in actual contact with each other. The potential space between them, called the intrapleural space, has a slightly negative pressure. Within this potential space, there is a small amount of serous fluid that reduces friction and allows the pleu-

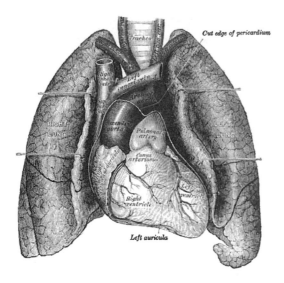

FIGURE 3-4. The lungs. (From Clemente, C [ed]: Gray's Anatomy, ed 30. Lea & Febiger, Philadelphia, 1985, with permission.)

rae to glide over each other during ventilation. The right and left pleural sacs are completely separated from each other by the mediastinum, which comprises the thoracic viscera (a mass of organs and tissues separating the lungs).[4]

The left lung has one fissure line, the oblique fissure, which separates the upper and the lower lobes. The right lung also has an oblique fissure; it separates the upper lobe from the lower lobe posteriorly. The right lung contains a horizontal or transverse fissure that divides the upper and the middle lobes anteriorly. The visceral pleurae are continuous along the fissure lines.

Each lobe of the lung is divided into segments. The right lung has three lobes and ten segments and the left lung has two lobes and eight segments (Fig. 3-6).

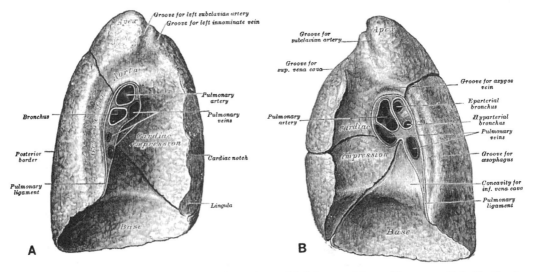

FIGURE 3-5. Mediastinal surfaces of the right and left lungs. (From Clemente, C [ed]: Gray's Anatomy, ed 30. Lea & Febiger, Philadelphia, 1985, with permission.)

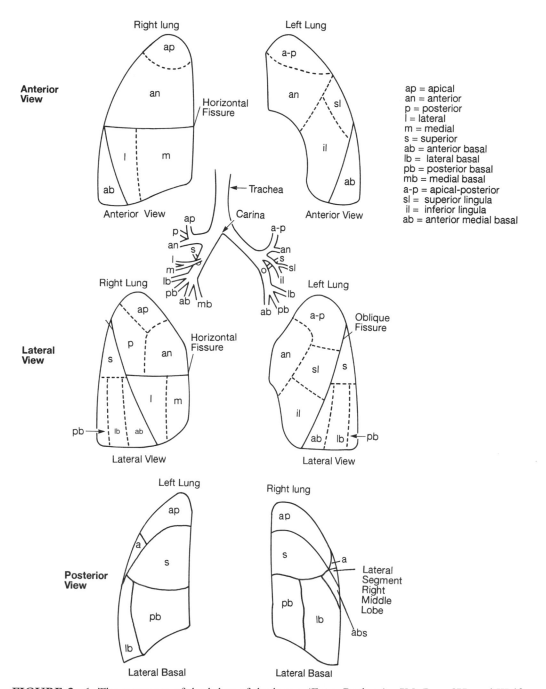

FIGURE 3–6. The segments of the lobes of the lungs. (From Rothstein, JM, Roy, SH, and Wolf, SL: The Rehabilitation Specialist's Handbook, ed. 2. FA Davis, Philadelphia, 1998, p. 497, with permission.)

CONDUCTING AIRWAYS

Air must be delivered from the atmosphere to the distal respiratory unit, where the actual gas exchange takes place. The conducting airways provide this transportation route.

Upper Conducting Airways

The upper airways of the respiratory system contain the nose, mouth, pharynx, and larynx (Fig. 3–7). The function of the nose is to filter, humidify, and warm the air before its delivery to the pharynx. The nose provides a large surface area that is lined with a respiratory mucous membrane. This membrane is comprised of ciliated epithelium, goblet cells, and mucous and serous glands. The mucous membrane filters the inhaled air by trapping foreign material in the mucus. The cilia sweep the mucus layer to the nasopharynx, where it is either swallowed or expectorated. The nose also contains sensory receptors that can initiate a sneeze, which is a forceful clearing mechanism.[1]

The pharynx includes the tonsils and adenoids. It is divided into three sections: the nasopharynx, oropharynx, and laryngopharynx. The nasopharynx contains a ciliated mucous membrane and continues to filter and humidify the inspired air. The oropharynx and laryngopharynx do not have cilia and mucous membranes. They conduct inspired air from the oral cavity into the trachea, but they are unable to humidify

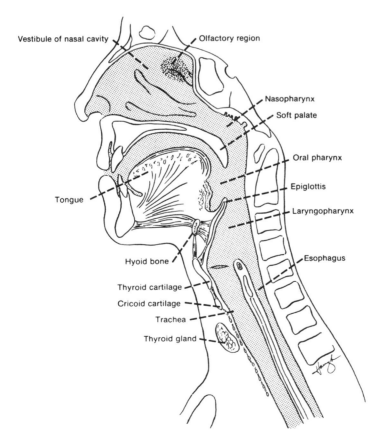

FIGURE 3–7. The upper airways. (From Frownfelter, D: Chest Physical Therapy and Pulmonary Rehabilitation: An Interdisciplinary Approach, ed 2. Mosby-Year Book, Inc., Chicago, 1987, p. 18, with permission.)

and filter the air. The oropharynx and the laryngopharynx also provide the passage-way from the oral cavity to the esophagus, so they are part of the digestive system as well.

The larynx connects the pharynx with the trachea. The entrance into the larynx is called the glottis. The epiglottis is a leaf-shaped elastic cartilage that covers and pro-tects the glottis during swallowing. The larynx also has sensory fibers that can stimu-late a cough: a forceful clearing mechanism of the lower airways. The larynx ensures that only air is inspired into the trachea and that only solids and liquids pass into the esophagus. Only a portion of the larynx contains a mucous membrane. Finally, the lar-ynx contains the vocal cords, which provide the mechanism for phonation. The larynx is the narrowest structure of the upper airway.[12]

Lower Conducting Airways

The lower conducting airways begin with the trachea, which branches into the right and left main stem bronchi. The bronchi further branch into lobar bronchi and segmental bronchi for generations until they terminate in the bronchioles. The most distal conducting airway is called the terminal bronchiole (Fig. 3–8).

The trachea is considered to be the first-generation ventilatory passageway; it is the continuation of the airway inferior to the larynx. It originates at the lower border of the cricoid cartilage at the level of the sixth cervical vertebra and terminates at the level of the sternal angle. It is about 12 cm in length and has a cylindrical 2-cm lumen. Support and protection are provided anteriorly and laterally by C-shaped cartilage. The posterior wall of the trachea, which is shared with the anterior wall of the esopha-gus, is made up of fibrous tissue and the smooth muscle of the trachealis.

The mucous membrane of the trachea contains both goblet cells (which provide a mucus layer lining the trachea) and ciliated epithelial cells (which beat and move the mucus layer upward to the pharynx). Once the mucus layer reaches the level of the pharynx, it is either swallowed or expectorated. A number of reserve cells that lie be-neath the ciliated and goblet cells can become either goblet cells or ciliated cells as needed. Below the reserve cells is a layer of gland cells that also help to produce mu-cus.

At the level of the sternal angle, the trachea bifurcates and creates the right and left main stem bronchi, which are the second generation of the ventilatory passageway. This point of bifurcation is called the carina.

Cartilage continues to support the smooth muscle and other tissues of the bronchial walls, although at this point it is shaped as flat plates rather than as rings.[14] The right main stem bronchus is shorter, less angular, and wider than the left main stem bronchus. It extends caudally into the right lung at the hilum. The left main stem bronchus angles more laterally at the tracheal bifurcation because of the presence of the heart. It enters caudally and laterally into the left lung at the hilum.

The main stem bronchi divide, on entering the lungs, into lobar bronchi (third-generation ventilatory passage). Each branch of the bronchi corresponds to a lobe of the lung. Branching continues into segmental bronchi (fourth generation), subsegmen-tal bronchi (fifth generation), and so on. The cartilaginous support within the smooth muscle of the airway decreases with each generation, as does the number of cilia.[15] The term "bronchiole" is used when there is no longer any cartilage or any cilia in the smooth muscle of the airway. The bronchioles continue to divide until they become

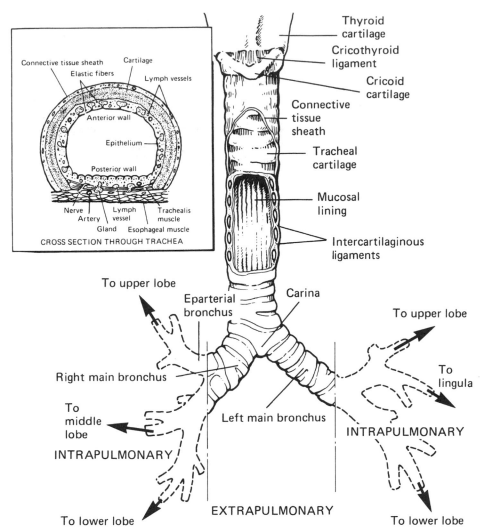

FIGURE 3–8. The lower airways. Anterior view of the trachea and primary bronchi. A cross-section through a part of the trachea shows the anterior and lateral support of the C-shaped cartilage. The trachealis muscle provides the necessary protective support posteriorly. (From Martin and Youtsey,[20] p. 27, with permission.)

the final generation of the conducting airways, the terminal bronchioles. A terminal bronchiole is 0.5 to 1.0 mm in diameter.[16] There are 20 to 25 generations of conducting passages in all.

THE RESPIRATORY UNIT

The inspired air travels from the conducting airways to the distal respiratory unit, which contains the respiratory bronchioles, alveolar ducts, alveolar sacs, and the alveoli and pulmonary capillary bed (Fig. 3–9). In an adult, there are an estimated 300 million alveoli available for gas exchange.[17] The alveolar membrane, the pulmonary capillary membrane, and the interstitial space are all that separate the alveolar air from the pulmonary capillary red blood cells (Fig. 3–10).

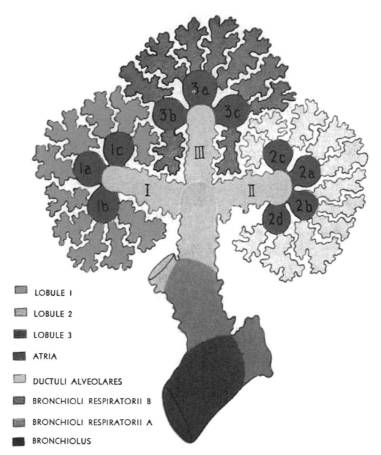

LOBULE 1

LOBULE 2

LOBULE 3

ATRIA

DUCTULI ALVEOLARES

BRONCHIOLI RESPIRATORII B

BRONCHIOLI RESPIRATORII A

BRONCHIOLUS

FIGURE 3–9. The respiratory unit, the acinus. (From Miller, WS: The Lung. Courtesy of Charles C. Thomas, Publisher, Springfield, Illinois, 1950, p. 42, with permission.)

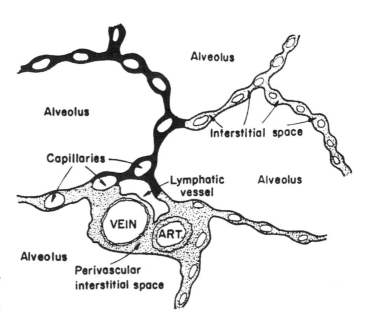

FIGURE 3–10. The alveolar capillary network. (From Guyton,[3] p. 487, with permission.)

VENTILATION

Air is inspired through the nose or mouth and through all of the conducting airways until it reaches the acinus. The act of moving air in and out of the lungs is termed "ventilation." The terminology surrounding the amount of air involved in ventilation is the topic of the next section.

Lung Volumes and Capacities

At full inspiration, the lungs contain their maximum amount of gas. This volume of air, called total lung capacity (TLC), can be divided into four separate volumes of air: (1) tidal volume, (2) inspiratory reserve volume, (3) expiratory reserve volume, and (4) residual volume (Fig. 3–11). The combination of two or more volumes yields a capacity. This section discusses inspiratory capacity (IC), functional residual capacity (FRC), and vital capacity (VC). Normative values for these volumes and capacities depend on the age, height, race, gender, and body position of the subject.[18]

TIDAL VOLUME

The amount of air that is inspired and expired during normal resting ventilation is called the tidal volume (VT). For a young, healthy man the VT is approximately 500

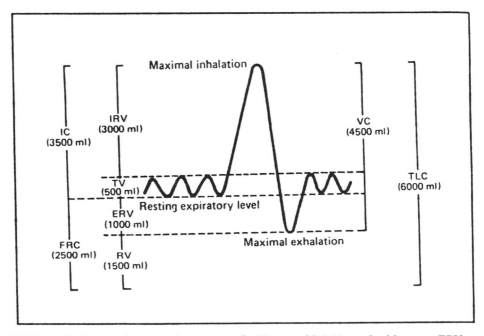

FIGURE 3–11. Lung volumes and capacities of a 23-year-old, 166-cm, healthy man. ERV = expiratory reserve volume; FRC = functional residual capacity; IC = inspiratory capacity; IRV = inspiratory reserve volume; TLC = total lung capacity; RV = residual volume; TV = tidal volume; VC = vital capacity. (From Youtsey,[18] p. 377, with permission.)

milliliters (see Fig. 3–11).[18] REEP, or the point during ventilation at which all forces about the rib cage are at equilibrium, occurs at the end of a tidal exhalation.

As the V_T (500 milliliters) enters the respiratory system, it travels through the conducting airways to reach the respiratory units. The amount of inspired air that actually reaches the respiratory unit and takes part in gas exchange is about 350 milliliters. The remaining 150 milliliters of the inhaled tidal breach remains in the conducting airways. This 150 milliliters of air is considered to be within the anatomic dead space of the lungs, since it does not take part in gas exchange. There is a numerical relation between the amount of air contained in the anatomic dead space (V_{DS}) and the total amount of air inhaled (V_T). The normal dead-space-to-tidal-volume ratio (V_{DS}/V_T) in the example (see Fig. 3–11) of a 23-year-old healthy man is 150 milliliters per 500 milliliters, or 30 percent.[18]

INSPIRATORY RESERVE VOLUME

When only a tidal breath occupies the lungs, there is "room" for additional air that can be further inhaled. This inspiratory volume, in excess of tidal breathing, is the inspiratory reserve volume (IRV). Aptly named, it is the volume of air that can be inspired when needed, but it is usually kept in reserve. Again referring to Figure 3–11, the IRV is approximately 3000 milliliters.[18]

EXPIRATORY RESERVE VOLUME

There is a quantity of air that can potentially be exhaled beyond the end of a tidal exhalation, or below REEP. Usually kept in reserve, this volume of air, called the expiratory reserve volume (ERV), is about 1000 milliliters in the example of a young man[18] (see Fig. 3–11).

RESIDUAL VOLUME

The lungs are not completely emptied of air after maximal exhalation of the ERV. The external forces of the rib cage do not allow the lungs to collapse fully. The volume of air that remains within the lungs when the ERV has been exhaled is called the residual volume (RV). The normal value of the RV in a young, healthy man is approximately 1500 milliliters.[18]

As previously stated, the total of the four lung volumes is the TLC; that is, TLC = IRV + V_T + ERV + RV. Combinations of two or more lung volumes are termed "capacities."

INSPIRATORY CAPACITY

The sum of TV and IRV is called the inspiratory capacity (IC). In a young, healthy man (see Fig. 3–11), the IC would be V_T + IRV, or 500 + 3000 = 3500 milliliters of air.

FUNCTIONAL RESIDUAL CAPACITY

The functional residual capacity (FRC) is the combined RV and ERV. Physiologically, it is the amount of air that is left in the lungs after a resting tidal exhalation. Thus, FRC = ERV + RV, or 1000 + 1500 = 2500 milliliters of air in the example (see Fig. 3–11).

VITAL CAPACITY

Vital capacity (VC) comprises the three volumes that are under volitional control; that is, VC = IRV + V_T + ERV. The common method of measuring VC is to achieve maximal inspiration and then forcibly exhale all of the air as hard and as fast as possible until the ERV has been exhausted. Because the exhalation is forced, it is called the forced vital capacity (FVC). An equation that is useful to predict VC in men is[19]:

$$VC = 0.0481 \times H - 0.020 \times A - 2.81$$

For women, the equation is[19]:

$$VC = 0.0404 \times H - 0.022 \times A - 2.35$$

where

H = height in centimeters
A = age in years

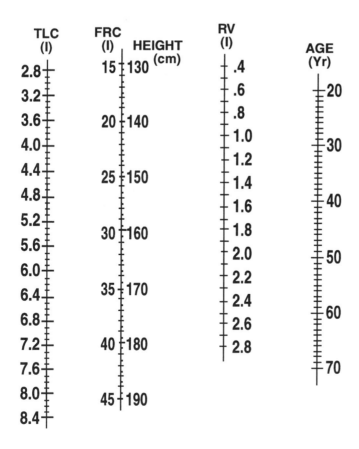

MALES

FIGURE 3–12. Nomograms for calculating lung volumes and capacities in healthy, nonsmoking men. FRC = functional residual capacity; RV = residual volume; TLC = total lung capacity. (From Cherniak, R: Pulmonary Function Testing. WB Saunders, Philadelphia, 1977, p. 247, with permission.)

In the continuing example, the maximum amount of air that could be exhaled after a maximal inhalation would be VC = IRV + TV + ERV or 3000 + 500 + 1000 milliliters = 4500.

Figures 3–12 and 3–13 are nomograms used for calculating lung volumes and capacities in healthy, nonsmoking men and women.

Volumes and capacities are dependent on the age, height, race, gender, and body position of a subject.[18,20] With increasing age, the lungs gradually lose their elastic properties and the thorax becomes stiffer.[21] Lung volumes reflect these changes with an increase in the FRC.[21] The increase in FRC is caused primarily by an increase in residual volume. With increasing age, there are also decreases in the IRV and VC.[12] Expiratory flow rates also are found to decrease as a result of the aging process.[22]

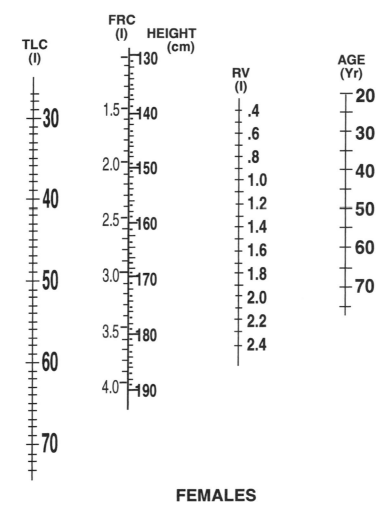

FEMALES

FIGURE 3–13. Nomograms for calculating lung volumes and capacities in healthy, nonsmoking women. FRC = functional residual capacity; RV = residual volume; TLC = total lung capacity. (From Cherniak, R: Pulmonary Function Testing. WB Saunders, Philadelphia, 1977, p. 248, with permission.)

There is a direct relationship between a person's height and that person's measured lung volumes and capacities.[23] Arm span can be used to predict lung volumes in patients with spinal deformities that alter their heights.[24]

Ethnicity and gender also play a role in the predicted values of the pulmonary function tests.[25-27] Black men have smaller lung volumes than white men of equal height and age.[23,25-27] Smaller lung volumes are found in women than in men when age and height are the same for both.[28] A quantitative measurement of thoracic size may be a more reliable predictor of lung volumes and capacities than height, race, or gender.

Body position also can alter lung volumes and capacities. Both FRC and VC decrease when a subject moves from the erect posture of sitting or standing to lying supine.[29] The effects of gravity on the thorax, diaphragm, and abdominal contents, as well as restriction of the supporting surface, are at least partly responsible for the changes. During conventional measurement of lung volumes and flow rates, the body position is erect, usually sitting.[30]

Any alteration in the properties of the lungs or chest wall will change lung volumes and capacities. A loss of the elastic properties of the lung parenchyma allows an unrestrained expansion of the chest. The result is an increase in RV, FRC, and TLC; vital capacity is decreased.[31] This can occur in certain obstructive disease states such as emphysema.

Fibrosis of the lung parenchyma increases the elastic properties of the lungs, resulting in the characteristic pattern observed in restrictive pulmonary disease: a decrease in vital capacity and TLC.[32] Pleural fibrosis and restriction of the chest wall as a result of disease or deformity can also restrict the lungs' ability to expand and structurally reduce VC and TLC.[33,34] Figure 3–14 shows the normal lung volumes and capacities as well as the changes that occur with obstructive and restrictive pulmonary disease.

LUNG VOLUMES AND CAPACITIES

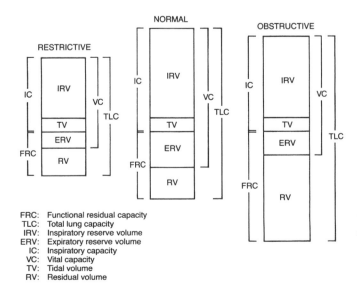

FRC: Functional residual capacity
TLC: Total lung capacity
IRV: Inspiratory reserve volume
ERV: Expiratory reserve volume
IC: Inspiratory capacity
VC: Vital capacity
TV: Tidal volume
RV: Residual volume

FIGURE 3–14. Lung volumes and capacities in normal as well as obstructive and restrictive pulmonary diseases. (From Rothstein, JM, Roy, SH, and Wolf, SL: The Rehabilitation Specialist's Handbook, ed. 2. FA Davis, Philadelphia, 1998, p. 509, with permission.)

Flow Rates and Mechanics

Flow rates are the measurements of gas volumes moved in a period of time. Expiratory flow rates, therefore, are measurements of exhaled gas volume divided by the amount of time of the exhalation. Flow rates reflect the ease with which the lungs can be ventilated, and they are related to the resistance to airflow, or the elasticity of the lung parenchyma.[20]

FORCED EXPIRATORY VOLUME IN ONE SECOND

An important airflow measurement is the volume of air that can be forcefully exhaled during the first second of a forced vital capacity maneuver. This is called the forced expiratory volume in one second, or FEV_1. In a healthy individual, the FEV_1 is greater than 75 percent of the total FVC. Using the example of a 70-kg man, a normal value of FEV_1 should be 3.4 liters per second or greater (4500 liters × 0.75). The expiratory flow rate in Figure 3–15 shows an FEV_1 of 3.8 liters per second, within the normal range. Nomograms for forced expiratory flow rates are given in Figures 3–16 and 3–17. Inspiratory flow rates can also be determined by measuring the amount of air inspired and the amount of time necessary for the inhalation.

FORCED EXPIRATORY FLOW FROM 25 TO 75 PERCENT OF VITAL CAPACITY

Forced expiratory flow from 25 to 75 percent of FVC ($FEF_{25\%-75\%}$) or mid maximal expiratory flow rate (MMEFR) is the flow rate found in the middle of the forced expiratory flow volume curve, Figure 3–18. This flow rate is thought to reflect the status of the smaller airways of the lung. These airways may be the first to show the presence of disease, and therefore may make it possible to protect the lungs from further deterioration by changes in lifestyle (smoking cessation) and appropriate medical management.

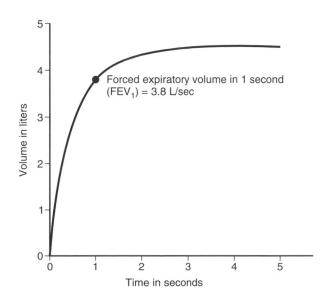

FIGURE 3–15. Forced expiratory volume in 1 second (FEV_1) assessed from a forced vital capacity curve.

MALES

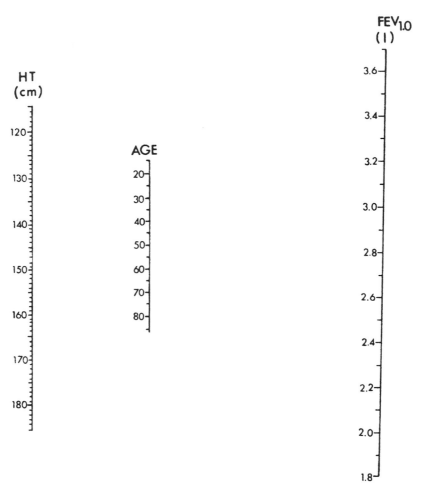

FIGURE 3–16. Nomogram for calculating FEV_1 in healthy nonsmoking men. (From Cherniak,[18] p. 245, with permission.)

Any alteration in the properties of the lungs or chest wall will also alter flow rates. Patients who present with obstructive pulmonary disease will have a VC that takes longer to exhale because of the loss of the elastic recoil of the lungs: the FEV_1 and $FEF_{25\%-75\%}$ will be decreased, less air will be exhaled in the time period. Patients who present with restrictive pulmonary disease may also have a volume of air exhaled in the first second that is less than would be predicted by their height, age, race, and gender. However, in the case of the patient with restrictive pulmonary disease, the decrease in FEV_1 is due to the overall lack of volume, not the ability to exhale it. Therefore, when corrected for vital capacity, FEV_1/FVC, the resulting percentage is within the normal range of greater than 75.

Measurement and interpretation of spirometric values are covered in greater detail in Chapters 6 and 10.

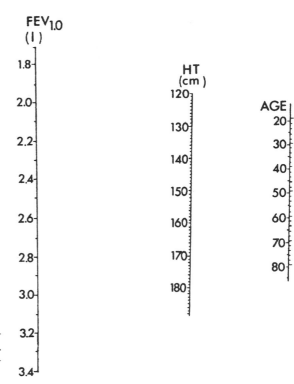

FEMALES

FEV$_{1.0}$
(l)

HT
(cm)

AGE

FIGURE 3-17. Nomogram for calculating FEV$_1$ in healthy nonsmoking women. (From Cherniak,[19] p. 246, with permission.)

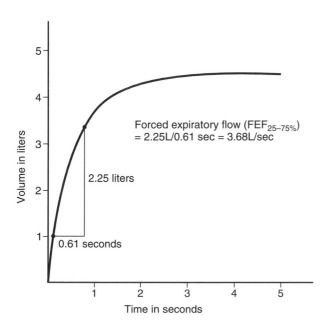

Forced expiratory flow (FEF$_{25-75\%}$)
= 2.25L/0.61 sec = 3.68L/sec

2.25 liters

0.61 seconds

Volume in liters

Time in seconds

FIGURE 3-18. Forced expiratory flow rate (FEF$_{25-75\%}$) assessed from a forced vital capacity curve. The total volume (4500 liters) is divided into quarters. The middle two quarters (2.25 liters) are divided by the time it takes to exhale that volume (0.61 second). FEF$_{25-75\%}$= 3.68 liters/second.

RESPIRATION

"Respiration" is a term used to describe the gaseous exchange that occurs between the atmospheric air and pulmonary capillaries or between the tissues and the surrounding capillaries. It should not be confused with ventilation, which describes only the movement of air. External respiration is the gaseous exchange that occurs at the alveolar/capillary membrane; internal respiration takes place at the tissue/capillary level. The following discussion describes the course of gas exchange, specifically, oxygen and carbon dioxide, during both external and internal respiration.

For external respiration to take place, there must first be an inhalation of air from the ambient environment, through the conducting airways, and into the alveoli. Oxygen diffuses through the alveolar wall, through the interstitial space, and through the pulmonary capillary wall. Most of the oxygen (98.5 percent) then travels through the blood plasma into the red blood cells and onto one of the gas-carrying sites of hemoglobin.[20] A small portion of oxygen (1.5 percent) is carried dissolved in the plasma.

The rate of diffusion of oxygen from the alveoli into the capillary is dependent on three factors that can vary with pulmonary pathologies: (1) the surface area of the respiratory units available for gas exchange (A), (2) the thickness of the alveolar capillary membranes (T), and (3) the pressure gradient (P_1-P_2) created between the partial pressure of oxygen within the alveoli (P_1) and that within the pulmonary capillary (P_2). Fick's law describes these relations as follows:

$$15_{V_{GAS}} \propto A/T \, D(P_1 - P_2)$$

where D is the diffusing constant for a specific gas, in this case, oxygen.

To better understand diffusion during respiration, a further discussion of the variables of Fick's law may be helpful. The lungs' approximately 300 million alveoli correspond to 160 m^2 of the alveolar surface area potentially available for gas diffusion.[3] The alveolar capillary membrane that must be permeated to permit the diffusion of oxygen consists of several layers. There is a thin layer of surfactant fluid that lines the inside of the alveoli, an alveolar epithelium, an alveolar epithelial basement membrane, an interstitial space, a pulmonary capillary basement membrane, and a capillary endothelial membrane. Although that seems like an abundance of layers, the approximate thickness of the combined layers is only 0.63 μm.[3]

Determining the partial pressure of oxygen in the ambient environment is the first step in understanding the pressure gradient created by oxygen for diffusion. The total pressure exerted by the atmospheric gases at sea level is 760 mm Hg. Oxygen makes up approximately 21 percent of all of the atmospheric gases; this is called the fraction of inspired oxygen: $F_{IO_2} = 0.21$. The fraction of inspired nitrogen is about 79 percent: $F_{IN_2} = 0.79$. All other gases make up less than 1 percent of atmospheric air. Because all gases combined exert a pressure of 760 mm Hg, the partial pressure exerted by oxygen (P_{O_2}) alone is 21 percent of 760 mm Hg, or 159 mm Hg. As atmospheric air enters the lungs, some oxygen becomes displaced by water vapor (P_{H_2O}) from the humidification process of the upper airway and diluted by carbon dioxide (P_{CO_2}), which is constantly diffusing into the alveoli. The partial pressure of oxygen is thus decreased. In the alveoli, P_{AO_2} (P_1 of Fick's law for oxygen diffusion) is 104 mm Hg[20] (Table 3–1).

The blood within the pulmonary capillary returns from the tissue level with a partial pressure of oxygen (P_{VO_2}) of 40 mm Hg; P_2 of Fick's law is 40 mm Hg (see Table

TABLE 3–1 The Approximate Partial Pressures of Atmospheric Air at Sea
Level and at Different Points During Ventilation and Respiration

	Dry Atmosphere, mm Hg	Moist Atmosphere, mm Hg	Tracheal, mm Hg	Alveolar, mm Hg	Arterial, mm Hg	Venous, mm Hg	Exhaled, mm Hg
P_{O_2}	159	159	149	104	95	40	120
P_{CO_2}	0.3	0.3	0.3	40	40	45	27
P_{H_2O}	0.0	47	47	47	47	47	47
P_{N_2}	600	597	563	569	569	569	566

*Although single numbers are given for clarity, ranges providing some variability would be more accurate.

3–1). Therefore, the pressure gradient for oxygen diffusion at the alveolar capillary membrane is from 104 mm Hg (arterial side) to 40 mm Hg (venous side).

The blood leaving a fully functioning alveolar capillary unit has a partial pressure of oxygen in the arterial blood (Pa_{O_2}) of 104 mm Hg.[3] Diffusion across the pressure gradient has occurred, and most of the blood (98 percent) that enters the left side of the heart has a Pa_{O_2} of 104 mm Hg.[3] The other 2 percent of blood entering the left atrium comes from the bronchial circulation system, which supplies the conducting airways. This blood is venous blood that does not take part in the external respiratory process and therefore has a P_{O_2} of 40 mm Hg. Mixing the newly oxygenated blood from the pulmonary veins with the venous blood from the bronchial vein causes the partial pressure of oxygen within the left heart to become slightly diluted: The blood within the left side of the heart has a Pa_{O_2} of 95 to 100 mm Hg. (Note that alveolar partial pressures of gas are denoted by "A" and arterial blood partial pressure by "a.")

The oxygenated blood travels out of the left side of the heart into the aorta and through a network of connecting arteries, arterioles, and capillaries until it reaches its destination, the tissue. Internal respiration takes place as the arterial blood reaches the tissue level. Oxygen now diffuses off the gas-carrying sites of hemoglobin, out of the red cells, out of the capillary through the membranes, and into the mitochondria of the working cells. Again, this process of diffusion is caused by differences in pressures. The capillary has a Pa_{O_2} of 95 to 100 mm Hg, since no oxygen has been given off. The interstitial fluid has a partial pressure of oxygen of between 5 and 40 mm Hg.[3] Therefore, the pressure gradient promotes oxygen diffusion from the capillary into the tissues—from an area of high pressure to an area of lower pressure. Blood leaving the cell and going into the venous system has a Pv_{O_2} of 40 mm Hg.

Carbon dioxide, which is produced at the tissue level as a by-product of metabolism, diffuses out of the cells and back into the capillaries. It is transported through the venous system into the right side of the heart. Once the carbon dioxide makes its way to the pulmonary capillary, it is released through the capillary membrane, through the interstitial space, and into the alveoli, where it is finally exhaled into the atmosphere. The rate of diffusion of carbon dioxide out of the cell, into the capillary, and then out of the capillary into the alveoli depends on all the variables of Fick's law:

$$V_{GAS} \propto A/T\ D(P_1 - P_2)$$

The surface areas (A) for diffusion of CO_2 are the same as those already described for oxygen. The thicknesses of the membranes T through which diffusion occurs also are the same as those for oxygen. The pressure gradient (T) (P_1-P_2) created by carbon dioxide are not, however, the same. Blood leaves the tissue and returns to the pulmonary artery and pulmonary capillary with a partial pressure of CO_2 of 46 mm Hg.[3] The alveoli have a partial pressure of CO_2 of 35 to 45 mm Hg. Carbon dioxide diffuses out of the pulmonary capillary and into the alveoli. As blood leaves a functioning alveolar-capillary unit, the partial pressure of CO_2 is 35 to 45 mm Hg. The pressure gradient created by the partial pressure of carbon dioxide is far less than the pressure gradient created by oxygen. The diffusion of CO_2 might not be so complete if the diffusion constant of CO_2 were not so great. In fact, the diffusion constant for CO_2 is 20 times greater than the diffusion constant for O_2. Carbon dioxide diffusion across the lower pressure gradients occurs rapidly and completely.

When the cycle of external and internal respiration has occurred, oxygen has been provided and carbon dioxide has been removed. Of course, this system is dependent on an intact cardiovascular system to pump the blood through the lungs, deliver it to the working cells, and then return it to the lungs—all in a timely fashion.

Perfusion

"Perfusion of the lung" is the term used to describe pulmonary circulation. Blood is ejected from the right ventricle into the pulmonary artery, through which it goes to the lungs. Blood returns to the left heart via the pulmonary veins. The pulmonary circulation is a low-pressure system as compared with the systemic circulation. Normal pulmonary artery pressure is 25/10 mm Hg as compared with the pressure in the aorta, which is 120/80 mm Hg. Gravity affects the low-pressure pulmonary vascular system more than the systemic high-pressure system. The lower areas of the lung, the gravity-dependent areas, obtain the greatest amount of the blood flow that is due to the effects of hydrostatic pressure (gravity). That is, when a person is in the standing position, the gravity-dependent areas of the lungs (the bases) receive the greatest amount of blood flow. The apices of the lungs in this position are the most gravity-independent and therefore receive the least amount of perfusion. When a person is in the supine position, the posterior aspect of the lungs is the most gravity-dependent area and receives the most blood flow, whereas the gravity-independent area, the anterior surface, receives the least amount of perfusion. Figure 3–19 shows the effect of body position on areas of gravity dependence and therefore areas of greatest perfusion.

The effects of local stimulation on the pulmonary system are usually opposite that of the systemic circulation. For example, the pulmonary system responds to hypoxemia by vasoconstriction whereas the systemic circulation responds by vasodilation. In the lung, this vasoconstriction acts to reroute (shunt) the pulmonary blood flow from underventilated alveoli (areas of hypoxia) to ventilated alveoli, thereby causing gas exchange to be nearly optimal. In the systemic circulation, hypoxia stimulates vasodilation to reverse the lack of oxygen the tissue is experiencing. Hypercapnea (an increase in carbon dioxide) causes pulmonary vasoconstriction but systemic vasodilation. Other stimuli that may cause opposite reactions are norepinephrine, serotonin, histamine, and acidemia.

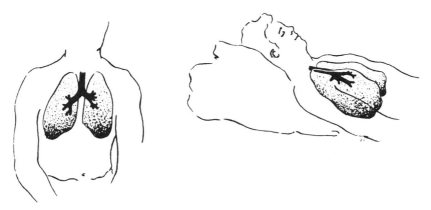

FIGURE 3–19. The effect of body position on pulmonary perfusion. (From Frownfelter, D: Chest Physical Therapy and Pulmonary Rehabilitation: An Interdisciplinary Approach, ed 2. Mosby-Year Book, Inc., Chicago, 1987, p. 51, with permission.)

Ventilation-Perfusion Relationship

At the alveolar capillary level, the ventilation (V) and the perfusion (Q) must be balanced so that optimal gas exchange can occur. Regional differences in pulmonary blood flow caused by the influence of hydrostatic pressure have been discussed in the section on pulmonary perfusion. Similar differences are found in the ventilatory aspect of the lungs.[35] The regional differences in ventilation are caused by an intrapleural pressure gradient that tends to be more negative at the upper part of the lung and less negative at the lower part of the lung. When a person is in the upright position, this pressure gradient results in a greater resting expansion in the apical areas of the lung than in the basalar areas. When air is inhaled, the apices, being almost full at the onset of inhalation, receive very little of the new volume of air. The bases, however, being almost empty, receive most of the inhaled volume of air. The greatest change in volume, and therefore the most ventilation, occurs at the bases of the lungs, whereas the least change in volume, and therefore the least ventilation, occurs in the apices. When the position is changed, the areas of greatest ventilation also change. For example, when a person is in the supine position, the area of greatest volume change is in the posterior aspect of the lungs and the least volume change is in the anterior aspect of the lungs.

The relation of pulmonary ventilation ($\dot{V}$) to perfusion ($\dot{Q}$) is written as the ratio $\dot{V}/\dot{Q}$. In a normal state of health, ventilation and perfusion are balanced. Knowing that ventilation is 4 liters of air per minute (on the average) and perfusion is 5 liters of blood per minute (again, on the average), the ventilation:perfusion relationship in health can be calculated: $\dot{V}/\dot{Q} = 4/5$, or 0.8.

Ventilation-perfusion inequalities occur in diseased states. Three examples of possible relations are shown in Figure 3–20. The first abnormality shows a normally aerated alveolus with no capillary perfusion; it is called a physiologic dead space ($\dot{V}/\dot{Q} = 4/0 = \infty$). The second abnormality shows a fully perfused capillary with no alveolar ventilation; it is referred to as a physiologic shunt ($\dot{V}/\dot{Q} = 0/5 = 0$). The final abnormality is an alveolus with no ventilation and a capillary with no perfusion, which is called a silent unit ($\dot{V}/\dot{Q} = 0/0 = 0$). In disease states the alveolar capillary

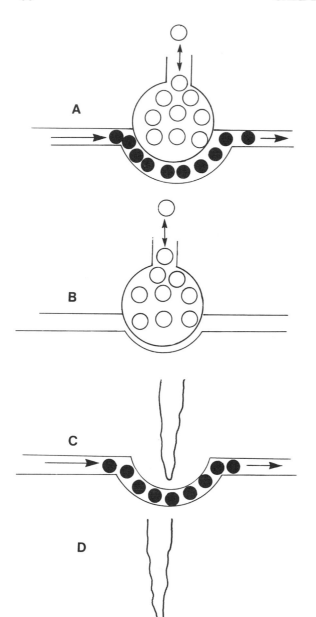

FIGURE 3–20. The ventilation-perfusion relationships that can exist in health and in pulmonary disease. *A,* Healthy alveolar capillary unit. *B,* Normally aerated alveoli with no capillary perfusion-physiologic dead space. *C,* Normally perfused capillary with no alveolar aeration-physiologic shunt. *D,* A nonaerated alveoli next to a nonperfused capillary = silent unit. (Adapted from Price, SA and Wilson, LM: Pathophysiology: Clinical Concepts and Disease Processes, ed 4. Mosby Year Book, Inc. St Louis, 1992, with permission.)

unit may have slight to severe alveolar capillary abnormalities. The result of these abnormalities can be detected and monitored with the use of arterial blood gas analyses, which are discussed later in this chapter.

REGULATION OF RESPIRATION

Neurologic control of ventilation and respiration is multifactorial. Breathing is primarily an involuntary act, and there is no need to cognitively take a breath. The autonomic nervous system has control over breathing, and there is volitional control over ventilation. Chemoreceptors, baroreceptors, and proprioceptors provide the necessary input to assist in the control of breathing.

The respiratory centers are located within the pons and the medulla oblongata.[36] The medulla seems to control the basic rhythm of inspiration and expiration.[20] The pons is divided into two centers that modulate the basic rhythm of the medulla. The apneustic center in the lower pons provides for greater inspiration effort, and the pneumotaxic center of the upper pons seems to inhibit or limit inspiration after it has reached a certain level, allowing exhalation to occur.

The autonomic nervous system is another entity involved in the neural control of ventilation. The sympathetic nervous system, when stimulated, increases both the depth and frequency of ventilation. It also increases the size of the bronchial lumen (bronchodilation) and decreases the production of pulmonary secretions. Stimulation of the parasympathetic nervous system will have the opposite effects.

Volitional control by the cerebral cortex, which can override the normal rhythm of breathing, is also present. This volition grants us the ability to phonate, sing a song, or even hold our breath until we "turn blue."

Involuntary stimulus-response types of breathing are also possible. Many types of sensory feedback elicit respiratory responses.[37] For example, imagine that you put your hand on a hot stove. Along with quickly removing your hand, you will find that you also take a quick inhalation.

Chemoreceptors respond to changes in the chemical concentration in the cerebral spinal fluid (CSF) and the blood. These are the main receptors for the neurologic control of breathing. The central chemoreceptors line the fourth ventricle of the brain and are sensitive to the changes in CO_2 and H^+ concentrations of the CSF. The peripheral chemoreceptors are located in the aortic arch and the carotid bodies; they sense changes in the circulating partial pressures of O_2 and CO_2 and the pH. The central chemoreceptors are responsible for the regulation of breathing. Slight variations in the body's Pa_{CO_2} begin the firing of the receptors, thereby changing the ventilatory pattern. The oxygen-sensitive aspect of the peripheral chemoreceptors seems to be more of a reserve or backup system because the partial pressure of oxygen must fall to approximately half of its normal value before the receptors respond and change the ventilatory pattern.

Receptors located within the lung can also exert some control over the ventilatory pattern. The Hering-Breuer inflation receptor is a stretch receptor mechanism that limits inhalation. J receptors, found in "juxtaposition" to the pulmonary capillaries, lie in the alveolar walls close to the pulmonary circulation. The stimulation of these receptors may cause rapid, shallow breathing and bradycardia and may be associated with the sensation of dyspnea. Irritant receptors within the airways can cause bronchoconstriction and hyperapnea.

There are also receptors located outside the lungs that can exert some control over ventilation. Baroreceptors within the aorta and carotid bodies can cause reflex hypoventilation or apnea during an episode of increased arterial pressure or hyperventilation during a period of decreased arterial pressure. Receptors within the respiratory muscles and proprioceptors in the joints of the thoracic cage or exercising limbs may activate a change in the ventilatory pattern.[38,39] The regulation of ventilation is a complex modulation of various stimuli from the receptors. Figure 3–21 integrates these complex interactions into a very simple diagram.

The three corners of the triangle in Figure 3–21 are labeled the sensors, the central

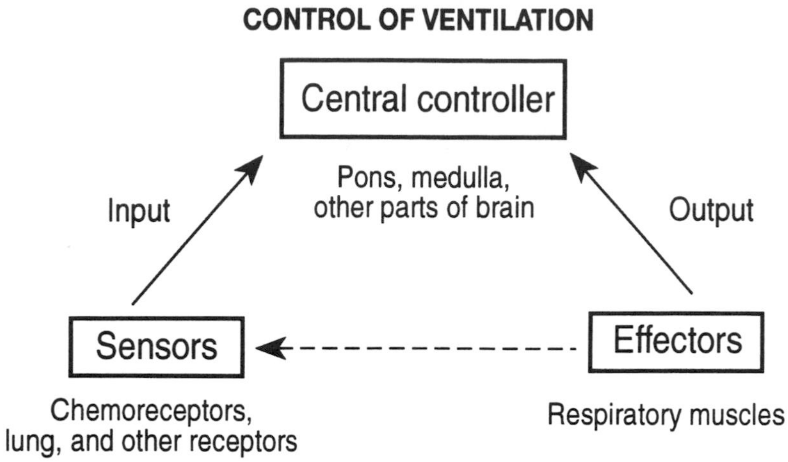

CONTROL OF VENTILATION

FIGURE 3-21. Schematic representation of the regulation of ventilation and respiration. Information from various sensors is fed to the central controller, the output of which goes to the ventilatory muscles. By changing ventilation, the ventilatory muscles reduce perturbations of the sensors (negative feedback). (From West, J: Respiratory Physiology: The Essential, ed 2. Williams & Wilkins, Baltimore, p. 115, with permission.)

controllers, and the effectors. The sensors are the chemoreceptors, the stretch receptors, the baroreceptors, and the proprioceptors. They send signals to the central controllers: the medulla oblongata, the pons, and the cortex. The central controllers respond by increasing or decreasing the impulses sent to the effectors, which are the muscles of ventilation. The breathing parameters are changed, and the sensors now evaluate the adequacy of the new breathing pattern. The cycle continues sensing and effecting the breathing pattern.

Each breath is initiated, evaluated, and adjusted when necessary to create a breathing pattern that maintains appropriate levels of oxygen and carbon dioxide and provides for hemodynamic stability throughout the body.

ACID-BASE BALANCE

Acid-base balance is of the utmost importance in the maintenance of the body's homeostasis. The acid-base balance of the body hinges on the amount of hydrogen ions (H^+) in the blood. The pH of the body is the negative logarithm of the concentration of the hydrogen ions in the body fluids. A normal range for arterial blood pH is 7.35 to 7.45. Any decrease in blood pH below 7.35 is called acidemia; that is, the blood is more acidic than is normal. Any increase in the blood pH above 7.45 is termed alkalemia; the blood is then more alkaline than is normal. A small change in the pH in either direction can cause depression or overexcitation of the nervous system; a substantial change in the pH can result in coma or convulsions.

The body has three buffer systems that attempt to maintain and normalize blood pH at all times. The blood buffers provide an immediate defense against an alteration in H^+ concentration. Hemoglobin and other blood proteins can act as buffers, as they have the ability to bind with H^+ and effectively negate its influence on the pH.

The second system that helps regulate the acid-base balance of the body is the respiratory system. By increasing or decreasing alveolar minute ventilation, the respiratory system has the ability to modulate the concentration of carbon dioxide and therefore effect a change in the amount of H^+ in the blood through the following equation:

$$H_2O + CO_2 \Leftrightarrow H_2CO_3 \Leftrightarrow H^+ + HCO_3^-$$

The respiratory system's ability to directly regulate $Paco_2$ and thereby indirectly regulate the H^+ concentration provides an influence on the pH of the body.[40] As previously stated in this chapter, the partial pressure of carbon dioxide in arterial blood ($Paco_2$) is 35 to 45 mm Hg. Hyperventilation is defined as a decrease in $Paco_2$, which decreases the available H^+. The blood is less acidic, resulting in a pH greater than 7.45. Hypoventilation is an increase in $Paco_2$, which causes an increase in available H^+. An acidemia results; it is reflected by a pH lower than 7.35. An inverse relation therefore exists between $Paco_2$ and the pH of the blood.

The final body system to be mentioned in the regulation of acid-base balance is the renal system. Serum bicarbonate (HCO_3^-), which is produced and retained by the kidneys, acts as a buffer. The normal level of HCO_3^- in arterial blood is 24 mEq per liter. Bicarbonate can combine with H^+ to form H_2CO_3, which effectively eliminates its influence over pH. If the kidneys produce more than the usual amount of bicarbonate, greater than 24 mEq per liter, the blood will be more buffered. The result will be an alkalemia. Any decrease in the amount of metabolic buffers results in a decrease in the body pH, and the result is an acidemia. A direct relation exists between the amount of HCO_3^- and the pH of the blood.

Both the respiratory and renal systems can cause a primary acidemia or alkalemia. Each system's ability to influence the pH can also be used to correct alterations in acid-base balance, and therefore either system can be a compensatory mechanism. Within 1 to 15 minutes, the respiratory system can compensate for an alteration in H^+ concentration and move the pH back toward the normal range of 7.35 to 7.45.[3] In contrast, several minutes to several days are required for a readjustment of the pH by the serum bicarbonate mechanism.[3]

ARTERIAL BLOOD GAS ANALYSIS

The analysis of the partial pressures of gases within the arterial blood indicates the effectiveness of alveolar ventilation and the role of the ventilation in acid-base balance.[40] Three factors from an arterial blood gas analysis are required to evaluate the acid-base status: (1) the blood pH, (2) the partial pressure of carbon dioxide, and (3) the amount of serum bicarbonate. The pH should be evaluated first. Any change from the normal range, 7.35 to 7.45, and also the direction of the change, should be noted. By determining the pH, an acidemia, alkalemia, or normal pH can be determined.

The next value to be evaluated in the assessment process is the $Paco_2$. Again, any change from the normal range, 35 to 45 mm Hg, should be noted. The direction of the change should be compared with the direction of change in the pH. It is important to remember that an inverse relation exists between the $Paco_2$ and the pH. For example, if all other body systems are stable and the $Paco_2$ becomes less than 35 mm Hg, the pH will rise: a respiratory alkalosis has occurred. An increase in $Paco_2$ will cause the pH to fall, producing a respiratory acidosis. An approximate numerical relation also exists between the Pa_{CO_2} and the pH. For every 10 mm Hg change in the Pa_{CO_2} value, there should be an approximate change (in the opposite direction) of 0.08 in the pH. For example (using the midrange of 40 mm Hg for Pa_{CO_2} and the midrange of 7.40 for pH), an increase in the Pa_{CO_2} to 50 mm Hg would result in a pH decrease to 7.32. Likewise, a decrease in the Pa_{CO_2} to 30 mm Hg would result in a rise in the pH to 7.48. If this inverse relationship between the Pa_{CO_2} and pH is evident, the alteration in pH is respiratory in origin. If the inverse relationship does not exist, further investigation into the cause of altered acid-base balance is necessary.

The third value to assess when determining acid-base balance is the concentration of the bicarbonate ion (HCO_3^-). Any deviation from 24 mEq per liter should be noted, as should be the direction of the change. There is a direct relation between bicarbonate and pH. An increase in bicarbonate concentration results in an increase in pH, and vice versa. When this direct relationship exists, the primary cause of the alteration in pH is of metabolic etiology.

Patients may present with signs and symptoms of alkalosis and acidosis from either a respiratory or metabolic etiology. Table 3–2 summarizes the alterations in the components of primary, uncompensated alterations in body pH as well as their causes, signs, and symptoms.

There are also compensatory mechanisms to be considered in the acid-base balance. For example, if the metabolic system causes a change in the pH, the respiratory system has the ability to compensate for that change. The reverse is also true. The respiratory system could be the cause of the pH disturbance, and the metabolic system could compensate. In this way, both the respiratory system and the renal system have the ability to create a compensating acidosis or alkalosis to normalize the original dysfunction.[41] It is helpful to know that the body never overcompensates for an acid-base disturbance.

The analysis of the arterial blood gas also offers insight into arterial oxygenation. The partial pressure of oxygen within the arterial system of a subject breathing room air ($F_{IO_2} = 0.21$) at sea level has been previously stated to be approximately 95 to 100 mm Hg. "Hypoxemia" is the term used when the amount of oxygen in the blood is below 80 mm

TABLE 3–2 Abnormalities of Acid-Base Balance

Type	pH	Pa_{CO_2}	HCO_3^-	Causes	Signs/Symptoms
Uncompensated respiratory alkalosis	↑	↓	—	Alveolar hyperventilation	Dizziness, tingling, syncopy, numbness, early tetany
Uncompensated respiratory acidosis	↓	↑	—	Alveolar hypoventilation	Early: Anxiety, restlessness, dyspnea, headache. Late: confusion, somnolence, and coma
Uncompensated metabolic alkalosis	↑	—	↑	Bicarbonate ingestion, vomiting, diuretics, steroids, adrenal disease	Vague symptoms: weakness, mental dullness, possibly early tetany
Uncompensated metabolic acidosis	↓	—	↓	Diabetic, lactic uremic acidosis, prolonged diarrhea	Nausea, vomiting, cardiac arrhythmias, lethargy, coma

Source: Adapted from Rothstein, JM, Roy, SH, and Wolf, SL: The Rehabilitation Specialist's Handbook, ed. 2. FA Davis, 1998, p 529, with permission

TABLE 3–3 Estimated Fractions of Inspired Oxygen FIO_2 with
Low-Flow Devices

Nasal Cannula, L/min	Estimated FIO_2	Oxygen Mask, L/min	Estimated FIO_2	Mask with Reservoir, L/min	Estimated FIO_2
1	0.24	5–6	0.40	7	0.70
2	0.28	6–7	0.50	8	0.80
3	0.32	7–8	0.60	9	0.90
4	0.36			10	0.99+

Source: Adapted from Rothstein, JM, Roy, SH, and Wolf, SL: The Rehabilitation Specialist's Handbook, ed. 2. FA Davis, 1998, p 532, with permission.

Hg.[20] In mild hypoxemia, the $PacO_2$ is less than 80 mm Hg; in moderate hypoxemia, it is less than 70 mm Hg; and in severe hypoxemia, it is less than 60 mm Hg.[20]

There is not a finite relation between the partial pressures of oxygen and CO_2 in the blood. Although it is true that if subjects decrease their minute ventilation, $PacO_2$ will rise and PaO_2 will fall, the reverse is not true. If minute ventilation is increased, $PacO_2$ will fall but the oxygen tension within the arterial system will stay approximately the same. This is partly because of the fixed pool of oxygen in the atmosphere and the efficiency of the system, which is difficult to "improve" upon.

To increase the $PacO_2$ above the normal range, an increase in the fraction of inspired oxygen is needed. Table 3–3 lists estimates of the fraction of inspired oxygen available through different types of oxygen delivery systems.[42]

The amount of oxygen available at the alveoli can be estimated from the FIO_2:

$$PAO_2 - FIO_2(PB \quad 47) \quad PacO_2(FIO_2 + 1 - FIO_2R)$$

where PB is the barometric pressure, which can be assumed to be at sea level, or 760 mm Hg, and R is the respiratory quotient, which can be assumed to be 0.8 in most instances.[1] Table 3–4 illustrates the partial pressure of oxygen available within the alveoli according to the FIO_2 present.

TABLE 3–4 Fraction
of Inspired Oxygen (FIO_2)
and the Corresponding
Alveolar Partial Pressure
of Oxygen (PAO_2)

FIO_2	Available PAO_2, mm Hg
0.21	104
0.30	167
0.40	239
0.50	311
0.60	384
0.70	456
0.80	528
0.90	601
1.00	673

CASE STUDIES

It may be helpful to study the following three examples of arterial blood gas analyses to determine their significance in patient diagnoses.

CASE 1

A 45-year-old man with asthma was in his usual state of health until he noticed shortness of breath and wheezing. The arterial blood gas values are shown below.

	Arterial Blood Gas Values	
	Normal	Case Study #1
F_{IO_2}	0.21	0.21
Pa_{O_2} (mm Hg)	95	70
Pa_{CO_2} (mm Hg)	40	25
pH	7.40	7.50
HCO_3^- (mEq/L)	24	24

To determine the acid-base balance, the pH was evaluated first. It was found to be 7.50, which is above the 7.45 upper limit of normal; therefore, there is an alkalemia. The next value assessed was the Pa_{CO_2}, which was 25 mm Hg: a 10 mm Hg decrease from the lower limit of normal. The pH and the Pa_{CO_2} have changed in opposite directions, so the respiratory system is determined to be the origin of the acid-base problem. (Clinical information also is important in making this conclusion.) For each change of 10 mm Hg in the Pa_{CO_2} there should be a change of approximately 0.08 in the pH (from midpoint 7.40), which results in a pH value of 7.50. Next, the HCO_3^- concentration was evaluated. It was found to be 24 mEq per liter. Compensation by the metabolic system has not yet occurred. Therefore, this man was diagnosed as having an alkalemia caused by a respiratory alkalosis with no compensation by the metabolic system. He is also moderately hypoxemic.

CASE 2

A 25-year-old woman with diabetes was in her usual state of health until 2 days ago, when she noted that her diabetes was no longer in control. She was admitted to the hospital in diabetic ketoacidosis with the arterial blood gas values shown below.

	Arterial Blood Gas Values	
	Normal	Case Study #2
F_{IO_2}	0.21	0.21
Pa_{O_2} (mm Hg)	95	95
Pa_{CO_2} (mm Hg)	40	25
pH	7.40	7.32
HCO_3^- (mEq/L)	24	18

Again, first her pH was evaluated. It was 7.32, a mild acidemia. Her $Paco_2$ has decreased to 25 mm Hg. There is a decrease in $Paco_2$ and a decrease in pH. The change in pH is not from a respiratory dysfunction. If the respiratory system were the cause of the abnormality, a $Paco_2$ of 25 should result in an alkalemia. The HCO_3 is 18 mEq per liter, less than the normal value of 24 mEq per liter. A decrease in HCO_3 and a decrease in pH mean that there is a metabolic cause for the acid-base disturbance. This ABG shows a metabolic acidosis caused by the diabetic ketoacidosis. For a moment, again consider the $Paco_2$ value. Why would the respiratory system decrease the $Paco_2$? It has effectively created a respiratory alkalosis to help compensate for the metabolic acidosis created by the diabetic ketoacidosis. If the respiratory system had not altered the $Paco_2$, the overall acidemia would be far worse. Summarizing this case study, the patient has a normal Pao_2 and a mild acidemia caused by a metabolic acidosis with a partially compensating respiratory alkalosis.

CASE 3

A 65-year-old man with a history of chronic obstructive pulmonary disease presents for a routine physical examination in his usual state of health. His arterial blood gas analysis is shown below.

Arterial Blood Gas Values

	Normal	Case Study #3
FIO_2	0.21	0.21
Pao_2 (mm Hg)	95	55
$Paco_2$ (mm Hg)	40	60
pH	7.40	7.40
HCO_3^- (mEq/L)	24	29

Again, first evaluate the pH: it is within the normal range of 7.40. His $Paco_2$ has increased to 60 mm Hg. The increase in $Paco_2$ is causing a respiratory acidosis that is not reflected in the pH. The HCO_3 is 29 mEq per liter, greater than the normal value of 24 mEq per liter. An increase in HCO_3 is causing a metabolic alkalosis that again is not reflected in the pH. From the clinical information, it can be assumed that the respiratory system is the primary cause for the acid-base disturbance. It can also be assumed that the metabolic alkalosis is the compensating mechanism that is trying to return the body's pH to normal. Summarizing this case study, the patient has severe hypoxemia, a normal pH, and a respiratory acidosis with a fully compensating metabolic alkalosis.

SUMMARY

This chapter has presented a brief review of respiratory anatomy and physiology. The anatomy of the respiratory system comprises the bony thorax (including the sternum, clavicle, humerus, scapula, ribs, and vertebral column), the lungs, the upper airways (nose, mouth, pharynx, and larynx), the lower airways (trachea, bronchi, and bronchioles), and the respiratory unit (respiratory bronchioles, alveolar ducts, alveolar sacs, and alveoli). The muscles of ventilation include both the muscles of inspiration and those of expiration.

The discussion of physiology includes both ventilation and respiration. Ventilation is the movement of air in and out of the pulmonary system. The ventilation topics discussed include lung volumes, capacities, flow rates, and the mechanics of ventilation. "Respiration" refers to the ability of the pulmonary system to diffuse gas. The respiration topics discussed include diffusion, ventilation-perfusion relations, acid-base balance, and arterial blood gas analysis.

Neurologic control of respiration is provided by a complex group of systems: the cerebral cortex, the pons, the medulla oblongata, the autonomic nervous system, mechanical receptors, and chemical receptors. Their contribution to the regulation of respiration has been presented.

Respiratory diseases can alter the anatomy and physiology of the respiratory system either acutely or chronically, and Chapter 6 will discuss the possible alterations of the respiratory system and the resulting effects.

REFERENCES

 1. Harper, R: A Guide to Respiratory Care: Physiology and Clinical Applications. JB Lippincott, Philadelphia, 1981.
 2. Loring, S and Mead, J: Action of the diaphragm and rib cage inferred from force-balance analysis. J Appl Physiol 53:756–760, 1982.
 3. Guyton, A: Textbook of Medical Physiology, ed 9. Saunders, Philadelphia, 1996.
 4. Williams, P (ed): Gray's Anatomy, the Anatomical Basis of Medicine and Surgery, ed 38. Churchill Livingstone, New York, 1995.
 5. Roussos, C: Function and fatigue of the respiratory muscles. Chest (suppl) 88:1245–1335, 1985.
 6. Roussos, C and Macklem, P: The respiratory muscles. N Engl J Med 307:786–796, 1982.
 7. DeTroyer, A, Kelly, S, and Zin, W: Mechanical action of the intercostal muscles on the ribs. Science 220:82–88, 1983.
 8. Luce, J and Culver, B: Respiratory muscle function in health and disease. Chest 81:82–89, 1982.
 9. Kigin, C: Breathing exercises for the medical patient: The art and science. Phys Ther 70:700–706, 1990.
10. Raper, A, et al: Scalene and sternomastoid muscle function. J Appl Physiol 21:497–502, 1966.
11. Woodburne, R: Essentials of Human Anatomy, ed 9. Oxford University Press, New York, 1994.
12. Loring, S and Mead, J: Abdominal muscle use during quiet breathing and hyperpnea in uniformed subjects. J Appl Physiol 52:700–704, 1982.
13. DeTroyer, A: Mechanical action of the abdominal muscles. Bulletin of European Physiopathology of Respiration 19:575–581, 1983.
14. Downie, P (ed): Cash's Textbook of Chest, Heart and Vascular Disorders for Physiotherapists, ed 4. JB Lippincott, Philadelphia, 1987.
15. Green, J: Fundamental Cardiovascular and Pulmonary Physiology, ed 2. Lea & Febiger, Philadelphia, 1987.
16. Hobson, L and Dean, E: Review of respiratory anatomy. In Frownfelter, D: Chest Physical Therapy and Pulmonary Rehabilitation: An Interdisciplinary Approach, ed 3. Year Book Medical Publishers, Chicago, 1996.
17. Moore, K: Clinically Oriented Anatomy, ed 3. Williams & Wilkins, Baltimore, 1992.
18. Youtsey, J: Basic pulmonary function measurements. In C Spearman (ed): Egan's Fundamentals of Respiratory Therapy, ed 4. Mosby, St Louis, 1982.
19. Cherniak, R: Pulmonary Function Testing, ed 2. Saunders, Philadelphia, 1992.
20. Martin, D and Youtsey, J: Respiratory Anatomy and Physiology. Mosby, St Louis, 1988.
21. Zadai, C: Pulmonary physiology of aging: The role of rehabilitation. Topics in Geriatric Rehabilitation 1:49–56, 1985.
22. Berry, R, Pai, U, and Fairshter, R: Effect of age of changes in flow rates and airway conductance after a deep breath. J Appl Physiol 68:635–643, 1990.
23. Rahman, M, Ullah, M, and Beguin, A: Lung function in teenage Bangladeshi boys and girls. Respir Med 84:47–55, 1990.
24. Hepper, N, Black, L, and Fowler, W: Relationship of lung volume to height and arm span in normal subjects and in patients with spinal deformities. Am Rev Respir Dis 91:356–362, 1965.

25. Sharp D, et al: Reference values for pulmonary function tests of Japanese-American men aged 71–90 years. Am J Respir Crit Care Med 153 (2):805–811, 1996.
26. Oscherwits, M, et al: Differences in pulmonary functions in various racial groups. Am J Epidemiol 96:319–327, 1972.
27. Dufetel, P, et al: Characteristics of lung volume and expiratory flow seen in black African adults. Rev Mal Respir 7:215–222, 1990.
28. Morris, J, Koski, A, and Johnson, L: Prediction nomograms (BTPS) spirometric values in normal males and females. Am Rev Respir Dis 163:57–67, 1971.
29. Craig, D, et al: Closing volume and its relationship to gas exchange in seated and supine positions. J Appl Physiol 31:717–721, 1971.
30. ATS Statement: Snowbird Workshop on Standardization of Spirometry. Am Rev Respir Dis 119:831–838, 1979.
31. Hodgkin, J and Petty, T: Chronic Obstructive Pulmonary Disease: Current Concepts. Saunders, Philadelphia, 1987.
32. Farzan, S: A Concise Handbook of Respiratory Diseases, ed 2. Reston Publishing, Reston, Va, 1985.
33. Kilburn, K and Warchaw, R: Pulmonary function impairment associated with pleural asbestos disease. Chest 98:965–972, 1990.
34. West, J: Pulmonary Pathophysiology: The Essentials, ed 4. Williams & Wilkins, Baltimore, 1992.
35. Attinger, E, Monroe, R, and Seagal, M: The mechanics of breathing in different body positions. I. In normal subjects. J Clin Invest 35:904–911, 1956.
36. West, J: Respiratory Physiology: The Essentials, ed 5. Williams & Wilkins, Baltimore, 1995.
37. McLaughlin, A: Essentials of Physiology for Advanced Respiratory Therapy. Mosby, St. Louis, 1977.
38. Cheeseman, M and Revelette, W: Phrenic afferent contribution to reflexes elicited by changes in diaphragm length. J Appl Physiol 69:640–647, 1990.
39. Tallarida, G, Pervzsi, G, and Raimondi, G: The role of chemosensitive muscle receptors in cardiorespiratory regulation during exercise. J Auton Nerv Syst (suppl) 30:155–161, 1990.
40. Flenley, D: Blood gas and acid-base interpretation. Respir Care 27:311–317, 1982.
41. Milhorn, H: Understanding arterial blood gases. Am Fam Physician 21:112–120, 1980.
42. Rothstein, J, Roy, S, and Wolf, S: The Rehabilitation Specialist's Handbook, ed. 2, FA Davis, Philadelphia, 1997.

CHAPTER 4

Physiologic Adaptations to Aerobic Exercise

Rehabilitation management of cardiopulmonary disease is designed to reduce the physical and psychologic impact of a disabling disease as well as to increase the individual's functional capacity. However, to meet increased demands for energy placed on the body during exercise, several physiologic adjustments must be made. Arm activity and muscular contractions of the isometric type may evoke the Valsalva maneuver and increase both muscle pressure on arteries and blood pressure, and do not benefit the cardiovascular system. When isometric contractions constrict arterioles, there is an increase in peripheral resistance, which causes an increase in heart rate, an increase in blood pressure, and a dramatic rise in the rate-pressure product (RPP) (Chapter 5). For these reasons, activities involving sustained contractions and dynamic overhead arm work are not generally recommended as a major part of cardiopulmonary rehabilitation programs or for older adults.[1-10] Although recent investigation indicates that low-intensity resistive exercise training, combined with aerobic activity, has beneficial effects on coronary heart disease (CHD) risk factors,[11] this discussion of physiologic adaptations to exercise (acute and chronic) is limited to changes that occur during dynamic, rhythmic, and continuous activities of an aerobic nature performed in the upright position.

ACUTE RESPONSES TO AEROBIC EXERCISE

The acute responses to exercise include the physiologic adjustments that normally occur in response to a single bout of exercise. The major adjustments that must be made include cardiac adaptations, coronary and systemic circulatory adjustments, blood pressure and volume changes, and metabolic adaptations.

Cardiac Adaptations

The rate of contraction of the heart begins to increase before exercise begins (anticipatory rise). As exercise commences and continues, the increase in heart rate is proportional to the intensity of the activity. If the intensity of the activity is too great, the maximum heart rate will be achieved, exhaustion will ensue, and the exercise will be anaerobic. Aerobically, there is a linear relationship between heart rate and oxygen consumption.[10,12,13] (See the section on metabolic adaptations.)

The cardiac muscle responds to exercise not only by increasing its rate of contraction but also by increasing its force of contraction. The increased force of contraction results in an increase in the stroke volume, or the amount of blood ejected by the heart per beat. The normal ejection fraction is 0.6 to 0.75 (60 to 75%) and it increases during exercise.[12-14] Stroke volume is equal to the difference between end-diastolic and end-systolic volume. End-diastolic volume is determined by (1) filling pressure and (2) ventricular compliance. Venous pressure is the most important factor in determining filling pressure and is a direct result of the amount of venous return. Ventricular compliance is determined by the ability of the ventricle to stretch in response to a given volume of blood (preload). End-systolic volume is a function of contractility and afterload. Contractility is the forcefulness of the contraction of the heart and afterload is the force resisting the ejection of blood by the heart. Increases in afterload caused by aortic pressure (or resistance) result in a decrease in ejection fraction. Increases in stroke volume during upright exercise result from a greater filling of the ventricles during diastole (end-diastolic volume) and a greater systolic emptying (end-systolic volume)[12-14] (see Chapter 2).

As a result of the increased heart rate and stroke volume that accompany dynamic exercise in the upright position, cardiac output increases. Cardiac output is equal to the volume of blood pumped by the heart per minute: it is a product of the stroke volume and the heart rate. As presented in Chapter 2, the rate and force of cardiac contraction are regulated by the autonomic system, chemoreceptors, baroreceptors, and body temperature.[15-17]

Two important aspects of heart rate and cardiac output should be noted. The first is that the maximal heart rate an individual can attain decreases with age; that is, there is an inverse relationship between maximum heart rate and age. The second is that both heart rate and stroke volume increase when an individual is exercising at 40 to 50 percent of his or her maximum capacity. At higher levels, however, increased cardiac output is accomplished by an increase in heart rate only; stroke volume does not appear to increase. Keeping in mind that coronary circulation (circulation to the heart muscle itself) occurs primarily during diastole, it is important to remember that, for people with limited ability to increase heart rates (coronary, pulmonary, and/or older patients), exercise must be at comparatively low heart rates.[1,12-14,18,19]

Coronary Circulation Adjustments

In response to exercise, the heart muscle must increase its work. It therefore needs more oxygen so that its metabolism can produce the energy for it to continue to contract. At rest, the cardiac muscle extracts approximately 70 to 75 percent of the oxygen that is delivered to it via the coronary circulation. That leaves little reserve for increasing oxygen delivery to the cardiac muscle by this mechanism. The increased coronary demands of exercise are met by increasing the rate at which blood flows through the coronary arteries and by increasing aortic blood pressure, both of which force more blood into the coronary arteries. Release of nitric oxide, an endothelial-derived relaxing factor (EDRF) by the endothelial cells in the coronary arteries appears to be an important factor in causing dilation of the coronary arteries with a resultant increase in coronary blood flow during exercise. Any obstruction to coronary blood flow decreases the amount of oxygen delivered to the cardiac tissues and could precipitate an ischemic condition. Literature suggests that high exercising heart rates in cardiopulmonary and older patients make it difficult for the myocardium to continue to receive adequate amounts of oxygen. Therefore, graded exercise testing with electrocardiogram (ECG) monitoring, a scientifically developed exercise prescription based on the exercise test, and careful monitoring during exercise sessions can help to avoid situations in which blood flow to the myocardium may be inadequate.[10,13,20-22]

Systemic Circulation Adjustments

During aerobic exercise, the muscles that are actively working need a greater oxygen supply to produce the energy needed for continuing muscular contraction. The increased need for oxygen by the working muscles is met not only by an increase in the cardiac output but also by an increase in blood flow to the active muscles. Because a limited amount of blood must supply all the tissues of the body, the amount of blood flowing to any specific tissue depends on the oxygen need of that tissue. Thus, during exercise, blood is shunted (directed away) from tissues, which are less active (such as those of digestive organs, kidneys, spleen), and directed to muscles, which are actively working and have increased metabolic activity. This redistribution, or shunting, is accomplished by a series of chemical (increased CO_2 and lower pH) and reflex adjustments (sympathetic nervous system firing) that cause the dilation of arterioles in the working muscles and a constriction of vessels in inactive regions of the body.[12,13,19] Recent research indicates that the release of nitrous oxide (or other relaxing factors) by the endothelium of smooth muscle may be an important factor in the vasodilation of the vasculature in muscle tissue.[23,24]

The increased blood flow to active muscles during exercise improves oxygen delivery to the active tissues. In addition, there are increases in the oxygen consumption (metabolism) of the muscle cells, and there is increased oxygen extraction by those cells. Nearly twice as many capillaries are open during exercise as during rest.[25]

Because blood is shunted to areas of increased activity during exercise, blood flow to the lungs is also increased. To meet the metabolic demands of the body, both the rate and depth of ventilation and the diffusion of oxygen from the alveoli into the pulmonary capillaries increase with increasing activity.[25]

To dissipate the heat produced during exercise, blood flow to the skin increases. The hypothalamus is responsive to changes in the temperature of the blood. When blood temperature increases, the hypothalamus signals the blood vessels that supply the skin to dilate. More blood can then flow to the surface of the skin so that perspiration can evaporate. The evaporation cools the skin and that, in turn, cools the blood. Exercising in an environment of high humidity impairs the cooling process because the environment's ability to evaporate sweat is decreased. Cardiopulmonary patients should be warned of the dangers of exercising in a highly humid environment, particularly when high humidity is combined with a high environmental temperature.[12]

Respiratory Adaptations

To supply adequate amounts of oxygen during exercise, there is an increase in all phases of respiration. Therefore, external, internal, and cellular respiration (Chapter 3) increase in response to increased oxygen demand. Because of an increase in tidal volume and respiratory frequency, the minute volume ($\dot{V}E$) may increase from a resting value of approximately 6 liters per minute to above 100 liters per minute during vigorous activity. The primary stimulus for the increase in $\dot{V}E$ seems to be the concentration of carbon dioxide (CO_2) in the arterial blood (Pa_{CO_2}). A linear relationship exists between pulmonary ventilation and increasing levels of activity. Increased ventilation during activity is combined with increased cardiac output, so adequate removal of CO_2, buffering of lactic acid, and maintenance of a constant pH are achieved. In patients with pulmonary disease, breathing rates during exercise increase more rapidly than in normal persons, partly because there is a smaller than normal increase in tidal volume. At minute ventilations of approximately 40 liters, the breathing rate of the individual with pulmonary disease may be twice that of a normal person and may approach the maximum voluntary ventilation (MVV). Exercise for the pulmonary patient is usually terminated at a relatively low heart rate because of ventilatory limitations.[7,26]

Blood-Pressure Adjustments

In the active muscles during aerobic exercise, the blood vessels dilate. The dilation decreases the resistance to blood flow and tends to cause a decrease in blood pressure. However, the trend toward lower blood pressure during exercise is negated by an increase in cardiac output. The net effect is that the systolic blood pressure increases in normotensive individuals. The increase in systolic blood pressure is normally proportional to the intensity and oxygen demand of the activity. In normotensive individuals, there is little or no increase in diastolic blood pressure with increased aerobic work.[12] Following aerobic exercise, blood pressure falls to below pre-exercise levels and may remain there for several hours. This decrease in postexercise blood pressure may be caused by a decrease in total and regional vascular resistance and a decrease in cardiac output.[27,28]

Dramatic declines in systolic blood pressure can be observed when an individual has been exercising intensively and suddenly stops. The resultant pooling of blood in the lower extremities decreases venous return and cardiac output. It may cause fainting associated with poor perfusion to the brain. To avoid this result, especially in cardiopulmonary patients, all aerobic exercise sessions should include a cool-down phase.[8,25,29]

Exercises involving the arms evoke a greater rise in blood pressure than exercises involving the legs. Apparently the difference is at least partially a result of the smaller muscles being used for the activity. Although there is dilation of the blood vessels in the arms, there is constriction of the vessels in the inactive, larger leg muscles, and blood pressure increases during arm exercises. For persons with cardiopulmonary disease and older individuals, aerobic activities involving the arms should be cautiously administered. Prolonged intense arm exercises are to be used with care, and patients should be cautioned about performing daily activities involving continued arm work such as shoveling, digging, raking, lifting, and carrying. However, because many leisure and vocational activities require arm activity, arm training is recommended as part of a comprehensive rehabilitation program. The central focus for rehabilitation programs should be aerobic activities that utilize the larger leg muscles: walking, jogging, and cycling.[12,27]

Blood and Fluid Adaptations

The body cools itself by the evaporation of perspiration. Continued aerobic exercise can cause significant loss of body fluid. Consequently, the plasma volume (approximately 90 percent water) may decrease while the protein and cellular components remain relatively unchanged. This state is referred to as hemoconcentration because the solid particles of the blood constitute a relatively higher percentage of whole blood. Hemoconcentration results in "thicker" blood, which can increase the resistance to blood flow and also increase blood pressure. Lower blood volume also decreases venous return of blood to the heart and impairs cardiac output. Exercises performed in an environment of high temperature and high humidity can promote further dehydration and fluid loss and should be avoided.[20,25,30,31]

Metabolic Adaptations

To meet the increased metabolic demands of exercise, the amount of oxygen delivered to the tissues increases as a result of increased cardiac output and increased blood flow to the working muscles. (This assumes that the hemoglobin concentration of the blood is normal and provides adequate oxygen transport.) On delivery to the individual cells, oxygen must be used by those cells to provide energy for continued muscle contraction. Oxygen utilization (oxygen uptake) is determined not only by delivery but also by the number of mitochondria in the cells, the amount of myoglobin, the enzymes of metabolism, the substrates available for metabolism, and probably many other factors. The maximal amount of oxygen ($\dot{V}O_2$max) that can be consumed by an individual is commonly considered to be the best and most accurate indication of cardiorespiratory fitness.[12,13] $\dot{V}O_2$max is usually expressed as milliliters of oxygen used per kilogram of body weight per minute. Direct measurements of $\dot{V}O_2$max can be made if the arterial-venous oxygen difference ($a - \bar{v}\ O_2$ difference) is found by sampling inspired and expired air. Because of the expense of the equipment needed for a direct measurement of $a - \bar{v}\ O_2$ difference, and depending on the circumstances, in many cases it is acceptable to predict $\dot{V}O_2$max. Predictions are based on heart-rate responses to a standard exercise workload as both $\dot{V}O_2$max and heart rate increase in a linear manner in response to increases in exercise intensities.[12,13]

A limiting factor in exercise performance is the ability of the tissues to utilize oxygen. Compared with the resting state, the $a - \bar{v}\ O_2$ difference during exercise increases by as much as three times. This ability of the active muscles to use more oxygen during exercise keeps the heart from having to work too hard to supply the necessary circulation for continued muscular contractions. Increased oxygen extraction by the tissues during exercise is enhanced by chemical, thermal, and hormonal changes in the blood.[12,13]

CHRONIC RESPONSES TO AEROBIC EXERCISE

In recent years, considerable interest has developed in the long-term physiologic benefits an individual derives from engaging in a program of dynamic, rhythmic, and continuous activities over a period of time. Although there is considerable controversy on the subject, many researchers feel that cardiopulmonary disease can be prevented and/or reversed by cessation of smoking, regular aerobic exercise (training), and elimination of, or reduction in, dietary fat, salt, caffeine, and the like.[32-38] Because of a lack of information, there seem to be different opinions about the constituents of a good training program.

Cardiac Adaptations to Aerobic Training

The individual fibers of cardiac muscle may adapt to aerobic training by becoming larger (hypertrophy) and stronger. This hypertrophy is caused by an increase in cellular protein causing an increase in the thickness of the myofibrils. Unlike skeletal muscle, cardiac tissues does not seem to respond to training by increasing the number of mitochondria or the oxidative capacity of the respiratory enzymes.[1,13,39]

The hypertrophy of cardiac muscle as a result of aerobic training is accompanied by a larger stroke volume, but maximal heart rate does not seem to change. As a result of aerobic training, increases in maximal cardiac output have been observed, but this increase seems to be a result of larger stroke volumes rather than increases in maximal heart rates. Thus, at any given workload, the heart does not have to beat as often to supply an adequate volume of blood. Endurance training also causes an increase in recovery heart rates from all levels of work.[39]

As yet, there is no clear explanation for the bradycardia that results from aerobic training. Bradycardia is observed at rest and at all levels of work. Bradycardia may be partially a result of the increased strength of the myocardial fibers, so that more blood is pumped per beat and the heart does not have to beat as often to supply the same amount of blood. Recent studies indicate an increased vagal tone in response to aerobic training. This results in a shift away from the sympathetic nervous system's influence (the catecholamines) on the heart in favor of the parasympathetic system, which enhances the influence of the vagus nerve and results in bradycardia. In cardiac patients, the bradycardia that results from training is a major factor in raising the angina threshold — the level of work at which angina occurs.[2,9,39-43]

Coronary Circulation Responses

Because aerobic training does not seem to increase the oxygen-extraction ability of the myocardium, the increased need of the myocardium for oxygen during exercise must be met by increases in coronary blood flow. These increases result from increases in heart rate, stroke volume, and vasodilation. Relatively speaking, however, the bradycardia and increased stroke volume that accompany training result in a longer period of diastole between beats, so there is enhanced perfusion in the coronary arteries as a result of training. These physiologic adaptations to aerobic training are major factors in the improvement of ischemic ECG changes in patients with coronary artery disease (CAD).[1,2,39-45]

There is considerable controversy as to whether there is an increase in the diameter of the coronary arteries and/or increased collateral circulation as a result of aerobic training. Such increases have been demonstrated to occur in animal experiments and in some studies with humans, but as yet no consistent results with humans have been reported. The finding that the rate-pressure product (RPP) increases in some patients before development of angina following aerobic training tends to support the theory that exercise training may improve myocardial perfusion by enhancing myocardial vascularity. It is possible that differences in training variables (such as frequency and intensity of exercise) and current methodologies to determine collateral circulation in humans may not be sensitive enough to detect improvements, should they occur.[32–38,45–55]

Pulmonary Responses

The effects of regular aerobic exercise on the pulmonary system are a decrease in the rate and an increase in the depth of ventilation. This training benefit apparently results partly from improved efficiency of the respiratory musculature. Increased pulmonary diffusion, not noted at rest or submaximal exercise, is increased during maximal work. It may be a result of increased pulmonary blood flow, which causes greater perfusion of the lung. Decreased lactic acid concentrations and an increased anaerobic threshold with improved functional capacity are other benefits of regular aerobic exercise.[39,41,56]

Whether or not aerobic activity improves pulmonary function, as measured by standardized tests, remains controversial. Some studies have reported improvements in lung volume; others have shown no improvements in lung function as a result of regular aerobic activity.[33,54,56–62] It may be that, at this time, the data are not available, since rehabilitation of the patient with pulmonary disease, as part of standard medical treatment for the pulmonary patient, is a fairly new concept.

Changes in Systemic Circulation

The capacity of blood flow to skeletal muscles is increased in response to aerobic training by an increase in the number of capillaries that supply the muscle fibers. There is also an increase in the number and size of the mitochondria and the enzyme systems in skeletal muscle that supply energy for contraction. Aerobic training is associated with a decrease in peripheral resistance (afterload) and an increase in vasodilation. These changes in skeletal muscle account for a greater arterial-venous oxygen difference in response to training. However, during submaximal work, blood flow to the active muscles does not seem to be as important as metabolism in the observed $a - \bar{v} \, O_2$ difference. During maximal work, blood flow and metabolism are considerably increased in response to aerobic training. These physiologic adaptations to training allow better delivery and utilization of oxygen at the tissue site so that, relatively speaking, the heart does not have to work as hard to deliver an adequate blood supply to the active muscles.[2,9,39,41,42,63,64]

Blood-Pressure Changes

Although there is considerable controversy about the long-term effects of aerobic exercise on blood pressure, recent studies have reported a decrease in both systolic and diastolic resting and working blood pressures following periods of consistent training. These changes have also been reported in individuals who are hypertensive and medicated.[65-71] The physiologic mechanisms whereby these changes occur are yet to be determined. It may be that aerobic training directly causes improvements in the smooth muscle of the circulatory system and increases circulating vasodilator substances, resulting in a decrease in total peripheral resistance. The sympathetic nervous system and plasma norepinephrine levels may also be altered by regular aerobic training, or the reported decreases in blood pressure may be a result of reduction of the risk factors that often accompany training—reduced body mass, cessation of smoking, higher HDL, and the like.[44,69,72]

Blood and Fluid Responses

Endurance training causes an increase in the total blood volume of the body. This increase is caused largely by an increase in the amount of the plasma portion of whole blood. As a result, aerobic training allows a person to adjust better to environments of high temperatures and high humidities by improving the sweating mechanism.[9,25,30,73]

Aerobic training slightly increases the number of red blood cells. Consequently, the amount of hemoglobin increases, although the hematocrit remains relatively unchanged. Aerobic training has also been found to decrease the aggregation of the platelets and to enhance fibrinolytic activity. These changes in response to aerobic training lessen the chance of forming an intravascular thrombosis.[9,25,41,42,45,54,74-77] Preliminary studies indicate that the increased fibrinolytic activity observed during aerobic training is influenced by the intensity of the activity (rather than duration) and time of day of the exercise (evening exercise seems to be better than morning exercise).[74-77]

Metabolic Adaptations

The increase in $\dot{V}O_2$max that results from aerobic training is caused by increases in cardiac output and in the arterial-venous oxygen difference. This increase in $a - \bar{v} O_2$ difference is caused by increases in blood volume, capillary density, and oxygen extraction from capillary blood during skeletal muscle contractions. Measurements of $\dot{V}O_2$max are used extensively in the diagnosis of cardiovascular diseases and in the prescription of appropriate exercise programs for persons with cardiovascular diseases. Tests for $\dot{V}O_2$max are discussed in Chapter 9.[45,59]

Training increases the number and size of mitochondria and the number of aerobic-system enzymes in the working muscles, resulting in an enhanced use of oxygen. Lipid and carbohydrate metabolism are also improved. During submaximal exercise, the lactic acid concentration of the blood does not increase as it does in maximal work because of adequate oxygen supply and utilization by the mitochondria (steady state). Exercise prescriptions for the cardiac patient should elicit work of a submaximal nature so that metabolic energy comes from aerobic metabolism (Krebs cycle) rather than from anaerobic sources.[19,59]

Body Composition Changes

It is well established that regular aerobic exercise can be an important factor in helping individuals lose and/or control body fat. Weight loss through exercise is accompanied by a decrease in the percentage of body fat and an increase in lean body mass. For best results, cardiopulmonary patients who need to lose body fat should combine an aerobic exercise program with restricted caloric intake.[78-82]

Changes in Blood Lipids

The lack of agreement in the literature about the effects of aerobic training on total blood cholesterol, triglycerides, and high-density lipoprotein cholesterol (HDL) is probably the result of lack of control over experimental variables. Several sources have reported that regular exercise is effective in lowering total blood cholesterol and triglyceride levels and increasing HDL levels. These results may be due to dietary modifications that reduce saturated fat intake rather than to exercise effects. Current thinking favors a combination of proper nutrition (with reduced fat intake) and proper exercise to reduce blood lipid concentrations and to prevent or reverse the atherosclerotic process that leads to heart disease.[35-38,82-90] Although more research is needed in this area, recent research indicates that intensity of aerobic activity may be as important as or more important than the distance or time of the aerobic activity in producing positive blood lipid profiles.[36,82,90-95]

Training and Stress

There is evidence of correlation between personality traits and incidence of ischemic heart disease, but the literature is inconclusive as to the traits and behaviors associated with increased risk for CHD. Individuals with type A personalities have been found to have higher levels of blood catecholamines, higher heart rates, and higher blood-pressure responses than those with type B personalities, when both types are subjected to the same stress situations. More recently, anger, hostility, anxiety, and depression have also been found to adversely affect the cardiovascular system. It is theorized that these emotional stresses can cause platelet aggregation, evoke an ischemic state, or even precipitate an acute attack. Persons subjected to prolonged adverse emotional states may be at higher risk for developing ischemic heart disease than nonstressed individuals.[96-104]

Although more research is needed in this area, aerobic exercise is valuable to some people in helping to relieve some personality and emotional tensions, perhaps as a result of a decreased catecholamine secretion. Speculations about the reason for "runner's high" include increased levels of endorphins in the blood in response to training. If for no other reason, the fact that aerobic activity undertaken on a regular basis gives individuals a sense of well-being may be sufficient justification for recommending training for persons in stressful situations or those with personality or emotional difficulties.[96,98,99,103,105] A current trend in cardiopulmonary rehabilitation programs is to identify patients with personality and emotional problems and to provide some formal type of program for treatment and management of stress.[98,99,102,106-108]

Training and Ischemic Heart Disease

Ischemia occurs when the myocardial demand for oxygen exceeds the supply and the muscle cells must rely on anaerobic metabolism (glycolysis) for their energy. Ischemia is usually thought to result from atherosclerosis of the coronary arteries, although coronary artery spasm may be responsible for ischemia in some individuals.

Angina occurs when an individual reaches his or her ischemic threshold—a phenomenon dependent on systolic blood pressure and heart rate or the RPP. Anything that causes an increase in either systolic blood pressure or heart rate can precipitate an attack of angina. Physical activity increases both of these parameters and can also cause an anginal attack. Regular aerobic activity, however, has been found to cause physiologic changes that lower the heart rate and systolic blood pressure for any given submaximal workload and thus raise the ischemic threshold.[5,33,45,109]

Other beneficial effects of regular exercise include a decreased catecholamine production, increased coronary perfusion, increased functional work capacity, decreased peripheral resistance, possible increased collateral circulation, increased fibrinolysis, and decreased ST wave changes. In some reported cases, there has been a reduction in the rate of disease progression and/or an apparent reversal of the symptoms of ischemic heart disease in individuals who exercise on a regular basis and restrict their dietary fat consumption. More research is needed in this area because it is becoming increasingly clear that aerobic training, in combination with risk-factor modification, is a viable adjunct to traditional medical therapy in the treatment of ischemic heart disease.*

SUMMARY

This chapter has presented the major physiologic adaptations made by the body in response to acute and chronic bouts of aerobic exercise. During an acute bout of activity, the heart rate rises in proportion to the intensity of the workload. Cardiac output, dilation of coronary arteries, and blood pressure all increase to allow increased coronary blood flow. Because coronary circulation occurs during diastole of the cardiac cycle, cardiopulmonary and/or older patients should exercise at relatively low heart rates to allow adequate coronary perfusion.

Blood flow during exercise is shunted (directed away) from less active tissues to the more active muscle tissues in which there is also dilation of the blood vessels. Increased rate and depth of ventilation and increased cellular metabolism also occur. The hypothalamus responds to increased heat production by stimulating the sweat glands to increase their output so that evaporation of sweat can promote the cooling process.

Exercise involving the arms and isometric activities should be used with caution in cardiopulmonary patients, because of the dramatic increases in blood pressure that may result. Rehabilitation programs should emphasize aerobic activities that use the larger leg muscles (walking, jogging, and cycling).

In response to chronic bouts of aerobic exercise, cardiac muscle fibers hypertrophy and become stronger. This results in a greater stroke volume and an increase in recovery heart rate. The bradycardia that also results from training seems to be a major factor in raising the angina threshold. It remains to be clearly demonstrated whether increased collateral circulation occurs.

Skeletal muscle capillarization and the number and size of skeletal muscle mitochondria all increase in response to aerobic training. As a result, there is better oxygen delivery and utilization with less lactic acid concentration in the working muscles, and the workload on the heart is reduced. Beneficial effects of aerobic training on both systolic and diastolic blood pressures and better adjustments to high temperatures have been reported.

---

*2,9,32–55,63,64,69,74–77,82–90,110,111

Aerobic exercise has been found to be very effective in helping individuals control body weight and in increasing the HDL cholesterol levels of the blood. It has also been shown to be beneficial to persons who are subjected to stress and similar tensions. Chronic aerobic activity has been found to raise the ischemic threshold, decrease catecholamine production, increase coronary perfusion, increase work capacity, decrease peripheral resistance, and decrease ST wave ECG changes. It has also been reported that regular aerobic activity can prevent, slow, or reverse the progression of atherosclerosis when combined with dietary and other risk-factor modifications and lifestyle changes.

REFERENCES

1. Brooks, GA, Fahey, TD, and White, TP: Exercise Physiology: Human Bioenergics and Its Applications, ed 2. Mayfield Publishing, Mountain View, Calif, 1996, pp 243–259.
2. Buttrick, PM and Scheuer, J: Exercise and the heart. In: Schlant, RC and Alexander, RW (eds): Hurst's The Heart, ed 8. McGraw-Hill, New York, 1995, pp 359–361.
3. deVries, HA and Housh, TJ: Physiology of Exercise, ed 5. Brown & Benchmark, Madison, Wis, 1994, pp 287–307.
4. Fletcher, GF, et al: Exercise standards: A statement for health professionals from the American Heart Association. Circulation 82(6):2286–2322, 1990.
5. Froelicher, VF, et al: Exercise and the Heart, ed 3. Mosby, St. Louis, 1993, pp 347–383.
6. Kass, JE and Castriotta, RJ: The effect of circuit weight training on cardiovascular function in healthy sedentary males. J Cardpulm Rehabil 14(6):378–383, 1994.
7. McArdle, WE, Katch, FI, and Katch, VL: Exercise Physiology, ed 4. Williams & Wilkins, Baltimore, 1996, pp 217–232.
8. Pollock, ML, Welsch, MA, and Graves, JE: Exercise prescription for cardiac rehabilitation. In: Pollock ML and Schmidt, DH (eds). Heart Disease and Rehabilitation, ed 3. Human Kinetics, Champaign, 1995, pp 243–276.
9. Sharkey, BJ and Graetzer, DG: Specificity of exercise, training and testing. In: ACSM's Resource Manual for Guidelines for Exercise Testing and Prescription, ed 2. Lea & Febiger, Philadelphia, 1993, pp 82–92.
10. Smith, JJ and Kampine, JP: Circulatory Physiology, ed 3. Williams & Wilkins, Baltimore, 1990, pp 236–276.
11. Goldberg, AP: Aerobic and resistive exercise modify risk factors for coronary heart disease. Med Sci Sports Exerc 21(6):669–674, 1989.
12. Brooks, GA, Fahey, TD, and White, TP: op cit, pp 281–299.
13. McArdle, WD, Katch, FI, and Katch, VL: op cit, pp 296–312.
14. Froehlicher, VF, et al: op cit, pp 1–10.
15. McArdle, WD, Katch, FI, and Katch, VL: op cit, pp 343–369.
16. Guyton, AC. Textbook of Medical Physiology, ed 8. Saunders, Philadelphia, 1992, pp 194–220.
17. West, JR (ed). Best and Taylor's Physiological Basis of Medical Practice, ed 12. Williams & Wilkins, Baltimore, 1991, pp 276–330.
18. Miller, HS and Fletcher, GF: Community-based cardiac rehabilitation outpatient programs. In: Pollock, ML and Schmidt, DH (eds): Heart Disease and Rehabilitation, ed 3. Human Kinetics, Champaign, 1995, pp 229–242.
19. Wasserman, K, et al: Principles of Exercise Testing and Interpretation, ed 2. Lea & Febiger, Philadelphia, 1994, pp 1–49.
20. Brooks, GA, Fahey, TD, and White, TP: op cit, pp 260–280.
21. McAllister, RM: Endothelial-mediated control of coronary and skeletal muscle blood flow during exercise: introduction. Med Sci Sports Exerc 27(8):1122–1124, 1995.
22. Shen, W, et al: Nitric oxide production and NO synthase gene expression contribute to vascular regulation during exercise. Med Sci Sports Exerc 27(8):1125–1133, 1995.
23. McAllister, RM, Hirai, T, and Musch, TI: Contribution of endothelium-derived nitric oxide (EDNO) to the skeletal muscle blood flow response to exercise. Med Sci Sports Exerc 27(8):1145–1151, 1995.
24. Segal, SS and Kurjiaka, DT: Coordination of blood flow control in the resistance vasculature of skeletal muscle. Med Sci Sports Exerc 27(8):1158–1164, 1995.
25. deVries, HA and Housh, TJ: op cit, pp 124–135.
26. Wyka, KA: Cardiopulmonary rehabilitation. In: Scanlan, CL, et al (eds): Egan's Fundamentals of Respiratory Care, ed 5. Mosby, St. Louis, 1990, pp 899–907.
27. McArdle, WD, Katch, FI, and Katch, VL: op cit, pp 267–283.

28. Rueckert, PA, et al: Hemodynamic patterns and duration of post-dynamic exercise hypotension in hypertensive humans. Med Sci Sports Exerc 28(1):24–32, 1996.
29. American College of Sports Medicine: ACSM's Guidelines for Exercise Testing and Prescription, ed. 5. Williams & Wilkins, Baltimore, 1995, pp 206–219.
30. Folinsbee, LJ: Heat and air pollution. In: Pollock, ML and Schmidt, DH (eds): Heart Disease and Rehabilitation, ed 3. Human Kinetics, Champaign, 1995, pp 327–342.
31. McArdle, WD, Katch, FI, and Katch, VL: op cit, pp 35–79.
32. Rosenson, RS: Reversing coronary artery disease. The Physician and Sportsmedicine 22(11):59–64, 1994.
33. Balady, GJ, et al: Cardiac rehabilitation programs: A statement for healthcare professionals from the American Heart Association. Circulation 90(3):1602–1610, 1994.
34. Hambrecht, R, et al: Various intensities of leisure time physical activity in patients with coronary artery disease: Effects of cardiorespiratory fitness and progression of coronary atherosclerotic lesions. J Am Coll Cardiol 22:468–477, 1993.
35. Ornish, D, et al: Can lifestyle changes reverse coronary heart disease? Lancet 336(8708):129–133, 1990.
36. Paffenberger, RS and Blair, SN: Exercise in the primary prevention of coronary artery disease. In: Pollock, ML and Schmidt, DH (eds): Heart Disease and Rehabilitation, ed 3. Human Kinetics, Champaign, 1995, pp 169–176.
37. Sherman, C: Reversing heart disease: Are lifestyle changes enough? The Physician and Sportsmedicine 22(1):91–95, 1994.
38. Schuler, G, et al: Regular physical exercise and low-fat diet: Effects on progression of coronary artery disease. Circulation 86:1–11, 1992.
39. Smith, ML and Mitchell, JH: Cardiorespiratory adaptations to exercise. In: ACSM's Resource Manual for Guidelines for Exercise Testing and Prescription, ed 2. Lea & Febiger, Philadelphia, 1993, pp 75–81.
40. Babcock, MA, Paterson, DH, and Cunningham, DA: Effects of aerobic endurance training gas exchange kinetics of older men. Med Sci Sports Exerc 26(4):447–452, 1994.
41. Balady, GJ and Weiner, DA: Physiology of exercise in normal individuals and patients with coronary heart disease. In: Wenger, NK and Hellerstein, HK (eds): Rehabilitation of the Coronary Patient, ed 3. Churchill Livingstone, New York, 1992, pp 103–122.
42. Kavanagh, T: Cardiac rehabilitation. In: Goldberg, L and Elliot, DL (eds): Exercise for Prevention and Treatment of Illness. FA Davis, Philadelphia, 1994, pp 48–74.
43. Seals, DR, et al. Exercise and aging: Autonomic control of circulation. Med Sci Sports Exerc 26(5):568–576, 1994.
44. American College of Sports Medicine: Position stand: exercise for patients with coronary artery disease. Med Sci Sports Exerc 26(3):i–iii, 1994.
45. Squires, RW: Mechanisms by which exercise training may improve the clinical status of cardiac patients. In: Pollock, ML and Schmidt, DH (eds): Heart Disease and Rehabilitation, ed 3. Human Kinetics, Champaign, 1995, pp 147–160.
46. Caspersen, CJ and Heath, GW: The risk factor concept of coronary heart disease. In: ACSM's Resource Manual for Exercise Training and Prescription, ed 2. Lea & Febiger, Philadelphia, 1993, pp 151–167.
47. Foster, C, Schrager, M, and Cohen, J: The value of cardiac rehabilitation: Secondary prevention. In: Pollock, ML and Schmidt, DH (eds): Heart Disease and Rehabilitation, ed 3. Human Kinetics, Champaign, 1995, pp 177–183.
48. Froelicher, et al: op cit, pp 347–383.
49. Hamm, LF and Leon, AS: Exercise training for the coronary patient. In: Wenger, NK and Hellerstein, HK (eds): Rehabilitation of the Coronary Patient, ed 3. Churchill Livingstone, New York, 1992, pp 367–402.
50. Laughlin, HM: Effects of exercise training on coronary circulation: introduction. Med Sci Sports Exerc 26(10):1226–1229, 1994.
51. McKirnan, MD and Bloor, CM: Clinical significance of coronary vascular adaptations to exercise training. Med Sci Sports Exerc 26(10):1262–1268, 1994.
52. Overholser, KA, Laughlin, HM, and Bhatte, MJ: Exercise training-induced increase in coronary transport capacity. Med Sci Sports Exerc 26(10):1239–1244, 1994.
53. Parker, JL, et al: Effects of exercise training on regulation of tone in coronary arteries and arterioles. Med Sci Sports Exerc 26(10):1252–1261, 1994.
54. Squires, RW, et al: Cardiovascular rehabilitation: status, 1990. May Clin Proc 65:731–765, 1990.
55. Tomanek, RJ: Exercise-induced coronary angiogenesis: A review. Med Sci Sports Exerc 26(10):1245–1251, 1994.
56. Badenhop, D, et al: Improvement in peak ventilatory parameters and 12:00 walk time after 36 pulmonary therapy sessions (pts). J Cardpulm Rehabil 14(5):323, 1994.
57. Badenhop, D, et al: Changes in conditioning and sub-maximal ventilatory parameters subsequent to participation in an outpatient pulmonary rehabilitation program. J Cardpulm Rehabil 14(5):324, 1994.
58. Joughin, HM, Digenio, AG, Daly, L, and Kgare, E: Physiological benefits of a prolonged moderate intensity endurance training programme in patients with coronary artery disease. J Cardpulm Rehabil 14(5):327, 1994.

59. McArdle, WD, Katch, FI, and Katch, VL: op cit, pp 390–413.
60. Perk, J, Boden, C, and Perk, L: Physical training of patients with chronic obstructive lung disease: On land or in water? J Cardpulm Rehabil 14(5):324, 1994.
61. Swerts, PMJ, et al: Exercise training as a mediator of increased exercise performance in patients with chronic obstructive pulmonary disease. J Cardpulm Rehabil 12(3):188–193, 1992.
62. Westerman, JH, et al: Improved exercise capacity following pulmonary rehabilitation in patients with severe obstructive lung disease. J Cardpulm Rehabil 14(5):325, 1994.
63. Babcock, MA, Paterson, DH, and Cunningham, DA: op cit, pp 447–452.
64. Essig, DA: Contractile activity-induced mitochondrial biogenesis in skeletal muscle. In: Holloszy, JO (ed): Exercise and Sport Sciences Reviews, Vol 24. Williams & Wilkins, Baltimore, 1996, pp 289–319.
65. Bittner, V and Oberman, A: Efficacy studies in coronary rehabilitation. Cardiol Clin 11:333–347, 1993.
66. Kelemen, MH, et al: Exercise training combined with antihypertensive drug therapy. Effects on lipids, blood pressure, and left ventricular mass. JAMA 263:2766–2771, 1990.
67. Martin, JE, Dubbert, PM, and Cushman, WC: Controlled trial of aerobic exercise in hypertension. Circulation 81:1560–1567, 1990.
68. Physical exericse in the management of hypertension: A consensus statement by the World Hypertension League. J Hypertens 9:283–287, 1993.
69. American College of Sports Medicine: Position stand: physical activity, physical fitness, and hypertension. Med Sci Sports Exerc 25(10):i–x, 1993.
70. Gordon, NF and Scott, CB. Exercise guidelines for patients with high blood pressure: An update. J Cardpulm Rehabil 14(2):93–96, 1994.
71. Hanson, P, and Rueckert, P: Hypertension. In: Pollock, ML and Schmidt, DH (eds): Heart Disease and Rehabilitation, ed 3. Human Kinetics, Champaign, 1995, pp 343–356.
72. Eaton, CB, et al: Physical activity, physical fitness, and coronary heart disease risk factors. Med Sci Sports Exerc 27(3):340–346, 1995.
73. Carroll, JF, et al: Effect of training on blood volume and plasma hormone concentrations in the elderly. Med Sci Sports Exerc 27(6):79–84, 1995.
74. Morris, JN: Exercise in the prevention of coronary heart disease: today's best buy in public health. Med Sci Sports Exerc 26(7):807–814, 1994.
75. Szymanski, LA and Pate, RR: Fibrinolytic responses to moderate intensity exercise: Comparison of physically active and inactive men. Arterioscler Thromb Vasc Biol 14:1746–1750, 1994.
76. Szymanski, LA and Pate, RR: Effects of exercise intensity, duration, and time of day on fibrinolytic activity in physically active men. Med Sci Sports Exerc 26(9):1102–1108, 1994.
77. Szymanski, LA and Pate, RR: Fibrinolytic responses to moderate intensity exercise: a comparison of physically active and inactive men. J Cardpulm Rehabil 14(5):333, 1994.
78. Ballor, DL, Harvey-Berino, J, and Ades, PA: A healthy lifestyle is the treatment of choice for obesity in coronary patients. J Cardpulm Rehabil 15(1):14–18, 1995.
79. Brooks, GA, Fahey, TD, and White, TP: op cit, pp 512–535.
80. Kannel, WB: Epidemiologic insights into atherosclerotic cardiovascular disease—from the Framingham study. In: Pollock, ML and Schmidt, DH (eds): Heart Disease and Rehabilitation, ed 3. Human Kinetics, Champaign, 1995, pp 3–16.
81. McArdle, WD, Katch, FI, and Katch, VL: op cit, pp 602–633.
82. Wood, PD: Physical activity, diet, and health: independent and interactive effects. Med Sci Sports Exerc 26(7):838–843, 1994.
83. Gordon, PM, et al: The acute effects of exercise intensity on HDL-C metabolism. Med Sci Sports Exerc 26(6):671–677, 1994.
84. Haskell, WL, et al: Effects of intensive multiple risk factor reduction on coronary atherosclerosis and clinical events in men and women with coronary artery disease: The Stanford Coronary Risk Intervention Project (SCRIP). Circulation 89:975–990, 1994.
85. Lawson, GJ and Hilgenberg, HA: Blood lipid profile changes with and without participation in outpatient cardiac rehab. J Cardpulm Rehabil 13(5):340, 1993.
86. Niebauer, J, et al: Five years of physical exercise and low fat diet: Effects on progression of coronary artery disease. J Cardpulm Rehabil 15(1):47–64, 1995.
87. Rauramaa, R, et al: Inverse relation of physical activity and apolipoprotein A1 to blood pressure in elderly women. Med Sci Sports Exerc 27(2):164–169, 1995.
88. Rifkind, BM and Rossouw, JE: Lowering cholesterol: The secondary prevention of coronary heart disease. J Cardpulm Rehabil 12(2):87–91, 1992.
89. Whaley, MH, et al: Change in total cholesterol after endurance training: a function of pretraining concentration. J Cardpulm Rehabil 12(1):42–50, 1992.
90. Wood, PD, et al: The effects on plasma lipoproteins of a prudent weight reducing diet, with or without exercise, in overweight men and women. N Engl J Med 325:461–466, 1991.
91. Andersen, LB and Haraldsdottir, J: Coronary heart disease risk factors, physical activity, and fitness in young Danes. Med Sci Sports Exerc 27(2):158–163, 1995.
92. DiPietro, L: The epidemiology of physical activity and physical function in older people. Med Sci Sports Exerc 28(5):596–600, 1996.

93. Gordon, NF, Kohl, HW, and Blair, SN: Life style exercise: A new strategy to promote physical activity for adults. J Cardpulm Rehabil 13(3):161–163, 1993.
94. Jackson, AS, et al: Changes in aerobic power of men, ages 25–70 yr. Med Sci Sports Exerc 27(1):113–120, 1995.
95. Kokkinos, PF, et al: Cardiorespiratory fitness and coronary heart disease risk factor association in women. J Am Coll Cardiol 26:358–364, 1995.
96. Benight, CC and Taylor, CB: Exercise, emotions, and type A behavior. In: Goldberg, L and Elliot, DL (eds): Exercise for Prevention and Treatment of Illness. FA Davis, Philadelphia, 1994, pp 319–331.
97. Kop, WJ and Krantz, DS: Hostility and anger in coronary artery disease: Identification and management. J Cardpulm Rehabil 14(3):153–156, 1994.
98. Lavie, CJ, Milani, RV, and Boykin, C: Effects of cardiac rehabilitation and exercise training on functional capacity, coronary risk factors and quality of life. J Cardpulm Rehabil 14(5):325, 1994.
99. Milani, RV, Littman, AB, and Lavie, CJ: Depressive symptoms predict functional improvement following cardiac rehabilitation and exercise program. J Cardpulm Rehabil 13(6):406–411, 1993.
100. Miller, NH, et al: Position paper of the American Association of cardiovascular and pulmonary rehabilitation: The efficacy of risk factor intervention and psychosocial aspects of cardiac rehabilitation. J Cardpulm Rehabil 10(6):198–209, 1990.
101. Siegler, IC: Hostility and risk: demographic and lifestyle variables. In: Siegman, AW and Smith, TW (eds): Anger, Hostility, and the Heart. Lawrence Erlbaum Associates, Hillsdale, NJ, 1994, pp 199–214.
102. Siegman, AW: From type A to hostility to anger: Reflections on the history of coronary-prone behavior. In: Siegman, AW and Smith, TW (eds): Anger, Hostility, and the Heart. Lawrence Erlbaum Associates, Hillsdale, NJ, 1994, pp 1–12.
103. Sime, WE, McGahan, M, and Eliot, RS: Stress management and coronary heart disease: risk assessment and intervention. In: ACSM's Resource Manual for Guidelines for Exercise, Testing and Prescription, ed 2. Lea & Febiger, Philadelphia, 1993, pp 489–506.
104. Frasure-Smith, N: The Montreal Heart Attack Readjustment Trial. J Cardpulm Rehabil 15(2):103–106, 1995.
105. Nicoloff, G and Schwenk, TL: Using exercise to ward off depression. The Physician and Sportsmedicine 23(9):44–58, 1995.
106. Galleske, SA, et al: Learning stress management in cardiac rehabilitation. J Cardpulm Rehabil 15(5):378, 1995.
107. Nelson, DV, et al: Six-month follow-up of stress management training versus cardiac education during hospitalization for acute myocardial infarction. J Cardpulm Rehabil 14(6):384–390, 1994.
108. Saini, NK, Cooper, P, Eichenauer, K, and Daggy, D: Correlation between low high-density lipoprotein (HDL-C) levels and stress in patients with known coronary heart disease. J Cardpulm Rehabil 13(5):339, 1993.
109. Franklin, DA. Exercise and angina. Relieving the pain. The Physician and Sportsmedicine 23(7):79 80, 1995.
110. LaFontaine, T and Roitman, J: Life style changes can prevent or reverse the progression of atherosclerosis: support for comprehensive cardiovascular rehabilitation. J Cardpulm Rehabil 12(3):159–162, 1992.
111. Lakka, TA, et al: Relation of leisure-time physical activity and cardiorespiratory fitness to the risk of acute myocardial infarction in men. N Engl J Med 330(22):1549–1554, 1994.

CHAPTER 5

Pathophysiology of Coronary Artery Disease

The American Heart Association estimates that in 1994, 489,970 individuals, or 1 of every 4.6 deaths, in the United States died of coronary heart disease and that approximately 13.5 million people have a history of some form of cardiovascular disease. It is estimated that annually, 1.5 million Americans will have a heart attack and 500,000 of those individuals will die. One fifth of those individuals will be less than 65 years old. Although the overall mortality as a result of coronary artery disease (CAD) has declined 29.7 percent from 1983 to 1993, CAD remains the number one cause of sudden death in adults.[1,2] The cost of cardiovascular disease in 1997 is estimated by the American Heart Association to be approximately 259.1 billion dollars including care, professional services, medications, and lost productivity.[1]

CAD is an atherosclerotic process characterized by a thickening in the intiminal layer of the blood-vessel wall caused by a localized accumulation of lipids. The onset and the process are insidious. As the plaque develops, the artery narrows and blood flow is reduced. Beginning as early as the second decade of life, atherosclerosis may affect any arterial system in the body, with the most common sites being the aorta, coronary arteries, and cerebral, femoral, and other middle-sized to large arteries.[3-6] CAD is most pronounced proximally in large-caliber vessels. The proximal segment of the left anterior descending (LAD) is the most severely affected because of its location, which is just distal to the largest bifurcation in the coronary system. Severity is also greatest in an individual's dominant coronary artery.[7] However, CAD is not inevitable; some octogenarians have been found to have no or minimal disease.[8]

The actual pathogenesis of atherosclerosis remains unknown at this time. Establishing cause and effect has been difficult because the disease begins and progresses insidiously; it exists months to years before the onset of symptoms.[4] Past and current research have closely tied the development of atherosclerotic plaque in the coronary arteries to a group of coronary risk factors. Risk factors, discussed in Chapter 13, are certain characteristics that, through systematic observation and clinical study, have shown a significant relationship between their presence and the subsequent development of CAD.[3,7] The major risk factors are high blood pressure, hyperlipidemia, and cigarette smoking. Obesity, diabetes mellitus, and a sedentary lifestyle have recently been considered major risk factors as well.[7] Risk factors are classified as either modifiable (smoking, blood lipid levels, obesity, inactivity) or nonmodifiable (age, sex, family history of CAD, previous medical history). The presence of more than one risk factor has a synergistic effect on the other risk factors in predicting an individual's risk of CAD.[5]

CAD manifests itself in one or more of four clinical syndromes—angina pectoris, myocardial infarction, sudden cardiac death, and/or heart failure. These manifestations each represent a diverse spectrum of disease with symptoms from progressive ischemia to myocardial necrosis to left ventricular dysfunction to death. Correlation between an individual's symptoms and his or her actual pathology are so imprecise that one cannot be predicted on the basis of the other.[8]

This chapter reviews the pathophysiology of CAD, beginning with the normal arterial wall structure, and describes the changes that occur with atherosclerosis. The hypothesized pathogenesis of atherosclerosis is briefly reviewed, with the majority of the chapter devoted to the clinical manifestations of coronary artery disease.

THE ARTERIAL WALL

The normal arterial wall is a smooth muscular wall made up of three distinct layers of tissue: the intima, media, and adventitia. The wall and the individual layers vary in thickness depending on the caliber of the vessel (the larger the inner diameter, the thicker the arterial wall). The layers become progressively less distinct as the vessels reach the level of the arteriole (Fig. 5–1).[9,10]

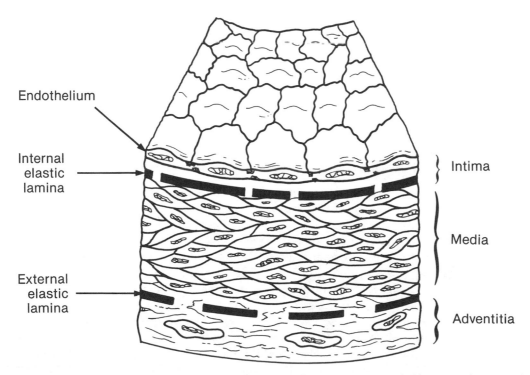

FIGURE 5–1. Structure of normal muscular artery. (From Ross, R and Glomset, JA. N Engl J Med 295:370, 1976, with permission.)

The intima is a single layer of endothelial cells lining the vascular lumen. It is impermeable to proteins circulating in the blood and is separated from the second layer, the media, by a continuous boundary of elastic fiber known as the internal elastic lamina. The media constitutes the bulk of the arterial wall and is composed almost entirely of smooth muscle cells, interspersed with collagen, elastin fibers, and proteoglycans. The media makes the dilation and contraction of the vessel wall possible. The outer layer, the adventitia, is separated from the media by a noncontinuous elastin fiber boundary called the external elastic lamina. The adventitia consists primarily of fibrous tissue that gives the arterial wall strength and at the same time provides for some dispensability to prevent rupture in the presence of hypertension.[6,10]

ATHEROSCLEROTIC LESIONS

Atherosclerosis, derived from the Greek words athero (gruel or paste) and sclerosis (hardness), is a multifaceted disease process affecting primarily the intimal and medial layers of the arterial wall. It occurs as a result of extensive proliferation of smooth muscle cells in the intima of the artery and the deposition of fatty substances, cholesterol, cellular wastes, calcium, and fibrin into the intimal layer.[11] The resulting buildup is called plaque or a lesion. The plaque then goes through what is hypothesized to be a series of changes that alter both arterial structure and functional capacity.[10,12-14] The intimal layer of the vessel wall is primarily affected by the atherosclerotic degeneration. The media undergoes some secondary changes as the atheromatous plaque extends into it, weakens the wall, and possibly causes localized dilatation or aneurysm formation.[3] These progressive lesions of CAD are classified into three morphologic types: fatty streak, fibrous plaque, and complicated plaque or lesion. The clinical manifestations accompanying these lesions are unpredictable at best and each individual's clinical course varies from periods of acute illness to periods when the individual is fully active without symptoms.[8]

Fatty Streak

The atherosclerotic process begins as a recognizable fatty streak in the intima of the blood vessel. The lesion does not impinge on the lumen of the artery and there are no symptoms at this time. Fatty streaks have been found throughout the arterial tree in individuals from infancy through late adulthood. They most commonly involve the aorta, the coronary and cerebral arteries, and the arteries of the lower extremities.[3] Microscopically, these intimal lesions consist of smooth muscle cells with varying proportions of lipid material and fat droplets. These are commonly referred to as "foam cells" because of their tendency to "balloon out."

The lipids are composed mainly of cholesterol, cholesterol ester, phospholipid, and neutral fat. Because of the predominant fatty content, they are often soft and yellow in appearance.[15] It remains controversial whether these lesions progress to raised fibrous lesions or are reversible.[9] Data supporting the progression of a lesion to a raised fibrous lesion include observations by Stary[12a] showing that the fatty streaks of early life are found at the same anatomic sites as the fibrous plaques of older age. McGill[12b] reviewed data demonstrating that the increased surface area involvement of fatty streaks precedes the formation of advanced lesions, adding support to the precursor-product relationship between these two types of lesions.

Raised Fibrous Plaque

The raised fibrous plaque is the characteristic lesion of atherosclerosis. This lesion is a yellowish-gray elevated lump that thickens and begins to impinge on the lumen of the vessel but rarely occludes it.[8] As the plaque develops, muscle cells from the intima and media proliferate, and lipids are deposited from the plasma into the lesions. A matrix of collagen, elastin, and connective tissue cells surrounds the plaque and gives it a fibrous cap.[3,10,12] The central core of the plaque remains mainly a lipid material with various plasma components including white blood cells, albumin, fibrin, fibrinogen, and cellular debris. The predominant cells in the central core are the smooth muscle cells, and their proliferation is a key event that determines how extensive the fibrous plaques will become and what clinical sequelae will occur[16] (Fig. 5–2). Although most pathologists believe this plaque is irreversible, some feel that its progression may be slowed by appropriate lifestyle modifications.[3,13,17] Recent angiographic studies have shown slower rates of progression and some evidence of regression in atherosclerotic lesions when people have significantly lowered their cholesterol levels.[18] It is possible that lowering the circulating cholesterol may decrease the fat-storing phenomenon of the plaque. With a decrease in the storage of fat in the plaque, the lesion "shrinks" and therefore occupies less space, and the patency of the vessel is increased. As yet, there is no evidence to suggest that the damage to the vessel wall structure itself is reversed.[7,11,17]

Complicated Plaques

The complicated plaque is a fibrous plaque that has undergone one or more of the following pathologic changes: calcification, necrosis, internal hemorrhage, rupture of the plaque, or thrombus formation over the plaque. The plaques impinge upon the lumen of the vessel, but it does not appear that flow is impaired until the stenosis exceeds 70 percent of the lumen.[8] At this point of impaired flow, the individual may often demonstrate symptoms of decreased or inadequate blood flow in the organ supplied by the affected arteries.

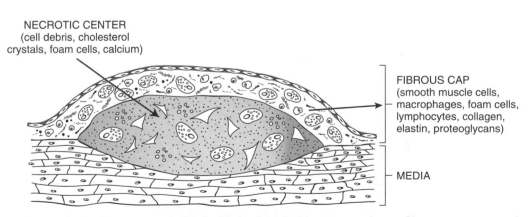

FIGURE 5–2. Major components of well-developed atheromatous plaque: fibrous cap composed of proliferating smooth muscle cells, macrophages, lymphocytes, foam cells, and extracellular matrix. The necrotic core consists of necrotic debris, extracellular lipid with cholesterol crystals and foamy macrophages. (From Cotran, RS, et al: Pathologic Basis of Disease, ed 5. WB Saunders, Philadelphia, 1994, p. 477, with permission.)

Structural changes in the intima may progress to affect the medial layer of the wall. Degeneration of a medial muscular layer further affects the arteries' ability to distend and meet the oxygen demand of the cells.[11,16] The weakened arterial wall may permit localized arterial dilatation or ballooning out, that is, an aneurysm, which may rupture and cause hemorrhage. Other complications arise if the plaque has broken through the intima and comes in contact with the flowing blood. The rough surface of the complicated plaque provides a site for platelet aggregation, fibrin deposition, and clot formation. The clot further impinges on the vessel's lumen and may either completely occlude the artery or embolize to occlude a more distal, smaller vessel, causing ischemia. Ischemia occurs when the supply of oxygen to the myocardium is inadequate to meet metabolic demands. It is caused by a functional constriction or actual obstruction of the coronary artery. If ischemia is prolonged, infarction or death of the adjacent muscle may occur.[8]

All three types of lesions may be present at the same time, at various sites in the arterial tree (Fig. 5–3). Except in young adults, single lesions of localized atherosclerosis is rare. Usually, severe atherosclerosis is accompanied by multiple lesions of varying severity.[7,10] Unaffected segments may be interspersed with diseases segments[16,19] and the plaque usually compromises only a portion of the circumference of the vessel.[10] Postmortem studies indicate that when the coronary arteries are affected, most lesions occur at proximal points in the three major coronary arteries at the points of bifurcation.[1,20] These proximal lesions are usually more severe and more prevalent. However, these lesions can be reached and bypassed or "ballooned" more easily.[1] In young adults (under 35 years of age), there is a high incidence of single-vessel disease, (usually of the left anterior descending [LAD]); in older adults and the elderly, there is a much greater prevalence of multivessel disease.[21]

The progression of CAD is neither linear nor predictable. New high-grade lesions often appear in segments of the artery that were relatively normal only months earlier. This type of abrupt progression in the plaque is most likely caused by a rupture or fissure, which changes the shape of the plaque. Pathologic studies show that rupture of the plaque complicated by an occlusive thrombus is the most fundamental mechanism in the development of acute ischemic syndrome.[22]

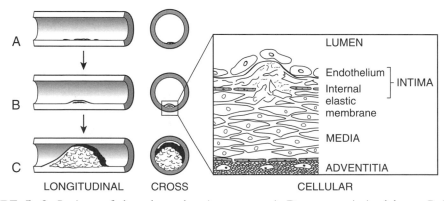

FIGURE 5–3. Lesions of the atherosclerotic process. *A,* Damage to intimal layer. *B,* Fibrous plaque. *C,* Complicated lesion. (From Huang, SH, et al: Coronary Care Nursing, ed 2. WB Saunders, Philadelphia, 1989, p. 133, with permission.)

PATHOGENESIS OF ATHEROSCLEROSIS

Although the pathogenesis of atherosclerosis is unknown, many hypotheses have been suggested. However, the three most common are the response-to-injury hypothesis, the monoclonal hypothesis, and the lipid-insudation hypothesis. Some factors of these hypotheses are interchangeable and have been combined with one another through years of speculation and research. These hypotheses are briefly discussed in the following sections, and the reader is referred to other sources for more in-depth explanations of these and other hypotheses.[4,5,8,10,11,13-15,23]

Response to Injury Hypothesis

The response-to-injury hypothesis is the most widely accepted explanation for the pathogenesis of atherosclerosis.[8] According to this theory, plaque formation begins in response to some type of trauma to the endothelial lining of the vessel wall. The damage may result from any one of a number of mechanical, chemical, hormonal, or immunologic stressors. The turbulence of arterial blood flow in an individual with hypertension, the hydrocarbons from cigarette smoke, Type 1 or 2 diabetes, and elevated levels of circulating cholesterol and triglycerides have all been hypothesized as causative agents.[1,10,12,15] Cigarette smoke, in particular, aggravates and accelerates the development of atherosclerosis in the coronary arteries, the aorta, and the arteries of the legs.[1] The damaged endothelium then becomes permeable to substances in the blood and provides a site for platelet aggregation. As the platelets aggregate, they release substances that may interact with plasma constituents and cause a proliferation of smooth muscle cells into the intima, forming new connective tissue. Also, in response to the injury, the endothelial cells proliferate to repair the damage. In limited injury, the regeneration of the endothelial layer may be a self-limiting event and, once endothelial function is restored, the proliferative lesions may be capable of regression.[10] However, in repeated injury, this relationship may be out of balance, and the plaques of atherosclerosis develop through continual proliferation of smooth muscle and connective tissue cells and additional lipid deposition into the intima.[4,10,12] Thus, this theory suggests that chronic injury to the endothelium leads to a long-standing inflammatory response, which becomes excessive over time, and the proliferation process becomes a disease process in itself.[10]

Monoclonal Hypothesis

The monoclonal hypothesis suggests that each lesion is a result of the proliferation of one smooth muscle cell that has acquired a selective advantage and may be equivalent to a benign monoclonal neoplastic growth. Benditt[15] suggests that this is a result of some mutagenic agent such as cigarette smoke or a virus. Microscopically, however, neither fibrous plaques nor fatty streaks are of one type of cell origin, and this raises serious questions as to the validity of this theory.[10,15]

Lipid-Insudation Hypothesis

The lipid-insudation hypothesis is closely related to the response-to-injury hypothesis and often considered a part of it. The lipid insudation theory suggests that elevation in the plasma low-density lipoproteins (LDL) results in the penetration of LDL into the intima of the arterial walls, which leads to lipid accumulation in the smooth muscle cells and macrophages (foam cells). The LDL then augments the smooth muscle cell hyperplasia that occurs in response to growth factors. Proliferating smooth muscle cells accumulate lipid and become sites for thrombi formation, setting up a cycle of further proliferation and platelet deposition.[1,10]

ATHEROSCLEROSIS AND CORONARY ARTERY DISEASE

Atherosclerosis is a disease that affects people in the middle-to-older-age brackets. Although it has been stated that the initial lesions can be isolated in infants, the onset of symptoms is usually in the fourth to fifth decade of life for men and approximately 10 years later for women.[8,24] The female sex hormone, estrogen, tends to increase levels of high-density lipoproteins, and this is thought to protect premenopausal women from heart disease.[1,25,26] Although atherosclerotic changes and plaque formation can occur in any artery, this text is specifically concerned about the effects of atherosclerotic changes on the coronary arteries and the clinical manifestations of atherosclerosis in CAD.

The atherosclerotic lesions develop in the intima of the coronary arteries. Although uncomplicated plaques rarely occlude arteries, these lesions may grow, thicken, and harden the walls of the artery, reducing arterial wall elasticity and impinging upon the lumen of the vessel. These plaques and structural changes in the wall result in a decrease in coronary-artery blood flow and a decrease in oxygen distribution to the myocardium. Atherosclerosis also affects vascular tone within the coronary system by interfering with the normal function of an endogenous vasodilator. Although the mechanism is unknown, it is believed to be associated with low-density lipoproteins.[17]

When the coronary circulation is compromised and the arteries are inelastic, the normal adaptive mechanism (local dilation of the coronary arteries) to increase blood flow through the coronary arteries in response to increasing oxygen requirements is diminished. The body's chronic compensatory mechanism is the development of collateral circulation. Collateral vessels, between the normal coronary artery and the affected artery distal to the stenosis, are found in practically all cases of severe stenosis.[8,22] As the lesions progressively occlude the vessels' lumen, if collateral circulation is inadequate to provide blood flow to the area by another vessel, the demands of the heart cannot be met. This causes an ischemic situation (an inadequate supply of oxygenated blood to the muscle).

Individuals with CAD may be initially asymptomatic but, as the atherosclerotic lesions progress, become symptomatic. Although there is considerable variation among individuals, clinical manifestations of CAD usually begin to appear when the vessel is 70 percent occluded. In angiographic and postmortem evaluations, the extent of CAD has never been predictive of clinical manifestations, because there is so much variation from one individual to another. Recent studies suggest that the measurement of blood flow across the lesion, comparing it to what the flow would be without the stenosis, may more accurately predict the relationship between the severity of the stenosis and incidence of thrombolic events.[27] Although symptomatology and the progress of the atherosclerotic disease process vary tremendously from one individual to the next, the functional inability of the artery to supply oxygenated blood remains the same. The resulting imbalance in myocardial oxygen demand versus supply is known as ischemia.

Ischemia and Infarction

Ischemia occurs when blood flow to the cell is insufficient to meet cellular needs. It may be the result of some obstruction to blood flow, an increased metabolic demand that the heart is unable to meet, inadequate hemoglobin content in the blood, or pulmonary disease. The duration and severity of ischemic imbalance determine the pathologic injury to the involved tissue. Transient ischemia is completely reversible. The ischemic tissues do not sustain any permanent damage. When ischemia is prolonged, the tissues undergo a series of changes, including a shift from aerobic to anaerobic metabolism. Prolonged ischemia may ultimately result in irreversible injury or infarction.[10]

Manifestations of ischemia and infarction include pain, elevated serum enzymes (enzymes that are released by the damaged cells into the circulation), and symptoms related to the function of the affected organ or tissues (angina with cardiovascular ischemia; decreased renal function with renal ischemia; intermittent claudication or muscle cramps with peripheral ischemia). Chronic ischemia may produce a dull pain, whereas acute occlusion causes an intense pain often followed by numbness or absence of sensation. The mechanism of ischemic pain is not fully understood and may be a result of one of two phenomena. The peripheral nerve endings may be stretched and stimulated by swelling of the cell caused by the ischemia, or the nerve endings may be stimulated by the localized release of kinins and other chemical mediators that result in the sensation of pain.[3,4,28]

The transition from ischemia to infarction is not inevitable. Several factors determine whether or not infarction will occur. These factors include the rate of onset of the ischemia, the ability of the iscehmic tissue to compensate for decreased blood flow, the oxygen requirements of the particular tissue, and the availability of oxygen in the blood.[25] Ischemia that has developed gradually is usually better tolerated because collateral circulation (communicating channels that serve as an alternate pathway to blood flow) may develop and supply the otherwise ischemic areas. Tissues also compensate for decreased oxygen supply by increasing their oxygen extraction from whatever blood flow is available. However, the heart is unable to compensate in this manner because at rest the heart muscle extracts 65 to 70 percent of the available oxygen, leaving little for reserve in response to decreased blood flow or increased oxygen demand.[28] The overall oxygen requirement of the affected tissue also determines its vulnerability to infarction. Some tissues, like the brain, are very sensitive to decreased oxygen supply. Cardiac cells can withstand ischemia for about 20 minutes before necrosis occurs, but cardiac tissue hypoxia causes visible electrocardiogram (ECG) changes in less than 1 minute.[28] Skeletal muscle, however, has a longer survival time in the presence of decreased oxygen. Finally, the quality of the individual's blood influences the ischemia-to-infarction progression. Anemia, decreased oxygen-carrying capacity, and decreased oxygen diffusion into the blood all reduce potential oxygen availability to the tissue and increase vulnerability to infarction.[29]

Infarction, or cellular death, is identified as a central core of necrotic cells that are electrically and functionally silent. Surrounding this core are cells with gradations of function dependent on the severity of the ischemia to the surrounding area.[11,28,30]

Treatment is aimed at reversing the ischemia and preventing further infarction by promoting oxygen supply to the affected area. This is achieved by removing any physical impedance to blood flow and any stimulus that may increase metabolic demands to the tissue. Oxygen and pharmacologic agents may be used, as appropriate, to relieve ischemia. If the individual is anemic, transfusion of red blood cells may be necessary to provide sufficient hemoglobin to transport oxygen adequately.

Despite all interventions, cell necrosis may still occur. When cells die, they release enzymes that initiate the inflammatory response and promote cellular destruction. Cellular debris is removed via phagocytosis, and the tissues undergo a series of changes ending in the formation of fibrous scar tissue.

Myocardial Ischemia and Infarction

Ischemia occurs when the oxygen demand of a tissue exceeds the oxygen supply. Myocardial ischemia results when an inadequate amount of oxygen is supplied to the heart.

The myocardial oxygen demand (MVO_2) is determined by the heart rate, the myocardial contractility, and the ventricular wall tension.[4,24,31] The heart rate is the frequency at which the heart pumps. The faster the heart rate, the greater the demand for oxygen. The myocardial contractility is the actual mechanical work of the heart. The workload is determined by the oxygen demands of the tissues. The heavier the workload, the harder the pump has to work and the greater its own demand for oxygen. Ventricular wall tension is directly influenced by preload (the ventricular volume or filling pressure) and afterload (the resistance, primarily the systemic blood pressure, against which the ventricle must pump to expel the blood). As the workload increases, the ventricular wall tension also increases, resulting in an increased myocardial oxygen demand.

The supply of oxygen to the myocardium depends on many factors, including the integrity of the pulmonary system, the hemoglobin content of the blood, the health of the coronary arteries, the heart rate, the blood pressure, and the resistance of the coronary arteries.[4,23,30]

An intact pulmonary system ensures that oxygen will diffuse from the lungs into the blood, where it binds to the hemoglobin and is carried to the tissues. If there is disease in the pulmonary system, the availability of oxygen is reduced. If the hemoglobin level is low (anemia), the oxygen-carrying capacity of the blood is reduced.

The health of the coronary arteries refers to their ability to dilate in response to demand. Because there is 65 to 70 percent oxygen extraction from the blood by the heart at rest, coronary artery blood flow must increase during periods of increased oxygen demand to meet the increased needs of the heart muscle at work. During exercise, the coronary arteries may need to carry four to five times their normal capacity. Coronary atherosclerosis not only impairs the vessels' patency and ability to dilate, but also affects redistribution of blood and oxygen within the heart.

Because the myocardium is perfused during diastole, the heart rate is a factor in myocardial oxygen supply and demand. The faster the heart rate, the greater the myocardial oxygen demand and the shorter the myocardial perfusion time during diastole. The increased myocardial demand associated with tachycardia is the most common cause of myocardial ischemia.

Hypotension (low blood pressure) inhibits adequate coronary artery perfusion. Hypertension (high blood pressure) affects the ventricular wall tension by increasing the afterload against which the heart must pump (increasing oxygen demand).

Resistance within the coronary circulation depends on the ventricular wall pressure. During systole, the ventricular wall pressure collapses the coronary arterial walls and occludes the blood flow to the myocardium. The greatest external wall pressure is on the subendocardial vessels, making the subendocardium particularly vulnerable to ischemia.[23,28]

The six factors previously discussed emphasize the interrelationship among factors that determine myocardial oxygen demand and supply. The heart's initial response to increased demand (increased heart rate) increases the oxygen supply as well as further increasing the oxygen demand. If the demand continues to exceed the supply, a vicious cycle is established.

When the oxygen demand is increased sixfold to eightfold, the healthy heart responds by increasing the coronary artery flow to four to five times its normal level and by increasing its oxygen extraction to make up for the relative deficiency.[23] In a heart with CAD, the diseased vessels are not able to dilate to provide an increased blood flow and therefore, the muscle supplied by the stenotic artery becomes ischemic.

Collateral circulation can play a role in preventing myocardial ischemia. In some people, chronic myocardial ischemia stimulates the growth of collateral vessels, which provide an alternative route for blood flow to the heart muscle. Collateral circulation development is unpredictable, further adding to the unpredictability of the relationship between the severity of disease and the severity of symptoms.[1,5]

CORONARY ARTERY DISEASE: CLINICAL MANIFESTATIONS

Coronary artery disease is manifested by any of four clinical syndromes: angina, myocardial infarction, sudden cardiac death, and congestive heart failure.[5,6] To varying degrees, the manifestations are results of the ischemia-infarction process on the myocardial muscle, which is extremely sensitive to decreased oxygen supply, particularly in the presence of coronary atherosclerosis. Interestingly, large variabilities exist between the severity of coronary atherosclerosis from one individual to another and the symptomatology they experience with similar extent of disease.

Angina Pectoris

Angina pectoris (literally "strangling of the chest") is a reversible ischemic process caused by a temporary inability of the coronary arteries to supply sufficient oxygenated blood to the heart muscle. There are four basic categories of angina: stable or chronic exertion angina, unstable angina, variant or Prinzmetal's angina, and asymptomatic or "silent" angina. All are a result of ischemia to the myocardium and, except for variant angina, occur secondarily to the arterial changes brought on by CAD.[5,28,32] Except for silent angina, all are characterized by the sudden onset of anterior chest pain that is relatively diffuse. The pain is usually described as a "squeezing" or pressure sensation. It can also manifest itself as burning in the throat or jaw, discomfort between the shoulder blades, shortness of breath, or other associated symptoms. The types of anginal episodes differ in their duration, intensity, pattern of occurrence, and precipitating factors.

As many as 3 to 4 million Americans may have silent or asymptomatic angina.[1,33] They experience ischemic episodes of which they are unaware. These individuals may also experience painful angina attacks.

STABLE ANGINA

Stable or chronic exertion angina is known as effort angina in that it is most often precipitated by exercise or stress. Individuals who experience stable angina quickly become aware of the specific activities that bring on the pain. Some of the most common precipitating events include exercise (particularly after a large meal), emotional stress, cigarette smoking, and exposure to cold temperatures.[5,11,18,30] The angina "attack" is characterized by substernal chest pain or pressure that may or may not radiate. The duration of pain is 5 to 10 minutes. Cessation of activity is often sufficient to relieve the pain; otherwise, rest and sublingual nitrates completely relieve the angina.[6] In stable angina, the episodes of pain are very similar in cause, character, and method of relief.[3,29] Angina brought on by emotional stress may last longer and be more difficult to relieve because the stressor itself is more difficult to eliminate.[18,30]

UNSTABLE ANGINA

Unstable angina is also effort related, but the episodes of pain occur with increased frequency, intensity, and duration. Angina pectoris at rest that occurs for the first time and is present less than 60 days and effort angina occurring with an accelerated change in pattern may also be classified as unstable angina. It is also known as crescendo or preinfarction angina. Crescendo angina may indicate progressive CAD and an increased risk of impending myocardial infarction.[34] Individuals with this type of angina are likely to have a mixture of severe, fixed-disease CAD, and coronary spasm.[4,6,10]

The symptoms are less responsive to rest and nitrates. Individuals may require hospitalization for rest and treatment with intravenous nitrates to prevent the myocardial ischemia from progressing to myocardial infarction. Unstable angina is a transient phase because it either progresses to a myocardial infarction, or the patient's condition stabilizes because the individual develops collateral circulation[20,23] or receives appropriate medical intervention.[30]

PRINZMETAL/VARIANT ANGINA

Prinzmetal/variant angina, commonly known as rest angina, is caused by coronary artery spasm.[5,10,29,30] The pain often occurs while the individual is at rest and most frequently in the early morning or on arising. The anginal episodes are cyclic and often occur at the same time each day. Variant angina is unaffected by exertion, but may be relieved by rest and nitrates. The pain is usually more intense and of longer duration than in stable angina. Variant angina more frequently leads to myocardial infarction.[8,24,31,34] Individuals with variant angina often present with both pain and related complaints of syncope and palpitations. Cardiac arrhythmias occur more frequently during episodes of variant angina than during effort angina.[24]

Although variant angina may be seen in individuals without CAD, it is often seen in the presence of significant CAD.[8,9] Variant angina is also more common in women than in men.[25] With the advent of coronary arteriography, actual coronary artery spasm has been visualized and documented. During cardiac catheterization, coronary artery spasm has been provoked by use of ergonovine, an ergot alkaloid that exerts a strong vasoconstricting effect on the coronary vascular system. The spasm of variant angina has been successfully relieved by use of nifedipine, a calcium channel blocker.

ASYMPTOMATIC "SILENT" ANGINA

As many as 70 percent of anginal episodes may be clinically silent.[16,33] The episodes are usually first observed via a 24-hour Holter monitor examination because the individual is unaware of their occurrence. Silent angina is common in individuals who have diabetes in which their neuropathies interfere with pain perception.[7,8] Although the individual is not aware that it is occurring, ischemia at the cellular level is documented via changes in the electrocardiogram (ECG).

Diagnosed silent angina is treated effectively with nitrates and beta blockers.

DIAGNOSIS AND TREATMENT

The frequency and characteristics of angina attacks vary. The attacks may depend upon the degree of coronary insufficiency, the collateral circulation, the response to treatment, and physical and emotional characteristics of the individual.[10,20,34] Angina provoked by emotional stress may last longer than episodes brought on by physical activity.

In CAD, the degree of stenosis (structural change) does not always correlate well with the functional impact of the disease because of individual variations in oxygen demand and workload tolerance. Predicting the extent of the coronary artery disease based on the anginal symptoms alone is difficult.[8,10,33]

The diagnosis of angina is usually by history alone because anginal episodes do not usually occur during a physical examination.[6,30] If an individual is examined during an episode of pain, tachycardia and hypertension will be found. During auscultation of the heart, an S3 or S4 gallop or a paradoxically split S2 heart sound may be noted. A mitral regurgitation murmur occurring secondarily to ischemia of the papillary muscle may be present.[29,30] ECG findings during episodes of pain reveal ST-segment elevation in variant angina and ST depression in unstable angina.[5,34] Exercise tolerance tests with cardiac radionuclide imaging may reveal areas of decreased perfusion and evidence of silent anginal episodes. Twenty-four-hour monitoring (24-Hour Holter Monitor) is used to document angina during normal daily activity. It is particularly useful in cases in which silent angina may be suspected, or it may present the initial evidence of angina. Cardiac catheterization provides a means of definitive diagnosis and treatment. It is used to assess atypical chest pain by allowing indirect visualization of coronary anatomy and left ventricular function. Cardiac catheterization is also used to document myocardial damage and LV function after myocardial infarction.

There are two fundamental goals in the treatment of angina. The first is directed toward symptom relief and diminishing the limitations of activity imposed by CAD. The second is arresting or reversing the progress of the disease and the anticipated worsening symptoms with medications, surgical procedures, and appropriate lifestyle modification. Chronic effort angina is treated pharmacologically with beta blockers, nitrates, and calcium channel blockers, specifically nifedipine. Beta blockers relieve angina by directly lowering myocardial oxygen demand but may aggravate coronary spasm and therefore should be avoided in individuals with rest/variant angina. Nitrates and calcium channel blockers are the drugs of choice in variant angina.[5,30,34] Pharmacologic trials with nitrates and beta blockers have shown them to be effective treatment for silent angina as well.[26] In addition, the use of lipid-lowering drugs (see Chapter 13) to slow the progression of CAD by lowering circulating cholesterol have produced positive results as well as being cost-effective treatments for coronary artery disease.[35]

Myocardial Infarction

Myocardial infarction (MI), the second manifestation of CAD, is the single largest killer of both men and women in the United States.[1] In a myocardial infarction, death or necrosis of some portion of the cardiac muscle occurs in response to sustained myocardial ischemia. Ischemia, secondary to reduced coronary artery blood flow, is most often caused by acute occlusion of coronary arteries. Evidence indicates that the acute occlusions are usually the result of a thrombotic event complicating existing atherosclerosis.[5,17,29,32] A coronary artery thrombus or a coronary artery spasm occludes the vessel at the site in the coronary artery where atherosclerotic plaques have significantly compromised the vessel's lumen.[8,23,36] Decreased blood flow associated with hemorrhage or profound shock (hypovolemia) may also result in decreased coronary artery perfusion and myocardial infarction.

Because the underlying pathology of angina and MI is similar, the initial clinical presentations may also be similar. The classic presenting symptom of MI is "viselike" retrosternal tightening of the chest. The tightening becomes progressively intense over a period of hours to days until the pain becomes absolutely unbearable. The pain typically radiates to any number of areas, the most common of which are the jaw, upper back, and down the inner aspects of both arms. The pain of the myocardial infarction usually begins at rest and is unrelieved by nitrates, rest, or any other method the individual typically uses to relieve anginal pain.[30] It is often accompanied by any, or all, of numerous symptoms that include dyspnea, nausea and/or vomiting, diaphoresis, and generalized weakness.

About 30 percent of myocardial infarctions are asymptomatic or silent. They usually occur as a result of decreased coronary artery blood flow as opposed to increased myocardial oxygen demand. These silent episodes have similar outcomes to symptomatic MIs in regard to damage to the myocardium, although the individual may not be at all aware that he or she has had a myocardial infarction. Some individuals seek treatment for the related symptoms that they are experiencing.[30,37] MIs, during which the individual experiences ischemic pain, are believed to be more severe and of longer duration than silent infarctions.[30,37]

ASSESSMENT AND DIAGNOSIS

The medical diagnosis of MI is based on the individual's history, current symptoms, serial serum enzymes, and electrocardiogram (ECG) changes. Positive findings in any two of these three diagnostic parameters are unequivocal evidence of MI.[30,37,38]

However, because of the vulnerability of the myocardium, even suspected MIs are treated as MIs until the diagnosis is ruled out.

HISTORY AND CURRENT SYMPTOMS

Individuals with suspected MIs often have histories of angina pectoris. However, a considerable number of individuals experience an acute infarct as the first indication of cardiovascular problems.[1,20,29,39] Other individuals, about 30 percent of those who have MIs, may experience no discomfort at all ("silent MI").[20,21,37,41] The silent MI is discovered on subsequent routine ECGs. About 50 percent of these MIs are truly silent because the individual is unable to recall any symptoms. In the other 50 percent, the individual is able to recall some episode of symptoms compatible with an infarct.[21]

The typical patient presents with complaints of severe substernal pressure or pain. He or she may appear to be in acute distress: dyspneic, diaphoretic, with pale, cool, and clammy skin and associated complaints of nausea and vomiting. The patient may also experience extreme weakness and an overwhelming feeling of impending doom.

Vital signs almost always reveal an elevated temperature and respiratory rate. The respiratory rate may be elevated because of pain and anxiety or in relation to a marked degree of cardiac failure. The blood pressure may be elevated (partially in response to pain and anxiety), but most individuals are normotensive even if they were hypertensive before the MI. In tachycardia, there may be a decreased systolic and increased diastolic pressure. If the LV function is severely compromised, the individual may have severe hypotension, secondary to decreased cardiac output.

On examination, the heart rate may vary from marked bradycardia to a rapid and regular or irregular tachycardia, depending on the underlying rhythm and the degree of left ventricular (LV) failure. Usually the pulse is regular and rapid, indicative of a sinus tachycardia (see Chapter 8). Premature ventricular contractions (PVCs) are common, secondary to an irritable ventricle. Almost 95 percent of individuals evaluated early in the course of the MI have PVCs.[39] Multiple arrhythmias are often observed.[23] Other common arrhythmias include atrial tachycardia, atrial fibrillation or flutter, paroxysmal atrial tachycardia, supraventricular tachycardia, conduction blocks, ventricular tachycardia, and ventricular fibrillation.

Life-threatening arrhythmias, ventricular tachycardia (VT), and ventricular fibrillation (VF) occur and are the most common cause of death after an MI. There are two particularly vulnerable periods when VT and VF are most likely to occur: within the first 10 minutes after the infarction and during a second period of cardiac irritability beginning 3 to 5 hours after the infarction and lasting for several days.[39]

On auscultation, an S4 heart sound is universally present. An S3 gallop, indicating decreased compliance of the myocardium and significant LV dysfunction, may be heard. A mitral murmur may indicate that a structural defect, such as an ischemic or ruptured papillary muscle or a ventricular septal defect, has occurred as a result of the MI.

ELECTROCARDIOGRAPHIC CHANGES

Typical ECG changes are observed in 88 percent of individuals having MIs.[8,30,32] Though myocardial cells can withstand ischemia for about 20 minutes before necrosis occurs, hypoxia causes electrical conduction changes in the cells in less than 1 minute. The ECG reflects these changes in myocardial electrical conduction in the area of the

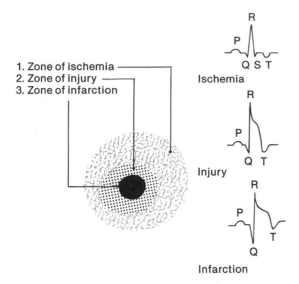

1. Zone of ischemia
2. Zone of injury
3. Zone of infarction

Ischemia

Injury

Infarction

FIGURE 5–4. ECG changes of infarction, injury, and ischemia as they correspond to the zones of infarction. (1) Ischemia causes inversion of T waves. (2) Injury causes ST-segment elevation. (3) Infarction causes permanent Q waves. (From Underhill, SL, et al: Cardiac Nursing. JB Lippincott, Philadelphia, 1983, p. 206, with permission.)

myocardial injury. Ischemia causes the T wave to become enlarged and symmetrically inverted because of late repolarization. With injury, cells depolarize normally but repolarize more rapidly, resulting in ST-segment elevation. An absence of current flow through the infarcted cells reveals unopposed currents from the myocardium diametrically opposite the infarcted side causing a permanent Q wave (Fig. 5–4). The appearance of pathologic Q waves is the classic ECG marker for a recent myocardial infarction, but Q waves do not always accompany an MI.[42] Non–Q wave infarcts tend to be smaller and usually not associated with total coronary artery occlusion. Interestingly, Q waves are associated with an initially low mortality rate, but have a higher mortality late in the postinfarction period and a higher rate of later reinfarction.[43] If the infarction is small, an abnormal Q wave may not appear. Approximately 30 percent of abnormal Q waves disappear or revert to borderline significance within 18 months after infarction.[29]

In the MI, the infarcted area is surrounded by a zone of injury, which in turn is surrounded by a zone of ischemia. As the areas of ischemia and injury resolve (usually within 1 to 2 weeks of the MI), the ECG changes associated with them return to normal. The area of infarction is permanent and therefore the Q wave may be permanent also.[42]

SERUM ENZYMES AND ISOENZYMES

Enzymes are groups of proteins found in all cells. The major cardiac enzymes are creatine kinase (CK), lactate dehydrogenase (LDH), and serum glutamic-oxaloacetic transaminase (SGOT). These particular enzymes are found in all cells, but specific forms of each, their isoenzymes, are found only in cardiac cells. With cellular ischemia and death, the enzymes and isoenzymes are released into the serum in a characteristic pattern over the ensuing hours to days following the infarct. Each enzyme has an individual pattern of increasing and decreasing. Serial blood samples can reveal patterns that are diagnostic of acute myocardial infarction (Fig. 5–5).[6,8,30,39] Enzyme-elevation

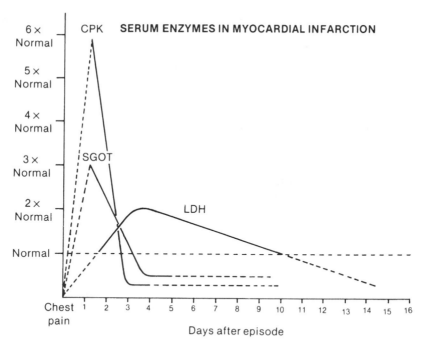

FIGURE 5–5. Serum enzymes in myocardial infarction. (From Vinsant, MO and Spence, MI,[6] p. 185, with permission.)

patterns may also be indicators of the prognosis following myocardial infarction. Laboratory studies for these specific enzymes (LDH, CK, and SGOT) are sensitive but may have a false-positive rate as high as 15 percent.[8,39] More accurate identification of the enzyme activity indicative of myocardial necrosis can be made from the separation of the total enzyme activity into subunits, called isoenzymes or enzyme fractionals. This separation is done by electrophoresis.

CK is found in high concentrations in skeletal muscle, the brain, and myocardium, and trauma to any of these tissues will cause an elevation in the total CK. The isoenzymes, subunits of CK, are different forms of the CK enzyme that have slight molecular differences but influence the same metabolic reactions. There are currently three recog- nized forms of CK isoenzymes: CK-MM, CK-BB, and CK-MB. On electrophoresis the three isoenzymes form separately colored bands that allow highly specific identification of the injured tissue. CK-MM is predominant in skeletal muscle, and CK-BB is predominant in brain tissue. Myocardial tissue is the only human tissue containing substantial amounts of CK-MB. Elevation in CK-MB is highly specific for myocardial necrosis. The level begins to rise 2 to 4 hours after the infarct, with an increase greater than 5 percent considered abnormal. Serial CK-MB levels have been correlated with infarct size, arrhythmic complications, and prognosis. CK-MB may also be elevated after cardiac surgery or cardiopulmonary resuscitation and in individuals with muscular dystrophy.[6,37,44]

LDH can be separated into five separate isoenzymes by electrophoresis. Cardiac tissue is rich in LDH_1 and LDH_2. Normally, LDH_2 activity exceeds LDH_1 activity. Myocardial infarction results in LDH_1 activity exceeding LDH_2 activity, which is referred to as a flipped LDH pattern. Elevated LDH_1 activity is seen within 24 hours and returns to normal in 7 to 10 days. An increase in LDH_1 activity is seen with hemolytic anemias, hemolysis of blood specimens, renal infarction, hyperthyroidism, and cancer of the stomach.

The flipped LDH pattern in combination with at least a 5 percent elevation of CK-MB provides objective evidence of myocardial necrosis.[6,39]

INFARCTION SITES AND MUSCULAR INVOLVEMENT

Myocardial infarcts are identified by their anatomic location and the layers of the myocardium involved. The location is identified by the surface or combination of surfaces of the ventricle that is infarcted: lateral, inferior, posterior and anterior, septal or anteroseptal, inferoposterior, and so forth. The location of the infarction depends on which coronary artery is occluded and the location of the occlusion within the arterial tree. Occlusions that occur in the large branches of the coronary circulation result in more extensive damage than those occurring in smaller arteries. Table 5–1 summarizes the areas of the heart that are supplied by the left and right coronary arteries. It is important to note that 70 to 80 percent of the vessel must be occluded before the myocardial blood flow is diminished.[5,8] Therefore, significant disease is usually present when symptoms begin to appear. Additional information on myocardial blood supply and MI location can be found in references[6,8,30,39] at the end of this chapter.

The myocardial infarction is also identified by the layers of myocardium involved. Transmural infarcts, in which necrosis extends through the full thickness of the wall of the myocardium, occur with 40 percent frequency and are usually associated with the occlusion of an epicardial artery. Transmural infarcts are the most commonly diagnosed infarcts.[6,18] Nontransmural infarcts occur in about 60 percent of infarcts. They may be limited to layers below the epicardium (subepicardial), in the middle of the heart muscle (intracardial), or the muscle below the endocardium (subendocardial). Because of its poor blood supply, greater ventricular wall pressure, and higher intravascular resistance, the subendocardial layer is the most vulnerable to ischemia.[6,23,28,39]

The location, size, and degree of myocardial involvement are determined by the patterns of ECG changes revealed in the various leads of the 12-lead ECG. Cardiac catheterization allows indirect visualization of the coronary arterial system and allows assessment of the damaged myocardium. Cardiac catheterization is also the means by

TABLE 5–1 Comparison of Right and Left Coronary Distribution

Right Coronary Artery Supplies	Left Coronary Artery Supplies
1. SA node (55%)	1. SA node (45%)
2. AV node	2. Anterosuperior division of left bundle
3. Bundle of His (a portion)	3. Right bundle branch (major portion)
4. Poterior one-third of septum	4. Anterior two-thirds of septum
5. Posteroinferior division of left bundle (a portion)	5. Posteroinferior division of left bundle (a portion)
6. Inferoposterior surface of left ventricle	6. Anterolateral surface of left ventricle

Source: From Vinsant, MO and Spence, MI,[6] p. 25, with permission.

which direct intracoronary antithrombolytic therapy (streptokinase, urokinase, tPA) and percutaneous transluminal angioplasty (PTCA) are initiated in the treatment of acute MI. The goal of both of these therapies is reperfusion of the ischemic area in an attempt to minimize the damage to the heart muscle. Knowledge of the location and amount of muscular damage enables health care providers to anticipate the clinical course, complications, and prognosis following the infarction.[39]

TREATMENT GOALS

The immediate goals of treatment for the individual who has experienced a myocardial infarction are:

1. Rapid management of myocardial ischemia/infarction and related symptoms (pain, dyspnea, nausea/vomiting) in order to limit the size of the infarction and promote comfort
2. Rapid reperfusion of the ischemic/infarcted area by the use of antithrombolytics and/or percutaneous transluminal coronary angioplasty (PTCA)
3. Prevention and/or early detection and treatment of arrhythmia
4. Prevention of complications of MI (see Complications of MI, p. 102)

Clinical Course

UNCOMPLICATED MYOCARDIAL INFARCTION

An uncomplicated MI is one in which the infarction is small and no complications arise during recovery.

Reperfusion with thrombolytic agents to reduce infarct size, improve myocardial performance, and reduce immediate and probably late mortality has been firmly established as the first line of treatment for the past 10 years. Successful treatment is that which provides the highest rate of reperfusion, the lowest rate of reocclusion, and the lowest rate of complications from bleeding.

All efforts are directed toward restoring coronary artery perfusion, decreasing myocardial workload, and decreasing myocardial oxygen demand.[23] Thrombolytic therapy (streptokinase, tPA) that is initiated within 6 to 12 hours of the onset of symptoms has shown progressively successful outcomes in reperfusion (see Chapter 7).[20] If thrombolytic therapy is unsuccessful or is contraindicated, PTCA or atherectomy may be used initially to attempt reperfusion of the myocardium. Individuals with non–Q wave infarcts have not been shown to benefit consistently from thrombolysis. Thrombolytics are contraindicated in individuals with uncontrolled hypertension, pregnancy, bleeding diatheses, recent trauma to the head and neck, and cerebrovascular disease.[38]

The patient is treated symptomatically. Oxygen, nitroglycerin, and/or morphine sulfate are given to reduce ischemic pain and improve myocardial perfusion via vasodilation. Although many people are hypotensive or normotensive after an MI,[20] antihypertensive medications are administered to treat hypertension. Other drugs like beta blockers or calcium channel blockers are given as necessary (see Chapter 7). Beta blockers reduce myocardial oxygen demand by decreasing the heart rate and contractility. Calcium channel blockers decrease the heart rate and also decrease the workload of the heart by systemic vasodilatation (decreased afterload).

Cardiac rhythm is observed for arrhythmias. Of all people who experience MIs, 90 percent have some type of arrhythmia. Early detection and treatment with appropriate pharmacologic agents have significantly reduced in hospital mortality.[23,29,30] The prophylactic use of lidocaine during the first 24 to 48 hours to prevent ventricular fibrillation is currently being advocated.[6,30]

The individual typically remains in the coronary care or intensive care unit 2 to 3 days postinfarction and remains in the hospital up to 1 week. During this time, activity is gradually increased and the patient is monitored for signs and symptoms of repeat ischemia. The rehabilitation process, which begins in intensive care with low-intensity exercise to prevent complications of bed rest, continues. Dietary restrictions usually limit sodium, fat, and caffeine. Education of the individual and his or her family centers on understanding the CAD process, dietary management, lifestyle modification, and risk-factor adjustment.

COMPLICATIONS OF MYOCARDIAL INFARCTION

Myocardial infarction has four major complications: arrhythmias, heart failure, thrombolytic complications, and damage to the heart structures.

Arrhythmias

Arrhythmias, caused by abnormalities in impulse generation, conduction or both, occur in 90 percent of individuals who have an MI. Although benign arrhythmias are often observed in healthy individuals, several, including VT, VF, and superventricular tachycardia (SVT), are dangerous or life threatening and require immediate treatment (see Chapters 7 and 8). Ventricular tachycardia and ventricular fibrillation occur frequently and are believed to be the cause of sudden cardiac death (SCD) and the cause of many fatalities post-MI. The types of arrhythmias seen as a result of MIs vary according to the surface of the heart infarcted and the point on the conduction pathway where the tissue is ischemic or infarcted.

Ischemia of a myocardial cell causes an alteration in the initiation and conduction of impulses throughout that area. Infarcted cells are electrically silent and neither initiate nor conduct impulses. Abnormalities in conduction may also result from the elongation of conduction pathways secondary to dilation of the infarcted ventricle. Arrhythmias are responsible for many deaths after MI, but, in many cases, prompt recognition and intervention by hospital personnel have succeeded in controlling potentially lethal arrhythmias.

Heart Failure

Heart failure is a syndrome with many different etiologies that reflects a fundamental abnormality in the effective mechanical performance of the heart muscle. It is characterized by the inability of the heart to maintain a cardiac output sufficient to meet the oxygen and nutritional needs of the tissues. Heart failure manifests itself in two ways. Acutely, the myocardial muscle that is ischemic does not contract normally and the infarcted myocardium does not contract at all. When the myocardium heals after an MI, the scar tissue that forms does not contract either. The presence of this abnormally functioning segment of the heart muscle results in asynchronous cardiac contraction and a low cardiac output. The second way in which heart failure is manifested is congestive heart failure (CHF). CHF is characterized by hypotension, retention of water and sodium from decreased renal perfusion, and the pooling of blood in either the pulmonary or systemic venous beds. It can be either an acute or chronic condition and usually requires treatment with diuretics, digoxin, and other medications.

Acutely, following an infarct, the cardiac output may be greatly reduced. Sympathetic stimulation increases the heart rate and the contractility within seconds of the infarct in an attempt to maintain cardiac output. (Cardiac output equals stroke volume times heart rate: $CO = SV \times HR$.) These compensatory mechanisms may be adequate to regain a normal cardiac output. If they are not, the kidneys, sensing the decreased renal blood flow, retain water and sodium in an attempt to increase the circulatory volume and venous return to the heart. If the heart is not damaged severely, these changes may be enough to compensate for the diminished pumping ability (even when the cardiac output is as low as 30 to 50 percent of normal) and bring the cardiac output back to normal.[46,47] However, if the heart is severely damaged and neither compensatory mechanisms nor medical intervention can return the cardiac output to normal, the patient deteriorates. When more than 40 percent of the left ventricle is infarcted, cardiogenic shock (low output failure) develops. This condition is associated with a 70 percent mortality rate.

As the myocardium heals, the scar contracts and becomes smaller. This allows progressively less systolic bulge at the sight of the scar. Systolic bulge is ballooning of the infarcted area of myocardium when left ventricular pressure increases during systole. Over time, the normal areas of the heart hypertrophy to compensate, at least partially, for the scarred musculature, and the heart at rest may have a normal cardiac output.[32,48] Individuals who continue to have symptoms of heart failure must be managed on daily diuretics, digitalis, and other cardiac drugs.

Thrombolytic Complications

Two types of thrombus formation, venous and mural thrombi, may occur after MI. Both are primarily triggered by venous stasis (stoppage of the flow of blood).

Deep vein thrombi usually form in the calf as a result of circulatory stasis imposed by activity restrictions. Mural thrombi form on the areas of relative stasis that are present in the ventricular wall after infarction. Both have the potential for embolism.

Emboli from a venous thrombus may result in a pulmonary embolism. Pulmonary embolism, once a major complication and cause of death after myocardial infarction, now accounts for less than 1 percent of total deaths.[39] Prophylactic antithrombolytic therapy with intravenous heparin, early ambulation for individuals with uncomplicated MIs, and in-bed exercises for patients who are confined to bed have decreased the incidence of deep vein thrombus and recurrent intracoronary thrombosis.

Emboli from a mural wall thrombus may lodge in visceral arteries and result in an infarction of the brain, kidney, spleen, or intestine, or an embolus may lodge in an extremity. The sudden onset of pain, numbness, and coldness in an extremity is indicative of an arterial clot and requires immediate intervention to prevent infarction in that extremity. An embolectomy may be required to remove the clot and restore the blood flow to the extremity.

Heart Structural Damage

Damage to the heart structures as a result of ischemia or infarction is a fourth major complication of MI. Structural damage includes papillary muscle rupture, ventricular free-wall rupture, intraventricular septal rupture, and ventricular aneurysm formation. With the exception of aneurysm formation, these complications can occur any time in the immediate post-MI period, but they usually occur 4 to 7 days after the initial infarct and often have immediate catastrophic consequences. Papillary muscle dysfunction or rupture occurs with papillary muscle ischemia or infarction and results in mitral-valve insufficiency. Ventricular free-wall rupture, with subsequent acute cardiac tamponade, occurs at the site where the myocardium is weakened because phagocytosis occurs earlier than collagen scar-tissue formation. Rupture of the intraventricular septum, although rare, may also occur as a result of necrosis and the inability of the infarcted area to withstand the repeated pressure generated by the left ventricle during systole.[29,32] The "rupture" is usually a tunnel-like lesion through the septum. Ventricular aneurysm is a late complication, usually the result of a transmural infarct that heals into a thin layer of scar tissue, which paradoxically bulges during systole. The aneurysm significantly affects myocardial performance and cardiac output. Any one of these structural problems may be fatal or result in mild to severe heart failure. Immediate surgical intervention may be required to repair the structural damage and restore adequate ventricular function.

Pericarditis, an inflammation of the pericardium, may also occur post-MI. Occurring the second to third day postinfarct, the characteristic symptom of pericarditis is pain over the precordium, aggravated by breathing and relieved by sitting up. Pericarditis accompanied by the accumulation of fluid in the pericardial sac is known as pericardial effusion. The accumulation of fluid may be sufficiently slow that the pericardium stretches and accommodates the fluid without interfering with cardiac performance. However, if the onset is abrupt and fluid accumulates rapidly in the pericardial sac, the heart is compressed and tamponade results. Cardiac tamponade is a life-threatening complication of pericarditis. The increased external pressure restricts diastolic filling and results in reduced ventricular volume, elevated ventricular diastolic pressure, and reduced ventricular diastolic compliance. Cardiac output and arterial blood pressure are decreased. The decreased cardiac output is not a result of mechanical pump failure but of the external restraint to cardiac filling and inadequate ventricular preload. This constitutes a severe cardiac emergency. A pericardial aspiration to remove fluid from the pericardial sac and relieve the restriction is necessary immediately. Once the accumulated fluid is removed and the tamponade is relieved, the symptoms should immediately abate and the heart function should return to "normal." Further treatment with analgesics, steroids, and antibiotics is usually indicated.

Prognosis After Myocardial Infarction

Sixty percent of deaths from myocardial infarction occur within the first hour, usually before the individual even reaches the hospital. These mortalities are believed to be caused by ventricular fibrillation. Hospital deaths after acute MI are usually attributed to heart failure and cardiogenic shock (shock occurring as a consequence of heart failure). Cardiogenic shock results from severe impairment of cardiac muscle contractility in which 40 percent or more of the myocardium is necrotic or injured and carries with it a high incidence of mortality.[6]

Infarct size and transmural extent are probably the greatest determinants of prognosis after MI. Prognosis can be modified favorably by early intervention or treatment; therefore, individuals who delay seeking treatment may be in control of the most important factor in determining their final outcome.[30,49] Occasionally, after the MI, the heart returns to its full functional capacity. More often, however, the functional capacity is decreased.[46] Exercise testing and other diagnostic tests provide valuable information about functional capacity, blood pressure response, and the potential for or presence of myocardial ischemia or arrhythmia after MI. Results of these tests provide information for treatment, including medical management or the need for surgical revascularization (see Chapter 7).[44] Although two-thirds of individuals never completely recover, 88 percent of those under 65 years of age are able to return to their previous employment.[1]

Women are more likely to suffer complications and reinfarction and also have a higher mortality associated with myocardial infarction than men. Women also require longer periods of recuperation, take longer to return to work, and suffer more psychologic distress and sexual dysfunction than men.[24,25,43,50]

The long-term prognosis depends on many factors, the most important of which are the extent of ventricular damage, the remaining cardiac reserve (the ability to respond to increased metabolic demands), the severity of the CAD, the potential for malignant arrhythmias, and coexisting morbid factors such as diabetes mellitus.[44] The medical and surgical management of the individual postinfarct is directed toward maximizing the existing cardiac function and minimizing any residual effects of the infarct. The introduction of angioplasty and thrombolytic therapy have significantly changed post-MI care. Myocardium that would have otherwise been infarcted can now be salvaged and low-risk individuals can safely resume activities earlier. Exercise tests have shown that low-risk individuals can safely resume activities as early as 3 to 4 weeks after infarct.[5] Cardiac rehabilitation programs, through exercise, vocational counseling, education on risk-factor reduction, and cholesterol-normalizing diet, facilitate lifestyle modifications that may reduce the risk of future infarctions. Increasing evidence of slowed progression and even regression of atherosclerotic plaques with significant cholesterol reduction should motivate individuals to make appropriate lifestyle changes after MI.

SUDDEN CARDIAC DEATH

A third clinical manifestation of CAD is sudden cardiac death. Sudden cardiac death (SCD) is commonly defined as an unexpected, witnessed cardiac death resulting from cardiac dysfunction and occurring in apparently healthy individuals engaging in their normal activities of daily living, without prior symptoms or with symptoms of less than 6 hours' duration.[26] The American Heart Association estimated that, in 1996, one of every three individuals who had a myocardial infarction died. Fifty percent of these individuals died within 1 hour from the onset of symptoms and before they reached the hospital.[1,23,39] It is estimated that, in 1 of every 5 persons who develop CAD, sudden cardiac death is the first and only symptom of the disease.[41] However, approximately half of all SCD occurs in individuals with known CAD.

The leading cause of SCD is cardiac arrhythmias, ventricular tachycardia, or ventricular fibrillation, often in the presence of severe but perhaps unrecognized CAD, and unrelated to an acute myocardial infarction.[1,19,26,39,41,52] About one-third of the individuals have seen a physician within the previous 2 weeks, often for symptoms that were misinterpreted or disregarded.[34] The majority of victims of SCD are men about 60 years of age.[26,53] Ventricular tachycardia, often a result of myocardial hypoxia, degenerates to ventricular fibrillation. Ventricular fibrillation is a rapid and chaotic heart rhythm in which the ventricle quivers rather than contracts. There is no effective cardiac output and, if fibrillation is sustained, death may occur within 4 minutes.[23,44,54]

Prompt initiation of cardiopulmonary resuscitation is the only proven means of preventing SCD.

Four characteristics are associated with an increased risk of SCD: ventricular electrical instability, extensive coronary artery narrowing, abnormal left ventricular function, and impulse conduction and repolarization abnormalities.

Four conditions contribute to the heart's tendency to fibrillate. Ischemia of the muscle cells causes the release of potassium into the extracellular fluid, which may increase myocardial irritability. Ischemic muscle remains negatively charged and can elicit abnormal impulses, which may cause fibrillation. Sympathetic stimulation resulting from low cardiac output may increase myocardial irritability. A previous myocardial infarction, resulting in a dilated ventricle, may cause stretching or changes in the conduction pathways or routing of impulses along abnormal pathways around the infarcted site. This abnormality in the conduction pathway allows for a cyclic state of myocardial cell excitation. In this situation, impulses re-enter muscle cells during the relative refractory period and set up a cycle of excitation that overrides the normal depolarization-repolarization cycle and allows the heart to fibrillate.[23,26,31] This is called a re-entry mechanism.

Antiarrhythmic drug therapy (Chapter 7) is always the first line of defense in suppressing recurrent ventricular arrhythmias. In individuals whose arrhythmias are refractory to all drug therapy as documented by electrophysiologic testing, an implantable cardioverter defibrillator (ICD) may be used. This implantable device, which detects and terminates life-threatening arrhythmias, is implanted in the abdomen and monitors the heart rate via epicardial leads. If the ICD senses VT or VF, it delivers a small charge directly to the myocardium to convert the arrhythmia. The use of ICDs has drastically lowered the incidence of repeat lethal arrhythmias in patients at high risk for SCD.[52,55] One study reports that the 1-year survival with an ICD is 97 percent.[56] Third-generation ICDs can also pace and store rhythms, as well as sense and defibrillate (see Chapter 8).

CONGESTIVE HEART FAILURE

Congestive heart failure (CHF) is a fourth manifestation of CAD. This syndrome is characterized by the inability of the heart to maintain a cardiac output that is adequate to meet the demands of the tissue due to an abnormality in the function of the heart muscle (the pump). CHF results in diminished blood flow to the tissues, abnormal retention of sodium and water, and congestion in the pulmonary and systemic circulation. The most common etiology is ischemic heart disease secondary to CAD. CHF may also be associated with hypertension, valvular disease, or congenital heart disease.[23]

The ability of the heart to maintain an adequate cardiac output depends on the heart rate and the stroke volume. The stroke volume is a function of: preload, the end-diastolic volume in the left ventricle; afterload, the systemic vascular resistance or the force against which the heart must pump; and contractility, the force of the contraction generated by the myocardium. Alterations in any one of these three factors result in decreased cardiac output. Changes in myocardial contractility are the most frequent cause of heart failure.[23,31]

In the person with CAD, decreases in normal coronary blood flow cause hypoxia and acidosis of the myocardial cells. Contractility is rapidly altered by these changes in the cellular environment. Even if blood flow is restored, contractile activity does not return to normal for hours or even days.[31] This is called myocardial stunning and may contribute to ventricular dysfunction and symptoms of heart failure. Myocardial infarction results in a loss of function in the area served by the occluded vessel. The scar from the MI may further contribute to ventricular dysfunction by restricting filling or by creating an aneurysm. Compensatory hypertrophy and dilatation of the myocardium, called ventricular remodeling, may result in marked impairment of the systolic function.[31,57]

When a reduction in cardiac output occurs, the body immediately brings compensatory mechanisms into play to restore the balance. Compensatory mechanisms are physiologic alterations in the body's functioning that maintain homeostasis or, in this case, cardiac output. These mechanisms include increased sympathetic nervous system stimulation, increased sodium and water retention by the kidneys, increased dilation of the cardiac muscle fibers to accommodate the increased volume, and ventricular hypertrophy. Increased sympathetic activity occurs immediately and causes increased heart rate and contractility. It also increases vascular tone, augmenting both venous return (preload) and systemic vascular resistance (afterload). The second compensatory mechanism is retention of water and sodium, triggered by a drop in kidney perfusion. Initially, the increased circulating volume augments preload, afterload, and contractility. The heart may also dilate or hypertrophy (increase its muscle mass) in response to increased workload.[41,46] These mechanisms may be successful in maintaining a normal cardiac output for some period of time, but they all increase myocardial oxygen demand. Over time, they are not adequate to sustain the cardiac output. Impaired cardiac function may be manifested initially only during exertion or significant stress, but with the progression of the syndrome, the contractile performance of the heart deteriorates and the signs and symptoms of CHF may even occur at rest.[31,46] Prognosis is based on left ventricular function, the incidence of ventricular arrhythmias, and the underlying disease process.

TYPES OF HEART FAILURE

There are several types of heart failure. Each is described briefly below.

Acute Versus Chronic Failure

Acute heart failure may characterize the initial manifestation of heart disease or may be an acute exacerbation of chronic cardiac failure. The events that precipitate the symptoms of acute heart failure occur rapidly. The rapid failure of the pump may result in an acute shift of blood from the systemic circulation to the pulmonary circulation before the compensatory mechanisms can be effective. The individual may experience a symptomatic fall in cardiac output and rapid onset of the associated symptoms, including dyspnea at rest, orthopnea, pulmonary congestion, and edema.[6,31,57]

Chronic heart failure develops gradually and is associated with the chronic retention of fluid and salt by the kidneys and other compensatory mechanisms. Pulmonary congestion or peripheral edema is usually the reason why an individual seeks medical attention. Chronic heart failure is the leading cause of hospital admission in individuals older than 65 years of age.[24] With time, the chronic overstimulation of compensatory mechanisms may lead to end-organ failure.

Compensated Versus Uncompensated Failure

In compensated failure, the heart has been able to maintain adequate cardiac output by means of the compensatory mechanisms described previously and perhaps some medical intervention. Sympathetic stimulation and renal retention of water and sodium have maintained the cardiac output at normal levels, except for a mild to moderately elevated right atrial pressure (+4 mm Hg to + 6 mm Hg). The end-diastolic volume and the end-diastolic pressure also remain elevated and the ejection fraction is reduced. Other compensatory mechanisms include increased vasoconstriction, cardiac dilatation, and hypertrophy.[31] Cardiac function at rest appears normal[23,57] and symptoms reappear when myocardial oxygen demand increases. A rapid heart rate, pallor, and diaphoresis all indicate that the cardiac output cannot meet the increased demand.

Uncompensated failure occurs when a severely damaged heart cannot regain normal cardiac output. Although compensatory mechanisms are at work, normal cardiac output is not attained. Fluid retention worsens because inadequate renal perfusion persists. Gradually the heart is stretched until it is unable to pump even moderate quantities of blood. The heart may fail completely and the individual may die. More often, the symptoms severely limit activity and the individual seeks medical attention for the uncompensated cardiac failure. Often this cyclical progression of worsening failure can be halted or slowed by appropriate pharmaceutical therapy. Diuretics and fluid and salt restriction may control circulating volume while cardiac glycosides (for example, digitalis) are given to improve contractility. In this way, an adequate cardiac output may be regained and maintained. Although digitalis has little effect on the contractility of the normal myocardium, in the failing heart it may double the strength of contraction.[23]

Intractable Heart Failure

Intractable heart failure occurs when the heart fails despite application of all therapies. Pulmonary and systemic congestion and a low cardiac output (ejection fraction less than 20 percent) exist even at rest.[31,58] The cause of pump failure is usually ischemic cardiomyopathy from CAD and idiopathic dilated cardiomyopathy. The current treatment of choice, for patients who meet specific medical criteria, is cardiac transplantation with the goal of improving survival, symptoms, and exercise capacity.[57-59]

Left Ventricular Failure Versus Right Ventricular Failure

The left and right sides of the heart may fail separately or together. Left-side failure is more common than right-sided failure and frequently leads to right-sided failure.[23,46,48] Because both are parts of a circuit, it is apparent that one side cannot pump significantly more blood for any length of time without significant impact on the other side.

Left-sided failure is most frequently seen after MI. When the heart is significantly damaged, it may not pump effectively, and blood can back up in the left ventricle. As the pressure from the increased volume builds, it is communicated in a retrograde fashion to the left atrium and on through the pulmonary capillary beds. Pulmonary capillary pressure builds and the fluid is forced from the capillaries into the interstitial spaces and then into the alveoli. The presence of fluid in the interstitial spaces and the alveoli produces edema, which interferes with the diffusion of gases. Clinically, the individual becomes increasingly dyspneic, progressing over time to dyspnea at rest, even when sitting upright. As pulmonary congestion increases, the lungs become stiff and less compliant and dyspnea worsens. A cough produces frothy pink (blood-tinged) sputum, and rales (abnormal breath sounds from the movement of air through fluid in the alveoli) are audible over the lungs. Signs and symptoms of left ventricular failure are included in Table 5–2. If this condition is left untreated, acute pulmonary edema ensues. This is a medical emergency, requiring immediate treatment with oxygen, bronchodilators, vasodilators, and diuretics.

Right ventricular failure may occur unilaterally. It can result from congenital heart problems or chronic obstructive pulmonary disease (COPD). In the latter, lung compliance decreases significantly, and pulmonary vascular resistance increases significantly. The most common cause of right ventricular failure, however, is left ventricular failure.[31,46,57] Right ventricular failure follows left ventricular failure when the increase of pressure through the pulmonary circulation overloads the right ventricle (Fig. 5–6). The first sign of right ventricular failure is elevated central venous pressure (CVP) and neck vein distension. Liver engorgement, ascites, and peripheral edema of the dependent portion of the body (feet and ankles) are also observed as the syndrome progresses.

All individuals with heart failure complain of fatigue and a decreased tolerance for activity. Treatment of the acute episode is directed toward decreasing circulatory overload, decreasing myocardial workload and oxygen demand, and increasing myocardial contractility. These goals may be accomplished with the judicious use of diuretics, water, and sodium restrictions, cardiac glycosides (to increase myocardial contractility), and oxygen therapy as necessary.

TABLE 5–2 Signs and Symptoms of Cardiac Failure

Left Ventricular Failure	Right Ventricular Failure
Subjective	
Dyspnea	Abdominal pain
Orthopnea	Anorexia/nausea
Paroxysmal nocturnal dyspnea	Bloating
Cough	Fatigue
Fatigue	Ankle swelling (bilateral)
Objective	
Rales	Distended neck veins
S3gallop	Decreased urine output
Pleural effusion	Hepatojugular reflux
Peripheral cyanosis	Hepatomegaly/splenomegaly
Increased respiratory rate	Ascites
Cheyne-Stokes respirations	Elevated CVP, right atrial pressure
Decreased urine output	S4 gallop
Pink frothy sputum	Peripheral edema

Source: From Patrick, ML, et al (eds): Medical-Surgical Nursing: Pathophysiological Concepts. JB Lippincott, Philadelphia, 1986, p. 548, with permission.

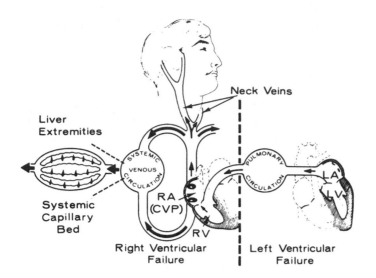

FIGURE 5–6. Retrograde failure of right ventricle from left ventricle. (From Vinsant, MO and Spence, MI,[6] p. 385, with permission.)

CHF is usually a recurring phenomenon characterized by repeated exacerbations of symptoms increasing in frequency and severity as the myocardial muscle becomes progressively weaker and distended.[3,5,31,60] Chronic management attempts to decrease the frequency and severity of the symptoms and the limitations imposed by the symptoms. Individuals are instructed as to the benefits of salt restriction, weight loss, and risk-factor reduction to slow the progress of atherosclerotic disease. Although historically individuals with CHF were instructed to lead a sedentary lifestyle, it is now recommended that they exercise to their symptomatic limits.[23,31,61]

PHYSIOLOGIC CHANGES IN INDIVIDUALS WITH CORONARY ARTERY DISEASE IN RESPONSE TO PHYSICAL CONDITIONING

There is no evidence that physical training alters coronary atherosclerotic lesions, increases coronary artery blood flow, or stimulates the growth of coronary collateral circulation, but regular moderate-intensity exercise does improve functional capacity and decrease activity-related symptoms in the individual with CAD.[60,62] The World Health Organization has concluded that regular vigorous exercise can enhance approaches to treatment and modify risk factors in patients with CAD.[63] The most beneficial physiologic change is an improvement in functional capacity, attributable to peripheral adaptations that include increased oxygen extraction and utilization by trained skeletal muscles, resulting in a decrease in myocardial oxygen demand and coronary blood flow requirements for a given level of exercise.[62,64] This allows the individual to perform higher workloads for longer periods of time without reaching his or her ischemic threshold.[60,61,65] There is also a more rapid return to resting heart rate after exercise. The workload can be expressed as the product of the heart rate (HR) and the systolic arterial blood pressure (SBP); this is known as the rate-pressure product (RPP) or double product (HR × SBP = RPP; for example, 70 × 100 = 7000 or 70 × 10(2)) (see Chapter 9). Both the heart rate and arterial BP are major determinants of the myocardial oxygen consumption during exercise. As they increase, so does the RPP. In the physically conditioned individual with CAD, heart rate and blood pressure are decreased at rest and with submaximal exercise. Therefore, the RPP, the myocardial oxygen demand, and the myocardial oxygen consumption are all lower.[64]

To date, physical conditioning has not been shown to facilitate the development of collateral coronary circulation,[60,66] but in a recent cumulative analysis by Shephard,[67] the data showed that individuals who had undergone physical conditioning not only experienced fewer repeat myocardial infarcts but also had a lower percentage of these events with fatal outcome.[60,61,67] Other studies have indicated that high-intensity, long-duration conditioning may improve myocardial function in a very select group of cardiac patients.[53,61,62,68,69] Coexisting health problems may limit, influence, or contraindicate the "normal" cardiac rehabilitation program for some individuals. Individuals who have had heart transplants do increase their work capacity with exercise therapy, but their heart rate increases more gradually during exercise and their peak exercise response is lower.[65] Individuals with chronic renal failure are usually anemic and may not be able to improve their tolerance for activity. Improvements in functional capacity may also be very slow or minimal for individuals with chronic respiratory disease because of their hypoxia, and rehabilitation must be significantly modified to best serve individuals with significant mobility limitations.[64]

In addition to the physiologic response to exercise, the psychologic satisfaction, the improved sense of well-being, and the decrease in cardiac risk factors that occur as a result of physical conditioning are of great benefit to the individual with CAD.

SUMMARY

In presenting the pathophysiology of coronary artery disease (CAD), particular attention was given to atherosclerosis and to the ischemia-infarction process that is the basis for all the related clinical manifestations of CAD.

The clinical manifestations of CAD, including angina, myocardial infarction, sudden cardiac death, and cardiac failure, were discussed in relation to the pathophysiology and the progression of CAD, their presenting symptoms, and their major complications.

The major physiologic changes in relation to training and physical conditioning of individuals with CAD were found to be improvement in functional capacity and the increased efficiency with which peripheral muscles use oxygen.

REFERENCES

1. 1997 Heart and Stroke: Statistical Update. American Heart Association, Dallas, 1996.
2. Years of Life Lost From Cardiovascular Disease. Morbidity and Mortality Weekly Report, Massachusetts Medical Society 35:42, 1986.
3. Generalized cardiovascular disease. In Berkow, R (ed): Merck Manual, ed 16. Merck, Sharp and Dohme, Rahway, NJ, 1992, p 409.
4. Zierler, BK and Cowan, MJ: Pathogenesis of atherosclerosis. In: Woods, SL, et al (eds): Cardiac Nursing, ed 2. JB Lippincott, Philadelphia, 1995, p 187.
5. Braun, LT, Murphy, MP, and Carlson, EV: Coronary artery disease. In: Kinney, MR, et al (eds): Comprehensive Cardiac Care, ed 7. Mosby, St. Louis, 1991, p 253.
6. Vinsant, MO and Spence, MI: Commonsense Approach to Coronary Care: A Program, ed 5. CV Mosby, St Louis, 1988, pp 178–210, 449, 498–500.

7. Stehbens, WE: Atherosclerosis and degenerative diseases of the blood vessels. In: Stehbens, WE and Lie, JT (eds): Vascular Pathology. Chapman and Hall Medical, London, 1995, p 175.
8. Cheitlin, MD, Sokolow, M, and McIlroy, MB: Clinical Cardiology. Lange Medical Publications, Los Altos, Calif, 1993, p 147.
9. Chaffee, EE and Greisheimer, EM: Basic Physiology and Anatomy, ed 2. JB Lippincott, Philadelphia, 1969, pp 343–391.
10. Davis, MJ: The pathology of coronary atherosclerosis. In: Schlant, RC and Alexander, RW (eds): Hurst's The Heart, Arteries and Veins, vol 2, ed 8. McGraw-Hill, New York, 1994.
11. Ross, R: Pathogenesis of atherosclerosis. In Braumwald, E: Heart Disease, ed 4. WB Saunders, Philadelphia, 1992, p 1106.
12. Ross, R: The pathogenesis of atherosclerosis–An update. N Engl J Med 314(8):488, 1986.
12a. Stary, HC: Evolution of atherosclerotic plaques in the coronary arteries of young adults. Arteriosclerosis (abstract) 3:471, 1983.
12b. McGill, HC: Persistent problems in the pathogenesis of atherosclerosis. Arteriosclerosis 4:443–451, 1984.
13. Ross, R and Glosmet, JA: The pathogenesis of atherosclerosis, Part I. N Engl J Med 295:369, 1976.
14. Ross, R and Glosmet, JA: Ibid, Part II. N Engl J Med 295:426, 1976.
15. Benditt, E: The origin of atherosclerosis. Sci Am 236:74, 1977.
16. Roberts, WC: Preventing and arresting coronary atherosclerosis. Am Heart J 130(3), pt 1:580, 1995.
17. Brown, BG, et al: Coronary angiographic changes, lipid-lowering therapy and their relationship to clinical cardiac events. In: Fuster, V (ed): Syndromes of Atherosclerosis: Correlation of Clinical Imaging to Pathology. Futura Publishing Company, Inc, Armonk, NY, 1996.
18. Froehlicher, ES, et al: Risk profile screening. J Cardiovasc Nurs; 10(1):30, 1995.
19. Schoen, F: Blood vessels. In: Cotran, RS, et al (eds): Pathologic Basis of Disease, ed 5. WB Saunders, Philadelphia, 1994, p 517.
20. Diseases of the heart and pericardium. In: Berkow, R (ed): Merck Manual, ed 16. Merck Research Laboratories, Rahway, NJ, 1992.
21. Corrado, D, et al: Sudden death in the young. Circulation 90(5):2315, 1994.
22. Wilson, RF: Assessing the severity of coronary artery stenosis. N Engl J Med 334(26):1735, 1996.
23. Guyton, AC and Hall, JE: Textbook of Medical Physiology, ed 9. WB Saunders, Philadelphia, 1996.
24. Wingate, S: Woman and coronary heart disease: Implications for the critical care setting. Focus on Critical Care 18:212, 1991.
25. Wenger, NK, Speroff, L, and Packard, B: Cardiovascular health and disease in women. N Engl J Med 329(4):247, 1993.
26. Fleury, J and Murdaugh, C: Patients with coronary artery disease. In: Clochesy, JM, et al: Critical Care Nursing. WB Saunders, Philadelphia, 1993.
27. Pijls, NH, et al: Measurement of fractional flow reserve to assess the functional severity of coronary-artery stenosis. N Engl J Med 334(26):1703, 1996.
28. Jensen, SK: Pathophysiology of myocardial ischemia and infarction. In: Woods, SL, et al (eds): Cardiac Nursing, ed 3. JB Lippincott, Philadelphia, 1995, p 212.
29. Factor, SM: Pathophysiology of myocardial ischemia. In Schlant, RC and Alexander, RW (eds): Hurst's The Heart, Arteries, and Veins, ed 8. McGraw-Hill, New York, 1994.
30. Osguthorpe, SG and Woods, SL: Myocardial ischemia and infarction. In: Woods, SL et al (eds): Cardiac Nursing, ed 3. JB Lippincott, Philadelphia, 1995, p 212.
31. Schlant, RC and Sonnenblick, EH: Pathophysiology of heart failure. In: Schlant, RC and Alexander, RW (eds): Hurst's The Heart, Arteries, and Veins, ed 8. McGraw-Hill, New York, 1994.
32. Woods, SL and Underhill, SL: Coronary heart disease: Myocardial ischemia and infarction. In Patrick, ML, et al (eds): Medical Surgical Nursing: Pathophysiological Concepts. JB Lippincott, Philadelphia, 1986.
33. Cutler, BC: Perioperative evaluation and management of cardiac disease. In: Dean, RH, et al (eds): Current Diagnosis and Treatment in Vascular Surgery. Appleton and Lange, Norwalk, Conn, 1995, p 45.
34. Matrisciano, L: Unstable angina. An overview. Critical Care Nursing 12:30, 1992.
35. Amsterdam, E, Hyson, D, and Kappagoda, CT: Non-pharmacologic therapy for coronary artery atherosclerosis: Results of primary and secondary prevention trials. Am Heart J (suppl)128(6) pt 2:1344, 1994.
36. Flugelman, MY, et al: Smooth muscle cell abundance and fibroblast growth factors in coronary lesions of patients with nonfatal unstable angina. Circulation 88(5-6):2493, 1993.
37. Tsunoda, D: Acute myocardial infarction. Am J Nurs 96(5):38, 1996.
38. Massie, BM: The heart. In Tierney, LM, McPhee, S, and Papadakis, MA (eds): Current Medical Diagnosis and Treatment, ed 35. Appleton and Lange, Stamford, Conn, p 295.
39. Pasternak, RC, Sobel, BE, and Braunwald, E: Acute myocardial infarction. In: Braumwald, E (ed): Heart Disease, ed 4. WB Saunders, Philadelphia, 1992, p 1200.
40. Waller, BF, et al: Cardiac pathology in 2007 consecutive forensic autopsies. Clin Cardiol 15:760, 1992.
41. Manolino, TA and Furbero, CD: Epidemiology of sudden cardiac death. In: Khtar, MA, Myerburg, RJ, and Ruskin, JN: Sudden Cardiac Death. Williams & Wilkins, Philadelphia, 1994, p 3.
42. Gilmore, SB and Woods, SL: Electrocardiography and vectorcardiography. In Woods, SL et al (eds): Cardiac Nursing, ed 3. JB Lippincott, Philadelphia, 1995, p 290.

43. Young, R and Kahana, E: Gender recovery from late-life heart attack and medical care. Women Health 20(1):11, 1993.
44. Ayers, SM: Cardiovascular. In: Ayers, SM: Textbook of Critical Care, ed 3. WB Saunders, Philadelphia, 1995, p 448.
45. Fuster, V, et al: The pathogenesis of coronary artery disease and the acute coronary syndrome. N Engl J Med 326 pt 1:242, pt 2:310, 1992.
46. Vinsant, MO and Spence, MI: Mechanical complications in coronary artery heart disease: Heart failure and shock. In: Vansant, MO and Spence MI: Commonsense Approach to Coronary Care: A Program, ed 5. Mosby, St. Louis, 1988, p 345.
47. Bopp, DL: Heart failure. In: Patrick, ML, et al (eds): Medical Surgical Nursing: Pathophysiological Concepts. Lippincott, Philadelphia, 1986.
48. Cochrane, BB: Complications of Acute Myocardial Infarction. In: Woods, SL, et al (eds): Cardiac Nursing, ed 3. Lippincott, Philadelphia, 1995, p 496.
49. Schoen, F: The heart. In: Cotran, RC, et al (eds): Pathologic Basis of Disease, ed 5. Saunders, Philadelphia, 1994, p 476.
50. Rankin, S: Differences in recovery from cardiac surgery: A profile of male and female patients. Heart Lung 19:481, 1990.
51. Miller, NH: Cardiac rehabilitation: Management of the patient after a myocardial infarction. In: Kinney, MR and Packa, DR: Andreoli's Comprehensive Cardiac Care, ed 8. Mosby, St Louis, 1996, p 402.
52. Lehmen, MH and Steinman, RT: Preventing sudden cardiac death. Postgrad Med 82:7, 1987.
53. Ehsani, AA, et al: Improvement of left ventricular function in patients with coronary artery disease. Circulation 74:350, 1986.
54. Davies, MJ: Anatomical features in victims of sudden cardiac death; coronary artery pathology. In: Khtar, MA, Myerburg, RJ, and Ruskin, JN: Sudden Cardiac Death. Williams & Wilkins, Philadelphia, 1994, p 21.
55. Cooper, DK, Valladares, BK, and Futterman, LG: Care of the patient with the automatic implantable cardioverter defibrillator: A guide for nurses. Heart Lung 16(6) pt 1:640, 1987.
56. Kelly, PA, Cannom, DS, and Garan, H: The automatic implantable cardioverter-defibrillator: Efficacy, complications and survival in patients with malignant ventricular arrhythmias. J Am Coll Cardiol 11:1278, 1988.
57. Cohn, JN and Sonnenblick, EH: Diagnosis and therapy of heart failure. In: Schlant, RC and Alexander, RW: Hurst's The Heart, Arteries and Veins, ed 8, Vol 1. McGraw-Hill, New York, 1994.
58. Squires, RW: Cardiac rehabilitation issues for heart transplant patients. J Cardpulm Rehabil 10:159, 1990.
59. Schroeder, JS and Hunt, S: Cardiac transplantation: Update 1987. JAMA 258:3142, 1987.
60. Hung, J, et al: Changes in rest and exercise and myocardial perfusion and left ventricular function 3 to 26 weeks after clinically uncomplicated acute myocardial infarction: Effects of exercise training. Am J Cardiol 54:943, 1984.
61. Hartley, LH: Exercise for the cardiac patient. Long term maintenance phase. Cardiol Clin 11(2):277, 1993.
62. Wenger, NK: Rehabilitation of the patient with coronary heart disease. In: Schlant, RC and Alexander, RW (eds): Hurst's The Heart, Arteries and Veins, ed 8, Vol 2. McGraw-Hill, New York, 1995.
63. Ritchie, DE: Exercise and activity. In: Woods, SL, et al (eds): Cardiac Nursing, ed 3. Lippincott, Philadelphia, 1995, p 708.
64. Oberman, A: Exercise and the primary prevention of cardiovascular disease. Am J Cardiol 55:100, 1985.
65. Hartley, LH: Exercise for the cardiac patient. Long term management. Cardiol Clin 11(2):270, 1993.
66. Wenger, NK: Rehabilitation of the patient with symptomatic coronary atherosclerotic heart disease: Part II. In: McIntosh, HD (ed): Cardiology Series, 3(3). Parke-Davis, Morris Plains, NJ, 1980.
67. Shephard, RJ: The value of exercise in ischemic heart disease: A cumulative analysis. J Cardiac Rehab 3:294, 1983.
68. Leon, AS, Casal, D, and Jacobs, D: Effects of 2,000Kcal per week of walking and stair climbing on physical fitness and risk factors for coronary heart disease. J Cardpulm Rehabil 16(3):183, 1996.
69. Oldridge, NB, et al: Cardiac rehabilitation after myocardial infarction: Combined experience of randomized clinical trials. JAMA 260:945, 1988.

CHAPTER 6

Chronic Lung Diseases

In this chapter, chronic obstructive pulmonary disease (COPD) (including chronic bronchitis and emphysema), asthma, bronchiectasis, cystic fibrosis, and restrictive lung disease are discussed. COPD and asthma are the most common chronic lung diseases for which pulmonary rehabilitation is needed. Patients with cystic fibrosis are surviving with increased pulmonary dysfunction, which makes them candidates for pulmonary rehabilitation. Patients with restrictive lung disease and bronchiectasis make up a relatively small percentage of all patients with chronic pulmonary diseases; however, there is support for the use of pulmonary rehabilitation programs with these patient populations.[1]

CHRONIC OBSTRUCTIVE PULMONARY DISEASE

Definition

In 1962, the American Thoracic Society (ATS) defined the clinical conditions of COPD as "damage to the alveolar walls and inflammation of the conducting airways."[2] Numerous revisions of this definition have been published since,[3-6] the most recent of which is taken from the 1995 position statement by the American Thoracic Society. This statement concluded that COPD is a disorder characterized by the presence of airflow obstruction that is generally progressive and may be accompanied by partially reversible airway hyperreactivity.[6] The individual pulmonary diseases that are currently included in the definition of COPD are chronic bronchitis and emphysema. Asthma, bronchiectasis, and cystic fibrosis have been excluded from the diseases termed COPD.[6]

The definition of COPD continues to evolve. Although little doubt exists that there is a reversible asymptomatic precursor to COPD,[5-9] it is not mentioned in the current ATS definition. The 1995 statement includes only the two components of the chronic pulmonary disease that cause symptoms and are irreversible: chronic bronchitis and emphysema.

Changes in peripheral airways have been found in asymptomatic smokers under 40 years of age.[10] In the 1987 version of the ATS statement, peripheral airways disease, the precursor to COPD, was described as a component of COPD. It was defined as a condition including inflammation, fibrosis, and narrowing of the terminal and respiratory bronchioles. The symptoms of peripheral airways disease were described as cough and expectoration. In a recent publication by Murray and Petty, asthmatic bronchitis is described as a condition including productive cough, exertional dyspnea, and airflow obstruction of a significantly reversible nature.[11] In both peripheral airway disease and asthmatic bronchitis, early detection may allow timely alteration in the patient's personal environment and therefore halt or even reverse the progression of these states and prevent the development of COPD.[10]

Controversy over definitions and terminology abound when describing this combination of pulmonary disorders. Even the acronym is in question. Chronic obstructive airways disease (COAD), chronic obstructive lung disease (COLD), chronic airflow or airways obstruction (CAO), and chronic airflow limitation (CAL) all refer to the same combination of pulmonary disorders.[12]

Etiology

COPD is the most commonly encountered chronic pulmonary disorder, and its prevalence is increasing. It has been estimated that between 14 and 16 million Americans have symptomatic COPD.[13,14] It is the fourth leading cause of death in the United States, and physical disability caused by COPD is second only to disability caused by heart disease.[14,15]

Although the primary cause of COPD is exposure to tobacco smoke, other environmental factors (air pollution and occupational exposures) and host factors (genetics, gender, and ethnicity) may also contribute to its development.[6,16–18]

Pathophysiology

The pathophysiology of COPD is a composite of individual components that contribute to the disease process. In the bronchi, there is enlargement of the mucous glands. Goblet cells proliferate, producing excessive secretions that obstruct the airway. The smooth muscle encircling the airway becomes hypertrophied, an increase in connective tissue can be observed, and the bronchioles show inflammation.[8] Airways that are less than 2 mm in diameter show inflammation, mucus plugging, and fibrosis. These obstructive changes lead to weakened bronchiolar walls, air trapping, and alveolar hyperinflation and destruction.[19] Airflow obstruction caused by the structural changes is irreversible. Bronchoconstriction from inflammation accounts for the limited amount of reversibility of airflow obstruction.[6]

Clinical Presentation of COPD

Patients with COPD present with a variety of symptoms. Chronic cough, expectoration, and exertional dyspnea may all be present in varying degrees. The symptoms are related to the unique combination of chronic bronchitis, emphysema, and peripheral airways disease. For example, if a patient has a large component of chronic bronchitis, the predominant presenting symptom may be chronic cough rather than shortness of breath. The intensity of symptoms relates to the severity of each component of COPD.

The hallmark of COPD is a significant and progressive decrease in expiratory flow rates as measured by pulmonary function tests, the most important of which is the forced expiratory volume in one second (FEV_1).[5] Pulmonary function studies also reveal that this airway obstruction does not show a major reversibility in response to pharmacologic agents.[6,14] Hyperinflation is demonstrated by an increase in total lung capacity (TLC), functional residual capacity (FRC), and residual volume (RV). Vital capacity may be decreased. The diffusing capacity of the lungs for carbon monoxide (DL_{CO}) is reduced proportionally to the severity of the disease.[20] (See Chapter 10 for more information relating to DL_{CO}.)

Arterial blood gas alterations occur in COPD. Ventilation and perfusion imbalances due to patchy areas of disease lead to hypoxemia. As the disease progresses and more areas of the lung become involved, hypoxemia worsens and hypercapnea develops. The chronicity of these changes in advanced disease allows the metabolic system to compensate for the developing respiratory acidosis by elevating the bicarbonate ion, which allows the arterial blood gas analysis to show a relatively normal pH.

Chest radiographs display regional hyperlucency and overinflation as measured by the anterioposterior diameter. Bullous lesions can be found on chest radiographs or high-resolution CT scans in some patients with COPD.[21]

Course and Prognosis

Most smokers have symptoms of chronic cough and expectoration for many years without developing any disability or complication. In some, but not all smokers, progression of the symptoms occurs and COPD is diagnosed.

The clinical course of COPD can run for 30 years or more,[12] and the progression of the disease can be monitored by pulmonary function studies.[22] The rate of decrease in FEV_1 for nonsmokers is approximately 25 to 30 milliliters per year. The rate of decline for smokers is approximately 54 milliliters per year.[23] Smoking cessation has been shown to delay this decline in function, and in one study, patients were able to regain some lung function.[24,25] In persons with an FEV_1 value less than 0.75 liters per second, the approximate mortality at the end of 1 year is 30 percent and at 5 years, 95 percent.[26] Chest radiograph do not usually depict the severity of the disease, nor do they indicate the prognosis of COPD.

The two components of COPD—chronic bronchitis and emphysema—are discussed individually in the following sections. Although separating COPD into its basic components allows a more organized discussion, it must be remembered that, in pulmonary rehabilitation programs, the components appear most often in combinations that are broadly referred to as COPD.

CHRONIC BRONCHITIS

Definition

Chronic bronchitis is defined by the American Thoracic Society in clinical terms as chronic cough and expectoration when other specific causes of cough can be excluded.[5] "Chronic" means that the cough and expectoration have persisted for at least 3 months and this pattern has been repeated for at least 2 consecutive years.[20]

Etiology

The incidence of chronic bronchitis in men is significantly different from that in women. Symptoms of chronic cough and expectoration are found in 25 to 35 percent of all men and 15 percent of all women.[13]

The most important etiologic factor in the development of chronic bronchitis is cigarette smoking. There is a direct relation between the amount and duration of cigarette smoking and the severity of the disease.[13] There is also significant individual variation in the susceptibility and effect of smoking on the lungs. The etiologic role of other factors, such as agents inhaled from occupational exposure without the effect of smoking, appears to be relatively insignificant.[13,15] Chronic bronchitis is rare in the nonsmoking population.

Pathophysiology

Pathophysiologic changes in chronic bronchitis are related to narrowing of the airways. Chronic exposure to irritants results in chronic inflammation of the bronchial mucosa, which is the major cause of airway narrowing. The airways are further narrowed by hyperplasia of the bronchial mucous glands, hypertrophy of the smooth muscle within the bronchial walls, and an increase in the number of goblet cells. These glands and cells produce an increased amount of mucus in response to chronic irritant exposure, leading to plugging of the smaller airways.[27] Decreases in ciliary function and an alteration in the physiochemical characteristics of bronchial secretions impair airway clearance and also affect the airway size.[15] Stagnant bronchial secretions predispose the patient to recurrent respiratory infections. Damaged and inflamed mucosa cause increased sensitivity of the irritant receptors within the bronchial walls, which in turn causes bronchial hyperreactivity.

During inhalation, airways are pulled open by the surrounding air sacs, which allows air to pass into the alveoli. Upon exhalation, the airways normally become narrowed. When incomplete obstruction caused by secretions occurs, exhalation becomes abnormal. Airways take longer to empty and often collapse before full exhalation has occurred. That type of incomplete obstruction acts like a ball valve. It lets air into the lungs, but does not let air out. The results of this pathology are a decreased expiratory flow rate, hyperinflation of the chest, and an altered ventilation-perfusion ratio, which cause abnormalities in the partial pressures of oxygen and carbon dioxide in arterial blood. In advanced stages of chronic bronchitis, destruction of the alveolar capillary membrane may also be present. Increased pulmonary vascular resistance caused by capillary destruction and reflex vasoconstriction in the presence of hypoxemia and hypercapnea results in right ventricular hypertrophy, or cor pulmonale. Polycythemia, an increase in the amount of circulating red blood cells, is another advanced complication of chronic bronchitis.[27]

Clinical Presentation

The major presenting symptoms in chronic bronchitis are cough and expectoration that appear slowly and insidiously. Dyspnea, another symptoms of chronic bronchitis, also begins slowly; it is first seen during exertion. Severely afflicted patients may appear dyspneic even at rest. Chronic bronchitis results in prolonged expiratory wheezing. Crackles may also be present and can be altered by coughing. Initially, chest radiographs may appear normal, but abnormalities of hyperinflation and increased lung markings may be found with disease progression.

Pulmonary function tests reveal a reduced FEV_1 that does not improve significantly following bronchodilator inhalation. Inspiratory flow rates are also reduced in chronic bronchitis. The narrowing of the airways causes air trapping. An increase in residual volume may be detectable, although the total lung capacity is usually normal or near normal. With advancing disease and increasing airway obstruction, ventilation-perfusion relations are altered and there are resulting changes in the arterial blood gas values of hypercapnea and hypoxemia. Because this is a chronic change, the metabolic system compensates for it by increasing the bicarbonate ion and thereby returning the arterial blood to a relatively normal pH value. The patient with advanced chronic bronchitis is in a chronic compensated respiratory acidosis.

Course and Prognosis

Patients have symptoms of chronic cough and expectoration for many years before developing signs or symptoms of airway obstruction. The progression of chronic bronchitis is evidenced by an increase in the severity of symptoms caused by increased airway obstruction, deterioration of pulmonary function, and more frequent respiratory tract infections.[28] Once patients show evidence of pulmonary function abnormalities, the prognosis becomes much less favorable, and they may advance to the point of severe respiratory insufficiency and failure. Pulmonary emphysema often develops; it complicates chronic bronchitis and adversely affects the prognosis. Proper medical management and patient compliance in smoking cessation can positively influence the prognosis of chronic bronchitis.[10,12]

EMPHYSEMA

Definition

Emphysema is defined in anatomic or pathologic terms as abnormal enlargement of the acinus, accompanied by destructive changes of the alveolar walls.[5] Overdistension of the air spaces without destruction of the alveolar walls, as normally seen in aging, is not included in the definition of emphysema.

Emphysema has been classified into three forms, according to the site of involvement in the distal respiratory unit or acinus: centriacinar, panacinar, and distal acinar.[6] Centriacinar emphysema often involves the upper lung fields and is almost always associated with chronic bronchitis. Panacinar emphysema is less common and affects the entire acinus. It is predominantly found in the lower and anterior aspects of the lungs and is more often associated with the alpha-1 antitrypsin deficiency form of emphysema. Finally, distal acinar emphysema affects the distal portion of the acinus, predominantly the alveolar ducts and alveolar sacs.

Etiology

The development of pulmonary emphysema has been linked to environmental pollutants. Because of a definite relation between cigarette smoking and chronic bronchitis and an association between chronic bronchitis and emphysema, it has been deduced that smoking is a major etiologic factor in the development of pulmonary emphysema. However, many patients with long-standing chronic bronchitis never develop emphysema. It is also true that emphysema occurs in individuals who have never smoked. Therefore, emphysema may not be caused by pollutants alone, and other as-yet unknown factors must be involved in the development of this disease.

A small number of patients with emphysema are known to have a genetically determined deficiency of alpha-1 antitrypsin. This serum enzyme normally inhibits the effects of trypsin, an enzyme that digests the proteins of the lung parenchyma, namely, elastin and collagen. Trypsin is present in the white blood cells and macrophages and may be released during an inflammatory process. Based on this theory, the alveolar destruction caused by emphysema is a result of the release of trypsin from the inflammatory cells, which remains unopposed by alpha-1 antitrypsin, its natural inhibitor.[15]

Not all individuals with a deficiency in alpha-1 antitrypsin enzyme develop emphysema in the same manner. Again, other factors must be present, factors that cause an inflammatory response and contribute to the development of emphysematous changes. The trypsin/antitrypsin imbalance may be exacerbated by the chronic inflammatory response to respiratory irritants, such as cigarette smoke, and infectious processes. Indeed, smoking appears to be implicated in the development of emphysema in patients with alpha-1 antitrypsin deficiency. In nonsmoking patients with alpha-1 antitrypsin deficiency, the mean age of onset of dyspnea has been reported to be 51. In smoking patients with alpha-1 antitrypsin deficiency, the mean age of onset of dyspnea has been found to be 32.[29] Pulmonary function abnormalities are also more pronounced in smokers than in nonsmokers who have the enzyme deficiency.[29,30]

Pathophysiology

Airflow obstruction in emphysema is caused by the destruction of pulmonary elastic tissues, which results in a loss of the normal elastic recoil properties of the lungs. During expiration, the airways collapse from a lack of support by the surrounding elastic parenchyma.[15] Premature airway collapse causes hyperinflation or air trapping and reduced expiratory flow rates. Inspiratory flow rates are normal except when associated obstructive bronchitis is present.[15]

Gas exchange is impaired as a result of the destruction of the alveolar-capillary membrane and ventilation-perfusion mismatches. A reduction in the diffusing capacity of carbon monoxide also occurs in emphysema (see Chapter 10).

In advanced stages of emphysema, destruction of the alveolar-capillary membrane is present. Increased pulmonary vascular resistance caused by capillary destruction and reflex vasoconstriction in the presence of hypoxemia and hypercapnea results in right ventricular hypertrophy, or cor pulmonale. Polycythemia, an increase in the amount of circulating red blood cells, is another advanced complication of emphysema.

Clinical Presentation

The major clinical symptom of emphysema is dyspnea. The onset of dyspnea is noted initially during physical exertion, but it can gradually progress so that it is present even when the patient is at rest. In patients who do not also have chronic bronchitis, the symptoms of cough and expectoration are absent.

On physical examination, the thorax appears enlarged because of the loss of lung elastic recoil. The anteroposterior diameter of the chest increases, a dorsal kyphosis is noted, the ribs are elevated, and there is flaring of costal margin and a widening of the costochondral angle.[15] Collectively, these anatomic changes give the patient a "barrel-chest" appearance. Consistent with hyperinflation of the lungs, breath sounds are usually distant and somewhat difficult to hear. Expiratory wheezing can sometimes be heard, and heart sounds may appear distant. Use of accessory muscles of ventilation, hypertrophy of the accessory muscles, pursed-lip breathing, cyanosis, and digital clubbing may be present in the advanced stages of emphysema.

Several radiographic changes occur with emphysema. They include depressed and flattened hemidiaphragms, alteration in pulmonary vascular markings, hyperinflation of the thorax evidenced by an increased anteroposterior diameter of the chest, and an increased retrosternal air space, hyperlucency, elongation of the heart, and right ventricular hypertrophy. Appearance of bullous lesions on x-ray is an unequivocal sign of emphysema.[31]

Pulmonary function tests show an irreversible decrease in FEV and in forced expiratory flow, midexpiratory phase (FEF_{25-75}). There is also an increase in residual volume, which may be several times the normal value.[20] As a result, functional residual capacity is also increased. Despite the reduction in vital capacity caused by emphysema, total lung capacity is generally increased.[20]

Reduction of diffusing capacity in emphysema usually differentiates the disease from chronic bronchitis and peripheral airways disease.[15] Arterial blood gas analyses may show a reduced arterial Pao_2, and arterial $Paco_2$ may be chronically elevated.

Course and Prognosis

Periods of increased symptoms, usually related to recurrent infections, frequently exacerbate pulmonary emphysema. Expiratory flow rates measured during stable periods are good indicators of the progression of emphysema. There is also a good correlation between the severity of airway obstruction, as judged by FEV_1, and mortality from emphysema. With an FEV_1 below 750 mL, few patients survive 5 years.[15]

Arterial blood gas changes are related to the severity of the disease, but the severity of dyspnea is not always correlated with the degree or pathologic and physiologic abnormalities caused by emphysema. Radiographic evidence appears later in the disease and does not relate well with the severity. It is therefore not useful as a prognostic indicator.[31]

ASTHMA

Definition

Asthma is a clinical syndrome characterized by an increase in the reactivity of the tracheobronchial tree to various stimuli. The most remarkable feature of asthma is the episodic attacks of wheezing and dyspnea that improve either spontaneously or with medical therapy and are interspersed with symptom-free intervals. Although asthma is considered an obstructive disease and is chronic in nature, it is not part of the definition of COPD.

Etiology

Asthma is a common respiratory disease of uncertain etiology. Depending on race, age, gender, and geographic differences, the prevalence of asthma has been reported to be from 1.1 to 26.9 percent.[32,33] During the last decade, the incidence of asthma has increased significantly in children, but not in adults.[34] Although the exact mechanism of airway hyperreactivity is unknown, genetic predisposition,[35-37] environmental contributions,[38] diet,[39] respiratory-tract infections, autonomic nervous system imbalance, and mucosal epithelial damage[15] have been implicated in the development of asthma.

The airways of people with asthma are hypersensitive to a variety of factors including allergens, respiratory irritants, cold air, exercise, emotional stresses, and chemical substances.[33,38,39] Any or all of these may precipitate or aggravate all forms of asthma.

Allergen exposure is the most important etiologic or precipitating factor in asthma, especially in children.[34,40] When there is clear association with allergy, asthma is referred to as extrinsic or allergic. Intrinsic or idiopathic asthma, usually found in older patients, seems to have no relation to allergens.

Common respiratory irritants in the atmosphere include sulfur dioxide, ozone, dust, pollen, and even perfume.[13] Primary and ambient tobacco smoke is a respiratory irritant that may cause asthma attacks in smokers and also in nonsmokers.[13,41]

Exercise and cold air are also known to provoke bronchospasm.[42,43] In fact, exercise-induced bronchospasm (EIB) may be the first manifestation of asthma. The conditions required to induce EIB are as follows:

1. Exercise has to be vigorous, and the intensity must be approximately 90 percent of the predicted maximum heart rate.
2. Exercise should last at least 8 minutes.
3. The exercise should be performed in a cold, dry environment.
4. Running is the mode of exercise most often associated with exercise-induced bronchospasm. Shortly after that type of activity, bronchospasm develops in susceptible persons. Pulmonary function tests show that the most impairment occurs 8 to 15 minutes after exercise.[44]

Although this description of EIB is "classic," bronchospasm that occurs any time during the exercise session and/or at any time following the exercise session should be considered exercise-induced.[45] As minute ventilation increases during exercise, the humidification and warming mechanisms of the nose may become inadequate and colder air is delivered to the tracheobronchial tree. The cooling of the airways appears to be the basic mechanism that causes bronchospasm during exercise.[44-48] To prevent bronchospasm, the inspired air should be 37°C in temperature and saturated with water vapor before reaching the alveoli.

Chemical substances such as histamine and methacholine are known to produce bronchospasm in persons with asthma. For diagnostic purposes, a solution containing methacholine can be nebulized and inhaled. A reduction of 20 percent in FEV_1 following the methacholine challenge is a positive diagnostic sign for asthma.[7]

Other chemical substances, such as those found in the workplace, are associated with occupational asthma and lung hypersensitivity. Among the chemical agents are cotton dust, toluene diisocyanate, aspergillus, and moldy hay.[15,49] Occupational asthma and hypersensitivity are characterized by respiratory symptoms of cough, chest tightness, and wheezing that are cyclical in occurrence and coincide with the work schedule. Symptoms may become chronic and somewhat continuous after many years of exposure.[49] In many patients, different etiologic agents in various combinations are responsible for asthma attacks.

Pathophysiology

The major physiologic manifestation of asthma is widespread narrowing of the airways. This is usually caused by a combination of bronchospasm, inflammation of the mucosa, and increased secretions. Inflammation of the airways is found even during periods of remission.[50] The narrowed airways increase the resistance to airflow and decrease forced expiratory flow rates, thereby causing hyperinflation. These narrowed airways provide an abnormal distribution of ventilation to the alveoli.

Clinical Presentation

The major clinical symptom of asthma is bronchoconstriction with varying degrees of dyspnea and wheezing. During an acute exacerbation, the chest is usually held in an expanded position, which indicates that hyperinflation of the lungs has occurred. Accessory muscles of ventilation are used for breathing, and expiratory wheezes can be heard over the entire chest. Sometimes crackles can be heard as well. With severe airway obstruction, breath sounds may become markedly diminished because of poor air movement. Wheezing may occur on inspiration as well as expiration and intercostal, supraclavicular, and substernal retractions may be present on inspiration.[15]

Chest radiographs taken during an exacerbation of asthma usually indicate hyperinflation, evidenced by an increase in the anteroposterior diameter of the chest with hyperlucency of the lung fields. Less commonly, chest x-rays may reveal areas of atelactasis or infiltrates from the bronchial obstruction. Normal chest x-rays can be seen between exacerbations.

The most consistent changes during episodes of bronchospasm are decreased expiratory flow rates that increase airway resistance. Residual volume and functional residual capacity are increased because of air trapping at the expense of vital capacity and inspiratory reserve volume, which are reduced. During an acute exacerbation, the results of pulmonary function studies appear somewhat similar to the results found in pulmonary emphysema. However, the reversibility of the abnormalities is distinctive of asthma. During remission, the patient with asthma may have normal or near normal FEV_1 values.

During an exacerbation of asthma, the most common arterial blood gas finding is mild to moderate hypoxemia. Usually some degree of hypocapnea is present because of hyperventilation, which causes an acute respiratory alkalosis. In severe attacks, hypoxemia may be more pronounced. With further clinical deterioration, arterial $Paco_2$ rises, indicating that the patient is exhausted and respiratory failure is imminent.[15,49,51] Even in severe exacerbations, diffusing capacity usually remains normal.[49]

Clinical Course and Prognosis

When asthma begins in childhood, 33 percent of those asthmatics are symptom-free by the time adulthood is reached.[15] When the onset of symptoms begins later in life, the clinical course is usually more progressive. Pulmonary function tests during periods of remission become less normal; yet asthma with no concomitant complicating disease has a relatively low mortality.[38]

BRONCHIECTASIS

Definition

Bronchiectasis is an anatomic abnormality characterized by abnormal, irreversible dilatation of the bronchial tree.[52] Associated inflammation and destruction of the bronchial walls are also present. There are three major morphologic types of dilatation of the airway: cylindrical, fusiform, and saccular. Again, although bronchiectasis is considered an obstructive disease and is chronic in nature, it is not part of the definition of COPD.

Etiology

Although the exact cause of the condition is not known, a number of mechanisms have been proposed to explain the dilatation of the bronchi.[53] Chronic inflammation and the eventual progression to destruction of the bronchial wall are the most likely causes. Bacterial infections have been implicated in the development of altered cilia.[52,54] With impaired ciliary function, infected secretions stagnate within the bronchi, causing further inflammation and eventually destroying the bronchial wall. Certainly, not all bacterial pulmonary infections result in bronchiectasis. With improved treatment of pulmonary infections, most newly diagnosed cases of bronchiectasis are the result of concomitant disease, cystic fibrosis, dyskinetic cilia syndrome, and immuno-deficiency states.[52,55] Tuberculosis, aspiration of a foreign body, and allergic bronchopulmonary aspergillosis have also been associated with the development of bronchiectasis.[15]

Pathophysiology

Bronchiectasis causes atrophy of the mucosa and loss of ciliated epithelium in the bronchi. Infiltration of inflammatory cells and squamous-cell metaplasia also are present. The dilated bronchial lumina are often filled with purulent material that causes ulcerations and abscess formation on the bronchial walls.[13,15] With progression of the disease, fibrosis occurs, with marked enlargement of the bronchial circulation and an increase in the systemic pulmonary anastomoses in the affected area of the lung.[56] There is also some evidence that bronchiectasis also presents with signs of chronic systemic inflammation.[57]

Clinical Presentation

The classic sign of bronchiectasis is cough with expectoration. Patients may have relatively small amounts of secretions ("dry bronchiectasis"), but more commonly the patient produces an extraordinary amount of mucopurulent sputum. Hemoptysis commonly occurs, although the amount and frequency of bleeding are variable and unpredictable. Dyspnea may be present in varying degrees.

Signs of bronchiectasis include diminished breath sounds, crackles that can be heard over the affected areas of the lung, cyanosis, and digital clubbing. These signs vary in intensity and are dependent on the amount of lung involvement.

Chest radiographs may show patchy infiltrates, increased lung markings caused by peribronchial thickening, segmental atelectasis, and occasional cystic changes with air-fluid levels. These changes occur more frequently in the lower lung fields. High-resolution computerized tomography (HRCT) scans are the diagnostic modality of choice for the identification and extent of the disease.

Bronchography is helpful in quantifying the extent of the disease in a patient pending surgical management. With the advent of HRCT, however, bronchography is no longer a frequently used diagnostic tool.[53]

Pulmonary function tests reveal no abnormality in mild and moderate cases of bronchiectasis. Patients with advanced disease may show both obstructive and restrictive changes. Expiratory flow rates such as FEV_1 are decreased and residual volume is increased. There is usually no alteration in diffusing capacity, but in severe cases the ventilatory impairment may cause hypoxemia.

Course and Prognosis

Variations in the severity, extent, and medical management of the disease affect the prognosis of bronchiectasis. In patients with minimal involvement, effects are minimal. Some patients in the second and third decades of life show spontaneous improvement.[53] However, the course of the disease is usually characterized by exacerbations. Chronic infections are common and pneumonia tends to recur at the same location. There is a slow decline in pulmonary function. Within several years, severely affected patients usually succumb to respiratory and/or infectious complications.

CYSTIC FIBROSIS

Definition

Cystic fibrosis (CF), or mucoviscidosis, is the most common lethal genetically inherited disease among white children.[58] The disease is characterized by an exocrine gland dysfunction that results in abnormally viscid secretions. Although any organ system can be involved, the most common presentation of the disease is involvement of the pulmonary and pancreatic systems.

Etiology

CF is a hereditary disease transmitted as an autosomal-recessive (Mendelian) trait. The pattern of inheritance results in a one-in-four chance of two carriers producing a child with the disease (homozygous), a two-in-four chance of producing a child who is a carrier of the disease (heterozygous), and a one-in-four chance of producing a child who is completely free of the trait. The incidence in white children is approximately 1 in 2500 live births.[59] Although the incidence is less common in the black population, 2.25 percent of all patients with CF identified by the Cystic Fibrosis Foundation in 1979 were black.[60] This disease is rare in the Asian population.[60]

Pathophysiology

The chronic pulmonary involvement seen in CF results from an abnormally viscous mucus secreted by the tracheobronchial tree and hyperplasia of the mucus-secreting glands. The function of the mucociliary transport is impaired by the altered secretions and the impairment results in airway obstruction, recurrent infection, bronchiectasis, and hyperinflation. Fibrotic changes are also found in the lung parenchyma.

Incomplete obstruction of the airways reduces ventilation to the alveolar units. A low ventilation-perfusion ratio is present with diffusion abnormalities in both oxygen and carbon dioxide. A "ball valve" situation, caused by incomplete obstruction of an airway, accounts for the hyperinflation seen in these patients. (Refer to the discussion of hyperinflation in the section on chronic bronchitis.) Complete obstruction of the airways results in absorption atelectasis.

Clinical Presentation

CF may be suspected in patients who present with a positive family history of the disease, with pneumonia or recurrent respiratory infections caused by *Staphylococcus aureus* or *Pseudomonas aeruginosa,* or with a diagnosis of malnutrition and/or failure to thrive.

The "sweat" test is diagnostic for CF. The sweat and saliva of patients with cystic fibrosis are not particularly viscid, but they do contain abnormally high amounts of sodium chloride. A sodium chloride concentration of greater than 60 mEq per liter in the perspiration of a patient is positive for the diagnosis of CF.

Acute pulmonary infections may be the first radiographic sign of the disease. Diffuse hyperinflation, increased lung marking, and atelectasis are common in advanced disease.

Pulmonary function studies show obstructive impairments, decreased FEV_1, a decreased forced vital capacity (FVC), and an increased residual volume and functional residual capacity (FRC).

Arterial blood gas values also show alterations caused by the abnormal ventilation-perfusion relation within the lungs. Hypoxemia and hypercapnea with a chronically compensated respiratory acidosis are present.

As the disease progresses, destruction of the alveolar capillary network, hypoxemia, and hypercapnea cause pulmonary hypertension and cor pulmonale.

Nonpulmonary manifestations of CF include pancreatic insufficiency, leading to possible diabetes mellitus; gastrointestinal dysfunction, leading to meconium ileus at birth; and gastroesophageal reflux, hepatobiliary disease, and malabsorption, leading to poor weight gain and failure to thrive. Reproductive problems are also reported. Obstructive azoospermia is present in 98 to 99 percent of male patients with CF.[59]

Course and Prognosis

The life expectancy of patients with CF has continued to increase because of advances in diagnosis and treatment. Although some patients still die in infancy and early childhood, most survive into adulthood.[61] In 1993, the mean survival rate was 29.6 years for men and 27.3 years for women.[62]

Gastrointestinal dysfunctions resulting from CF can be improved by proper diet, vitamin supplements, and replacement of pancreatic enzymes. Treatment of the pulmonary dysfunction centers around the removal of the abnormal pulmonary secretions and prompt treatment of pulmonary infections. In 95 percent of cases, pulmonary involvement is the primary cause of death.[59]

RESTRICTIVE LUNG DISEASE

Definition

Restrictive lung disease is actually a group of diseases with differing etiologies. The common link among these disorders is a difficulty in expanding the lungs and a reduction in lung volume. The restrictions can come from changes in the chest wall such as thoracic burns and scoliosis, or in the neuromuscular apparatus, such as Guillain-Barré syndrome or muscular dystrophy.[63] For the purpose of this text, the diseases most likely to be encountered in a pulmonary rehabilitation setting are presented, that is, restrictive diseases of the lung parenchyma and/or the pleura. Diseases of the chest wall and neuromuscular diseases are not discussed.

Etiology

Interstitial lung disease has over 200 causes.[64] Bacterial, viral, fungal, or parasitic infections; radiation therapy; inorganic dust; inhalation of noxious gases; oxygen toxicity; asbestos exposure; and beryllium can damage the pulmonary parenchyma and pleura. Petty[65] categorizes the etiology of pulmonary parenchymal restriction in four ways:

1. The pneumoconioses (the dust diseases leading to pulmonary fibrosis)
2. The immunologically mediated cryptogenic fibrosing alveolitis

3. The collagen diseases
4. Pulmonary fibrosis of unknown etiology

Pleural thickening and fibrosis can restrict the movement between the lung and the thoracic wall and thereby cause another type of restrictive disease. Radiation therapy and asbestos exposure are two of the most common causes of pleural thickening.

Pathophysiology

The particular changes occurring within the lungs depend on the etiologic factors of restrictive disease. Parenchymal changes result in fibrosis of the alveoli, small airways, and pulmonary vasculature, whereas pleural disease causes pleural thickening and fibrosis.

Parenchymal changes often begin with chronic inflammation and a thickening of the alveoli and interstitium. As the disease progresses, distal air spaces are destroyed and replaced by fibrotic tissue, resulting in an increase in the elastic recoil property of the lungs. Consequently, lung volumes are reduced. A reduced pulmonary vascular bed eventually leads to hypoxemia and cor pulmonale.

In pleural diseases, thickened plaques of collagen fibers cause fibrosis that may be found in various locations. In asbestos exposure, for example, the plaques are found on the parietal pleura. The mechanism responsible for plaque development is not completely clear. There may also be parenchymal alterations that accompany pleural diseases. These changes may be the result of injury or inflammatory reactions that lead to fibrosis.

Clinical Presentation

Dyspnea is the classic symptom of restrictive lung diseases, beginning with dyspnea on exertion and progressing to shortness of breath at rest.[64] A nonproductive cough is often encountered, and weakness and easy fatigue are common.

Signs of restrictive lung disease include rapid, shallow breathing, limited chest expansion, fine-end expiratory crackles (especially over the lower lung fields), digital clubbing, and cyanosis.

In the early stages of parenchymal restrictive disease, chest x-ray changes may be the first abnormal objective finding.[64] Conventional chest radiographs reveal fine interstitial markings that look like ground glass. Long-standing fibrosis has radiographic evidence of diffuse infiltrates and has been likened to a honeycomb. Reduction in lung volumes can be seen serially on the chest x-ray. Radiographic evidence of pleural thickening can also be seen, especially on oblique films. HRCT is helpful in differentiating between reversible and irreversible changes in the lung parenchyma and the extent of the disease.[66]

Pulmonary function tests reveal a reduction in vital capacity, functional residual capacity, and total lung capacity. Residual volume may be normal or near normal, and expiratory flow rates remain normal in pulmonary fibrosis. Lung compliance is significantly reduced, and diffusing capacity is diminished. Arterial blood studies show varying degrees of hypoxemia and hypocapnia. Hypoxemia is usually exacerbated by exercise. Exercise may significantly lower Pa_{O_2}, even in patients with normal resting Pa_{O_2}. Hyperventilation, which results in a lower-than-normal Pa_{CO_2}, often occurs.

Course and Prognosis

Some restrictive pulmonary diseases may have self-limiting courses, but most are progressive and fatal in nature. Survival depends on the type of restrictive disease, the etiologic factor, and the treatment.

A reliable prognostic test for idiopathic pulmonary fibrosis is histology study from an open lung biopsy.[67] HRCT is also a good predictor of the extent of the disease.[66] Finally, survival rates have been linked to the FEV_1/FVC ratio.[68] The most important prognostic information remains an evaluation of simple tests over time: serial pulmonary function tests of volumes and flow rates, serial arterial blood gas samples, and serial chest x-rays.[68] Arterial blood gas values showing hypercapnea are, however, an ominous sign of the terminal stage of pulmonary fibrosis.[65]

SUMMARY

The etiology, pathophysiology, clinical presentation, and prognosis for several diseases of the lungs were presented in this chapter.

All types of obstructive lung diseases are associated with hyperinflation of the chest caused by air trapping, increases in pulmonary volumes and capacities, abnormal ventilation-perfusion ratios, abnormal radiographs, and abnormal arterial blood gas values. These diseases include COPD, asthma, cystic fibrosis, and bronchiectasis.

Restrictive pulmonary disease results in reduced lung volumes and capacities from a variety of causes: parenchymal disease, pleural disease, and chest wall deformities. Changes can be seen in the pulmonary volumes and capacities, radiograph, and arterial blood gas values.

An understanding of the underlying lung disease and its severity allows development of realistic patient goals and appropriate treatment programs.

REFERENCES

1. Foster, S and Thomas, H: Pulmonary rehabilitation in lung disease other than chronic obstructive pulmonary disease. American Review of Respiratory Diseases 141:601–604, 1990.
2. American Thoracic Society: Definitions and classification of chronic bronchitis, asthma, and pulmonary emphysema. American Review of Respiratory Diseases 85:762–768, 1962.
3. Petty, T (ed): Management of Chronic Obstructive Lung Diseases. Conclusion of the Eighth Aspen Emphysema Conference. US Public Health Service Publication No 1457, May 1966.
4. National Heart, Lung and Blood Institute, Division of Lung Diseases Workshop Report: The definition of emphysema. American Review of Respiratory Diseases 132:182–185, 1985.
5. American Thoracic Society: Standards for the diagnosis and care of patients with chronic obstructive pulmonary disease (COPD) and asthma, 1987. American Review of Respiratory Diseases 136:225–244, 1987.
6. ATS Statement: Standards for the diagnosis and care of patients with chronic obstructive pulmonary disease. Am J Respir Crit Care Med 152:S78–S121, 1995.
7. Thurlbeck, ZW: Chronic airflow obstruction in lung disease. In Major Problems in Pathology, Vol V. Saunders, Philadelphia 1978.
8. Niewoehner, D, Kleinerman, J, and Rice, D: Pathologic changes in the peripheral airways of young cigarette smokers. N Engl J Med 291:755–758, 1974.
9. Wright, J, et al: The detection of small airways disease. American Review of Respiratory Diseases 129:989–994, 1984.
10. Cosio, M, et al: The relationship between structural changes in small airways and pulmonary function tests. N Engl J Med 298:1277–1281, 1977.
11. Petty, T: Pulmonary Rehabilitation: A personal historical perspective. In Casaburi, R and Petty, T (eds): Principles and Practice of Pulmonary Rehabilitation. Saunders, Philadelphia, 1993.

12. Hodgkin, J and Petty, T: Chronic Obstructive Pulmonary Disease. Current Concepts. Saunders, Philadelphia, 1987.
13. Sharma, O and Balchum, O: Key Facts in Pulmonary Disease. Churchill Livingstone, New York, 1983.
14. Petty, T: The worldwide epidemiology of chronic obstructive pulmonary disease. Current Opinion in Pulmonary Medicine 2:84–89, 1996.
15. Farzan, S: A Concise Handbook of Respiratory Diseases, ed 2. Reston Publishing, Reston, Va, 1985.
16. Prince, S and Wilson, L: Pathophysiology: Clinical Concepts of Disease Processes, ed 3. McGraw-Hill, New York, 1986.
17. Buist, A, et al: Effects of cigarette smoking on lung function in four population samples in the People's Republic of China: The PRC-US cardiovascular and cardiopulmonary epidemiology research group. Am J Respir Crit Care Med 151:1393–1400, 1995.
18. Chen Y, Horne S, and Dosman J: Increased susceptibility to lung dysfunction in female smokers. American Review of Respiratory Diseases 143:1224–1230, 1991.
19. Chronic Obstructive Pulmonary Disease: A Manual for Physicians, ed 3. National Tuberculosis and Respiratory Disease Association, 1972.
20. Morris, J (chairman): Chronic Obstructive Pulmonary Disease. American Lung Association Publication, 1981.
21. Teramoto, S and Fukuchi, Y: Bullous emphysema. Current Opinion in Pulmonary Medicine 2:90–96, 1996.
22. Burrows, B: Prognostic factors in chronic obstructive pulmonary disease. Practical Cardiology 6:61–69, 1980.
23. Travers, G, Cline, M, and Burrows, B: Predictors of mortality in chronic obstructive pulmonary disease. American Review of Respiratory Diseases 119:895–902, 1979.
24. Nemeny, B, et al: Changes in lung function after smoking cessation: An assessment from a cross-sectional survey. American Review of Respiratory Diseases 125:122–124, 1982.
25. Anthonisen, N, et al: Effects of smoking intervention and the use of an inhaled anticholinergic bronchodilator on the rate of decline of FEV_1: The lung health study. JAMA 272:1497–1505, 1994.
26. Hodgkin, J: Prognosis in chronic obstructive pulmonary disease. Clin Chest Med 11:555–569, 1990.
27. Sheldon, J: Boyd's Introduction to the Study of Disease, ed 10. Lea & Febiger, Philadelphia, 1988.
28. The fate of the chronic bronchitic: A report of the 10-year follow-up in the Canadian Department of Veterans' Affairs coordinated study of chronic bronchitis. American Review of Respiratory Diseases 108:1043–1065, 1973.
29. Hutchinson, D, et al: Longitudinal studies in alpha-1 antitrypsin deficiency: A survey by the British Thoracic Society. In Taylor, J and Mittman, C: Pulmonary Emphysema and Proteolysis: 1986. Academic Press, London, 1987.
30. Janis, E, Phillips, N, and Cartell, R: Smoking alpha-1 antitrypsin deficiency and emphysema. In Taylor, J and Mittman, C: Pulmonary Emphysema and Proteolysis: 1986. Academic Press, London, 1987.
31. Pugatch, R: The radiology of emphysema. Clin Chest Med 3:433–442, 1983.
32. Robertson, C, et al: International comparison of asthma prevalence in children: Australia, Switzerland, Chile. Pediatr Pulmonol 16:219–226, 1993.
33. Leung, R and Jenkins, M: Asthma, allergy and atopy in southern Chinese school students. Clin Exp Allergy 24:353–358, 1994.
34. Peat, J: The epidemiology of asthma. Current Opinion in Pulmonary Medicine 2:7–15, 1996.
35. Sibbald, B, et al: Genetic factors in childhood asthma. Thorax 35:671–674, 1980.
36. Donohue, J: Asthma, editorial overview. Current Opinion in Pulmonary Medicine 1:3–8, 1995.
37. Sanford, A, Weir, T, and Pare, P: The genetics of asthma. Am J Respir Crit Care Med 153:1749–1765, 1996.
38. Burney, P: Prevalence and mortality from asthma. In P Vermeeire, M Demedts, and J Vernault (eds): Progress in Asthma and COPD. Elsevier, Amsterdam, 1989.
39. Peat, J: The rising trend in allergic illness: Which environmental factors are important? Clin Exp Allergy 24:797–800, 1994.
40. Stevensen, D, et al: Provoking factors in bronchial asthma. Arch Intern Med 135:777–783, 1975.
41. Fielding, J: Smoking: Health effects and control, Part I. N Engl J Med 313(8), 491–498, 1985.
42. Anderson, S, et al: Exercise-induced asthma: A review. British Journal of Diseases of the Chest 69:1–39, 1975.
43. Tat, A, et al: Response to cold air hyperventilation in normal and asthmatic children. J Pediatr 104:516–521, 1984.
44. Gilbert, I, Fouke, J, and McFadden, E: Heat and water flux in the intrathoracic airways and exercise-induced asthma. J Appl Physiol 63:1681–1691, 1987.
45. Berman, B and Ross, R: Exercise induced bronchospasm: Is it a unique clinical entity? Ann Allerg 65(2):81–83, 1990.
46. Anderson, S: Current concepts of exercise induced asthma. Allergy 38:289–302, 1983.
47. Strauss, R, et al: Influence of heat and humidity on the airway obstruction induced by exercise in asthma. J Clin Invest 61:433–440, 1978.
48. Noviski, N, et al: Exercise intensity determines and climatic conditions modify the severity of exercise-induced asthma. American Review of Respiratory Diseases 136:592–594, 1987.
49. Burki, N: Pulmonary Diseases. Medical Examination Publishing, Garden City, NY, 1982.

50. Foresi A, Bertorelli G, Pesci A, et al: Inflammatory markers in bronchioalveolar lavage and in bronchial biopsy in asthma during remission. Chest 98:528–535, 1990.
51. Berte, J: Critical Care: The Lungs, ed 2. Appleton-Century Crofts, Norwalk, Conn, 1986.
52. Moreschi, M and Fiel S: An update on bronchiectasis. Current Opinion in Pulmonary Medicine 1:119–124, 1995.
53. Daves, P, et al: Familial bronchiectasis. J Pediatr 102:177–185, 1983.
54. Corbeel, L, et al: Ultrastructural abnormalities of bronchial cilia in children with recurrent airway infections and bronchiectasis. Arch Dis Child 56:929–933, 1981.
55. Barker, AF and Bardana, EJ: Bronchiectasis, an update of an orphan disease. Am Rev Respir Dis 127:969–978, 1988.
56. Williams, M: Essentials of Pulmonary Medicine. Saunders, Philadelphia, 1982.
57. Ip, M, et al: Systemic effects of inflammation in bronchiectasis. Respir Med 85:521–525, 1991.
58. Wood, R, Boat, T, and Doershuk, C: State of the art: Cystic fibrosis. American Review of Respiratory Diseases 113:833, 1976.
59. Aitken, Moira: Cystic fibrosis, editorial view. Current Opinion in Pulmonary Medicine 1:425–434, 1995.
60. Tecklin, J: Pediatric Physical Therapy. Lippincott, Philadelphia, 1989.
61. Murphy, S: Cystic fibrosis in adults: Diagnosis and management. Clin Chest Med 8:695, 1987.
62. Cystic Fibrosis Foundation: Patient registry 1993 annual data report, Bethesda, Md, 1994.
63. West, J: Pulmonary Pathophysiology: The Essentials. Williams & Wilkins, Baltimore, 1977.
64. Sharma, O: Interstitial lung disease: Commentary. Current Opinion in Pulmonary Medicine 1:345–350, 1995.
65. Petty, T: Chronic Lung Disease: A Practical Office Approach to Early Diagnosis and Management. Breon Laboratories, New York, 1975.
66. Greaves, S and Batra, P: High-resolution computed tomography, magnetic resonance imaging and positron emission tomography in interstitial lung disease. Current Opinion in Pulmonary Medicine 1:351–357, 1995.
67. Winterbauer, R: Current concepts in and modes for measurement of activity in interstitial lung disease. Current Opinion in Pulmonary Medicine 1:358–362, 1995.
68. Schwartz, D, et al: Determinants of survival in ideopathic pulmonary fibrosis. Am J Respir Crit Care Med 149:450–454, 1994.

CHAPTER 7

The Medical and Surgical Management of Cardiopulmonary Disease

In this chapter, the pharmacologic agents commonly used in the medical management of acute and chronic coronary artery disease (CAD) are reviewed. Interventional cardiologic procedures are also discussed, including percutaneous transluminal coronary angioplasty (PTCA), directional coronary atherectomy, laser angioplasty, coronary stents, and coronary artery bypass graft surgery. Surgical interventions such as myocardial revascularization, heart and heart-lung transplantation, and cardiac myoplasty are included and the importance of cardiac rehabilitation as an adjunct to therapy is addressed. Finally, pharmacologic management of pulmonary disease and surgical intervention for the patient with pulmonary disease, including tumor resection, bullae resection, pneumonectomy, and lung transplantation are presented.

CORONARY ARTERY DISEASE

The medical and surgical management of CAD offers individuals a choice of various treatment options appropriate for their disease processes. In all cases, treatment is aimed at relieving symptoms and slowing the progression of the disease. With the combination of any of these interventions and risk factor modification, individuals with CAD can continue to live active and healthy lives.

Pharmacologic Management

The mainstay of the medical management of CAD relies on the various pharmacologic agents specifically used in the acute and long-term treatment of CAD and its symptoms: nitrates, beta-blocking agents, antiarrhythmics, cardiac glycosides, calcium channel blockers, angiotensin-converting enzyme (ACE) inhibitors, thrombolytics, and antithrombic agents. Treatment is directed toward preventing myocardial ischemia and infarction while maximizing and improving existing cardiac function.

NITRATES

Actions and Uses

Nitrates are most commonly used to treat angina caused by myocardial ischemia (Table 7–1). In addition, nitrates are prescribed for individuals with heart failure, acute myocardial infarction (AMI), and hypertension.[1] Nitrates belong to a class of drugs that vasodilate by relaxing smooth muscles in coronary and peripheral arteries, veins, bronchioles, the biliary system, the gastrointestinal (GI) tract, and the uterus. These agents can be administered orally, sublingually, intravenously, and topically. Thus peripheral vasodilation results in venous pooling, causing a decreased venous return to the heart (decreased preload). This decreased preload reduces ventricular dimensions and diastolic filling pressures. The vasodilating effects of nitrates on the arteries decrease peripheral vascular resistance (decreased afterload), which significantly reduced myocardial oxygen demand. This combined reduction in preload and afterload results in decreased myocardial oxygen demand, thereby relieving angina or delaying its onset.[2] Nitrates may cause redistribution of blood flow to subendocardial areas by vasodilation of the epicardial coronary arteries.[3]

Contraindications and Side Effects

The side effects of nitrates include reflex tachycardia, orthostatic hypotension, flushing, and headache, all related to generalized vasodilation. Topical preparations may cause dermatitis.[1]

Effects on Exercise in Individuals with Coronary Artery Disease

Anginal pain, often experienced at low levels of exercise by individuals with CAD, results from inadequate cardiac reserve. The heart cannot meet the increased oxygen demand of exercise. Nitrates, given before exercise or administered chronically, reduce cardiac workload and improve exercise performance. This is evidenced by an increased tolerance for activity before the onset of anginal pain and/or ischemic electrocardiographic changes. Probable explanations for these effects are a decrease in myocardial oxygen consumption and an increase in coronary artery perfusion to ischemic areas.[3]

Nitrate Therapy Management

Careful consideration should be given to the following:

1. Administer sublingual nitrate at the onset of chest pain. Obtain a blood pressure (BP) reading before administration.

TABLE 7–1 Nitrates: Acute and Chronic Management[1,4,18]

Generic Name (Trade Name)	Mode of Administration and Dosage	a. Onset b. Peak Action	Duration of Action	Implications for Individual with CAD
Acute Management				
Nitroglycerin (Nitrostat)	Sublingual: 1/100–1/400 g prn (for acute anginal pain)	a. 1–3 min b. 3–5 min	30–60 min	Should be taken with onset of pain; may repeat every 5 min × 3 doses. Additional medical attention should be obtained if pain is not relieved after 15 min.
	IV dosage: Titrated to relieve pain	a. Immediate	3–5 min	
Isosorbide dinitrate (Isordil)	Sublingual: 2.5–10 mg Chewable: 5.0–10 mg	a. 3–5 min b. 15–30 min	1–2 hr	Individual should be seated to prevent light-headedness. Keep nitroglycerin in dark-glass bottle.
Chronic Management				
Isosorbide dinitrate (Isordil, Sorbitrate)	(Extended release) 20–40 mg PO q 8 to 12 hr	a. 4 hr b. 30–45 min	6–8 hr	Tolerance may develop.
Isosorbide mononitrate (Imdur, Ismo)	20 mg BID PO first dose when wakening then in 7 hrs	a. 30–60 min	Not determined	Take on empty stomach.
Nitroglycerin (sustained-release tablets) (Nitro-Bid, Nitrospan)	2.6–9 mg PO q8–12 hr	a. 30 min b. 3–4 hr	8–12 hr	
Nitroglycerin (Transdermal) (Nitrodisc, Nitro-Dur, Transderm-Nitro)	2.5–15 mg QD	a. 30–60 min	Up to 24 hr when on patient	Apply to nonhairy site.
Nitroglycerin (Topical) (Nitro-Bid, Nitrol)	Topical: 1–3 inches (15–30 mg) of ointment TID or BID	a. 30 min	2–12 hr	Ointment may be placed on any nonhairy body part. Ointment should be covered with plastic wrap for correct absorption.[18]

2. Have patients lie down before drug administration to prevent hypotension. Monitor blood pressure frequently and observe for symptoms of hypotension (lightheadedness, dizziness, decreased urine output).
3. To decrease any incidence of postural hypotension, instruct patients to assume an upright position slowly.
4. If pain is unrelieved by three doses of nitroglycerin (one tablet every 5 minutes), institute the appropriate procedure for obtaining emergency medical care.[1]

BETA-BLOCKING AGENTS

Actions and Uses

Beta-adrenergic blocking agents (beta blockers, Table 7–2) reduce myocardial oxygen requirements by decreasing heart rate, blood pressure, and myocardial contractility, both at rest and during exercise.[3] By decreasing heart rate, beta blockers prolong diastole, which promotes an increased blood supply to the myocardium.[4] The primary mechanism of action in beta blockers is to diminish the actions of the sympathetic nervous system (i.e., catecholamine release) on beta-receptors. Normally, the catecholamines, epinephrine and norepinephrine, bind with beta-receptors to initiate responses to sympathetic nervous system adrenergic stimulation. Beta-blockers compete with epinephrine and norepinephrine for available beta-receptor sites in the heart and other tissues, thus inhibiting normal response to adrenergic stimuli. There are beta$_1$ and beta$_2$ receptor sites.[3] Beta$_1$ sites are located primarily in the heart, and beta$_2$ sites in the lungs and throughout the body. Inhibition of beta$_1$ receptors decreases the heart rate, decreases conduction through the atrioventricular (AV) node, decreases myocardial contractility, and decreases automaticity in the heart. Inhibition of beta$_2$ receptors causes bronchoconstriction, vasoconstriction, and decreased glycogenolysis (conversion of glycogen in the liver into glucose).[5,6]

Beta-blockers that act specifically on beta$_1$ sites (found in the heart) are referred to as cardioselective and beta-blockers that inhibit both beta$_1$ and beta$_2$ sites are categorized as nonselective.[5]

Beta-blockers are used in combination with nitrates for the treatment of chest pain in effort angina. The primary effect of beta-blockers is to reduce the resting heart rate and the heart rate response to exercise.[7] Following an AMI, beta-blockers can be used to salvage ischemic myocardium by decreasing myocardial oxygen demand. Various research trials have shown short- and long-term benefit with the use of beta-blockers in the setting of AMI. In most of the trials, an initial intravenous (IV) loading dose was administered usually during the first 6 to 8 hours of MI onset. This initial IV dose was followed by oral medication for the rest of the trial duration (varying from 27 hours to 1 year). One such trial was the International Study of Infarct Survival (ISIS), which reported a statistically significant 14 percent reduction in mortality of AMI patients acutely treated with IV and subsequent oral atenolol (Tenormin). Data from all trials indicate that beta-blockers, given acutely or over the long term, reduce mortality and nonfatal reinfarction.[5]

Beta-blockers are used in the treatment of mild hypertension and of atrial and ventricular arrhythmias because they decrease automaticity of myocardial cells and slow conduction through the AV node. The antiarrhythmic effects of beta-blockers may be the result of a property called membrane-stabilizing activity, meaning the ability of

TABLE 7–2 Beta-Blocking Agents[3,5–7,18,22,29]

Generic Name (Trade Name)	Dosage	Therapeutic Uses	Implications
Propranolol hydrochloride (Inderal)	10–80 mg PO BID to QID (Variable doses and varied uses)	Hypertension, angina, supraventricular tachyarrhythmias, postinfarct to prevent reinfarction, migraine headaches	Caution individual that sudden cessation of drugs may cause an exacerbation of angina.
Metoprolol (Lopressor)	100–450 mg/day PO single dose or TID (Cardioselective at lower doses)	Hypertension, angina, some arrhythmias	Cardioselective; may be administered to individuals with lung disease.
Nadolol (Corgard)	40–320 mg/day PO single dose	Hypertension, angina, some arrhythmias	Benefit of once-a-day dosing
Timolol (Blocadren)	15–45 mg PO TID or QID	Postinfarction to prevent reinfarction	Adult dosage to maintain clinical response.
Atenelol (Tenormin)	50–100 mg/day PO single dose (cardioselective at low doses)	Hypertension, angina	Cardioselect
Pindolol (Visken)	10–60 mg PO TID or QID	Hypertension, some arrhythmias	This beta-blocker possesses some intrinsic sympathetic activity (ISA), which is most apparent at rest, producing less resting bradycardia.[3]
Labetalol (Trandate/ Normodyne)	IV: 40–80 mg q 10 minutes (maximum dose 300 mg)	Hypertensive crisis	Possesses ISA property. Alpha-blockade causes vasodilation; does not decrease HR.[18]
Sotalol (Betaplace)	80–320 mg PO BID	Arrhythmias (SVT/VT), hypertension	Possesses both Class II and Class III properties, both beta-blockade and antiarrhythmic properties.[21]
Esmolol (Brevibloc)	IV only; titrated to desired effect	Intra- or post-operative atrial fibrillation and atrial flutter	Cardioselect. Very brief half-life (<10 min)[25]
Acebutolol (Sectral)	200–600 mg PO BID	Ventricular arrhythmias	Cardioselect with ISA; causes less slowing of heart rate.[6]

a drug to have a direct anesthetic effect on the myocardium, thereby reducing the potential for arrhythmias.[5] Many of the beta-blockers currently available are listed in Table 7–2. Another property of some beta-blockers is intrinsic sympathomimetic activity (ISA), meaning the ability of some beta-blockers to partially stimulate the beta-receptor sites. Pindolol (Visken) possesses some ISA. Beta-blockers with ISA may be advantageous in that little, if any, slowing of the heart rate, depression of contractility, or slowing of AV conduction occur at rest when sympathetic activity is low.[3] Stimulation of the sympathetic nervous system and the subsequent increase in catecholamines is a predominant pathophysiologic response to heart failure. Sympathetic nervous system stimulation in patients with chronic heart failure is a major factor in contributing to the severity and progression of this disease.[8] Previously, beta-blockers were contraindicated in heart failure because of their adverse effects on myocardial function. However, controlled trials have shown that beta-blockers in the setting of heart failure can produce hemodynamic improvement and reduction in morbidity and mortality. They improve the symptoms of heart failure by their ability to reduce the effects of sympathetic stimulation.[9] Additional beta-blockers, such as carvedilol, are available that block both alpha$_1$-receptors (causing vasodilation) and beta-receptors.[10]

Contraindications and Side Effects

Beta-blockers are relatively contraindicated in hypotension, congestive heart failure (CHF), bradycardia, AV blocks, and chronic obstructive pulmonary disease (COPD). At all times the risk-to-benefit ratio of these drugs should be evaluated. Beta-blockers must be used cautiously in patients with chronic lung disease because blockade of beta$_2$ receptor sites in the lung may cause bronchospasm. Beta-blockers with cardioselectivity, ISA, and alpha-adrenergic blocking actions (ability to block vasoconstriction) are less likely to cause airway resistance in individuals with asthma. However, a general rule is to avoid all beta-blockers in individuals with bronchospastic disease.[7] Beta-blockers (nonselective) can cause hypoglycemic reactions in diabetic and nondiabetic patients because of their effects on the beta$_2$ receptors' control of glucose release. Cardioselective beta-blockers may be preferred for individuals with insulin-dependent diabetes but may mask signs of hypoglycemia such as tachycardia. Patients with mild CHF may benefit from the decreased heart rate caused by beta-blockers but these drugs may be contraindicated in individuals with more severe CHF. The dose of beta-blockers must be gradually increased and the patient carefully monitored[11] because these agents can further decrease contractility and cardiac output, contributing to increasing heart failure.[7]

Side effects of beta-blockers include bronchospasm, hypotension, bradycardia, AV block, nausea, constipation, transient thrombocytopenia, fatigue, cold extremities, sleep disorders, depression, and impotence.[5] Abrupt cessation of beta-blockers may bring on a recurrence of anginal pain or AMI, arrhythmias, or sudden death. Individuals should be cautioned about the importance of titrating the drug when it is to be discontinued.[7]

Effects on Exercise in Individuals with Coronary Artery Disease

Therapy with beta-blockers results in increased exercise tolerance and increased aerobic capacity. The individual taking beta-blockers experiences a decrease in both resting and submaximal heart rate and blood pressure. This results in a decrease in the rate pressure product (the cardiac workload) and myocardial oxygen demand. Higher levels of activity are attained before the individual's ischemic threshold is reached and anginal pain or electrocardiographic (ECG) changes occur.[3]

Beta-Adrenergic Blockade Therapy Management

Careful consideration should be given to the following:

1. Patients should be cautioned not to abruptly stop taking beta-blockers unless bronchospasm occurs.
2. Increases in heart rate normally seen with exercise are lower in individuals on beta blockers.
3. Changes in beta-blockade therapy may necessitate a repeat graded exercise test and reassessment of the exercise prescription.
4. Observe patients for any change in respiratory effort or dyspnea.

CALCIUM CHANNEL BLOCKERS

Calcium channel blockers (Table 7–3) inhibit the flow of calcium ions across the membranes of myocardial and vascular smooth muscle cells. Calcium plays an important role in myocardial contractility, vasomotor tone, and cardiac electrical activity[7a] (see Chapter 2).

Calcium channel blockers have been categorized into four major groups:

1. Type 1 agents, which have myocardial and electrophysiologic effects
2. Type 2 agents (dihydropyridines), which have predominant vascular effects
3. Type 3 agents, which have selective vascular properties and are not presently being used in the United States
4. Type 4 agents, which have rather complex pharmacologic properties

Calcium channel blockers currently approved for clinical use in the United States are verapamil and diltiazem (type 1); nicardipine, nifedipine, isradipine, amlodipine, felodipine, and nimodipine (type 2); and bepridil (type 4).[12,13]

Verapamil decreases myocardial oxygen demand in three ways: it decreases afterload by peripheral vasodilation, decreases heart rate (negative chronotropic effect), and decreases contractility (negative inotropic effect). Verapamil is used in the treatment of hypertension, angina, and arrhythmias, specifically supraventricular tachycardias. Diltiazem acts through these same mechanisms, but the effects are not as strong as with verapamil.[3,13]

Nifedipine is a strong peripheral vasodilator. It decreases myocardial oxygen demand by that mechanism. However, it has no direct effect on heart rate and no antiarrhythmic properties. Moreover, nifedipine may cause a reflex increase in heart rate in response to vasodilation.[13] The potent vasodilating effects of nifedipine and other dihydropyridines make them beneficial in the treatment of heart failure and variant angina. Although nifedipine has a negative inotropic effect on myocardium, its ability to vasodilate, which reduces afterload, improves cardiac function.[7a] The newer-

TABLE 7-3 Calcium Channel Blockers[4,7,12,18]

Generic Name (Trade Name)	Dosage	Therapeutic Uses	Effects on Cardiovascular System
Diltiazem (Cardizem)	IV dose in acute care setting. Oral dose: 30 mg TID or QID (to maximum of 240 mg/24 hr)	Angina and hypertension, supraventricular arrhythmias	Dilates coronary arteries; antiarrhythmic action; causes some decrease in contractility (negative inotropic effect).
Diltiazem SR Diltiazem CD	60–120 mg PO q 12 hr 180–360 mg PO q day		
Nifedipine (Procardia)	Oral dose: Initially 10 mg TID Maintenance: 10–30 mg TID or QID	Angina, hypertension	Potent peripheral vasodilator; dilates coronary arteries. Increases resting heart rate; negative inotropic effects.
Bepridil (Vascor)	200–400 mg PO QD	Angina	Dilates peripheral and coronary arteries. Minimal or no decrease in heart rate and contractility.
Amlodipine (Norvasc)	2.5–10 mg PO QD	Angina, hypertension	Dilates peripheral and coronary arteries. Increases exercise tolerance and improves heart failure symptoms.
Felodipine (Plendil)	5–20 mg PO QD	Hypertension	Decreases peripheral vascular resistance.
Isradipine (DynaCirc)	5–10 mg PO QD or BID	Hypertension	Decreases peripheral vascular resistance.
Nicardipine (Cardene)	20–40 mg PO TID	Hypertension, angina	Dilates peripheral and coronary arteries. Increases resting heart rate.
Verapamil (Calan, Isoptin, Verelan)	IV dose in acute care setting. Oral dose: Initially 80 mg q 6–8 hr; 320–480 mg in divided doses.	Angina, supraventricular tachyarrhythmias	Slows AV conduction and decreases ventricular response to tachyarrhythmias; negative inotropic effects.
Verapamil SR	240–480 mg PO q 12–24 hr		

generation dihydropyridines are considered vasoselective. The term "vasoselectivity" refers to their selective action on vascular smooth muscle versus cardiac muscle. The potential benefits of these agents is a reduction in the negative inotropic effects that can occur with other calcium channel blockers.[12]

Calcium channel blockers are also used in the treatment of hypertension. They can be used in combination with nitrates to treat effort angina and are prescribed for angina caused by coronary artery vasospasm.[3] They may also be used in combination with beta-blockers in the treatment of effort angina because they permit the use of lower doses of the beta-blockers and avoid the undesirable effects of beta-blockade.[7a]

There is no evidence that calcium channel blockers alone are beneficial in treating AMI. In numerous trials, higher doses of nifedipine appeared to cause a higher mortality, probably secondary to reflex tachycardia.[14] However, diltiazem has been shown to reduce reinfarction rates in patients with non-Q wave infarctions who have also received nitrates or beta-blockers.[13] Calcium channel blocker therapy results in decreased myocardial contractility, vasomotor tone, peripheral vascular resistance, and heart rate, the latter because of slower impulse conduction resulting in a decrease in myocardial oxygen demand.[3]

Contraindications and Side Effects

Calcium channel blockers are contraindicated in moderate to severe CHF, significant hypotension, aortic stenosis, and sick sinus syndrome. Side effects of calcium channel blockers include headache, hypotension, flushing, peripheral edema, and worsening of sinus node dysfunction. Central nervous system (CNS) side effects include tremors, mood changes, and fatigue. Gastrointestinal distress and skin reactions have also been reported. Nifedipine can cause significant noncardiac pedal edema and reflex tachycardia. Bepridil has the potential to cause malignant ventricular arrhythmias.[7a,13]

Effects on Exercise in Individuals with Coronary Artery Disease

The ability of calcium channel blockers to decrease myocardial oxygen demand and improve myocardial blood supply may enhance an individual's tolerance for activity.[13]

Calcium Channel Blockade Therapy Management

Careful consideration should be given to the following:

1. Observe patients for symptoms of postural hypotension (lightheadedness upon arising, tachycardia, and pallor).
2. Assess patients for potential aggravation of myocardial ischemia with the dihydropyridine agents secondary to hypotension and decreased coronary perfusion.[13]
3. Monitor blood pressure and cardiac rhythm changes.

CARDIAC GLYCOSIDES

Digitalis is a term used to describe the entire group of cardiac glycosides. The most commonly utilized cardiac glycoside is digoxin; a less common preparation is digitoxin.[15]

Actions and Uses

The exact mechanism of action of cardiac glycosides is unknown. They are believed to increase the influx of calcium into the myocardial cell. They also alter the electrochemical properties of the cell by their effect on the active transport of sodium and potassium.[3] Digitalis has two major indications: (1) treatment of congestive heart failure, and (2) prevention of supraventricular arrhythmias, especially in the presence of heart failure.[16]

Cardiac glycosides are indicated in individuals with mild to moderate heart failure who continue to be symptomatic despite therapeutic doses of ACE inhibitors and diuretics.[17] The increased contractility improves oxygen delivery to all tissues. Increased renal perfusion results in a diuretic effect, decreasing circulating blood volume. Circulatory volume is further decreased by diuretic therapy administered in conjunction with cardiac glycosides in the treatment of heart failure. Cardiac glycosides have both a positive inotropic effect (increasing the contractility) and a negative chronotropic effect (decreasing the heart rate). The associated decreased heart rate may result from the vagal stimulation initiated by carotid baroreceptors when increased systolic pressure is sensed.[16]

Although these effects are seen in the healthy heart, they are more significant in the failing heart. Increased contractility increases the cardiac output and decreases preload, cardiac workload, and myocardial oxygen demand. This, in turn, reduces the clinical effects of congestive heart failure. Most clinicians do not rely on digitalis alone for the treatment of heart failure, but also include diuretics, ACE inhibitors, and nitrates.[16]

Cardiac glycosides also possess electrophysiologic effects. By decreasing conduction velocity through the AV node, cardiac glycosides can decrease ventricular response to supraventricular tachyarrhythmias such as atrial fibrillation and atrial flutter. In addition, digitalis can terminate paroxysmal supraventricular tachycardias (PSVTs) caused by re-entry involving the AV node. Digitalis alters the critical relationship between conduction time and the refractory period within the AV node; this can result in termination of a PSVT.[16]

Contraindications and Side Effects

In general, cardiac glycosides have a relatively narrow margin of safety between the therapeutic range and the toxic range. Levels near or in the toxic range may be very poorly tolerated.[3] Toxicity is generally associated with increased blood levels. Characteristic ECG changes associated with toxicity include bradycardia, prolongation of the PR interval (first-degree heart block), and a shortening of the QT interval. Other arrhythmias may be observed as the conduction blockade at the AV node increases. Premature ventricular contractions, ventricular tachycardia, excessively slow ventricular response to atrial fibrillation, and supraventricular tachycardia may all be a result of the alteration in conduction caused by digitalis toxicity.[15] Because it can precipitate almost any arrhythmia, digoxin must always be viewed as suspect when an individual taking this drug suddenly develops an arrhythmia. Other side effects include nausea, vomiting, anorexia, drowsiness, fatigue, and confusion. Visual disturbances, such as seeing yellow or green dots and experiencing double vision, are common with toxic blood levels. Risk factors for the development of toxicity are reduced renal clearance and old age. Hypokalemia in individuals on digoxin can predispose to arrhythmias.[16]

Cardiac glycoside therapy is used with extreme caution in individuals with hypertrophic cardiomyopathy, constrictive pericarditis, and incomplete AV block. In acute MI, cardiac glycoside therapy may be contraindicated because the increased contractility increases myocardial oxygen demand and may extend an infarction.[18]

Effects on Exercise in Individuals with Coronary Artery Disease

The individual with CHF receiving cardiac glycoside therapy will demonstrate increased exercise tolerance because of the increased efficiency of the ventricular function and oxygen utilization. The ST and T-wave changes associated with cardiac glycoside therapy may mimic the ECG changes of ischemia. Evaluation of the individual's rhythm strip or 12-lead ECG at rest and with exercise will permit definitive diagnosis.[3]

Cardiac Glycosides Therapy Management

Careful consideration should be given to the following:[18]

1. Familiarity with the effect of cardiac glycosides on the ECG is essential. The sagging ST segment may be mistaken for the ST depression seen in ischemia.
2. Arrhythmias associated with cardiac glycosides may be precipitated by exercise, especially if the patient is hypokalemic.
3. Patients should learn to check their peripheral pulse daily and report significant bradycardia or sustained tachycardia.
4. Classic early signs of toxicity include nausea, vomiting, anorexia, and visual disturbances.
5. Maintenance doses of digoxin, the most commonly prescribed cardiac glycoside, are 0.125 mg to 0.25 mg QD. Frail or underweight elderly individuals often require smaller doses.

ANTIARRHYTHMICS

Antiarrhythmic drugs alter the conductivity and automaticity of the myocardium to correct abnormalities in electrical activity. Generally, they suppress ectopic stimuli (impulses arising outside of the sinoatrial node, the normal pacemaker of the heart), slow the rate of impulse generation and conduction, and decrease myocardial irritability.[19]

There are four recognized classes of antiarrhythmics (Table 7–4). They are classified according to their mechanism of action on the action potential of cardiac cells.[19,20]

TABLE 7-4 Common Antiarrhythmics[6,21-23]

Generic Name (Trade Name)	Dosage	Class	ECG Changes	Implications/Side Effects
Quinidine sulfate (Cin-Quin, Quine, Quinidex Extentabs)	Tablets: 200 mg PO q 6 hr Extended release: 300 mg	IA	Prolongs QRS, QT, and PR.	Nausea and diarrhea may make drug intolerable; may cause VT or TdP.
Procainamide Hydrochloride (Pronestyl)	250–500 mg PO q 3–4 hr	IA	Prolongs QRS, QT, and PR.	Hypotension, lupuslike symptoms (rash, fever, chills, joint pain); GI symptoms.
Sustained release (Procan SR)	250–1250 mg PO q 6 hr			
Disopyramide (Norpace)	100–200 mg PO q 6 hr	IA	Prolongs QRS, QT, and PR.	Anticholinergic effects, heart block, hypotension, CHF.
Lidocaine (Xylocaine)	1 mg/kg IV bolus; may repeat with 0.5 mg/kg	IB	None; decreases or suppresses ventricular ectopy	Drowsiness, confusion, impaired coordination, tremors, seizures.
Mexiletine (Mexitil)	200–400 mg PO q 6–8 hr	IB	Usually none.	Unsteady gait, dizziness, tremors. To minimize GI symptoms, give with food.
Moricizine (Ethmozine)	600–900 mg PO q 8 hr	IC	Prolongs PR and QRS intervals.	Heart block, bradycardia, exacerbation of ventricular arrhythmias, dizziness, headache, nausea, drug-induced fever. Observe for signs of CHF.
Propafenone (Rhythmol)	150–300 mg PO q 8–12 hr	IC	Prolongs PR and QRS.	Nausea, hypotension, increased ventricular arrhythmias, bitter taste.
Flecainide (Tambocor)	100–200 mg PO BID	IC	Prolongs QRS, PR; slight increase of QT interval.	Dizziness, blurred vision, GI symptoms. Watch for signs of CHF.

142

Drug	Dose	Class	ECG Effects	Side Effects/Comments
Propranolol (Inderal)	10–30 mg PO TID or QID	II	Increases PR interval; slight increase in QT interval.	Hypotension, bronchoconstriction, drowsiness, impotence, hypoglycemia in patients with diabetes. Check for signs of CHF: edema, cough, decreased exercise tolerance.
Bretylium (Bretylol)	5–10 mg/kg IV bolus; followed by infusion (acute care setting only)	III	None	GI symptoms, orthostatic hypotension, arrhythmias.
Sotalol (Betapace)	80 mg PO BID or TID; up to 160 mg BID	Both Class II and Class III properties.	Prolongs QT.	Bradycardia, hypotension, fatigue. Does not cause myocardial depression, but may precipitate CHF in patients with past history of heart failure. Prolonged QT can lead to TdP.
Amiodarone (Cordarone)	Initial 1- to 3-week loading dose, then 400–800 mg PO QD	III	Prolongs QRS, QT intervals; may slightly increase PR interval.	CNS (tremor, headache, ataxia), GI, hyper/hypothyroidism, pulmonary fibrosis, corneal deposits, blue skin discoloration.
Verapamil (Calan, Isoptin)	5–10 mg IV bolus; may repeat with 10 mg in 30 min (acute care setting) 80 mg PO TID or QID; may receive up to 480 mg/day Available in sustained release	IV	Increases PR interval. Used for SVT. Slows conduction across AV node; decreases HR.	Hypotension, nausea, constipation. May cause reflex tachycardia. Check for bruising or purpura—can cause platelet dysfunction. May cause CHF.
Adenosine	6 mg rapid IV bolus over 1–2 sec; may repeat in 1–2 min with 12 mg	Unclassified	Prolongs PR.	Facial flushing, transient heart block, bradycardia, hypotension, nausea, dyspnea.

Class I agents suppress sodium (Na$^+$) channels and reduce conduction velocity. These drugs have "local anesthetic" or "membrane-stabilizing" activity.[21] Class I drugs are further divided into three subgroups[19]:

IA:　Quinidine-like drugs: depress cell membrane responsiveness by depressing the voltage-dependent sodium current; delay repolarization and lengthen action potential

IB:　Inhibit the current in the fast sodium ion channels; accelerate repolarization and shorten action potential duration

IC:　Inhibit the fast inward sodium current and inhibit conduction to the His-Purkinje system; prolong PR and QRS

Class II agents are beta-blocking agents. They block sympathetic receptors, causing a decrease in heart rate and AV conduction.[22] *Class III* agents act selectively on repolarization and re-entry circuits and are most effective in abolishing ventricular fibrillation. They prolong action potential.[19] *Class IV* agents are calcium channel blockers. They depress slow calcium (Ca^{2+}) channels and sinus and AV node conduction and are effective in terminating AV nodal re-entrant supraventricular tachycardia.[19]

Antiarrhythmics are used to restore normal heart rhythm. This benefits the individual hemodynamically by allowing the heart to work efficiently, resulting in improved activity tolerance. Asymptomatic arrhythmias or those that do not leave the individual at substantial risk for a life-threatening arrhythmia are usually left untreated. It should be remembered that all antiarrhythmics are cardiac depressants and must be administered with caution when either electrical or mechanical depression of the myocardium is present.[3] In addition, all antiarrhythmics may potentiate or generate the very arrhythmias they are designed to suppress. This is known as their proarrhythmic effect.[19]

Multitudinous antiarrhythmic agents are currently being developed and tested, many for the treatment of ventricular arrhythmias. The agents discussed in this chapter are only those currently approved for use in clinical situations.

Class I

All Class I antiarrhythmics suppress sodium (Na$^+$) channels but differ in regard to depolarization and repolarization. They are therefore divided into classes IA, IB, and IC.[19,21]

CLASS IA

Class IA drugs are effective in the treatment of both atrial and ventricular arrhythmias, including atrial fibrillation, premature ventricular contractions, and ventricular tachycardia. Because they have little or no effect on the sinoatrial (SA) node, they are not effective against disturbances in SA node function. These drugs slow conduction and prolong repolarization.[19,22,23]

Two marked ECG changes seen with class IA antiarrhythmics are (1) a prolongation of the QRS complex and (2) a prolongation of the QT interval. Therapy with Class IA antiarrhythmics should be discontinued if these ECG changes are observed. The increase in the QT interval can lead to the development of an atypical ventricular tachycardia called torsade de pointes (TdP). Characterized by bursts of VT and an undulating QRS axis that cannot be converted by conventional antiarrhythmics, torsade de pointes is usually associated with bradycardia, prolongation of the QT interval, and hypokalemia. Progression to ventricular fibrillation can occur and is life-threatening. Class IA antiarrhythmics are administered with caution to patients with congestive heart failure because of their negative inotropic affects.[19] Table 7–4 includes some of the common class IA antiarrhythmics.

Quinidine is one of the best-known class IA antiarrhythmics. This drug is frequently used to treat atrial arrhythmias, although it is also effective for ventricular arrhythmias. Quinidine is contraindicated in patients who are hypersensitive to it or who have conduction defects of the AV node, digitalis toxicity, or potassium imbalance. The most common side effects are nausea, diarrhea, and arrhythmias, including torsade de pointes. Quinidine is now used less often in the treatment of certain arrhythmias because of the development of other equally effective drugs with less significant side effects.[6,21]

Procainamide (Pronestyl, Procan SR) is another class IA antiarrhythmic used in the treatment of both atrial and ventricular arrhythmias. It is, however, more commonly used to treat ventricular arrhythmias. It controls cardiac arrhythmias by decreasing myocardial automaticity and conduction velocity and increasing the relative refractory period of the myocardial cells. As a result, procainamide decreases conduction through the heart and can prolong the QRS duration and QT interval. This drug's prolongation of the QT interval can lead to torsade de pointes in 1 to 2 percent of patients.[6,24] Common side effects with oral procainamide preparations include nausea, vomiting, and diarrhea. Procainamide may also cause myocardial depression. Chronic therapy may result in systemic lupus erythematosus (SLE) syndrome characterized by elevated antinuclear antibody titers, arthralgia, myalgia, fever, and pleuropericarditis. Discontinuation of the drug usually reverses these symptoms.[6,23]

Another Class IA drug is disopyramide (Norpace), which has actions similar to those of quinidine and procainamide but different adverse effects. Disopyramide is indicated for maintaining sinus rhythm in individuals with atrial fibrillation and atrial flutter and for preventing reappearance of ventricular tachyarrhythmias.[25] Like other Class IA drugs, disopyramide prolongs the QT interval and can be proarrhythmic, predisposing to torsades de pointes. This drug has significant anticholinergic effects, which can precipitate glaucoma, dry mouth, urinary retention (more commonly in men), and constipation. In addition, disopyramide also has negative inotropic effects on the myocardium that can precipitate or worsen heart failure. Contraindications to this drug include refractory heart failure, glaucoma, and obstructive uropathy.[21]

Class IA Antiarrhythmic Management[3]
Careful consideration should be given to the following:

1. Observe the ECG for prolongation of the QRS or QT interval.
2. Observe the ECG for the development of new or recurrent arrhythmias. Continue observation during the recovery period because arrhythmias often occur during recovery instead of peak exercise.
3. Negative inotropic effects of some of these drugs may decrease BP or exercise performance.
4. With procainamide, arthritic-like joint pains may be the first sign of SLE syndrome.
5. Observe for CHF because class IA antiarrhythmics are myocardial depressants.

CLASS IB

Class IB agents accelerate repolarization as well as shorten action potential duration. The QT segment is therefore not prolonged. The agents are used specifically for ventricular arrhythmias. Lidocaine, mexiletine (Mexitil), and tocainide (Tonocard) are class IB agents[19] (Table 7–4).

Lidocaine is the antiarrhythmic most commonly used in the treatment of acute premature ventricular contractions and ventricular arrhythmias. Lidocaine is administered only IV; it acts specifically on the Purkinje fibers. The sinus rate and atrial arrhythmias do not appear to be affected by lidocaine.[23]

Mexiletine, given orally, acts similarly to lidocaine and is used in the chronic management of ventricular arrhythmias. Tocainide is rarely prescribed because of the significant side effect of agranulocytosis. Although class IB agents rarely cause adverse cardiac effects, they may cause numerous neurologic and GI side effects, including nausea, vomiting, tremors, confusion, and seizures.[6]

Class IB Antiarrhythmic Management

Careful consideration should be given to the following:

1. Give mexiletine and tocainide with food to minimize GI upset.
2. Tocainide and mexiletene may cause agranulocytosis (decreased white blood cell count). Periodic blood counts should be monitored.[6]
3. Monitor BP in patients taking lidocaine because the drug may cause severe hypotension.
4. Do not give lidocaine for idioventricular rhythm because it may cause asystole.
5. In the cardiac rehabilitation setting, parameters for administration of lidocaine should be identified for each individual depending on his or her individual rhythm and pattern of ectopy. (A dose of 1 mg/kg IV push or 50 to 100 mg will suppress ventricular ectopy for about 20 minutes.[6])

CLASS IC

Class IC agents inhibit His-Purkinje conduction and cause a widening of both the PR interval and the QRS complex, but they have little effect on repolarization. Included in this class of drugs are flecainide (Tambocor), encainide (Enkaid), moricizine (Ethmozine), and propafenone (Rythmol). They are the most potent class I antiarrhythmics. The Cardiac Arrhythmia Suppression Trial (CAST) indicated that encainide, flecainide, and moricizine caused increased mortality and nonfatal cardiac arrest in AMI patients with non-life-threatening arrhythmias. These drugs have been found to have a proarrhythmic effect (worsening of ventricular arrhythmias). The results of CAST have led to encainide being no longer available and moricizine and flecainide being used only in patients with life-threatening arrhythmias. In addition, flecainide is also sometimes prescribed for the maintenance of sinus rhythm in individuals with supraventricular arrhythmias.[21,22,25–27]

Propafenone is approved for treatment of life-threatening ventricular arrhythmias. Its major effect is to slow conduction. In addition to its Class IC properties, propafenone also has the effects of beta blockade and calcium channel blockade. These latter effects can lower heart rate and depress myocardial contractility. It affects the ECG by prolonging the PR interval and QRS duration. As with other Class IC agents, propafenone is proarrhythmic.[25]

Side effects of the Class IC drugs include CNS effects (visual disturbances, dizziness and headache), GI disturbances (nausea), negative inotropy, and arrhythmia.[25]

Class IC Antiarrhythmic Management[18]

Careful consideration should be given to the following:

1. Monitor patients for proarrhythmic effects (increased ventricular ectopy).
2. Administer with caution to patients with CHF.
3. Assess patients for any neurologic symptoms.
4. Administer oral doses with meals to lessen GI side effects.

Class II

Antiarrhythmics in class II are the beta-blockers. They block sympathetic stimulation at the SA node, increase the effective refractory period of the AV node, and reduce automaticity in the Purkinje fibers. Beta-blockers are effective in the treatment of ventricular and supraventricular arrhythmias; however, they have not shown effectiveness in the treatment of recurrent ventricular tachycardia.[21] Currently, the beta-blockers approved for treatment of arrhythmias are propranolol (Inderal), acebutolol (Sectral), esmolol (Brevibloc), and sotalol (Betapace).[19,22]

Propranolol effectively slows ventricular response in individuals with supraventricular tachycardias (SVTs). The drug is effective in the treatment of SVT precipitated by CAD or exercise. Side effects of propranolol include potential exacerbation of congestive heart failure secondary to the negative inotropic effects and all other side effects previously identified for beta blockers. As with all beta-blockers, propranolol should be given with caution to diabetic patients because their sympathetic response to hypoglycemia may be masked.[6]

Acebutolol is a beta-blocker with cardioselectivity that is used to treat ventricular arrhythmias. This Class II drug also has intrinsic sympathomimetic activity (ISA), which essentially causes it to have a reduced effect on slowing of the heart rate and depression of myocardial function. Side effects include bradycardia, hypotension, CHF, dizziness, anxiety, abdominal discomfort, and nausea.[6]

Esmolol, a cardioselective IV beta-blocker, is effective when immediate beta blockade is required for rate control of supraventricular tacharrhythmias such as rapid atrial fibrillation and atrial flutter.[25] This drug is used frequently in the surgical or critical care setting because of its short half-life (about 9 minutes). Side effects include bradycardia, hypotension, and pulmonary edema.[6]

Sotalol has properties of both Class II and Class III antiarrhythmics and will be mentioned with Class III antiarrhythmics.

CLASS II ANTIARRHYTHMIC THERAPY MANAGEMENT[22]

Careful consideration should be given to the following:

1. An abrupt cessation of beta-blockers may exacerbate anginal pain in individuals with CAD or after an MI.
2. Observe ECG for bradyarrhythmias and heart block associated with beta-blockade therapy.

3. There is a decrease in resting and submaximal heart rate and blood pressure with beta blockers.
4. Assess patients for any signs of heart failure.
5. Avoid postural hypotension by instructing patients to change position slowly.

Class III

The only class III drugs that are currently available are bretylium tosylate (Brety-lol), amiodarone (Cordarone), sotalol (Betapace), and ibutilide (Corvert). Class III drugs slow the rate of repolarization, which increases the effective refractory period and the action potential duration. Bretylium, an intravenous sympathetic blocking agent, is used in the emergency treatment of ventricular arrhythmias refractory to treatment with other antiarrhythmics. Bretylium may potentiate digitalis toxicity because it causes a transient increase in norepinephrine release. Therefore it should be administered with caution to individuals receiving digitalis. Side effects of bretylium include severe hypotension and the related symptoms of lightheadedness, dizziness, and vertigo.[18,21,22]

Amiodarone is an antiarrhythmic that is effective in the treatment of both supraventricular and ventricular arrhythmias, but its potential for toxicity of multiple organ systems has thus far limited its use to life-threatening arrhythmias refractory to other antiarrhythmic therapy. It has a very slow onset of action (4 to 10 days) and therefore is not appropriate for the acute management of ventricular arrhythmias. Moreover, it has a prolonged duration of action with a half-life of 14 to 52 days.[6] Amiodarone prolongs the action potential duration and causes increased refractoriness of the conduction system. The ECG changes with amiodarone include prolonged PR and QT intervals with no change in the QRS complex. The ECG changes are usually seen before the therapeutic effects are evident. Amiodarone is associated with many severe but usually reversible side effects. These include corneal microdeposits in almost all patients, which may lead to impaired vision; thyroid dysfunction (hypothyroidism or hyperthyroidism); peripheral neuropathy; photosensitivity; slate-gray or bluish pigmentation of the skin; and elevated liver enzymes. The most potentially dangerous side effect is pulmonary fibrosis, which occurs in about 15 percent of patients on high chronic oral doses; this fibrosis may regress with discontinuation of the drug or progress to respiratory impairment and death. Side effects are slow to resolve, often taking more than 6 months after the drug is discontinued because of the extended half-life of amiodarone.[6,21,25]

As mentioned previously, sotalol is an antiarrhythmic agent that possesses both Class II (blocking beta-adrenergic receptors) and Class III (prolonging cardiac repolarization) properties. Unlike Class II agents, sotalol does not cause depression of myocardial function. It is effective in the treatment of supraventricular and ventricular arrhythmias. An ECG change associated with sotalol is a prolonged QT interval that can lead to an arrhythmia, specifically TdP in the presence of hypokalemia or hypomagnesemia. The drug does not affect the PR interval and QRS duration.[23] Side effects of sotalol are similar to those of other beta-blocking agents: bradycardia, hypotension, dizziness, fatigue, and dyspnea.[21,28,29]

A more recent addition to the Class III antiarrhythmics is ibutilide (Corvert). This agent is given IV for rapid termination of recent onset atrial fibrillation and atrial flutter; it is not as effective with atrial arrhythmias of longer duration (greater than 90 days). Ibutilide prolongs the action potential duration and increases the refractory period in atrial and ventricular tissue. This produces mild slowing of the sinus rate and AV conduction, thereby prolonging the QT interval without prolongation of the QRS duration. The usual dosage is 1 mg over 10 minutes for patients weighing more than 60 kg; patients weighing less than 60 kg should be given 0.1 mg/kg. Like other antiarrhythmic agents, ibutilide can be proarrhythmic, causing ventricular arrhythmias including polymorphic VT or TdP. Patients with a history of congestive heart failure are more at risk for this proarrhythmic effect. Other adverse effects include nausea, hypotension, AV block, and bundle branch block.[30]

CLASS III ANTIARRHYTHMIC THERAPY MANAGEMENT[21]

Careful attention should be given to the following:

A. Amiodarone

  1. Observe patients for pulmonary symptoms. Encourage them to inform physician of new onset of fever, cough, or shortness of breath. Many patients have a chest x-ray done every 3 months.
  2. Be alert for visual difficulties that are a result of corneal microdeposits.
  3. Encourage use of sunscreen; amiodarone causes skin photosensitivity and a gray-blue discoloration of the skin.
  4. Be alert for sings of hypo- or hyperthyroidism, heat and cold intolerance, fatigue, and so forth.

B. Sotalol

  1. Observe cardiac monitor for arrhythmias such as bradycardia or TdP.
  2. Monitor serum electrolyte levels, particularly for hypokalemia or hypomagnesemia.
  3. Assess patients for signs of dyspnea, fatigue, and congestive heart failure.

Class IV

Class IV antiarrhythmics are the calcium channel blockers, of which only verapamil (Calan, Isoptin, Verelan) and diltiazem (Cardizem) have been approved for the treatment of supraventricular tachycardias. These two drugs are used to decrease ventricular rate in atrial fibrillation and atrial flutter and to prevent nodal re-entrant tachycardia.[21] Class IV agents block the influx of calcium into cardiac cells resulting in a slowing of conduction through the AV node and prolongation of the PR interval.[22] Verapamil has a powerful depressant effect on the AV node; therefore it slows conduction and prolongs the effective refractory period in the AV node. In its IV form, verapamil is frequently able to terminate reentrant supraventricular tachyarrhythmias, such as PSVT, and can cause conversion to normal sinus rhythm. It is not effective, however, in converting atrial fibrillation or atrial flutter into sinus rhythm but may be used alone or with digoxin to decrease the ventricular rate response to atrial fibrillation or atrial flutter. Diltiazem is another calcium channel blocker that is approved for treatment of supraventricular arrhythmias. This drug is similar to its ability to slow ventricular response to atrial fibrillation and flutter and convert PSVT to sinus rhythm.[6]

The major side effect of IV verapamil and diltiazem is hypotension, especially when the drugs are given as IV boluses. Both verapamil and diltiazem can worsen sinus node dysfunction and impair AV nodal conduction. Verapamil can cause constipation and may exacerbate congestive heart failure especially when used with beta-blockers. In addition to arrhythmias and conduction abnormalities, diltiazem can also cause headache and GI disturbances.[6,23]

CLASS IV ANTIARRHYTHMIC THERAPY MANAGEMENT

Careful attention should be given to the following:

1. Observe patients for signs of hypotension: lightheadedness, dizziness, fatigue.
2. Monitor blood pressure.
3. Observe patients for symptoms of CHF (dyspnea, cough, decreased activity tolerance, peripheral edema).
4. In absence of CHF, encourage increased intake of fluid and fiber to reduce risk of constipation.

ADENOSINE

Adenosine (Adenocard) is an unclassified antiarrhythmic medication that is administered as a rapid IV bolus. This agent slows AV nodal conduction and causes transient AV block. Adenosine is used to convert re-entrant supraventricular arrhythmias and to assist in differentiating narrow and wide QRS complex tachycardias. The most common side effect of adenosine is transient asystole or ventricular standstill, which generally lasts less than 5 seconds and may even assist in the assessment of any underlying atrial rhythm. Other side effects include facial flushing, chest pressure, and dyspnea. Side effects are transient because of the drug's short half-life, which is approximately 1.5 to 10 seconds.[19,21,23]

Angiotensin-Converting Enzyme Inhibitors

ACE inhibitors are in the class of drugs called vasodilators. These drugs improve cardiac function by varying ability to dilate arteries or veins or both.[19] ACE inhibitors were originally indicated for treatment of hypertension. More recently, they are being used in the treatment of individuals with congestive heart failure or acute MI patients with left ventricular dysfunction (i.e., an ejection fraction less than 40 percent).[31] ACE inhibitors prevent conversion of angiotensin I to angiotensin II (a potent vasoconstrictor). Reduction in formation of angiotensin II decreases peripheral vasoconstriction and diminishes release of aldosterone, resulting in a decrease in sodium and water retention. Because ACE inhibitors cause both venous and arterial dilation, which reduces both preload and afterload, they have also been found beneficial in limiting infarct expansion and chamber dilation caused by ventricular remodeling.[32–34] In addition, these drugs decrease renal vascular resistance thereby increasing renal blood flow. ACE inhibitors also enhance levels of bradykinin, an endogenous and potent vasodilator. They lower total peripheral vascular resistance without appreciable change in cardiac output or heart rate. In the setting of congestive heart failure, ACE inhibitors improve cardiac output by decreasing afterload.

The most common ACE inhibitors are captopril (Capoten), enalapril (Vasotec), lisinopril (Zestril, Prinivil), ramipril (Altace), and moexipril (Univasc). These drugs should be used cautiously in patients with renal impairment, autoimmune diseases such as SLE, or who are taking other drugs known to affect the immune response.[18] Common side effects of ACE inhibitors include cough, hypotension, rash, angioedema (swelling of face, lips, and tongue), GI disturbances, headache, dizziness, lightheadedness, and fatigue. Coughing occurs in about 7 to 10 percent of patients on ACE inhibitors; severe, intolerable coughing occurs only in 2 to 3 percent of patients but may necessitate discontinuation of the drug. Symptomatic hypotension, although infrequent, often occurs in patients with CHF who are on high-dose diuretics.[35] Less common side effects include hyperkalemia, renal insufficiency, neutropenia, and agranulocytosis.[18,32,36]

ANGIOTENSIN-CONVERTING ENZYME INHIBITOR THERAPY MANAGEMENT

Careful attention should be given to the following:

1. Assess blood pressure response to ACE inhibitors. Patients on diuretic therapy may be more prone to hypotension.
2. Lightheadedness can occur during initial therapy; instruct patients to change positions slowly.
3. Emphasize the importance of maintaining adequate fluid intake and using caution in warm weather and during exercise.
4. Monitor patients for elevations of potassium (especially in patients on potassium-sparing diuretics or with underlying renal dysfunction), serum creatinine levels, and proteinuria.

THROMBOLYTIC THERAPY FOR MYOCARDIAL INFARCTION

In 1990, the American College of Cardiology (ACC) and the American Heart Association (AHA) recommended that thrombolytic therapy become a standard first-line therapy for eligible patients presenting with symptoms of acute MI.[37] The National Heart Attack Alert Program (NHAAP) set the goal of 30 to 60 minutes as a time frame ("door to drug") for rapid assessment of the patient with subsequent administration of thrombolytic therapy.

A landmark study in 1980 by DeWood et al.[39] revealed the presence of occlusive coronary thrombi within 1 hour of symptom onset in 90 percent of patients with acute MI. The "open-artery" hypothesis, a basis of many research trials, proposes that early opening of an occluded coronary artery in a patient with acute MI improves morbidity and mortality.[40] Many clinical trials have shown that thrombolytic therapy, when given within 6 hours after onset of symptoms of acute MI, is beneficial in reducing infarct size, preserving ventricular function, and reducing mortality.[41] Currently, three thrombolytic agents are approved for clinical use in acute MI: streptokinase (Kabikinase, Streptase), anisoylated plasminogen activator complex (APSAC, Eminase), and recombinant tissue plasminogen activator (TPA, Activase). A fourth thrombolytic agent, urokinase (UK) is primarily used as an intracoronary thrombolytic during percutaneous transluminal coronary angioplasty.[42] All four drugs activate the body's fibrinolytic or clot lysis system by directly or indirectly activating plasminogen to form plasmin.[40] Inclusion criteria for thrombolysis has expanded as a result of findings from various clinical trials. These criteria include patients with at least one-half hour of ischemic cardiac pain and a minimum of 1 mm of ST segment elevation in two adjacent ECG leads (or new complete bundle branch block) who have presented within 12 hours of symptom onset.[41,47] Historically, indication for thrombolysis required patient presentation within 6 hours of symptom onset. Recent studies, however, indicate a benefit in "late" administration of thrombolytic agents.[43] New indications for the use of thrombolytics include pulmonary embolism, subclavian vein thrombosis, and acute thrombotic strokes.[44] Patients should have a thorough risk assessment before initiation of thrombolytic drugs. Absolute contraindications to thrombolysis include aortic dissection, acute pericarditis, active bleeding, previous hemorrhage, intracerebral aneurysm, AV malformation, and cerebral neoplasm. Relative contraindications include cerebrovascular accident (CVA), diabetic retinopathy, severe uncontrolled hypertension (systolic ≥ 200 mm Hg and/or diastolic ≥ 120 mm Hg), GI or genitourinary (GU) hemorrhage, bleeding tendency, hepatic disease, cancer and/or pregnancy, and if having occured in the past 2 to 4 weeks, major surgery, organ biopsy, puncture of a noncompressible vessel, prolonged CPR, major trauma, or minor head trauma.

Streptokinase

Streptokinase (SK) is a systemic, thrombolytic enzyme derived from beta-hemolytic streptococcal bacteria. This drug is effective in dissolving thrombi and restoring patency to an occluded coronary artery during the early hours of acute MI. It can be administered indirectly by the IV route or directly to the occluded artery by cardiac catheterization. SK therapy activates both fibrin-bound and circulating plasminogen; it is not clot-specific and therefore has more systemic fibrinolytic effects.[37,40] In coronary artery occlusion, the goal of SK therapy is to restore coronary perfusion and minimize the size of the myocardial infarction. In the Gruppo Italiano per lo Studio della Streptochinasi nell'Infarcto miocardio (GISSI) Trial, researchers randomized 11,806 patients to intravenous SK therapy or routine coronary care. Results at 21 days showed that mortality was 10.7 percent in patients who received SK versus 13 percent in the control group.[37] Most guidelines suggest that, to be effective, thrombolytics should be initiated within 3 to 6 hours after the onset of chest pain. A delay in therapy significantly decreases the potential to salvage myocardium. SK effectively lyses new clots for approximately 12 hours,[45] with patients remaining in a fibrinolytic state for 24 to 36 hours.[37]

A specific contraindication to SK is previous SK or anisoylated plasminogen streptokinase activator (APSAC) therapy in less than 1 year or a streptococcal infection in less than 6 months.[6] Because SK is produced from streptococcal bacteria, it is antigenic and can cause an allergic reaction (fever, chills, rash, bronchospasm) in patients with streptococcal antibodies from previous infections. The major side effects of SK therapy include hemorrhage, arrhythmias, recurrent thrombosis, severe hypotension, and allergic reaction. Arrhythmias are a result of a reperfusion phenomenon from the alteration in electrical conduction in ischemic cells.[19,40,47]

ANISOYLATED PLASMINOGEN STREPTOKINASE ACTIVATOR

APSAC is an inactive form of plasminogen bound to streptokinase which has a sustained release of activity. Given as an IV bolus, APSAC also has a long half-life (100 minutes), which produces a prolonged fibrinolytic effect. One study indicated a higher reinfarction rate with APSAC versus tissue plasminogen activator (TPA) or SK. Like SK, APSAC is antigenic and can cause an allergic reaction.[37,46]

RECOMBINANT TISSUE PLASMINOGEN ACTIVATOR

Recombinant tissue plasminogen activator (Activase, TPA) is a naturally occurring protein produced from recombinant DNA technology and is therefore nonantigenic.[47] Administered IV, this drug is clot-specific and activates plasminogen, a fibrinolytic enzyme, only after binding to the plasminogen bound to fibrin that is contained in the existing thrombus. It has a very short half-life of about 5 to 10 minutes. As with other thrombolytics, the primary indication for TPA is an acute myocardial infarction. Expanded indications include pulmonary embolism, peripheral arterial occlusions, and thrombotic stroke.[19,44,45] Studies[46] have shown TPA to be more effective than APSAC and SK. In the Global Utilization of Streptokinase and Tissue Plasminogen Activator for Occluded Coronary Arteries (GUSTO) trial, 41,021 patients with AMI presenting less than 6 hours after symptom onset were randomized to various protocols of SK and TPA. TPA was given as an accelerated dose over 90 minutes (in contrast to the FDA-approved 3-hour regimen). Patients randomized to TPA had a 14 percent lower mortality rate than the patients who received SK.[48,49]

Urokinase

Urokinase is another systemic thrombolytic agent with a half-life of approximately 14 minutes. It is a naturally occurring human enzyme derived from kidney cells and acts in a similar manner to TPA, streptokinase and APSAC. Like TPA, urokinase is nonantigenic, but like streptokinase and APSAC, it is not specific for fibrin-bound clots. Clinically, it is administered most frequently as an intracoronary infusion during cardiac catheterization procedures or intra-arterially for peripheral vascular occlusions.[19,45]

The most common adverse effect of thrombolytic therapy is bleeding, which is caused by both the systemic effects of thrombolysis and concomitant anticoagulation therapy. Patients receiving thrombolysis are also on anticoagulation therapy for several days to decrease the possibility of rethrombosis (reocclusion by a thrombus). Mild bleeding is more common and includes bruising, oozing at venipuncture sites, and gingival bleeding. Less common but more serious sites of bleeding include the GI, GU, retroperitoneal, and intracranial areas. Although rare, intracranial bleeding can result in serious morbidity or even mortality.[19,45]

Successful thrombolysis, also referred to as reperfusion, can be suggested by noninvasive clinical markers. Reliable clinical indicators include sudden cessation of ischemic pain, appearance of reperfusion arrhythmias (frequently accelerated idioventricular rhythm), rapid resolution of ST segments back to the baseline, and marked and rapid elevation of creatine kinase caused by a "washout" phenomenon of rapid enzyme release into the circulation.[19] To maintain coronary artery patency, acetylsalicylic acid (aspirin, ASA) and IV heparin are recommended during and after thrombolytic therapy.[37]

ANTITHROMBOTIC AGENTS

After thrombolysis, significant obstruction and potential residual thrombus often occur. This unstable condition influences potential platelet deposition, rethrombosis, and possible vasospasm.[50] The most common antithrombotic drugs include the antiplatelet agents aspirin and ticlopidine (Ticlid) and the anticoagulants heparin and warfarin (Coumadin). The role of antithrombotic drugs is to prevent acute MI and myocardial ischemia and treat the acute and early phases of myocardial infarction. After thrombolysis, antithrombotic drugs may limit infarct size by preventing platelet aggregation and possible reocclusion.[51] Other indications for antithrombotic therapy after myocardial infarction include prevention of embolic stroke and secondary prevention of recurrent MI and death.[32] As with all antithrombotic agents, the most common adverse effect is bleeding.

Aspirin

Aspirin is an antiplatelet agent that is able to inhibit the platelet-aggregating substance thromboxae A_2.[53] The Physicians' Health Study showed a 44 percent reduction in risk of first MI in the aspirin-treated group (325 mg every other day); there was, however, an increase in the rate of hemorrhagic stroke. The current recommendation for prevention of MI with aspirin is to treat patients on an individual basis. A dose of 160 to 325 mg a day should be considered for those patients with cardiovascular risk factors.[51] Another major trial (ISIS-2 [Second International Study of Infarct Survival]) showed that aspirin alone reduced vascular mortality, nonfatal reinfarction and stroke rates. Whether thrombolytic therapy is administered or not, all eligible patients with acute MI should immediately receive nonenteric coated aspirin (160 to 325 mg) followed by daily doses. If patients receive heparin, aspirin may be given concomitantly; it should not, however, be given concurrently with warfarin.[42] With unstable angina and after MI, aspirin (325 mg daily) has demonstrated a preventive effect for further coronary or cerebrovascular events.[51]

Ticlopidine

Ticlopidine (Ticlid) is one of the more recent antiplatelet agents to be approved by the Food and Drug Administration (FDA) for prevention of thrombotic stroke. This drug is a more potent platelet inhibitor than aspirin and is known to inhibit the formation of arterial thrombi. Ticlopidine is an alternative agent for those patients who cannot tolerate aspirin. Clinical trials indicate that ticlopidine may be more effective than aspirin in reducing the occurrence of stroke and myocardial infarction.[54] Like aspirin, ticlopidine is also effective in unstable angina, PTCA, coronary artery bypass graft surgery, and cerebrovascular disease. In patients who have had stent placement during PTCA, ticlopidine is used long term along *with* aspirin. The usual dosage of ticlopidine is 250 mg twice daily. The most significant side effects are bleeding, diarrhea, rash, and reversible neutropenia, the last occurring in about 2 percent of patients.[53,54]

Heparin

Following an MI, the antithrombotic effects of heparin, an IV anticoagulant, are beneficial in acute MI in preventing further thrombosis and reducing thrombotic complications (mural thrombi, deep vein thrombosis, and pulmonary embolism). Other indications for heparin include its use as adjunctive therapy in patients with acute MI, unstable angina, and after interventional cardiology procedures.[51] In addition, early initiation of heparin after TPA (within 60 to 90 minutes) is important to maintain early coronary artery patency.[55] Heparin accelerates the formation of antithrombin III-thrombin complex and prevents conversion of fibrinogen to fibrin by deactivating thrombin.[18] Standard dosage is an initial bolus loading dose (5,000 to 10,000 units) followed by a continuous IV infusion (15 to 20 units/kg per hour). The dose is titrated by frequent monitoring of the blood lab test called activated partial thromboplastin time (APTT).[53]

Recent clinical trials are evaluating another antithrombotic agent called hirudin, which is derived from the saliva of the medicinal leech. Data from the TIMI-5 (Thrombolysis in Myocardial Ischemia phase 5) study indicated that hirudin had advantages over heparin and aspirin in reducing reocclusion rates in patients with acute MI treated with thrombolytics without an increase in bleeding.[51]

Abciximab

A recently approved and genetically engineered antithrombotic agent is abciximab (ReoPro). This drug inhibits platelet aggregation and is used to decrease ischemic complications in patients after PTCA or atherectomy. A specific indication for this drug is prevention of abrupt coronary vessel closure in patients who are at high risk after PTCA. The recommended dosage is an IV bolus of 0.25 mg/kg given within an hour before the interventional procedure, followed by a continuous infusion of 10 µg/min for about 12 hours. Heparin and aspirin are also given concurrently with abciximab. The most common complication to this drug is bleeding, which in rare circumstances may include intracranial hemorrhage. Other side effects include hypotension, bradycardia, nausea, and vomiting, and pain in the extremities. Contraindications to this agent are similar to those for thrombolytic drugs.[56]

Warfarin

Warfarin (Coumadin) is an oral anticoagulant that inhibits vitamin K-dependent activation of clotting factors formed in the liver.[10] Warfarin reduces the risk for systemic or cerebral embolism in the following conditions: left ventricular thrombosis, atrial fibrillation, mechanical prosthetic cardiac valves, venous thrombosis, and after acute MI.[53] The usual daily dose of coumadin is 2 to 10 mg with dosage dependent on patient response and results of the blood test prothrombin time (PT).[18,53] For patients at increased risk for systemic or pulmonary embolism after AMI, warfarin is frequently initiated before discontinuation of heparin therapy and maintained for up to 3 months.[42]

Antithrombotic Therapy Management

Careful attention should be given to the following:

1. Instruct patients to monitor self for bleeding and notify physician for bleeding gums, nosebleeds, bruises on arms or legs, petechiae, GI bleeding, hematuria.
2. Advise patients to take aspirin, if recommended by their physicians, or ticlopidine with food or milk to reduce GI side effects.
3. Advise patients to avoid aspirin-containing products and check with physician before taking any over-the-counter medications. (An exception to this are individuals who have had a stent placement; they are frequently on both aspirin and ticlopidine.)
4. Advise patients to tell all physicians and dentists that they are on antithrombotic drugs.
5. Inform patients of foods rich in vitamin K and their interactions with warfarin. A high intake of alcohol and foods rich in vitamin K (such as leafy green vegetables) inhibit warfarin's anticoagulant effect.[57]

MEDICAL AND SURGICAL INTERVENTION IN CORONARY ARTERY DISEASE

Medical and surgical interventional procedures in CAD do not alter the atherosclerotic disease process. However, they improve the quality of life by relieving the symptoms of CAD (angina) and restoring myocardial perfusion. Both types of intervention help to improve the individual's tolerance for activity. Coronary artery disease is treated medically with interventional techniques used both acutely and electively to alter structural changes contributing to coronary stenosis. These interventional procedures include PTCA, laser angioplasty, directional coronary atherectomy, and coronary stents. Surgical intervention incorporates myocardial revascularization by coronary artery bypass grafting or heart transplant.

Percutaneous Transluminal Coronary Angioplasty

PTCA, also referred to as balloon angioplasty, is an invasive but nonsurgical procedure used to dilate coronary arteries (Fig. 7–1). First performed in 1977 by Dr. Andreas Gruentzig, PTCA is now considered an adjunct to medical therapy for CAD and an alternative to coronary artery bypass graft (CABG) surgery. Initially, PTCA was performed for discrete, proximal, noncalcific, subtotal lesions that were evident in a single coronary artery. With advanced technology, the procedure has experienced rapid growth. Smaller balloon designs, steerable guide wires, and more advanced skill on the part of the practitioners have advanced this technique so that it can be used to

CORONARY ANGIOPLASTY

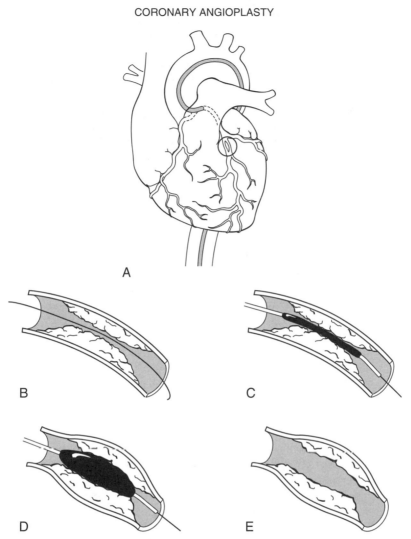

FIGURE 7–1. Intracoronary balloon angioplasty. *A*, A balloon catheter is inserted into the coronary artery through a guide catheter in the aorta. *B*, A guide wire is advanced through the area of narrowing. *C*, The balloon catheter is placed over the wire across the lesion. *D*, The balloon is inflated. *E*, Coronary artery after dilation. (From Schneider USA, Inc., Minneapolis, MN, with permission.)

treat multiple lesions almost anywhere in the coronary circulation.[6] Other methods that have been developed to expand the field of coronary intervention include atherectomy, lasers, and stents.[58]

Before performing a PTCA, coronary arteriography with a cardiac catheterization is required to evaluate coronary artery anatomy and the location of the stenotic lesions. Under fluoroscopy, a small balloon-tipped catheter is inserted via the femoral artery and advanced in a retrograde fashion to the coronary arteries. The catheter is advanced across the identified stenotic area and the balloon is inflated. Balloon inflation pressure is measured in pounds per square inch (psi) or in atmospheres (atm). The inflations usually last 1 to 3 minutes, with the average initial inflation between 60 to 80 psi or 4 to 6 atm. With the advent of perfusion catheters that can both dilate and perfuse at the same time, longer balloon inflations of up to 30 minutes can be safely performed. The benefit of longer balloon inflations is that they promote smoother and more regular vessel walls. Long inflations have often been used for treatment of major dissections or abrupt closure.[6] It was originally thought that balloon angioplasty compressed the soft noncalcified plaque into the intima of the coronary artery; more recent studies, however, reveal two hypotheses that explain immediate and long-term effects. The primary mechanism is intimal disruption or a controlled intimal tear with a secondary mechanism of stretching of the vascular media and adventitia, resulting in a localized ballooning or aneurysm formation.[6,59]

PTCA is performed only in patients who have at least a 50 percent or greater narrowing of the coronary artery. Individuals with complex coronary anatomy, multivessel lesions, post-CABG and bifurcated lesions have been successfully treated with PTCA. Individuals with total occlusions who have adequate resting collateral circulation but who cannot tolerate physical activity without developing anginal symptoms can also benefit from PTCA. Angioplasty is also being used in the acute treatment of unstable angina refractory to medical therapy and in conjunction with thrombolytic therapy in an AMI to recanalize the occluded vessels and prevent rethrombosis and reocclusion. Primary PTCA is a term used when performing an emergent PTCA (without prior thrombolytic therapy) for AMI. Rescue (or direct) PTCA is done after thrombolytic therapy for individuals with ongoing myocardial ischemia caused by a persistently occluded infarct-related artery. Patients with AMI complicated by cardiogenic shock have shown increased survival with direct PTCA as compared to conventional medical and thrombolytic therapy.[6,60]

The success of PTCA procedures ranges from 80 to 95 percent and is defined as a 40 to 50 percent reduction in stenosis of the luminal diameter with clinical improvement and no significant complications.[6] In-hospital mortality rate with PTCA is about 1 percent; mortality rate after 2 to 3 years is about 6 to 7 percent.[61] After the procedure, the individual is observed in a specialized care unit for 24 to 48 hours for any sign of arterial reocclusion or other complications. Patients usually remain on bed rest for 4 to 8 hours after femoral sheath removal to avoid any postprocedure bleeding.[62] Upon discharge, individuals generally have minimal activity restrictions and often return to work within 6 weeks after the procedure. McGee and colleagues[63] found that return to work rates were similar in patients who had either CABG surgery or coronary angioplasty (59 and 68 percent, respectively).

Contraindications to PTCA include absence of a significant lesion, multivessel diffuse disease in which CABG would be of more benefit, and left main disease of the left coronary artery (LCA) without the benefit of a prior patent bypass graft. The latter contraindication for PTCA is necessary because patients with left main disease are at risk for severe left ventricular dysfunction if abrupt closure or spasm of the LCA occurs.[50] High-risk patients may be able to undergo PTCA if supported with adjunct devices such as intra-aortic balloon pumping (IABP) or cardiopulmonary support (CPS).[6]

Complications during and immediately following PTCA include acute occlusion of the coronary artery by spasm, clot, or collapse, coronary artery dissection, MI, bleeding at the arterial puncture site, internal hemorrhage from systemic anticoagulation, and compromise of the circulation distal to the catheter insertion site. Immediate open-heart surgery may be necessary if there is significant coronary artery dissection.[6] Increasingly, dissections are being treated with placement of a coronary stent.

PTCA results in improved myocardial blood flow, and individuals have reported immediate relief of their anginal pain while experiencing minimal interventional discomfort. It should be emphasized that PTCA does not change or arrest the atherosclerotic process and that appropriate risk reduction techniques must be encouraged. Long-term efficacy of PTCA is limited by the problem of restenosis of the dilated coronary artery. Restenosis occurs in 25 to 50 percent of individuals, usually within the first 2 to 6 months after PTCA. The mechanism for restenosis is not fully understood but is believed to be caused by an "excessive healing" response by the dilated artery called fibrocellular intimal proliferation. This fibrocellular process causes migration, proliferation, and modification of the smooth muscle cells of the media, resulting in a narrowed vessel lumen. Restenosis is usually seen as a return of stable anginal symptoms, indicating slow progression of the restenotic process. Some of the predictors for restenosis are recent onset of angina, unstable angina, variant angina, diabetes mellitus, proximal LAD lesions, and multivessel disease. Innovative interventions for restenosis include repeat angioplasty, directional coronary atherectomy, laser angioplasty, and stent placement.[6,58]

Directional Coronary Atherectomy

Directional coronary atherectomy (DCA) is an interventional procedure designed to enlarge a coronary artery by excising and removing atheromatous plaque from the vessel walls.[65] This procedure can be used in conjunction with balloon angioplasty. A variety of devices have been developed, with one device having a cutter that, when activated, moves forward within the vessel and shaves the atherosclerotic lesion, collecting it into a nose cone. Another device uses high-speed rotation of a metal burr that pulverizes the plaque and allows minute particles to pass distally into the circulation.[64,66] The DCA procedure provides an alternative approach for stenotic lesions such as eccentric and ostial LAD lesions that are unable to be dilated by conventional angioplasty. The goal of atherectomy is a residual stenosis of less than 30 percent with a success rate reported at 85 to 90 percent.[64] The proposed benefits of DCA are smoother vessel wall lumens, ability to approach more difficult lesions that are anatomically unsuitable for PTCA, and reduction in abrupt vessel reclosure.[65]

Laser Angioplasty

Another interventional procedure developed as an alternative or adjunct to PTCA is laser angioplasty. The word laser is an acronym for "light amplification through stimulated emission of radiation." Lasers are devices that produce a monochromatic beam light. They became more widely used in the 1980s with the success of PTCA and the advancement of fiberoptic technology. Laser angioplasty is recommended for lesions that are long and diffuse, have an ostial location, are extremely calcified, are located in vein grafts, or are totally occluded.[67] Because of the different attributes of various laser devices, there are several techniques of laser angioplasty. The basic mechanism of laser angioplasty, however, is to deliver high temperatures to vascular tissue for the purpose of smoothing vessel wall irregularities, securing intimal dissections that may have occurred from standard PTCA or inhibiting the elastic recoil that can occur with balloon deflation.[66] The risks involved with laser angioplasty include blood clots, vessel perforation, intimal dissections, aneurysm, and thermal damage to the vessel wall.[67] With the advent of coronary stents, the use of laser angioplasty has decreased.

Coronary Stents

The primary goal of coronary stents is to prevent elastic recoil and enhance the mechanical dilation caused by balloon angioplasty. Coronary stenting was initially used as a "bailout procedure" for the complication of abrupt closure of the coronary vessel immediately after balloon deflation during a PTCA or atherectomy. Before the availability of coronary stents, patients with abrupt closure required emergency CABG surgery.[68] First used in 1987, coronary stents are rapidly becoming the intervention of choice to reduce the risk of abrupt closure and improve the long-term patency rates.[69] Developed by a variety of companies, coronary stents are usually made of wire mesh that is self-expanding or balloon-expandable (Fig. 7–2).[70] Stents are deployed during balloon angioplasty; they act as a "scaffold," maintaining intraluminal structure and

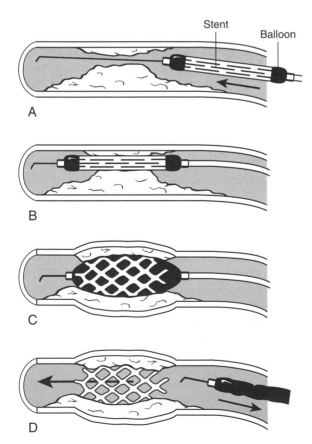

FIGURE 7–2. A coronary stent placed inside the coronary artery. *A,* To place a stent within a vessel narrowing, a special catheter is used that has a deflated balloon and the stent at the tip. *B,* The catheter is positioned so that the stent is within the narrowed region of the coronary artery. *C,* The balloon is inflated, causing the stent to expand and stretch the artery. *D,* The catheter is then withdrawn, leaving the stent behind to keep the artery open. (From Dracup,[31] with permission.)

patency by limiting formation of blood clots and reducing blood flow alterations.[69] The success of coronary artery stents is dependent on minimal thrombosis followed by rapid development of endothelialization (within days) over a thin layer of fibrin and thrombus. Early complications that can occur from coronary stents include acute thrombosis and reocclusion; intimal hyperplasia is a later complication. Therefore, anticoagulation and/or antiplatelet therapy is initiated both before and up to 6 weeks after the procedure to control thrombus formation. Patient education is essential because patients may be on any combination of heparin, aspirin, warfarin, or ticlopidine.[68-70]

Coronary Artery Bypass Grafting

CABG is surgical revascularization of the myocardium performed primarily to relieve anginal symptoms and improve survival.[71] Revascularization is commonly established by using either a saphenous vein graft (SVG) or internal mammary artery (IMA) graft (Fig. 7–3). One or both of the following methods are commonly used: (1) anastomosing grafts, usually the individual's own saphenous vein (SVG), to the aortic root and to the coronary artery distal to the stenosis, and/or (2) direct revascularization by anastomosing the distal end of the right or left internal mammary artery (RIMA or LIMA) to the coronary artery distal to the lesion. The IMA grafts have demonstrated excellent early and late graft patency rates compared with saphenous vein grafts. Patency rates of IMA grafts have approached 96 percent at 10 years after surgery com-

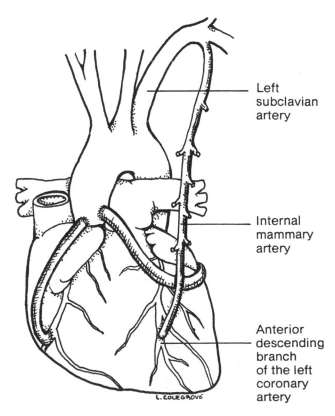

Left
subclavian
artery

Internal
mammary
artery

Anterior
descending
branch
of the left
coronary
artery

FIGURE 7–3. Coronary artery bypass graft using the SVG and IMA.

L. COLEGROVE

pared with 81 percent patency of saphenous vein grafts.[72,73] In many medical centers, 15 to 20 percent of CABG surgeries are reoperations, frequently secondary to graft failure. The risk of intraoperative mortality increases with a second CABG surgery.[71]

About a month after surgery, the wall of the saphenous vein graft begins to show progressive intimal proliferation and can cause graft failure within the first year. By 10 years, 44 percent of saphenous vein grafts reveal atherosclerosis.[71] In contrast, the IMA graft rarely develops atherosclerosis and does not develop intimal hyperplasia.[74] Because of its superior long-term patency, a left IMA is frequently used to bypass the left anterior descending (LAD) branch of the left coronary artery. The right IMA is used to bypass the right coronary artery (RCA), the posterior descending branch of the RCA, or the circumflex branch of the left coronary artery (LCA). A disadvantage of using the IMA is that it is limited by its length and anatomic position, is more difficult to dissect from the chest wall, and may extend the length of surgery. Postoperatively, patients may have persistent chest pain for many weeks.[72-74]

Alternative conduits include cephalic or basilic veins harvested from the arms or the gastroepiploic (GEA) artery from the abdomen. Vessels from the arm are not favored because they have a small caliber and tendency for increased aneurysm formation. Harvesting the GEA extends the length of surgery and requires opening the abdominal cavity.[73,75]

There are many indications for CABG surgery with criteria for patient selection varying among institutions. The use of CABG surgery is changing as PTCA has become increasingly more popular as an alternative intervention for select patient populations. Angioplasty allows patients with single or multiple high-grade lesions to undergo a less traumatic procedure to relieve coronary artery occlusion. The criteria for patient selection for CABG generally include[73,74]:

1. Left main coronary artery stenosis greater than 50 percent
2. Severe triple vessel coronary disease
3. Two-vessel CAD with left ventricular dysfunction
4. Chronic stable angina unresponsive to medical therapy
5. Unstable angina
6. Emergency surgery after acute MI for residual high-grade stenosis after thrombolysis, postinfarction angina, or complications of ventricular septal defect or papillary muscle rupture

When evaluating the need for surgical intervention, consider the location and degree of stenosis caused by the lesion, the amount of myocardium served by the affected artery, and whether the individual has had a previous myocardial infarction.[73]

Individuals are evaluated for surgery on the basis of their presenting symptoms, the coexistence of other chronic disease, and a battery of medical tests. The tests include blood studies, pulmonary function studies (for patients with COPD), ECGs, and, most importantly, coronary arteriography and a left ventriculogram. During coronary arteriography, contrast material is injected under fluoroscopy which allows direct visualization of coronary lesions and assessment of the coronary circulation distal to the obstruction. The cardiologist and the surgeon view the films and determine if bypassing the lesion will permit effective revascularization or if the disease process is so diffuse that grafting would have little value. The ventriculogram allows for visualization of the left ventricular function, wall motion abnormalities such as akinesis (immobile segments) or dyskinesis (paradoxical wall motion), heart valve defects, septal defects, or ventricular aneurysms. In addition, a ventriculogram allows measurement of pressures in the heart chambers, all of which provide vital information regarding the heart's effectiveness as a pump.[76]

In CABG surgery, with the patient under anesthesia, a median sternotomy is performed. This allows direct visualization of the heart. The circulation is supported by means of an extracorporeal oxygenation pump (cardiopulmonary bypass pump) that allows the blood to bypass the heart, become oxygenated, and then flow to the systemic circulation. To decrease metabolic demands during surgery, the patient's core body temperature is lowered during bypass to approximately 28 to 32°C. After the aorta is cross-clamped, the heart is put into asystole by administration of a cold, potassium-concentrated solution (cardioplegia) injected into the aortic root. The motionless heart allows the surgery to be performed more easily. Following the procedure, the heart is rewarmed and the blood is again circulated through it. The heartbeat either begins spontaneously or is initiated by means of internal defibrillation or cardiac pacing.[72,75]

In the 1980s, operative mortality was about 1 percent. Improvements in surgical techniques, coronary bypass pumps, cardioplegia, and myocardial preservation have decreased perioperative morbidity and mortality. The same improvements have safely allowed extended operative time to do more complete revascularizations. Despite these improvements, operative mortality rates have been up to 3 percent in the 1990s. The possible reasons for this increase in mortality may be the expansion of interventional cardiology and improved medical therapy, resulting in patients who are referred for CABG being older and having more chronic illnesses and more extensive coronary artery disease.[73] Elderly patients are increasingly undergoing CABG surgery, and in 1990 7.4 million patients over the age of 80 years underwent this surgery.[74] Postoperative complications include bleeding, alterations in blood pressure, cardiac arrhythmias, fluid and electrolyte imbalances, hemodynamic instability, pulmonary dysfunction, renal dysfunction, neurologic events, and infection.[72]

Following uncomplicated CABG surgery, individuals recover rapidly. Patients are frequently transferred out of the intensive care unit 18 to 24 hours after surgery. Before transfer, patients usually are given inpatient rehabilitation (see Chapter 1), which begins with the patient sitting on the side of the bed. This low-level activity is followed by allowing the patient to sit in a chair. Ambulation in the hallways usually occurs at time of transfer to the step-down unit, with discharge to home as early as 4 to 7 days after surgery. Cardiac rehabilitation often begins within the first 24 hours and includes in-hospital ambulation, exercises, and education followed by participation in a formal cardiac rehabilitation program after discharge (Chapter 1). A walking program is advised for those patients who are not involved with a formal outpatient cardiac rehabilitation program. Activities, particularly lifting, are restricted for 6 weeks to 3 months. Return to work is usually dictated by the patient's occupation, rate of recuperation, and duration of unemployment before surgery. Postoperative congestive heart failure, recurrence of angina, or arrhythmias may delay the return to work for some individuals. Return-to-work rates are lower in individuals who had a long period between preoperative work and surgery or are of older age or lower educational level. Depression and transient cognitive deficits are common after CABG and usually resolve in 6 to 8 weeks after surgery.[77]

CABG surgery has been shown to increase survival for patients with greater than 70 percent stenosis of the left main coronary artery and chronic, stable angina. Several large clinical trials have clarified indications for CABG and evaluated long-term survival. The Coronary Artery Surgery Study (CASS) compared the clinical efficacy of medical management with surgical management. This study randomized patients less than 65 years old with exertional angina who had greater than 70 percent stenosis of at least one vessel to either CABG surgery or medical therapy. At 7 years of follow-up, the CASS group showed an 88 percent survival in the surgical group as compared with a 65 percent survival in the medically treated group. In addition, CASS demonstrated that the patients also had a 20 to 50 percent increase in peak exercise performance following surgery.[74]

Other clinical trials agree that patients with severe angina unresponsive to medical therapy gain benefit from surgery as demonstrated by greater relief of symptoms and reduced need for antianginal drugs.[74] Jenkins and colleagues[76] quantified and predicted recovery after CABG surgery based on frequency of preoperative measures. Absence of cardiac symptoms 6 months after surgery correlated with decreased levels of many preoperative variables. The six most significant variables were shortness of breath, sleeping difficulties, lifetime use of cigarettes, preoperative hospitalization for cardiac care, anxiety, and social support. The Bypass Angioplasty Revascularization Investigation (BARI) study assigned 1829 patients with multivessel CAD to either PTCA or CABG surgery. These patients were followed for 5 years and preliminary results revealed that 5-year survival rates were similar for CABG and PTCA. Patients in the PTCA group, however, required subsequent revascularization (repeat PTCA). In addition, diabetic patients appeared to have a lower mortality risk with CABG surgery.[78]

It is important to remember that CABG surgery does not cure coronary artery disease; rigorous risk factor modification (specifically of hyperlipidemia and smoking) is required to deter progression of the disease process.[79]

Coronary Artery Bypass Graft Surgery Without Cardiopulmonary Bypass

A new surgical technique, direct coronary artery bypass surgery without cardiopulmonary bypass, is being explored as a possible alternative to conventional CABG surgery. Adapting the technology of laparoscopy and thoracoscopy, this surgical technique is able to bypass the LAD or RCA using an SVG or IMA without the need for cardiopulmonary bypass. Intravenous beta blockade is used to slow the rate of the beating heart and decrease myocardial oxygen consumption.[80] Benetti and colleagues[81] performed this surgery on 32 patients with acute myocardial infarction. There were no in-hospital deaths, with follow-up at 5 years revealing a 97 percent survival rate, 90.4 percent freedom of symptoms, and 96.9 percent freedom of reoperation. Potential advantages of this procedure include minimal surgical intervention, reduction of postoperative morbidity, and decreased hospital stay.[82]

Heart Transplantation

Heart transplantation is now the treatment of choice in end-stage myocardial disease in which the left ventricular ejection fraction is less than 20 percent, medical therapies are ineffective, and the patient's prognosis for survival is 6 to 12 months without transplantation.[83] The underlying disease processes are idiopathic, viral, or valvular cardiomyopathy, and ischemic heart disease.[73] Patient selection is done carefully because the surgery and postoperative management are complex and the risk is high. The maximum and minimum age limit varies according to each transplant center. Physiologic age of the patient is more important; the customary trend is for the upper age limit to be between 60 and 65 years.[73,83] Patients should also be free of donor-specific antibodies, irreversible hepatic or renal dysfunction, active infection, active peptic ulcer disease, and advanced peripheral and cerebral vascular disease.[72] In addition, patients should be emotionally stable, compliant with medical regimen, and have a strong psychosocial support system.[83] Some centers are beginning to accept patients with mild diabetes and patients with nonmetastatic cancer who are considered cured. In addition, the transplant recipient should not have irreversible pulmonary hypertension (greater than 6 to 8 Wood units or greater than 480 to 640 dynes/sec/cm^{-}5)[72] because this may cause right ventricular failure in the transplanted heart.[73] The recipient and donor must be comparable in body size and weight and have identical ABO blood groups.[72]

Transplantation is performed through a median sternotomy. The heart is removed, leaving the atrial posterior walls, the two venae cavae and pulmonary veins intact. The recipient's heart is removed while he or she is maintained on cardiopulmonary bypass. The donor heart is then anastomosed in the appropriate anatomical position.[73]

The two major postoperative complications are rejection and infection. Rejection of the transplanted heart is activated by antigens located on the surface of the cells of the transplanted heart.[73] Immunosuppressive therapy is used to minimize rejection and protective isolation is used to minimize the risk of infection. Ongoing improvements in immunosuppressive therapy is used to minimize rejection and protective isolation is used to minimize the risk of infection. Ongoing improvements in immunosuppressive therapy and the advent of transvenous endomyocardial biopsy have allowed early and more aggressive treatment of acute rejection. Acute rejection takes place within the first 3 months after surgery and is cell-mediated; this asymptomatic rejection is life threatening and may require retransplantation. Chronic rejection occurs from 3 months to years after transplantation and is caused by immune-mediated damage to the coronary arteries resulting in ischemic myocardial damage and loss of heart function. The clinical manifestations are the same as with CAD except that with a denervated heart there is no chest pain. A decrease in exercise tolerance during stress testing and coronary angiography assist in diagnosis.[72,73] Because the lesions are usually diffuse, bypass surgery or angioplasty are rarely appropriate. Retransplant is the only definitive treatment. In the first 3 months after transplantation, infection (commonly in the lungs) is a major cause of morbidity and mortality secondary to immunosuppressive therapy. Early detection is essential to prevent morbidity and mortality.[72] The survival rate at the end of 1 year is greater than 90 percent and at the end of 10 years is 72 percent.[72,73]

Rehabilitation is an important adjunct to medical therapy after transplant, and in some centers is a mandatory component of the pretransplant contract. Although the heart itself is healthy, the individual benefits from a prudent cardiac lifestyle. Rehabilitation is similar to that of any patient with CAD except for the heart's response to exercise. The response of the denervated heart is very different from that of the normal heart. Transplanted hearts depend on circulating catecholamines to increase heart rate, contractility, and cardiac output. With the cessation of exercise, the heart rate gradually returns to baseline as the plasma catecholamine levels decrease. Because of this lack of heart rate response to exercise, patients are taught to use perception of dyspnea as a guide for activity intensity.[73] Regular exercise programs are beneficial for increasing collateral circulation and counteracting the side effects of corticosteroids (weight gain and bone loss).[73]

The lack of available donor organs has been the impetus for development of other surgical techniques for severe congestive heart failure and cardiomyopathy; one such technique is cardiac myoplasty.

Dynamic Cardiac Myoplasty

Dynamic cardiac myoplasty is a surgical technique, approved for clinical trial by the FDA, in which the patient's left or right latissimus dorsi muscle is wrapped around the failing ventricle to augment left ventricular function (Fig. 7–4).[84,85] First developed in 1985 by Carpentier and Chachques, dynamic myoplasty involves surgical dissection of the native latissimus muscle while preserving the integrity of the neurovascular pedicle.[86] Exposure of the heart is then done through a median sternotomy and the muscle flap is wrapped around the ventricle. Muscle stimulation of the latissimus dorsi muscle is achieved by placing stimulating electrodes at the thoracodorsal nerve; these electrodes are then connected to a myostimulator. This device is placed in a small pocket in the rectus abdominal muscle.[85] Cardiac dynamic myoplasty is not considered a bridge to transplant but instead is used as a primary intervention for severe congestive heart failure, although subsequent heart transplantation may be necessary.[87] Indications for dynamic myoplasty are dilated or ischemic cardiomyopathy. Criteria for patient selection includes a diagnosis of New York Heart Association (NYHA) Functional Class III or IV cardiac disease, an age of 18 to 80 years, a left ventricular ejection fraction between 15 to 40 percent, and functional neuromuscular, hepatic, renal and pulmonary systems.[84] Patients are excluded from consideration if they have an extremely dilated ventricle, mitral insufficiency, refractory arrhythmias, severe biventric-

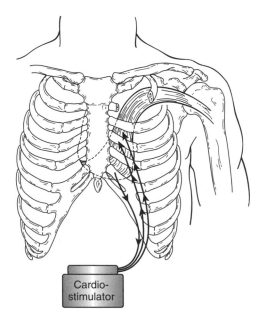

Cardio-stimulator

FIGURE 7–4. Completed dynamic cardiomyoplasty procedure with the cardiomyostimulator intact. (From Dimengo, JM,[88] with permission.)

ular failure, pulmonary hypertension with high lung pressures, severe renal failure, or an implanted pacemaker.[85] A frequent complication of this procedure is formation of subcutaneous seroma at the area of muscle dissection.[86] A potentially serious postoperative complication is ischemic and bacterial myonecrosis of the latissimus muscle flap. Although rare, this complication is associated with a high mortality rate.[88]

Stimulation of the latissimus dorsi muscle by a cardiomyostimulator is initiated 2 weeks after surgery. This time delay allows the latissimus dorsi muscle to adhere to the myocardium and promote the development of collateral circulation. The stimulator has both pacing and sensing electrodes that synchronize with myocardial contraction. Electrical stimulation of the muscle is continued over a 7-week period[85]; patients have reported no discomfort with the actual stimulation and conditioning process.[86] A slow progression of graded stimulation is required to transform the easily fatigued skeletal muscle (latissimus dorsi) into fatigue-resistant muscle.[88] Therapeutic hemodynamic benefits of cardiomyoplasty are not apparent until about 6 to 8 weeks after surgery. Cardiac rehabilitation of these patients should be initiated slowly and at a low intensity. Benefits of this procedure include improved LV function, improved ejection fraction, augmented systolic function, decreased ventricular stroke work, diminished pulmonary pressures, and reduced myocardial oxygen consumption.[84] Improvements continue over 6 to 12 months after surgery, which has been attributed to a phenomenon called "conformation change." This change is manifested by an adaptation of the flap so that it becomes another layer of the myocardium.[86]

One-year survival rates are better in patients with NYHA class III than patients with class IV heart disease.[84] In 1991, Magovern and associates reported a 47 percent 5-year survival rate. Future considerations include changes in wrap techniques and utilization of graft material to create a new ventricle.[85]

Heart-Lung Transplant

Patients with irreversible, disabling end-stage cardiopulmonary and pulmonary disease are candidates for heart-lung transplantation. This includes such diseases as primary or secondary pulmonary hypertension, bronchiectasis, and cystic fibrosis.[89,90]

The criteria for patient selection are essentially the same as for heart transplant. Absolute contraindications to a heart-lung transplant also include active pulmonary infection, cachexia, obesity, and continued cigarette smoking. In addition, relative contraindications include preoperative corticosteroid therapy because these drugs may cause early postoperative tracheal and bronchial dehiscence, and previous cardiothoracic surgery because the presence of pleural adhesions increases the risk of bleeding.[89] The patients suffer from the same set of problems as heart transplant patients because of similar long-term immunosuppressive therapy. In addition, three problems are specific to the lung transplant patients: (1) problems with the healing of the tracheal anastomosis site, (2) reversible pulmonary gas exchange deficit similar to pulmonary edema, and (3) obliterate bronchiolitis (OB), a major long-term complication and possibly the pulmonary equivalent of late chronic rejection in the heart. Characteristics of obliterative bronchiolitis include bronchitic symptoms followed by early appearance of dyspnea, severe obstructive and restrictive disease, and decreased total lung capacity. Obliterative bronchiolitis seems to be caused by infection, primarily by cytomegalovirus and adenovirus. Retransplantation is the primary intervention for end-stage obliterative bronchiolitis but has a high risk for complications.[90] One-year survival for heart-lung transplantation is about 57 percent. As with heart transplantation, a major limitation of heart-lung transplants is the availability of donor organs.[89]

CARDIAC REHABILITATION
AND CORONARY ARTERY DISEASE

Cardiac rehabilitation has been described as "the process of development and maintenance of a desirable level of physical, social, and psychologic functioning after the onset of a cardiovascular illness."[91] After a myocardial infarction or revascularization procedures, cardiac rehabilitation for the patient frequently begins in the acute care setting and may continue for 6 months to 1 year after discharge. Cardiac rehabilitation is an important adjunctive therapy in both the medical and surgical management of CAD and a mandatory adjunct after transplant. Medical and surgical interventions are designed to relieve the symptoms an individual experiences as a result of atherosclerosis. They do not alter the cause or the progression of the atherosclerotic process unless CAD patients concurrently recognize their risk factors and modify their lifestyles to reduce risk. With a suitable exercise prescription, intense education, and appropriate professional support, individuals are able to make and maintain specific changes in their lifestyles in the general areas of diet, exercise, stress management, and compliance with medical therapy in order to reduce their own cardiac risk factors.[92,93]

PHARMACOLOGIC MANAGEMENT OF
PULMONARY DISEASE

Pharmacologic management of chronic pulmonary disease includes a variety of drugs specifically used to optimize the ventilatory capacity of the respiratory system. The goal is to maximize the patient's functional abilities while minimizing the drug's possible side effects. The three major categories of these drugs are bronchodilators, anti-inflammatory agents, and cromolyn sodium.

Bronchodilators

There are neural and chemical influences on the contractile property of the bronchial smooth muscle. Neural control is mediated by the autonomic nervous system (ANS). Both sympathetic (adrenergic) and parasympathetic (cholinergic) receptors have been identified in the bronchial smooth muscle. These two branches of the ANS have antagonistic effects over the size of the airway lumen.

Stimulation of the sympathetic portion of the ANS causes relaxation of the bronchial smooth muscle, which results in bronchodilation. The postganglionic $beta_2$-adrenergic receptors of the sympathetic nervous system release the chemical norepinephrine, which results in an increased amount of cyclic adenosine 3'5' monophosphate (cAMP). An increase in cAMP is associated with bronchial smooth muscle relaxation.[94]

Stimulation of the parasympathetic system results in bronchoconstriction. The postganglionic cholinergic receptors of the parasympathetic nervous system release the chemical acetylecholine, which increases the level of cyclic 3'5' guanosine monophosphate (cGMP). An increase in cGMP is associated with contraction of the bronchial smooth muscle.[95]

The parasympathetic nervous system innervates the bronchial smooth muscle, and the sympathetic system indirectly affects the bronchial smooth muscle. The airways normally demonstrate intrinsic tone, suggesting that parasympathetic control is more dominant.[96]

Bronchospasm occurs when there is a greater than normal contraction of the bronchial smooth muscle. Pharmacologic therapy of chronic obstructive pulmonary disease is directed toward relieving the bronchospasm.[97] Pharmacologic enhancement of bronchodilation can be accomplished by stimulating the sympathetic nervous system to promote the relaxation of the bronchial smooth muscle or by blocking the influence of the parasympathetic nervous system, which also will promote relaxation of the bronchial smooth muscle. The drugs that assist the sympathetic nervous system are of two types: sympathomimetics and methylxanthines. The drugs that block the parasympathetic nervous system are called anticholinergics.

SYMPATHOMIMETICS

Actions and Uses

Sympathomimetic drugs are the most widely used first-line agents in the management of obstructive pulmonary disorders.[97] Sympathomimetics mimic the action of the sympathetic nervous system and stimulate the beta$_2$ receptors of the bronchial smooth muscle. This increases the activity of the enzyme adenyl cyclase, which causes adenosine 5'-triphosphate (ATP) to be converted to cAMP. Sympathomimetics, also called beta-adrenergic agonists, produce relaxation of the bronchial smooth muscle by increasing the amount of cAMP.

Contraindications and Side Effects

The side effects of sympathomimetics depend on the drugs' selectivity of beta$_2$ receptors and the route of administration. As indicated earlier in the section on cardiac beta-blocking agents, there are beta$_1$ and beta$_2$ receptor sites in the heart and lungs. Stimulation of beta$_1$ receptors affects cardiac parameters, whereas stimulation of beta receptors is responsible for alterations in the pulmonary system. The more beta$_2$ selective a drug is, the fewer cardiac side effects are observed. The ingestion of sympathomimetics, especially the nonselective sympathomimetics, produces the systemic side effects of tachycardia, palpitations, angina, GI distress, nervousness, muscle tremor, headache, dizziness, anxiety, sweating, and insomnia. Inhaled beta-adrenergic agonists may cause bronchial irritation with prolonged use but minimize the systemic side effects. The metered dose inhaler (MDI), with its ability to deliver sympathomimetics topically with minimal side effects, has gained acceptance as the best route for administration of sympathomimetic drugs.[97]

The cardiovascular side effects are the most dangerous of the reactions. Caution should be exercised in older patients, particularly those with hypertension, diabetes, and CAD.[98] Patients with hypoxemia from their pulmonary disease or those with an irritable myocardium from associated heart disease are at higher risk for tachycardia, arrhythmias, angina, and myocardial necrosis.[94]

Effects of Sympathomimetics on Exercise in Individuals with Pulmonary Disease

There is often an elevated resting heart rate in patients who are taking systemic sympathomimetics. By using the Karvonen formula for calculation of target heart rate

(THR), this heart rate elevation is taken into consideration. When a heart rate increase is observed, it is important to use the rate of perceived shortness of breath scale as an indicator of exercise intensity (see Chapter 11, Exercise Prescription).

By using an MDI of a sympathomimetic prior to exercise, the symptoms of exercise-induced bronchospasm can be minimized.

Sympathomimetic Therapy Management
Careful consideration should be given to the following:

1. Administration of sympathomimetics is based on relief of symptoms while minimizing side effects. Careful examination of symptomatic relief and untoward effects is important in determining the amount of drug required.
2. When inhalation is the route of administration, the mouth should be rinsed with water after each dose to minimize both oral irritation and ingestion of the drug.

METHYLXANTHINES

Actions and Uses
Methylxanthines also produce bronchodilation, and there are a number of theories to explain their action. The most widely held postulate is that methylxanthines block the enzyme phosphodiesterase, which converts cAMP into cGMP.[95] There is a resultant accumulation of cAMP that promotes relaxation of the bronchial smooth muscle. Current research suggests that drugs of the xanthine group block the binding of adenosine to the smooth muscle and thus block smooth muscle contraction.[99] Other theories are that the xanthines inhibit intracellular calcium release, which does not allow constriction of the smooth muscle, and/or that xanthines may be responsible for prostaglandin inhibition. Regardless of the action of drugs of the xanthine group, bronchodilation, increased ciliary action, and stabilization of the mast cells are accomplished with their use.[99]

Methylxanthines have been observed to increase the contractility of skeletal muscles, including the diaphragm.[96] An increase in the amount of work performed by the skeletal muscle has also been found under the influence of methylxanthines, that is, a resistance to muscle fatigue.[96]

Contraindications and Side Effects
Methylxanthines are not inhaled; they are given systemically, by ingestion, injection, or rectal absorption. The systemic effects of methylxanthines (theophyllin preparations) produce bronchodilation but also affect other organ systems, namely, the central nervous, cardiovascular, renal, musculoskeletal, and gastrointestinal systems.

The therapeutic effects of theophyllin are directly related to the serum concentration of the drug. Improvement in pulmonary function begins at a blood level as low as 5 μg per milliliter. Even at those low levels of serum theophyllin, headache, restlessness, anxiety, insomnia, and hyperactivity may all be reported.[96]

Improvement in pulmonary function increases in proportion to the serum concentration. The therapeutic range for theophyllin is 10 to 20 μg per milliliter, but toxicity may appear at the upper level of the therapeutic range, that is, 15 to 20 μg per milliliter. Gastrointestinal signs appear as the upper level of therapeutic range is reached; among them are anorexia, nausea, vomiting, and abdominal discomfort.[96]

Serious central nervous system (CNS) effects (e.g., grand mal seizures) and serious cardiovascular effects (e.g., palpitations, tachycardia, and arrythmias) may occur when the serum level exceeds 20 μg per milliliter.[96,99]

Effects on Exercise in Individuals with Pulmonary Disease

There is often an elevated resting heart rate in patients who are taking methylxanthines. By using the Karvonen formula for calculation of the THR, the heart rate elevation is taken into account. When a heart rate increase is observed, it is important to use the rate of perceived shortness of breath scale as an indicator of exercise intensity (see Chapter 11, Exercise Prescription).

Methylxanthine Therapy Management

Careful consideration should be given to the following:

1. The mean plasma half-life of theophyllin in adults ranges from 3 to 9½ hours. (Pediatric plasma half-life ranges from 1 to 9½ hours.) Therefore, the variability of serum plasma levels requires that serum drug levels be individually titrated and closely monitored to ensure that the drug is at a therapeutic level. Attention to signs and symptoms of theophyllin toxicity by health professionals involved in the patient's care may prevent untoward effects.
2. Methylxanthines are metabolized in the liver; therefore, alcohol consumption and liver disease increase the half-life of the drug.
3. Cigarette smoking has been shown to decrease the metabolism of the drug. It is important to carefully monitor any patient who changes smoking habits during the course of pulmonary rehabilitation for signs and symptoms of theophyllin toxicity.

ANTICHOLINERGICS

Actions and Uses

The parasympathetic nervous system contains cholinergic receptors. The subcategory of cholinergic receptors specific to airway smooth muscle is termed *muscarinic*. Anticholinergic pharmacologic agents block the muscarinic cholinergic receptors and thereby decrease the parasympathetic tone within the airway smooth muscle.[99] The result is bronchodilation. There is also a decrease in the secretion of the mucous glands with the use of anticholinergic agents.

Contraindications and Side Effects

The severity of side effects from anticholinergic drugs depends on the route of administration and the preparation of the drug. Atropine sulfate, even though used by respiratory patients as an inhalant, has significant systemic absorption. The side effects include dry mouth, throat irritation, constipation, urinary retention, tachycardia, blurred vision, photophobia, and confusion. Ipratropium bromide (Atrovent) is an inhaled agent with little systemic absorption and is therefore relatively free from side effects.

Effects on Exercise in Individuals with Pulmonary Disease

Inhaled ipratropium, which inhibits bronchoconstriction and mucus production, may assist the patient in prolonging the exercise session.

Anticholinergic Therapy Management

Because inhalation is the route of administration, after use the mouth should be rinsed with water to minimize irritation of the mouth and throat and any possible ingestion of the drug.

Anti-inflammatory Agents

The integrity of the airways is also affected by the inflammatory cells within the lungs.[100] Histamine, slow-reacting substance of anaphylaxis (SRS-A) from the mast cells, neutrophils, lymphocytes, eosinophils, macrophages, plasma cells, and monocytes can all take part in the inflammatory response within the airways. An increase in reactivity of the inflammatory response within the airways is commonly seen in asthma and other obstructive pulmonary diseases. The inflammatory response results in vascular engorgement and in swelling and hypersecretion of the mucous glands.[94] All these contribute to a decrease in the size of the airway lumen. With reduction of the amount of inflammation within the airways, relief of symptoms and improved ventilation can be obtained.

CORTICOSTEROIDS

Actions and Uses

Corticosteroids are the most potent anti-inflammatory drugs available.[101] They have many possible actions, including stabilizing the leukocyte lysosomal membranes, inhibiting the accumulation of macrophages, preventing the release of acid hydolases, reducing leukocyte adhesion to capillary endothelium, reducing capillary wall permeability, and depressing tissue reactivity to antigen-antibody interactions.[98] Reducing this inflammatory response within the airways discourages bronchoconstriction. There are also reduced capillary engorgement, a decrease in mucosal edema, and a decrease in secretion production. These collectively increase the inner diameter of the airways and decrease airway obstruction.

Contraindications and Side Effects

The side effects of corticosteroids are dependent on dosage and duration of therapy and the route of administration. Short-term use of systemic steroids, even in high doses, is unlikely to produce harmful effects.[98] However, prolonged systemic use of the drug can result in hypertension, nausea, GI irritation, headache, hypercholesterolemia, moon face, skin breakdown, bruising, muscle atrophy, osteoporosis, delayed wound healing, and an increased susceptibility to, and masking of, infection. Aerosolized corticosteroid preparations (metered dose inhalers) have become a mainstay in the treatment of airway reactivity because they effectively treat the cause topically while avoiding the serious adverse systemic side effects.[102]

Effects of Exercise in Individuals with Pulmonary Disease

The side effects of corticosteroids may affect the type of exercise chosen for patients who are receiving systemic corticosteroids. Long-term steroid use can alter the musculoskeletal system, and pathologic fractures secondary to osteoporosis are possible. Activities that produce excessive stress to skeletal structures should be avoided.

Corticosteroid Therapy Management

Careful consideration should be given to the following:

1. Patients should be advised that steroid dosages must always be tapered, not stopped abruptly. Rebound effects and tachyphylaxis are possible when proper tapering is not performed.

2. When the route of administration of corticosteroids is by inhalation, the mouth should be rinsed with water after each dose to minimize fungal growth and irritation.

Cromolyn Sodium

Cromolyn sodium is neither an anti-inflammatory agent nor a bronchodilator. It seems to be, so far, in a category all by itself.

ACTIONS AND USES

Histamine and SRS-A are chemical mediators of bronchoconstriction found within the mast cell. When an antigen is exposed to the body, these mediators are released from the mast cell and cause bronchoconstriction.

Cromolyn sodium acts to stabilize the mast cell membrane and prevent the release of histamine and SRS-A when an antigen is exposed to the body.[95] Because of its action, the drug is used prophylactically rather than reactively in the treatment of bronchospasm. That is, once bronchoconstriction has occurred, stabilizing the membrane is of no therapeutic value.

Cromolyn sodium seems to be most effective in the treatment of children or young adults with allergic asthma and exercise-induced bronchospasm.[95]

CONTRAINDICATIONS AND SIDE EFFECTS

Cromolyn sodium, in powder form, is used in a device called a Spinhaler for inhalation. This powder can actually produce bronchospasm, irritation of the bronchi, cough, and nausea. More recently, cromolyn sodium is available in a metered-dose inhaler (Intal). Contraindications are drug hypersensitivity and lactase deficiency.[98]

EFFECTS ON EXERCISE IN INDIVIDUALS WITH PULMONARY DISEASE

Patients can use an inhalant of cromolyn sodium before the initiation of exercise in an effort to avert exercise-induced bronchospasm.

CROMOLYN SODIUM THERAPY MANAGEMENT

Careful consideration should be given to the following:

1. Because cromolyn sodium is used to prevent bronchoconstriction, patients should be advised to continue its prophylactic use, especially when feeling well.
2. Improvement may take from 1 to 4 weeks from initiation of the drug, so patience is in order.
3. Cromolyn sodium should not be instituted during an acute period of bronchospasm because it may increase the bronchospasm.[95]

Additional Medications

Many other drugs are used in the management of lung disease. Some of the additional pharmacologic agents that may be used in the management of a patient with pulmonary disease are described below.

Infection is a contributory cause of bronchospasm and respiration dysfunction.[103] Antibiotics are used in the prevention as well as the treatment of pulmonary infections. They can be classified into different types: penicillins, tetracyclines, cephalosporins, aminoglycosides, sulfonamides, and erythromycins. The penicillin group includes such antibiotics as penicillin C, ampicillin, ticarcillin, amoxicillin, and carbenicillin. Although the penicillin group of antibiotics rarely has side effects, hypersensitivity reactions from skin rashes to anaphylactic reactions have been reported. Tetracyclines include such drugs as tetracycline, doxycycline, and methacycline. The most common side effects of the tetracyclines are GI disturbances such as nausea, vomiting, and diarrhea. The cephalosporin drugs, such as ceftazidine, ceftriaxone, cefaclor (Ceclor), cephalexin (Keflex), and cefamandole, have few side effects. They include pain from injection site, transient elevation of liver enzymes, and superinfections with prolonged use. Aminoglycosides include the antibiotics amikacin, gentamicin, tobramycin, streptomycin, and neomycin. Some of the side effects found with the use of aminoglycosides are nephrotoxicity, ototoxicity, and damage to cranial nerve VII resulting in partial or complete hearing loss. Finally, erythromycin is in a category practically by itself even though there are other drugs in the family (estolate, ethylsuccinate, gluceptate) that are rarely prescribed. The side effects of erythromycin most usually seen are GI cramping, nausea, vomiting, and diarrhea. Additional antibiotics used to treat infections that do not fit into the aforementioned categories include clindamycin, polymixin B, and cloramphenicol. These antimicrobial drugs decrease the morbidity and mortality of patients with pulmonary dysfunction. Laboratory sensitivity studies on the infecting organism(s) are necessary to ensure that the appropriate antibiotic will be selected and will be effective.

Anti-infection agents that are not antibiotics are also prescribed to treat various infections. Antifungals are used to treat fungal infections such as *Aspergillus* and *Candida*. The most commonly used antifungal agent is amphotericin B. Antituberculins are used in the treatment of tuberculosis. The most commonly used drugs in this category are streptomycin, ethambutol, isoniazid (INH), and rifampin. Two or more of these drugs are usually prescribed concurrently for long durations (6 months to 2 years) to combat the disease. Alcohol consumption causes a drug interaction that may increase the risk of hepatotoxicity. An antiprotozoal agent, aerosolized pentamidine isoethionate, is used in the treatment of pneumocystis carinii pneumonia (PCP). Some of the side effects of aerosolized pentamidine are fatigue, a metallic taste, and possible shortness of breath, presumably caused by bronchospasm. It is not uncommon to prescribe a sympathomimetic MDI (e.g., Ventolin) along with aerosolized pentamidine to relieve any shortness of breath that the pentamidine may cause.

Antitussive drugs, decongestants, antihistamines, mucolytics, and expectorants are available as over-the-counter preparations. They may have interactions with prescription drugs, and some of them have unwanted effects for patients in pulmonary rehabilitation programs. It is important that patients (and pulmonary rehabilitation personnel) be aware of and cautioned about the possible interactions and side effects.

SURGICAL INTERVENTION IN PULMONARY DISEASE

Surgical intervention for the pulmonary patient includes tumor resection, bullae resection, pneumectomy (lung volume reduction), and lung transplantation. Midsternal or thoracotomy incisions are used for most lung surgeries. Temporary decreases in lung function from the surgical procedure alone are to be expected, giving rise to potential postoperative pulmonary complications. Intervention such as secretion removal techniques, incentive spirometry, breathing exercises, and early ambulation may help to reduce these risks. See Chapter 14 for more information on these interventions.

Tumor resection is generally performed so that the smallest amount of viable lung tissue is lost during the removal of the tumor. A wedge resection removes the least amount of lung tissue resulting in a 0 to 10 percent permanent postoperative lung function decrease. A segmental resection or segmentectomy removes a segment of a lobe of a lung, resulting in a 5 to 10 percent permanent loss of lung function. Lobectomy removes an entire lobe of the lung resulting in a 10 to 20 percent permanent loss of lung function. Pneumonectomy is the removal of an entire lung, resulting in a 40 to 50 percent loss of function.[104] However, if the portion of the lung that is removed was functionally impaired before surgery, the amount of permanent loss will be less.

Large bullae are thin-walled, air-filled cavities on the lung surface or in the lung parenchyma. Bullae that occupy more than one-third of the hemithorax will compress otherwise intact lung parenchyma, rendering it nonfunctional. The surgical removal of large bullae has been effective in improving lung function and relieving dyspnea.[105] The diseased tissue is usually resected through a surgical incision, although the use of lasers during thoracoscopy is currently being evaluated.[106]

Pneumectomy, or lung volume reduction surgery, is a new surgical procedure being evaluated for the functional and symptomatic improvement of patients with pulmonary emphysema.[107] In emphysema, the lung tissue has lost its elastic recoil and therefore the thorax distends into the typical barrel chest. The altered ventilatory pump disrupts the thoracic mechanics, alters the length tension relationship of the ventilatory muscles, and flattens the diaphragm. The goal of the procedure is to remove some of the severely diseased, emphysematous tissue to allow the thorax to be reconfigured into a more mechanically efficient pump, regaining some thoracic mobility, returning the diaphragm to a more dome shaped resting position, and allowing the accessory muscles of respiration to return to a more feasible length-tension relationship. This procedure is in the beginning stages of development, although the preliminary studies have shown improvements in pulmonary function test results, arterial blood gas values and symptoms in selected patients.[108,109]

Lung transplantation may be performed for patients with end-stage diseases such as pulmonary vascular disease (pulmonary hypertension), obstructive pulmonary disease (emphysema or cystic fibrosis), and restrictive pulmonary disease (ideopathic pulmonary fibrosis).[110] The procedure can be either single-lung or double-lung allographs, depending on the recipient's underlying pulmonary disease. The 1-year survival rate is 61 percent overall and the 2-year survival rate for single-lung transplants is 56 percent.[111] The small number of donor organs, large number of appropriate potential recipients, and extensive long-term medical and pharmacologic follow-up require that this procedure remain extremely selective.

SUMMARY

Medical and surgical management of the individual with coronary artery disease has been presented. Emphasis was placed on the following classes of drugs: nitrates, beta-blockers, calcium channel blockers, cardiac glycosides, antiarrhythmics, ACE inhibitors, and antithrombotic agents. Various combinations of these are used to control the symptoms of CAD, including pain, arrhythmias, congestive heart failure, and thrombus formation. Actions of the medications as well as common side effects were reviewed. The use of thrombolytic agents in acute coronary artery occlusion was discussed.

Interventional techniques such as PTCA, laser angioplasty, atherectomy, coronary stents, and CABG surgery were explained, and it was emphasized that these techniques are not cures for the progression of atherosclerosis. Organ transplantation was discussed as a recognized treatment of end-stage cardiac and cardiopulmonary disease. Advanced surgical techniques of CABG without cardiopulmonary bypass grafting and dynamic cardiac myoplasty were described as potential alternatives for cardiac surgery and heart transplant.

Cardiac rehabilitation and risk factor reduction were briefly identified as important adjuncts to both medical and surgical management of coronary artery disease.

The discussion of pharmacologic agents commonly used to treat patients with pulmonary disease emphasized the medications that increase the ventilatory capacity of the respiratory system while minimizing side effects. Three major categories of medications were discussed: (1) bronchodilators, including sympathomimetics, methylxanthines, and anticholinergics; (2) anti-inflammatory agents (corticosteroids); and (3) cromolyn sodium. Actions, side effects, and effects of these drugs on exercise were presented. Finally, surgical intervention for the pulmonary patient, including tumor resection, bullae resection, pneumonectomy and lung transplantation, was discussed.

REFERENCES

1. Yacone-Morton, LA: Inotropic agents and nitrates. Registered Nurse 58:22, 1995.
2. Ziegler, MG and Ruiz-Ramon, PF: Antihypertensive therapy. In: Chernow, B. (ed): The Pharmacologic Approach to the Critically Ill Patient. Williams & Wilkins, Baltimore, 1994, p 405.
3. Peel, C and Mossberg, KA: Effects of cardiovascular medications on exercise responses. Phys Ther 75:387, 1995.
4. Cody, RJ, Conti, CR, and Samet, P: Managing angina and concomitant disease. Patient Care 27:45, 1993.
5. Byington, RP and Furberg, CD: Beta blockers during and after acute myocardial infarction. In: Francis, GS and Alpert, JS (eds): Coronary Care, ed 2. Little, Brown and Co., Boston, 1995, p 543.
6. Hudak, CM and Gallo, BM: Management Modalities: Cardiovascular System. In: Critical Care Nursing—A Holistic Approach, ed 6. (Benz, J Special Ed.) Lippincott, Philadelphia, 1994, p 213.
7. Frishman, WH and Sonnenblick, EH. Beta-adrenergic blocking drugs. In: Schlant, WH and Alexander, RW (eds): The Heart—Arteries and Veins. McGraw-Hill, New York, 1994, p 1271.
7a. Frishman, WH and Sonnenblick, EH. Calcium channel blockers. In: Schlant, WH and Alexander, RW (eds): The Heart—Arteries and Veins. McGraw-Hill, New York, 1994, p. 1291.
8. Sackner-Bernstein, JD and Mancini, DM: Rationale for treatment of patients with chronic heart failure with adrenergic blockade. JAMA 274:1462, 1995.
9. Adams, KF: Current perspectives on beta-receptor antagonists in the treatment of symptomatic ventricular dysfunction. Pharmacotherapy (suppl) 16:69S, 1996.
10. Packer, M et al: The effect of carvedilol on morbidity and mortality in patients with chronic heart failure. N Engl J Med 334:1349, 1996.
11. Ikram, H, Fitzpatrick, D, and Crozier, IG: Therapeutic controversies with use of beta-adrenoceptor blockade in heart failure. Am J Cardiol 71:54C, 1993.
12. Kayser, SR: Calcium channel blockers—Is vasoselectivity relevant? Prog Cardiovasc Nurs 10:35, 1995.
13. Robertson, RM and Robertson, D: Drugs used for the treatment of myocardial ischemia. In: Hardman, JG, et al (eds): Goodman and Gilman's The Pharmacological Basis of Therapeutics, ed 9. McGraw-Hill, New York, 1996, p 759.
14. Prisant, IM et al: Unstable angina—pharmaceutical versus invasive therapy. Postgrad Med 96:88, 1994.
15. Kelly, RA and Smith, TW: Pharmacologic treatment of heart failure. In: Hardman, JG, et al. (eds): Goodman and Gilman's The Pharmacological Basis of Therapeutics, ed 9. McGraw-Hill, New York, 1996, p 809.

16. Marcus, FI: Drugs and procedures used to treat patients with heart failure. In: Schlant, WH and Alexander, RW (eds): Hurst's The Heart—Arteries and Veins. McGraw-Hill, New York, 1994, p 573.
17. Williamson, KM: Is there a role for digoxin in patients with systolic dysfunction? Pharmacotherapy (suppl) 16:37S, 1996.
18. Nursing 95 Drug Handbook. Springhouse Corporation, Springhouse, PA, 1995.
19. Thelan, LA et al: Cardiovascular Therapeutic Management in Critical Care Nursing—Diagnosis and Management, ed 2. Mosby, St. Louis, 1993, 313.
20. Gold, MR and Balke, CW: The cellular action of antiarrhythmic drugs. Heart Disease and Stroke 2:434, 1993.
21. Woosley, RL: Antiarrhythmic drugs. In: Schlant, WH and Alexander, RW (eds): Hurst's The Heart—Arteries and Veins. McGraw-Hill, New York, 1994, p 775.
22. Yacone-Morton, LA: Antiarrhythmics. RN 58:26, 1995.
23. Colucci, RD and Somberg, JC: Treatment of Cardiac Arrhythmias. In: Chernow, B (ed): The Pharmacologic Approach to the Critically Ill Patient, ed 3. Williams & Wilkins, Baltimore, 1994, p 445.
24. Ellenbogen, KA, Wood, MA, and Stambler, BS: Procainamide: A perspective on its value and danger. Heart Disease and Stroke 2:473, 1993.
25. Roden, DM: Antiarrhythmic Drugs. In: Hardman, JG, et al (eds): Goodman & Gilman's The Pharmacological Basis of Therapeutics, ed 9. McGraw-Hill, New York, 1996, p 839.
26. Malik, R et al: Flecainide: Its value and danger. Heart Disease and Stroke 3:85, 1994.
27. Khan, AH: Management of chronic ventricular arrhythmias. Am Fam Physician 49:1805, 1994.
28. Meyer, C: New drugs in the cardiovascular arena. Am J Nurs 93:55, 1993.
29. Hussar, DA: New drugs. Nursing 23:52, 1993.
30. AHFS Drug Information 96—Current developments. In: McEvoy, GK (ed): American Hospital Formulary Service—Drug Information. American Society of Health-System Pharmacists, Bethesda, Maryland 1996, p 23A.
31. Dracup, K: Meltzer's Intensive Coronary Care—A manual for nurses, ed 5. Appleton & Lange, Norwalk, Connecticut, 1995.
32. Brown, EJ and Pfeffer, MA: Ventricular remodeling after myocardial infarction: a modifiable process. Heart Disease and Stroke 3:164, 1994.
33. Fara, AM: The role of angiotensin-converting enzyme inhibitors in reducing ventricular remodeling after myocardial infarction. J Cardiovasc Nurs 8:32, 1993.
34. Kelly, RA and Smith TW: op cit p 809.
35. Chatterjee, K: Use of angiotensin converting enzyme inhibitors. Heart Disease and Stroke 1:128, 1992.
36. Ziegler, MG and Ruiz-Ramon, PF: op cit p 405.
37. Toothill, CM: Thrombolytic therapy: Nursing strategies for successful patient outcomes. Prog Cardiovasc Nurs 10:3, 1995.
38. National Heart Attack Alert Program Coordinating Committee, 60 Minutes to Treatment Working Group: Emergency Department: Rapid identification and treatment of patients with acute myocardial infarction. Ann Emerg Med 23:311, 1994.
39. DeWood MA et al: Prevalence of total coronary occlusion during the early hours of transmural myocardial infarction. N Engl J Med 303:897, 1980.
40. Figueredo, VM, Amidon, TM, and Wolfe, CL: Thrombolysis after acute myocardial infarction. Postgrad Med 96:30, 1994.
41. Van de Werf, F and Verstraete, DP: Thrombolytic treatment of acute myocardial infarction. J Intern Med 236:439, 1994.
42. Cairns, IA et al. Antithrombotic agents in coronary artery disease. Chest 108:380S, 1995.
43. Late Study Group: Late assessment of thrombolytic efficacy (LATE) with altephase 6–24 hours after onset of acute myocardial infarction. Lancet 343:759, 1993.
44. Apple, S: New trends in thrombolytic therapy. Registered Nurse 59:30, 1996.
45. Weiner, B: Thrombolytic agents in critical care. Critical Care Nursing Clinics of North America 5:355, 1993.
46. ISIS-3 (Third International Study of Infarct Survival) Collaborative Group: ISIS-3: A randomized comparison of streptokinase vs tissue plasminogen activator vs anistreplase and of aspirin plus heparin vs aspirin alone among 41,299 cases of suspected acute myocardial infarction. Lancet 339:753, 1992.
47. Carins, JA et al: Coronary thrombolysis. Chest (suppl) 108:401S, 1995.
48. Habib, GB: Current status of thrombolysis in acute myocardial infarction. I. Optimal selection and delivery of a thrombolytic drug. Chest 107:225, 1995.
49. Holmes, DR, Califf, RM, and Topol, EJ: Lessons we have learned from the GUSTO Trial. J Am Coll Cardiol (suppl) 25:10S, 1995.
50. Cheitlin, M, Sokolow, M, and McIlroy, M: Coronary heart disease. In: Clinical Cardiology, ed 2. Appleton & Lange, Norwalk, Conn, 1993, p 147.
51. Fernandez-Ortiz, A, Ik-Kyung, J, and Fuster, V: Anticoagulant and platelet inhibitory agents for myocardial infarction. In: Francis, GS and Alpert, JS (eds): Coronary Care, ed. 2. Little, Brown and Co., Boston, 1995, p 569.
52. Vaitkus, PT: Indications for antithrombotic therapy after myocardial infarction. Heart Disease and Stroke 3:24, 1994.

53. Stein, B and Fuster, V: Pharmacology of anticoagulants and platelet inhibitor drugs. In: Schlant, WH and Alexander, RW (eds): Hurst's The Heart—Arteries and Veins. McGraw-Hill, New York, 1994, p 1309.
54. Rakel, RE. Use of antiplatelet medication for prevention of myocardial infarction and stroke. Heart Disease and Stroke 1:2, 1992.
55. Bowlby, H, Hisle, K, and Clifton, GD: Heparin as adjunctive therapy to coronary thrombolysis in acute myocardial infarction. Heart Lung 24:292, 1995.
56. Chase, SL: Critical care drug update. Part 1. Registered Nurse 59:46, 1996.
57. Hirsh, J: Use of warfarin (coumarin). Heart Disease and Stroke 2:209, 1993.
58. King, SB and Douglas, JS: Indications for percutaneous transluminal coronary angioplasty and atherectomy. In: Schlant, WH and Alexander, RW (eds): The Heart—Arteries and Veins. McGraw-Hill, New York, 1994, p 1339.
59. Snyder, ML and Deelstra, MH: Interventional cardiology techniques. In: Woods, SL, et al (eds): Cardiac Nursing, ed 3. Lippincott, Philadelphia, 1995, p 506.
60. Ryan, TJ and Skolnick, AE: Indications for coronary angioplasty. Heart Disease and Stroke 3:29, 1994.
61. Garratt, KN: Percutaneous revascularization strategies. Postgrad Med 99:125, 1996.
62. Callahan, LL and Frohlich, GC: Understanding nonsurgical coronary revascularization procedures. Am J Nurs 95:52H, 1995.
63. McGhee, HM, Crowe, T, and Horgan, JH: Return to work following coronary artery bypass surgery or percutaneous transluminal coronary angioplasty. Eur Heart J 14:623, 1993.
64. Hudgins, C and Sorenson, G: Directional coronary atherectomy: A new treatment for coronary artery disease. Critical Care Nurse 14:61, 1994.
65. Perra, BM: Managing coronary atherectomy patients in a special procedure unit. Crit Care Nursing 15:57, 1995.
66. Baim, DS: New devices for coronary revascularization. Hosp Pract (Off Ed) 28:41, 1993.
67. Goodkind, J, Coombs, V, and Golobic, R: Excimer laser angioplasty. Heart Lung 22:26, 1993.
68. Strimike, CL: Caring for a patient with an intracoronary stent. Am J Nurs 95:40, 1995.
69. Gardner, E et al: Intracoronary stent update: Focus on patient education. Critical Care Nurse 16:65, 1996.
70. Snyder, ML and Deelstra, MH: op cit.
71. Beattie, S: CABG surgery: The second time around. Am J Nurs 93:42, 1993.
72. Hudak, CM and Gallo, BM: Cardiac surgery and heart transplantation. In: Critical Care Nursing—A Holistic Approach. ed 6. (Benz, J Special Ed.) Lippincott, Philadelphia, 1994, p 213.
73. LeDoux, D and Shinn, J: Cardiac surgery. In: Woods, SL, et al (eds): Cardiac Nursing, ed 3. Lippincott, Philadelphia, 1995, p 524.
74. Shinn, IA: Management of a patient undergoing myocardial revascularization—Coronary artery bypass graft surgery. Nursing Clinics of North America 27:243, 1992.
75. Gallegos-Alvarez, M and O'Brien, M: Right gastroepiploic artery conduit use in myocardial revascularization. AORN J 60:763, 1994.
76. Vitello-Cicciu, J, and Eaga, JS: Data acquisition from the cardiovascular system. In: Kinney, MR, Packa, DR, and Dunbar, SB (eds): AACN's Clinical Reference for Critical-Care Nursing. ed. 3. Mosby, St. Louis, 1993, p 471.
77. Jenaans, D, Stanton, B, and Fono, RT: Quantifying and predicting recovery after heart surgery. Psychosom Med S6:203, 1994.
78. The Bypass Angioplasty Revascularization Investigation (BARI) Investigators: Comparison of coronary bypass surgery with angioplasty in patients with multivessel disease. N Engl J Med 335:217, 1996.
79. Kahn, JK: Caring for patients after coronary bypass surgery. Postgrad Med 93:249, 1993.
80. Arom, KV, Emery, RW, Nicoloff, DM: Mini-sternotomy for coronary artery bypass grafting. Ann Thorac Surg 61:1271, 1996.
81. Bennetti, FJ, Mariani, MA, Ballester, C: Direct coronary surgery without cardiopulmonary bypass in acute myocardial infarction. J Cardiovasc Surg 37:391, 1996.
82. Calafiore, AM et al: Left anterior descending coronary artery grafting via left anterior small thoracotomy without cardiopulmonary bypass. Ann Thorac Surg 61:1658, 1996.
83. Schroeder, JS: Indications for cardiac transplantation. Heart Disease and Stroke 3:345, 1994.
84. Vollman, MW: Dynamic cardiomyoplasty: Perspectives on nursing care and collaborative management. Prog Cardiovasc Nurs 10:15, 1995.
85. Bove, LA et al: Nursing care of patients undergoing dynamic cardiomyoplasty. Critical Care Nurse 15:96, 1995.
86. Pettrey, LJ and LeFlar-DiLeva, KM: Preparing for cardiomyoplasty: A new horizon in cardiac surgery. Dimensions in Critical Care Nursing 13:226, 1994.
87. Letsou, GV et al: Dynamic cardiomyoplasty. Cardiol Clin 13:121, 1995.
88. Dimengo, JM: Dynamic cardiomyoplasty and its use in patients with chronic heart failure. Critical Care Nursing Clinics of North America 5:627, 1993.
89. Thelan, LA et al: Transplantation. In: Thelan, LA et al (eds): Critical Care Nursing—Diagnosis and Management. ed 2. Mosby, St. Louis, 1994, p. 840.

90. Shumway, SJ: Specific critical care problems in heart, heart-lung, and lung transplants. In: Rippe, JM et al (eds): Intensive Care Medicine. ed 3. Little, Brown and Company, Boston, 1996, p 2083.
91. Squires, RW et al: Cardiovascular rehabilitation: status, 1990. Mayo Clin Proc 65:731, 1990.
92. Levy, JK: Standard and alternative adjunctive treatments in cardiac rehabilitation. Tex Heart Inst J 20:198, 1993.
93. Hellman, EA and Williams, MA: Outpatient cardiac rehabilitation in elderly patients. Heart Lung 23:506, 1994.
94. Zadai, C: Pulmonary pharmacology. In: Malone, T (ed): Physical and Occupational Therapy: Drug Implications for Practice. Lippincott, Philadelphia, 1989.
95. Yee, A, Connors, G, and Cress, D: Pharmacology and the respiratory patient. In: Hodgkin, J, Zorn, E, and Connors, G: Pulmonary Rehabilitation: Guidelines to Success. Butterworth Publishers, Boston, 1984.
96. Lehnert, B and Schachter, E: The Pharmacology of Respiratory Care. Mosby, St. Louis, 1980, pp 117–171.
97. Ziment, I: Pharmacologic therapy of COPD. In Hodgkin, J, and Petty, T (eds): Chronic Obstructive Pulmonary Disease: Current Concepts. Saunders, Philadelphia, 1987.
98. Benson, D and Conte, R: 89/90 Nursing Meds. Appleton & Lange, Norwalk, CT, 1989.
99. Ciccone, C: Pharmacology in Rehabilitation. FA Davis, Philadelphia, 1990, pp 290–307.
100. Sertl, K, Clark, T, and Kaliner, M: Inflammation and airway function: The asthma syndrome. American Review of Respiratory Diseases (Suppl)141:1–2, 1990 (Editorial).
101. Svedmyr, N: Action or corticosteroids on beta adrenergic receptors. American Review of Respiratory Diseases (Suppl)141:31–38.
102. Check, W and Kaliner, M: Pharmacology and pharmacokinetics of topical corticosteroid derivatives used for asthma therapy. American Review of Respiratory Diseases (Suppl) 141:44–51, 1990.
103. Berte, J: Critical Care: The Lung, ed 2. Appleton-Century-Crofts, Norwalk, CT, 1986, p 127.
104. American Thoracic Society: Standards for the diagnosis and care of patients with chronic obstructive pulmonary disease. Am J Respir Crit Care Med 152:S77–S120, 1995.
105. Nickoladze, G: Functional results of surgery for bullous emphysema. Chest 101:119–122, 1992.
106. Wakabayashi, A et al: Thoracoscopic carbon dioxide laser treatment of bullous emphysema. Lancet 337:881–883, 1991.
107. Snider, G: Health care technology assessment of surgical procedures: The case of reduction pneumoplasty for emphysema. Am J Respir Crit Care Med 153:1208–1213, 1996.
108. Cooper, J et al: Bilateral pneumectomy (volume reduction) for chronic obstructive pulmonary disease. J Thorac Cardiovasc Surg 109:106–119, 1995.
109. Cooper, J and Lefrak, S: Is volume reduction surgery appropriate in the treatment of emphysema? Yes. Am J Respir Crit Care Med 153:120–124, 1996.
110. American Thoracic Society: Statement on lung transplantation. American Review of Respiratory Diseases 147:772–776, 1993.
111. US Public Health Service: Single and Double Lung Transplantation. Health Technology Assessment Reports. Washington DC: Agency for Health Care Policy and Research Publications Clearinghouse. 1991. DHHS Publication No PB92-156793.

CHAPTER **8**

The Electrocardiogram

An electrocardiogram (ECG) is a graphic representation of the electrical activity generated by the atria and ventricles. Impulse formation and impulse conduction in the cardiac muscle generate weak electrical currents throughout the body.[1,2] The electrical impulses progressively depolarize the cardiac muscle and cause cardiac contraction.[1] By means of a galvanometer, the difference in potential between a positive and negative area in the body is detected, amplified, and recorded. The ECG allows indirect observation of the sequence of cardiac muscle excitation over any given period of time.

As electrical activity passes through the myocardium, it is detected by external skin electrodes placed at specific points on the body surface and recorded as a series of deflections on the ECG. The deflections or waves are known arbitrarily as P, Q, R, S, and T (Fig. 8–1). The upward deflections are positive, representing an electrical current moving toward the skin electrode. The downward deflections are negative, representing an electrical current moving away from the skin electrode. In both instances, the magnitude of the deflection represents the thickness of the muscle mass through which the current is being conducted (see section on waves, complexes, and intervals).

Each deflection, or wave, represents an aspect of the depolarization or repolarization of the cardiac muscle cells. Although this progressive wave of electrical current is infinitesimal, it can be detected by the skin electrodes as it passes through the heart. The wave of depolarization flows from the base of the heart to the apex. Depolarization, the change of the internal electrical potential of the cell from negative to positive, causes almost immediate myocardial contraction. Depolarization is followed by repolarization. During repolarization, the cells regain their electronegative state and the heart is physically quiet. Although the change in electrical potential during repolarization is seen on the ECG, no physical activity accompanies this electrical activity.

It is important to note that the ECG is a recording of the electrical activity of the heart (depolarization and repolarization of the muscle cells) and not a recording of the actual contraction and relaxation of the myocardium that should occur a split second after the deflection is observed. The ECG is a composite of the total electrical activity of the heart at any given moment; therefore, every aspect of electrical activity is not discernible. Most notably, atrial repolarization, occurring in conjunction with ventricular depolarization, is "lost" in the QRS complex because of the greater voltage of the latter.

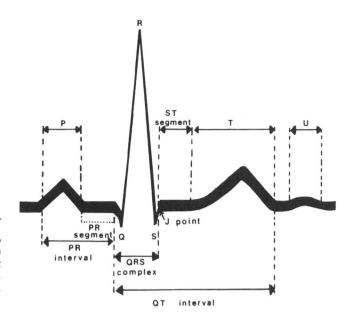

FIGURE 8-1. Normal PQRST wave configuration. ECG waves, complexes, and intervals. (From Underhill, SL, et al: Cardiac Nursing. JB Lippincott, Philadelphia, 1983, p. 204, with permission.)

THE CARDIAC CYCLE AND IMPULSE CONDUCTION

The cardiac cycle is one complete period of depolarization and repolarization of the cardiac muscle cells. Because of the heart cells' unique properties of automaticity, rhythmicity, and conductivity, the heart may regularly initiate and propagate an impulse along its conduction pathway without nervous system influence (Chapter 2). Every myocardial cell can initiate and propagate an impulse, but the sinoatrial (SA) node is the "natural pacemaker" of the heart. It serves this function because the SA node cells maintain the lowest resting membrane potential in the heart's conduction system. They depolarize first and thereby initiate the impulse (at a rate of 60 to 100 beats per minute [bpm]) that is propagated throughout the conduction system by the heart's "all-or-nothing" conduction property. If the SA node does not initiate an impulse at appropriate intervals (60 to 100 bpm), another ectopic focus in the atria may initiate the heartbeat. An ectopic focus is a site outside the SA node that initiates an impulse. In the normal sequence of events, once the impulse leaves the SA node, it traverses the atria and ventricles in a progressive wave of depolarization. The atria have not been determined to have any specialized conduction pathways; therefore, the impulse is propagated from cell to cell within the muscle. Almost immediately, simultaneous contraction of the left and right atria occur. The impulse is relayed from the atria to the ventricles via a specialized conduction pathway known as the atrioventricular (AV) node.

The AV node also has the capacity to perform the pacemaker function (at a rate of 40 to 70 bpm) if it does not receive any stimulation from the SA node. In normal conduction, the impulse is slowed as it passes through the AV node. Ventricular depolarization rapidly proceeds as the impulse moves via the bundle of His to the left and right bundle branches and through the Purkinje fibers, terminating in the subendocardium. The ventricular septum is depolarized first, followed by almost simultaneous depolarization of the left and right ventricles. Despite the fact that the left ventricle is depolarized just a fraction of a second before the right, the ECG records all of the electrical activity of the ventricles as a composite, the QRS complex (see Fig. 8–1). Contraction of the ventricles normally occurs within a split second of depolarization of the myocardium and then ventricular recovery (cellular repolarization) begins immediately. The repolarization of the atrium occurs simultaneously with ventricular depolarization. After ventricular repolarization occurs, the entire myocardium is returned to its electronegative state, and one cardiac cycle is completed.

WAVES, COMPLEXES, AND INTERVALS

The ECG is composed of a series of waves, complexes, and intervals, including the P wave, QRS complex, T wave, ST segment, and PR interval (see Fig. 8–1).

P Wave

The P wave is the first positive deflection on the ECG. It represents the depolarization of the atrial muscle cells following the release of an impulse from the SA node or some other focus in the atrium. The wave is symmetric in appearance, usually 2.5 mm or less in height, and of 0.08- to 0.11-second duration (Fig. 8–2).

PR Interval

The PR interval is measured from the beginning of the P wave to the beginning of the QRS complex. It represents the time required for the impulse to travel from the SA node through the conduction system to the Purkinje fibers. The pause of the impulse at

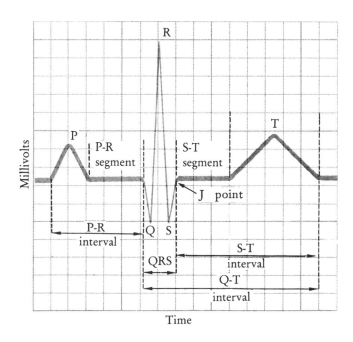

FIGURE 8–2. Normal electrocardiography and timing. Graphic representation of the normal electrocardiogram. Vertical lines represent 0.04 second, and each five-square block represents 0.2 second. The normal PR interval is less than 0.2 second; the average is 0.16 second. The average duration of the P wave is 0.08 second; the QRS complex is 0.08 second; the ST segment is 0.12 second; the T wave is 0.16 second; and the QT interval is 1.36 seconds. Each horizontal line represents voltage; each five-square block equals 0.5 millivolt (mV). (From McHenry, LM and Salerno, E: Pharmacology in Nursing, ed 17. CV Mosby, St. Louis 1989, p. 445, with permission.)

the AV node is within the PR interval. The entire atrial-AV node activity is 0.12 to 0.20 second in duration (Fig. 8–2).

QRS Complex

The first negative deflection of the QRS complex is known as the Q wave; it is followed by the upward R wave. Small Q waves seen in leads I, II, V_4, and V_5 are usually insignificant. A large Q wave is not often present, and, if present, may indicate a recent infarction. A diagnostically significant Q wave is usually 0.04 second in duration and one third the size of the QRS complex. The R wave is the first upward deflection followed by a downward deflection, the S wave. There are several variations of the QRS complex, but despite the variations, all represent ventricular depolarization (Fig. 8–3). The Q, R, and S waves, collectively, are known as the QRS complex.[3,4] The QRS complex has an amplitude of 20 to 30 mm and a duration of 0.06 to 0.10 second. An increase in duration is a sign of delayed conduction through the ventricle. An amplitude of greater than 35 mm indicates ventricular hypertrophy. An amplitude of less than 5 mm may indicate coronary artery disease (CAD), emphysema, marked obesity, generalized edema, or pericardial effusion.

ST Segment

The ST segment begins at the end of the QRS complex and represents the beginning of ventricular muscle repolarization. It is generally isoelectric (returns to the baseline) but may rise above the isoelectric line 1 mm in normal individuals. (In healthy black men, the ST segment may be elevated as much as 2 mm.) The point at which the ST segment begins is known as the J (meaning junction) point (Fig. 8–4). In evaluation of the cardiac patient, the J point is significant, as ST-segment depression greater than

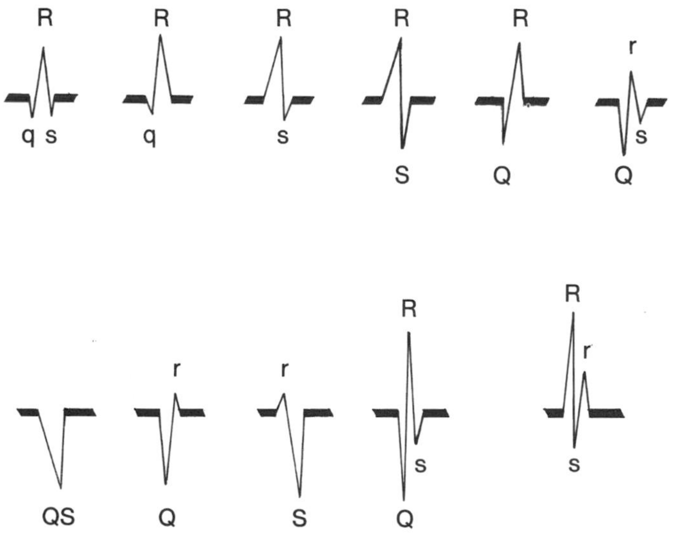

FIGURE 8–3. Variations in the QRS complex. Note that capital letters are assigned to large waves and that lowercase letters are assigned to small waves. (From Bernreiter, M: Electrocardiography. JB Lippincott, Philadelphia, 1963, p. 15, with permission.)

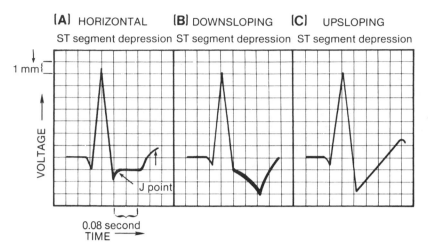

FIGURE 8–4. ST segment patterns: *A*, Horizontal ST segment depression; *B*, downsloping ST segment depression; *C*, upsloping ST segment depression. (From Vinsant and Spence,[10] p. 255, with permission.)

1 mm occurring 0.08 second after the J point is indicative of ischemia and diagnostic of CAD (Fig. 8–4).[5,6]

In an acute infarction, the ST segment is elevated, suggesting myocardial injury. Over time (weeks to months), the ST segment returns to the baseline. Prolonged ST-segment elevation suggests ventricular aneurysm. Generally, the ST segment is an average of 0.12 second in duration and slopes gently upward to the isoelectric line and beginning of the T wave.

T Wave

Representing ventricular repolarization, the T wave is slightly rounded and slightly asymmetric. The deflection is in the same direction as the QRS, and the duration is about 0.16 second.

The time elapsed during the ST segment through the first half of the T wave is known as the absolute refractory period of the cardiac cycle. During this time, no impulse, no matter how strong, is propagated through the ventricles. The second half of the T wave is referred to as the relative refractory period. During the relative refractory period, the vulnerable period of the cardiac cycle, a "stronger-than-normal" stimulus may initiate depolarization of the heart earlier than would normally be expected. A contraction resulting from this early impulse is known as a premature contraction. When premature ventricular depolarization occurs on the second half of the T wave, a lethal arrhythmia, ventricular tachycardia (VT) or ventricular fibrillation (VF), could be precipitated. This phenomenon is known as the R-on-T phenomenon.

QT Interval

The QT interval represents electrical systole; and extends from the beginning of the QRS complex to the end of the T wave.

Standard Electrocardiogram Paper

ECG paper is standardized. Time is measured horizontally, with each small block equal to 0.04 second and each bold block 0.2 second (Fig. 8–5). Amplitude is measured vertically. Each small block equals 0.1 mV and is equivalent to 1 mm. The paper progresses through the cardiograph at a standard rate of 22 mm/second.

Standardization

Each electrocardiograph machine contains a 1-mV standard for calibration purposes that should appear on ever ECG recording. The standard mark provides a manual check on the instrument's calibration. One millivolt of cardiac impulse should deflect the stylus exactly 1 cm (10 mm). The standard mark that appears on the ECG should be precisely 10 mm (1 cm) high, with a sharp upper left-hand corner. A slight sloping downward toward the right is normal. The shape and size of the standardization mark are significant because lack of calibration may distort the ECG recording.

Electrocardiogram Leads

Measurement of the normal ECG requires the use of 12 leads or reference points from which the electrical activity of the heart can be detected and subsequently viewed. Six leads (I, II, III, aVR, aVL, and aVF) are known as the limb leads and six (V_1 through V_6) are known as the precordial or chest leads. Leads I, II, and III are formed by three sides of a triangle connecting the right arm, left arm, and left foot. The heart is located approximately at the center of the triangle (Einthoven's triangle) formed by these three points (Fig. 8–6). At 80 to 90 percent accuracy in diagnosis can be ensured by correct interpretation of these three leads alone.

The limb leads I, II, and III are bipolar. They represent the difference in electrical potential between two specific points in the body. Lead I is the difference of potential between the left arm (LA) and the right arm (RA). Lead II is the difference in potential between the left leg (LL) and the right arm. Lead III is the difference in potential between the left leg and the left arm. The unipolar leads, aVF, aVL, and aVR, represent a

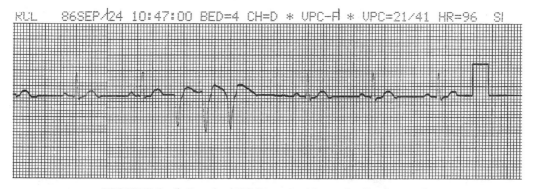

FIGURE 8–5. Standard ECG paper with standardization mark.

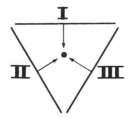

FIGURE 8-6. Vectors of leads I, II, and III. When these three lines are pushed to the center of the triangle, there are three intersecting lines of reference. (From Dubin,[7] p. 33, with permission.)

difference in electrical potential between one positive lead and the average of the potential between the other two leads. Lead aVR (meaning augmented voltage right) is the difference in potential between the right arm and the average of the potential of the left arm and left leg (Fig. 8–7). Lead aVL (meaning augmented voltage left) is the difference in potential between the left arm and the average of the potential between the left leg and the right arm. Lead aVF (meaning augmented voltage foot) is the difference in potential between the left leg and the average of the potential between the left arm and right arm (Fig. 8–7).[3,7] The waveforms of the aV leads are augmented (increased in size) to obtain waveforms of ample magnitude for evaluation.

The six limb leads intersect at 30-degree angles to form six intersecting reference lines in the frontal plane of the heart (Fig. 8–8). the six chest, or precordial, leads (V_1 through V_6) reflect the limb leads and are marked at six different positions, right to left, across the chest (Fig. 8–9); all the leads are positive. Normally, on an ECG the QRS becomes progressively more positive from V_1 to V_6 (right to left across the chest) because the chest leads follow the same vectors as the electrical activity of the heart

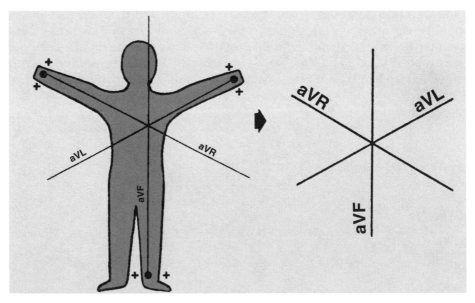

FIGURE 8-7. The unipolar limb leads. The aVR, aVL, and aVF leads interesect at different angles and produce three other intersecting lines of reference. (From Dubin,[7] p. 36, with permission.)

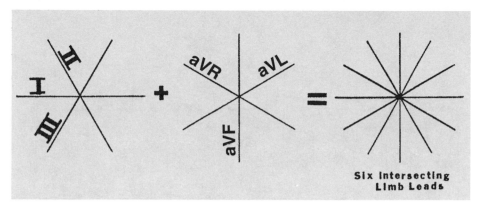

FIGURE 8–8. The limb leads. All six leads, I, II, III, aVR, aVL, and aVF, meet to form six neatly intersecting reference lines that lie in a flat plane on the patient's chest. (From Dubin,[7] p. 37, with permission.)

(Fig. 8–10). The chest leads record the electrical potential under each electrode compared to the central terminal connection, or V, that is made by connecting wires from the right arm, left arm, and left leg. The electrical potential of the V does not vary significantly throughout the cardiac cycle. Therefore, the recordings made with the V connections show the electrical activity that is occurring under each precordial electrode. In all 12 leads, the right leg serves as the ground or indifferent lead. Extraneous electrical activity is minimized by utilizing a ground lead.[3,7]

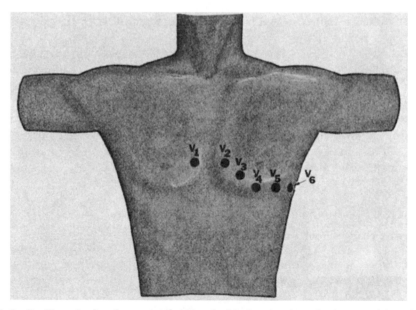

FIGURE 8–9. Chest-lead reference sites. To obtain the six chest leads, a positive electrode is placed at six different positions around the chest. (From Dubin,[7] p. 41, with permission.)

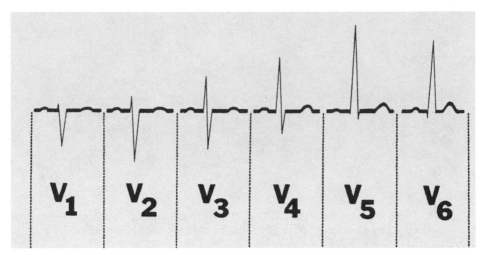

FIGURE 8-10. Progression of positive amplitude from V1 to V6. The ECG tracing will thus show progressive changes from V1 to V6. (From Dubin,[7] p. 43, with permission.)

Lead Placement

ECGs of the highest quality are necessary for meaningful interpretation. The quality of an ECG depends on both the equipment and proper technique in recording the electrical events.[8,9] Proper skin preparation (cleansing the skin with acetone or alcohol to reduce skin resistance and shaving the electrode site to ensure secure lead placement), as well as the selection of appropriate lead sites, ensures a definitive tracing. The limb leads are placed on the extremities. To ensure maintenance of good contact, they may be placed proximally when doing ECGs or monitoring during exercise testing and therapy (Fig. 8-11).

Although the 12-lead ECG gives the most complete view of the heart, it may be inappropriate during exercise therapy. Modified lead placement for exercise is effective. It is not cumbersome to the individual and does not impede activity. In most cases, one lead alone is sufficient to observe for arrhythmias.

A modified chest lead V_5 (CMV_5) may be recommended for exercise monitoring. It minimizes interference and permits ease of defibrillation should an emergency arise (Fig. 8-12). Of all the rhythm disturbances, 98 percent are thought to be detected by CMV_5 during exercise testing and therapy.[5,10,11]

The 12-Lead Electrocardiogram

The interpreter of the ECG can gain a great deal of information from the 12-lead composite. Particular alterations in the depolarization and repolarization patterns reflect myocardial pathology. By carefully reviewing the 12 different views of the heart, the pathologic problem can be localized.[12-14] Of course, the ECG must always be interpreted in conjunction with the total clinical picture, including laboratory results and other diagnostic tests and the individual's activity tolerance and state of well-being.

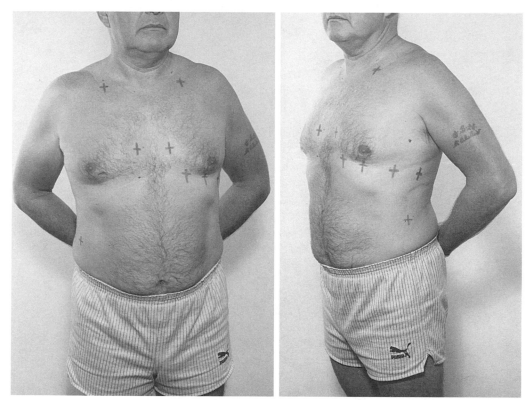

FIGURE 8–11. Electrode placement for a 12-lead exercise ECG recording. Electrode location and identification is as follows: (1) RL (right leg): just above the right iliac crest on the midaxillary line. (2) LL (left leg): just above the left iliac crest on the midaxillary line. (3) RA (right arm): just below the right clavicle medial to the deltoid muscle. (4) LA (left arm): just below the left clavicle medial to the deltoid muscle. (5) V_1: fourth interspace at the right sternal margin. (6) V_2: fourth interspace at the left sternal margin. (7) V_3: midway between V_2 and V_4. (8) V_4: fifth interspace at the midclavicular line just below the nipple. (9) V_5: midway between V_4 and V_6 on the anterior axillary line. (10) V_6: same transverse line as V_4 at the midaxillary line. (From Brannon,[8] p. 101, with permission.)

Table 8–1 describes the characteristics of wave configuration for each lead of a normal 12-lead ECG, and Figure 8–13 represents a normal ECG. The reader is referred to any of the many excellent ECG interpretation texts for more in-depth interpretation of the ECG.[2,3,7,15–18] In this text, information reviewed is in regard to the basic interpretation of the most commonly occurring cardiac arrhythmias.

A standard 12-lead ECG tracing is normally used for diagnostic purposes. Arrhythmia detection in both the hospital and the outpatient cardiac rehabilitation settings can be accomplished easily and accurately by monitoring a single lead (lead I, II, or CMV_5 may be used). In cardiac rehabilitation settings, telemetry systems, in which the individual's ECG is transmitted via radio waves to a remote observer, are most often used to free the patient from the hard-wire connection of the oscilloscope and to allow unencumbered exercise.

A true understanding of the normal range and the normal variation of the ECG

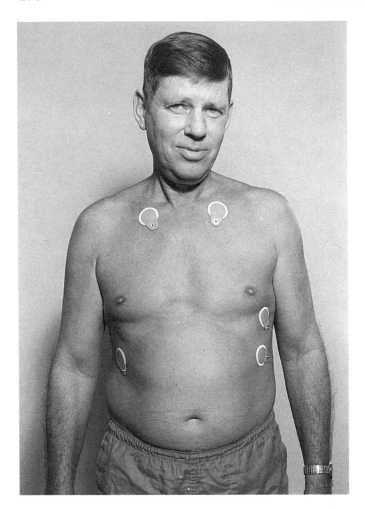

FIGURE 8–12. A modified chest lead V_5 (CMV5). RL = right leg; LL = left leg; RA = right arm; LA = left arm; V_5 = left fifth intercostal space on the anterior axillary line.

depends on a basic understanding of both normal and abnormal cardiac electrophysiology. It must be remembered that many of the configurations tabulated below may represent cardiac abnormalities when interpreted in the context of the entire tracing and in light of the clinical history and physical examination. Therefore the information contained in Table 8–1 is intended to be used only as a rough preliminary guide to the interpretation of ambiguous and borderline tracings.

INTERPRETING THE ELECTROCARDIOGRAM

Learning to interpret the 12-lead ECG takes a great deal of time and practice. In this text the primary focus is the basic interpretation of single-lead ECGs, or rhythm strips. Evaluation of the rate, rhythm, individual waveform, and their relationships to one another will prepare the reader for basic interpretation. This skill is necessary for safely monitoring patients during exercise testing and exercise therapy. Individuals involved in cardiac rehabilitation programs most frequently have atherosclerosis of the

TABLE 8–1 Normal Ranges and Variations in the Adult 12-Lead Electrocardiogram

Lead	P	Q	R	S	T	ST
I	Upright deflection	Small <0.04 s <25% of R	Dominant Largest deflection of the QRS complex	<R, or none	Upright deflection	Usually isoelectric; may vary from +1 to −0.5 mm
II	Upright deflection	Small or none	Dominant	<R, or none	Upright deflection	Usually isoelectric; may vary from +1 to −0.5 mm
III	Upright, flat, diphasic, or inverted, depending on frontal plane axis	Small or none depending on frontal plane axis; or large (0.04–0.05 s or >25% of R)	None to dominant depending on frontal plane axis	None to dominant depending on frontal plane axis	Upright, flat, diphasic, or inverted, depending on frontal plane axis	Usually isoelectric; may vary from +1 to −0.5 mm
aVR	Inverted deflection	Small, none, or large	Small or none depending on frontal plane axis	Dominant (may be QS)	Inverted deflection	Usually isoelectric; may vary from +1 to −0.5 mm
aVL	Upright, flat, diphasic, or inverted, depending on frontal plane axis	Small, none, or large depending on frontal plane axis	Small, none, or dominant depending on frontal plane axis	None to dominant depending on frontal plane axis	Upright, flat, diphasic, or inverted, depending on frontal plane axis	Usually isoelectric; may vary from +1 to −0.5 mm
aVF	Upright deflection	Small or none	Small, none, or dominant depending on frontal plane axis	None to dominant depending on frontal plane axis	Upright, flat, diphasic, or inverted, depending on frontal plane axis	Usually isoelectric; may vary from +1 to −0.5 mm
V_1	Inverted, flat, upright, or diphasic	None (may be QS)	<S or none (QS); small r' may be present	Dominant (may be QS)	Upright, flat, diphasic, or inverted*	0 to +3 mm
V_2	Upright; less commonly, diphasic or inverted	None (may be QS)	<S or none (QS); small r' may be present	Dominant (may be QS)	Upright; less commonly flat, diphasic, or inverted*	0 to +3 mm
V_3	Upright	Small or none	R<,>, or = S	S>,<, or = R	Upright*	0 to +3 mm
V_4	Upright	Small or none	R > S	S < R	Upright*	
V_5	Upright	Small	Dominant (<26 mm)	S SV_4	Upright	Usually isoelectric; may vary from +1 to −0.5 mm
V_6	Upright	Upright	Dominant (<26 mm)	S < SV_5	Upright	

*Inverted in infants, children, and occasionally young adults.
Source: From Goldman, MJ: Principles of Clinical Electrocardiography, ed 12. Lange Medical Publications, Los Altos, California, 1986, with permission.

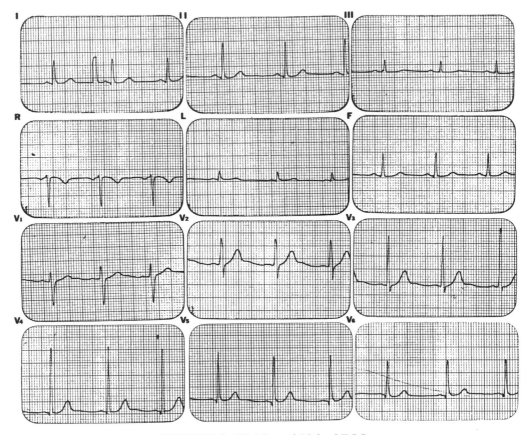

FIGURE 8–13. Normal 12-lead ECG.

coronary arteries. This condition interferes with the heart's normal response to exercise and increased myocardial oxygen demand. The individual is most likely to have a lower ischemic threshold and a more limited activity tolerance than individuals with healthy coronary arteries. Therefore, the clinician must be alert to the possibility of rate-dependent blocks and rhythm disturbances at low levels of activity.

In order to properly interpret an ECG strip, the clinician must answer five questions:

1. What is the rate?
2. What is the rhythm? Is it regular or irregular?
3. Are there P waves?
4. What is the QRS duration?
5. By evaluating the PR interval, what is the relationship between the P waves and the QRS complexes?[3,4,19]

The following discussion describes how to answer these five questions and will enable the reader to identify common cardiac arrhythmias.

Calculating the Rate

As already noted, the SA node is the natural pacemaker of the heart. It has an intrinsic rate of 60 to 100 bpm. When, for some reason, the SA node does not fire, there are many other pacemakers in the atria (ectopic foci) that can take over the pacemaker function. An ectopic focus is a potential pacemaker site somewhere outside the SA node that can take over as the pacemaker if the SA node is not effective.[7] Ectopic atrial pacemakers discharge at a rate of approximately 75 bpm, but this rate may increase to 150 to 250 bpm in pathologic situations. The intrinsic rate of the AV node is approximately 60 bpm, and the AV node may assume pacemaker activity when no impulse is received from the atria. Pathologic conditions may cause an ectopic focus in the ventricle to fire at a rate of 150 to 250 bpm, although the intrinsic rate of the ventricle is 20 to 40 bpm.

The heart rate is the first determination to be made in interpreting an ECG. One of the simplest methods used is to count the number of QRS complexes in a 6-second strip and multiply by 10 (chart speed = 25 mm per second). A second method is looking at consecutive R waves. Find an R wave that falls on heavy black vertical line on the ECG paper. Count off 300, 150, 100 on each of the heavy black lines that follow in succession. (Do not count the initial R wave that was selected.) Continue to count off 75, 60, 50 on the next three successive dark lines. (These numbers must be memorized.) Now, look for the next R wave by scanning to the right of the initial R wave identified. Where the next R wave falls will estimate the rate. If the second R wave falls between two heavy black lines, the location of its position between the two lines will affect the estimation of the rate (Fig. 8–14). This method allows the reader to quickly look at an ECG strip and roughly estimate the heart rate.[7,10] The two methods can be used to cal-

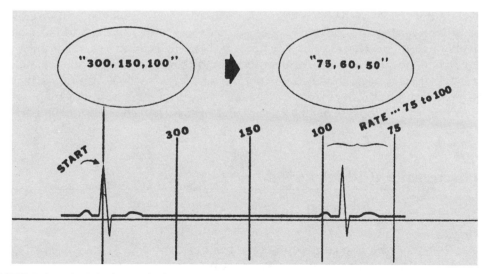

FIGURE 8–14. Calculating the heart rate. Note that the series of numbers assigned to the successive heavy black lines must be memorized: 300, 150, 100, 75, 60, 50. This figure represents an approximate rate of 90 bpm. (From Dubin,[7] p. 62, with permission.)

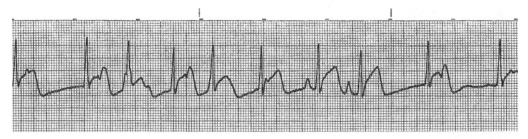

FIGURE 8–15. Ventricular response is irregularly irregular. There is no pattern to the occurrence of the R waves. Note the 3-second marks across the ECG paper.

culate the rate of regular rhythm in which there is constant interval between similar waves. Irregularly occurring rhythms are best estimated by counting the R waves that occur within a minute. Rates greater than 100 bpm are, by definition, tachycardias, and rates below 60 bpm are bradycardias.

Determining the Rhythm

In regular rhythm, there is a consistent distance between similar waves. The normal sinus rhythm (NSR) of the heart is a regular rhythm occurring at a rate of 60 to 100 bpm. Irregular rhythms may be regularly irregular, with patterns of irregularity that are identified and repeated, or they may be completely chaotic and termed irregularly irregular (Fig. 8–15). Disturbances in rhythm, cardiac arrhythmias, are caused by an abnormality in automaticity (initiation of the impulse), an abnormality in conduction (propagation of the impulse), or both. Disturbances in automaticity may be either decreased automaticity of the SA node, which may force an ectopic focus to take over or "escape," or enhanced automaticity of an ectopic focus, in which the ectopic focus may actively "usurp" or override the sinus pacemaker. The ectopic focus may be a point anywhere in the atria, AV node, or ventricles. Disturbances in conduction are the result of a block at some point in the conduction system that may be a result of ischemia to that area.[3,18–20] Identification of arrhythmias is based on the location of the origins of the arrhythmias in the conduction system and by the characteristics of the particular rhythm.

Characteristics of Rhythms

NORMAL SINUS RHYTHM

Definition and Cause

NSR is the conventional rhythm of the healthy heart (Fig. 8–16, Table 8–2). Arising from the SA node, the impulse follows normal conduction pathways. It is a regular rhythm, although there may be some phasic variation with respiration, that increases with inspiration and decreases with expiration. This is frequently seen in young adults. The rate may also be influenced by exercise, emotions, environmental and body temperature, drugs, and various disease states.

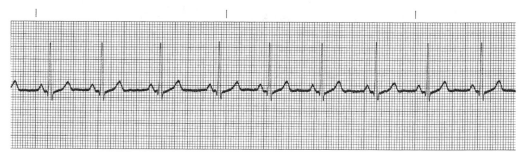

FIGURE 8–16. Normal sinus rhythm.

Hemodynamic Implications
    None.

Treatment
    No treatment is necessary.

SINUS BRADYCARDIA

Definition and Cause
    A sinus bradycardia is a slow rhythm of less than 60 bpm originating from a supraventricular source. It occurs normally during sleep and is commonly seen in individuals who are physically fit. It also occurs in response to increased vagal tone due to gastrointestinal (GI) distress, pain, carotid sinus pressure, ocular pressure, increased intracranial pressure, and acute myocardial infarction (AMI). Administration of digoxin, beta-adrenergic blocking agents, and calcium ion antagonists may also cause bradycardia.

ECG Appearance
    All waves (Fig. 8–17) are of normal configuration with a rate of less than 60 bpm.

Hemodynamic Implications
    Unless bradycardia is profound (less than 40 bpm), it is well tolerated. However, if cardiac output is not adequate, the individual is compromised hemodynamically and

TABLE 8–2 Normal Configuration of ECG Waves

Waves and Complexes	Duration	Amplitude
P wave	0.8–1.2 s	1–3 mm
PR interval	0.12–0.20 s	Isoelectric after the P wave deflection
QRS	0.06–0.10 s	25–30 mm (maximum)
ST segment	0.12 s	$-\frac{1}{2}$ to $+1$ mm
T wave	0.16 s	5–10 mm

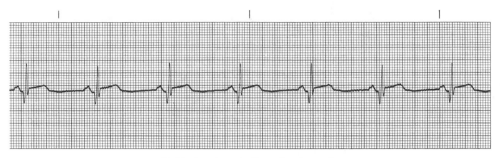

FIGURE 8–17. Sinus bradycardia.

exhibits signs of decreased cardiac output (cold, clammy skin, low blood pressure, syncope).

Treatment

Uncomplicated bradycardia requires no treatment. If the individual is compromised by the slow rate, atropine administered intravenously rapidly and dramatically increases the heart rate. If atropine is not successful in increasing the rate or the maximum dose has been reached, intravenous isoproterenol may be used.[21,22] Temporary or permanent pacing may be necessary if there is profound, poorly tolerated bradycardia.

SINUS TACHYCARDIA

Definition and Cause

Tachycardia is a rapid sinus rhythm of greater than 100 bpm. A sinus rhythm originates in the sinoatrial node. Sinus tachycardia is usually caused by something other than increased automaticity of the SA node. Anything that increases sympathetic activity, such as excitement, pain, fever, hypovolemia, hypoxia, strenuous exercise, and the consumption of caffeine and nicotine, are frequent causes of tachycardia. Cardiac failure, myocardial infarction, and many other diseases of the heart are accompanied by sinus tachycardia. It may also be induced by administration of drugs, including Isuprel, atropine, epinephrine, and alcohol.

ECG Appearance

Wave forms are normal (Fig. 8–18). The rate is greater than 100 bpm.

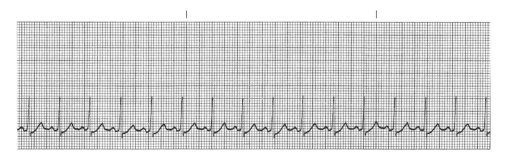

FIGURE 8–18. Sinus tachycardia.

Hemodynamic Implications

Unless associated with a pathologic state, sinus tachycardia is usually inconsequential and of brief duration. The rapid heart rate, however, increases myocardial oxygen demand and may decrease coronary artery perfusion, resulting in angina in the individual with CAD. Symptoms of low cardiac output might also be exhibited in those cases in which the decreased diastolic time prevents adequate ventricular filling.

Treatment

Intervention should include rest and treatment of the underlying pathologic state. Oxygen and sublingual nitroglycerin may be necessary if the individual experiences angina. Digoxin may be administered to increase contractility, slow AV conduction, and decrease the heart rate if the patient is symptomatic.

SINUS ARRHYTHMIA

Definition and Cause

A sinus arrhythmia is a varying irregular rhythm with all impulses originating in the SA node. Sinus arrhythmia may be normal, especially in young and elderly people. In a healthy individual, the sinus rate is noted to vary about 10 percent in its pattern, over time. Sinus arrhythmias occur in response to enhanced vagal tone, digitalis, or morphine.[19] The arrhythmia may be related to respiration, with the rate increasing with inspiration and decreasing with expiration.

ECG Appearance

All waves are normal in size and shape (Fig. 8–19), but the timing of the cycles is irregular. The rate is usually between 60 and 100 bpm.

Hemodynamic Implications

There are usually no hemodynamic consequences of sinus arrhythmia.

Treatment

No treatment necessary. If related to digitalis toxicity, the drug is discontinued.

Atrial Arrhythmias

Atrial arrhythmias are caused by the rapid and repetitive firing of one or more foci in the atria outside the sinus node. They override the slower SA node pacemaker

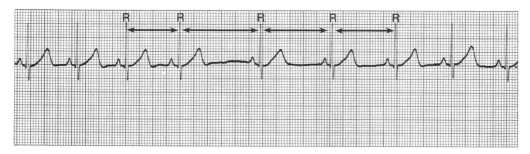

FIGURE 8–19. Sinus arrhythmia.

and take control of the rhythm of the heart. In atrial arrhythmias with rates of less than 200, every impulse may be conducted throughout the AV node to the ventricles (1:1 conduction). At rates greater than 200, the physiologic refractory period of the AV node introduces a block to conduction and therefore the conduction ratio (atrial:ventricular impulses) may be 2:1, 3:1, or greater. On the ECG, the P waves are variable in shape and rhythm, depending on the location of the ectopic focus. The configuration of the QRS may be normal because the conduction pathways below the AV node are normal. However, the rhythm may be very irregular because the atrial impulses are often conducted in an irregular pattern. Atrial arrhythmia frequently occur following coronary artery bypass surgery or heart valve replacement and as a result of age-related changes in the cardiac anatomy. Although they are usually transient, they can have significant hemodynamic implications and often require additional in-hospital time.[23-25]

WANDERING ATRIAL PACEMAKERS

Definition and Cause

The wandering atrial pacemaker is a varying rhythm caused by the changing focus of the pacemaker. It occurs when there is a change in vagal tone, change in sympathetic stimulation to the heart, inflammation of the SA node from rheumatic carditis, digitalis toxicity, and sick sinus syndrome. It is not uncommon and is most likely to be observed in athletes and in young and elderly people.

ECG Appearance

The atrial rate is very irregular. There is no consistent pattern to the rhythm (Fig. 8-20). The shape of the P waves and length of the PR intervals vary, with the pacemaker firing and the proximity of the ectopic pacemaker to the AV node. When the pacemaker site is closer to the AV node, the PR interval is shorter and the P wave becomes flatter. The ventricular rate is equal in rate and rhythm to the atrial rate, as all atrial impulses are conducted to the ventricle. The QRS is normal in appearance because ventricular conduction is normal.

Hemodynamic Implications

There are no hemodynamic consequences because the rate is usually 60 to 100 bpm and cardiac output is maintained.

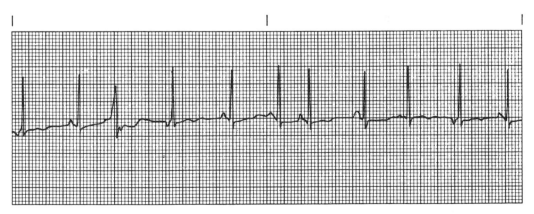

FIGURE 8-20. Wandering atrial pacemaker.

Treatment

No treatment is necessary unless the individual is symptomatic. Treatment of the underlying cause of the rhythm disturbance is initiated. Bradycardia is treated with a sympathomimetic drug (isoproterenol hydrochloride [Isuprel].) Sympathomimetic drugs are synthetic substances of similar chemical structure, and they have many effects similar to those of adrenergic neurohormones. They act on the alpha and beta receptors, increase heart rate and contractility, and accelerate conduction. If the rate is over 100 bpm, treatment is directed toward eliminating the cause and decreasing the heart rate with a beta-blocker such as propranolol.

PREMATURE ATRIAL CONTRACTIONS

Definition and Cause

A premature atrial conduction (PAC) is an earlier-than-expected depolarization from an ectopic focus in the atrial. The impulse travels through the atria by an unusual pathway and creates a P wave of a different configuration. If the ventricle is not in the absolute refractory period at the time the impulse reaches the AV node, the impulse will be conducted normally through the ventricles and produce a normal QRS complex. If the ventricle is refractory, only the P wave is seen on the ECG. PACs are usually conducted retrograde to the SA node, causing the SA node to depolarize prematurely and resetting the sinus rhythm. Therefore, the PP interval including the PAC is less than twice the normal PP interval; this is a noncompensatory pause. PACs are normal and are seen in healthy hearts as well as in those with CAD. Many other pathologic conditions may cause the development of PACs, including rheumatic heart disease, MI, hypertension, and hyperthyroidism. Stress, fatigue, and anxiety may cause PACs, as may the administration of epinephrine or digoxin, and/or the ingestion of stimulants (e.g., caffeine, nicotine).

ECG Appearance

NSR is present except for the PAC, which occurs earlier than expected (Fig. 8–21). The P wave of the PAC is abnormal, but all other waves are normal in configuration.

Hemodynamic Implications

PACs are usually well tolerated, as cardiac output is not altered.

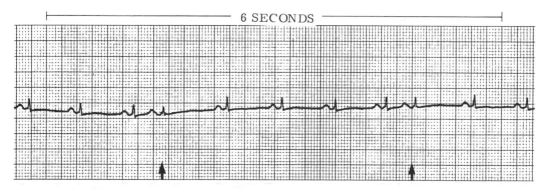

6 SECONDS

FIGURE 8–21. Normal sinus rhythm with a premature atrial contraction. Note that the fourth complex from the left and the third complex from the right occur early in the cycle; the P waves are of a slightly different configuration from the other P waves.

TREATMENT

The only treatment is to omit the stimulus that may be precipitating the PACs (e.g., digoxin, caffeine, nicotine). However, if the individual's clinical picture indicates that the PACs may be a precursor to some persistent atrial arrhythmia, with hemodynamic consequences, prophylactic treatment with antiarrhythmics may be indicated.[24,25]

PAROXYSMAL ATRIAL TACHYCARDIA

Definition and Cause

Paroxysmal atrial tachycardia (PAT) is rapid atrial rhythm characterized by abrupt onset and abrupt cessation. It is caused by increased automaticity and may be triggered by emotions, tobacco, fatigue, caffeine, alcohol, sympathomimetic drugs (Isuprel), or digitalis. It may also be related to congenital heart disease, hypoxia, hypokalemia, cardiomyopathy, MI, cor pulmonale, or systemic hypertension. The rhythm may be sustained for seconds, minutes, or hours, and the patient's tolerance for this arrhythmia may depend on the underlying pathology. The rate is usually 150 to 250 bpm, and there is a 1:1 atrial to ventricular conduction.

ECG Appearance

The P wave is slightly to grossly abnormal and may often be found in the preceding T wave (Fig. 8–22). The PR interval may be shortened (less than 0.12 second). QRS-complex and T-wave configurations are normal. In rapid rhythms, the T wave may not be discernible.

Hemodynamic Implications

PAT of short duration is of little consequence to the healthy heart. However, in the presence of an impaired left ventricle, sustained PAT may precipitate left ventricular failure. Angina may also occur as a result of decreased coronary artery blood flow.

Treatment

Treatment is directed at eliminating the cause of the tachycardia and decreasing the heart rate. Carotid sinus massage or Valsalva maneuvers are usually the first measures instituted. Pharmacologically, intravenous adenosine is the most effective agent

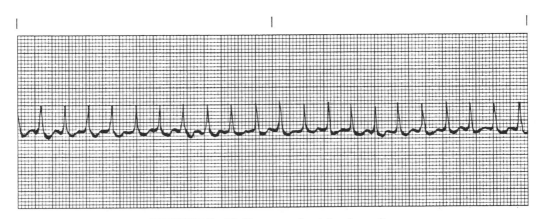

FIGURE 8–22. Paroxysmal atrial tachycardia.

for acute termination. PAT is also treated with verapamil, propranolol, quinidine, or edrophonium and, in some cases, beta-blocking agents or amiodarone.[26,27] If drug therapy is not successful in converting PAT to normal sinus rhythm, cardioversion may be used to terminate the rapid rhythm and restore NSR. Cardioversion is the delivery of an electrical charge to the heart, synchronized with the R wave, that results in complete depolarization of the myocardium. The charge has the potential to interrupt certain arrhythmias, which allows the SA node, the normal pacemaker of the heart, to resume control of the rhythm.

ATRIAL FLUTTER

Definition and Cause

Atrial flutter is a rapid, regular, atrial arrhythmia arising from one atrial focus with a rate of 250 to 350 bpm but most commonly 300 bpm. It is easily recognizable because of the regular "saw-toothed" baseline (called "F" or flutter waves). The refractory time of the AV nodal tissue prevents conduction of more than 200 impulses/minute through the AV node. The rate of impulses conducted to the ventricles is normally an even-numbered ratio to the atrial impulses initiated (2:1 and 4:1). Seen less frequently than atrial fibrillation, atrial flutter may convert to atrial fibrillation spontaneously or during treatment. Individuals with normal hearts experience occasional atrial flutter precipitated by anxiety, caffeine, alcohol, or nicotine. Persistent atrial flutter is usually associated with rheumatic heart disease, chronic obstructive pulmonary disease (COPD), decompensated heart failure, MI, digitalis toxicity, valvular disease, CAD, or pulmonary emboli.

ECG Appearance

The rhythm is recognizable by the regular saw-toothed baseline (Fig. 8–23). The configuration of the QRS complex is normal. Ventricular conduction follows the normal pathways. T waves are usually not identifiable because of the overriding F waves. When calculating the atrial rate, the F wave that falls within the QRS complex is also counted.

Hemodynamic Implications

The individual may experience a fluttering sensation in the chest or throat. If it is short-lived, there is probably minimal or no hemodynamic consequence. If the cardiac

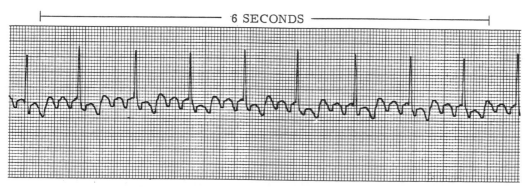

FIGURE 8–23. Atrial flutter (4:1). Note the saw-toothed baseline, known as F waves.

output is compromised by a rapid ventricular response, the individual will experience symptoms of decreased cardiac output.

Treatment

The goals of therapy are to terminate the rhythm or control ventricular response, as well as to identify and treat the cause. Verapamil or vagal stimulation may be used to slow the ventricular response temporarily and to permit clear identification of flutter waves. Digitalis is the drug of choice to convert AF and may restore NSR within 24 hours. If digitalis alone does not control the ventricular rate, the addition of verapamil, propranolol, quinidine, or amiodarone may slow the ventricular rate. Emergency synchronized cardioversion may be the treatment of choice when there is significant hemodynamic compromise. Long-term management may include the use of quinidine, procainamide, and disopyramide in conjunction with digitalis. Many patients require overdrive atrial pacing or cardioversion because chemical conversion is often unsuccessful.[26]

One potential side effect of terminating atrial flutter is that the patient's rhythm may spontaneously convert to atrial fibrillation, requiring further treatment.

ATRIAL FIBRILLATION

Definition and Cause

Atrial fibrillation is a rapid, chaotic atrial arrhythmia caused by the firing of multiple ectopic foci in the atria. The atrial rate may be 350 to 600 bpm. The conduction through the atrial tissue and AV node are random. The ventricular response may be very rapid or controlled, but is usually irregularly irregular (Fig. 8–24) owing to the refractory period of AV nodal cells.[28,29] The atrial activity does not support complete atrial contraction and is out of sequence with ventricular activity. This causes a loss of the atrial contribution to ventricular filling (atrial "kick"). The etiology of atrial fibrillation is varied, but systemic hypertension is the most common cause.[22] AF may occur paroxysmally (occurring and recurring suddenly) in the healthy heart. Chronic atrial fibrillation usually indicates heart disease and is seen in patients with CHF, CAD, pulmonary embolism, and following coronary artery bypass graft surgery or valve re-

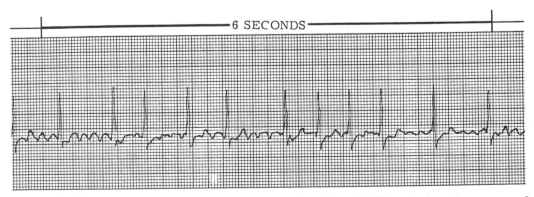

FIGURE 8–24. Atrial fibrillation with rapid ventricular response. (Note the irregular pattern of the ventricular response. There is no pattern to the irregularity, and therefore it is referred to as irregularly irregular.)

placement surgery.[23] AF may also occur following chest trauma or with an acute exacerbation of bronchitis in individuals with COPD.[28] Some drugs may precipitate atrial fibrillation; including alcohol, caffeine, and aminophylline. Atrial fibrillation occurs frequently in the elderly with or without underlying cardiac disease. It is considered to be an arrhythmia of old age.[24]

ECG Appearance

P waves are not identifiable. There is an undulating baseline or fine fibrillatory waves, representing the erratic atrial activity (Figs. 8–24 and 8–25). The ventricular response is irregularly irregular and occurs at a rate of 100 to 150 bpm in the untreated patient. The configuration of the QRS is normal. In atrial fibrillation with a controlled ventricular response, the ventricular rate is less than 100 bpm and, because of the irregular baseline, the T waves are usually unrecognizable.

Hemodynamic Implications

In atrial fibrillation with a controlled ventricular response (less than 100 bpm), the cardiac output is often adequate. However, at higher rates of ventricular response, there may be a decrease in cardiac output because ventricular fill time is decreased and coordination of atrial and ventricular systole is lost. There is a loss of the atrial "kick" that normally contributes as much as 20 to 30 percent to the left ventricular volume. Since this loss is within the normal cardiac reserve, it is tolerable for individuals with a healthy heart, but it may be very significant in a diseased heart.[28] Angina may result from decreased perfusion and increased oxygen requirements of tachycardia.[26,28] Chaotic motion of the atria may also predispose the individual to the development of mural thrombi. This is frequently a concern when attempting to convert atrial fibrillation to NSR, particularly when the atrial fibrillation has been present for longer than 6 months. The more vigorous motion of the myocardium in NSR may dislodge a thrombus, and pulmonary or cerebral emboli may result.

Treatment

Atrial fibrillation may be chronic or occur paroxysmally. Drugs that block AV node conduction (i.e., digitalis, verapamil, and propranolol) are the treatment of choice to convert the rhythm to NSR. If verapamil is ineffective, quinidine or diltiazem may be used. Qunidine decreases myocardial excitability, slows the ventricular rate, and en-

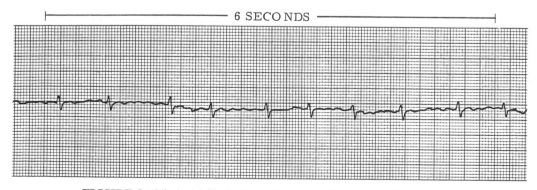

|————————————————— 6 SECONDS ——————————————————|

FIGURE 8–25. Atrial fibrillation with a controlled ventricular response.

hances the effectiveness of digitalis. No treatment is indicated when the ventricular response is controlled and the individual is asymptomatic. Individuals with chronic atrial fibrillation may be placed on anticoagulant therapy because the major concern is thrombus formation and subsequent embolization. Synchronized cardioversion may also be successfully used, especially when atrial fibrillation is new and the patient is hemodynamically compromised.

SUPRAVENTRICULAR TACHYCARDIA

Definition and Cause

Supraventricular tachycardia (SVT) is any tachycardia in which the impulse initiating the rhythm arises from a location above the ventricles. Examples include sinus, atrial, and junctional tachycardias. The onset is usually abrupt and initiated by a premature complex. Termination of the rhythm is also usually abrupt. The extremely rapid rates often make it difficult to identify the origin of the rhythm. Differentiation from ventricular tachycardia may be difficult, especially if the impulse is aberrantly conducted (other than normal pathways) and results in a QRS complex of greater than 0.12 second. In SVT, the ventricular rate is regular and is usually 150 to 200 bpm. SVT may be a sustained rhythm or may last only a few seconds. Although it may be seen in an individual with no underlying cardiac disease, SVT is most often observed in an individual with ischemic heart disease or as a complication of MI.

ECG Appearance

The origin of the arrhythmia determines the ECG appearance. If it is a sinus or atrial tachycardia, a P wave and PR interval should precede each QRS complex (Fig. 8–26). If it is junctional tachycardia, P waves may appear before or after or be buried within the QRS complex. The QRS complex is of normal configuration in the absence of a preexisting bundle branch block of intraventricular conduction delay.[24] A T wave is usually not observed.

Hemodynamic Implications

Usually the rapid rate is poorly tolerated. There is inadequate ventricular fill time, decreased cardiac output, and inadequate myocardial perfusion time. The individual often experiences dizziness or even syncope.

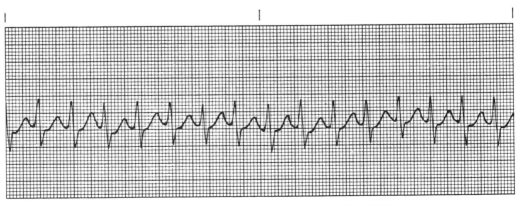

FIGURE 8–26. Supraventricular tachycardia (SVT).

Treatment

Treatment is aimed at controlling the ventricular rate and preventing CHF. The Valsalva maneuver is used first to stimulate a vagal response. The physician may cautiously apply carotid sinus massage or supraorbital pressure to stimulate a vagal response.[26,30] Carotid massage does present a number of risks to the patient, including embolization from a carotid artery plaque, bradycardia, or asystole.[22] Because of its fast rate of action, adenosine, administered rapidly, is very effective in terminating SVT.[22,26] Other drugs that may be used include beta-blockers, digitalis, antiarrhythmics, edrophonium, and vasopressors. Emergency cardioversion or atrial or ventricular pacing may terminate SVT.

AV Nodal Rhythms/Junctional Rhythms

AV nodal or junctional rhythms originate in the AV node when the SA node fails to initiate an impulse. The AV node fires intrinsically at a rate of 35 to 60 bpm. On the ECG (Fig. 8–27), the P wave may be absent or inverted, appearing before or after or buried within the QRS, because conduction in the atria occurs in a retrograde fashion. If the conduction pathways are healthy below the AV node, the QRS will be normal in configuration. With the loss of the synchronized cardiac contraction, the atrial contribution to the ventricular systolic volume (atrial kick) is lost and cardiac output may be decreased 20 to 30 percent.[28] Treatment is not indicated unless the cardiac output is compromised.

PREMATURE NODAL/JUNCTIONAL CONTRACTIONS

Definition and Cause

Premature nodal contractions (PNCs) or premature junctional contractions (PJCs) are premature beats originating in the AV node. They occur in conditions that cause sinus bradycardia or in digitalis toxicity, in which there is increased automaticity of the AV node. Several drugs, including Isuprel, atropine, amphetamines, and excessive caffeine may precipitate PNCs.

ECG Appearance

There is NSR or sinus bradycardia except for premature beats (Fig. 8–28). The abnormal P wave of the premature beat may precede, be buried in, or come after the QRS

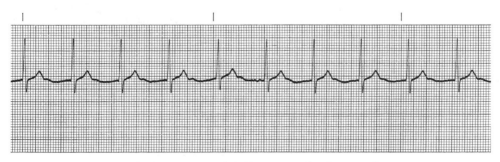

FIGURE 8–27. Junctional rhythm. Note the absence of P waves.

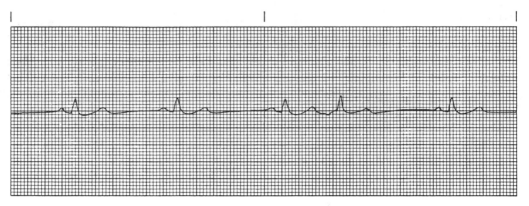

FIGURE 8–28. Normal sinus rhythm with one premature nodal contraction.

complex. If the PNC stimulates retrograde conduction through the atria, it will interrupt the sinus mechanism and produce a noncompensatory pause as the sinus mechanism is reset. If there is no retrograde conduction, the sinus mechanism is not interrupted and a compensatory pause will appear. (See the following section on premature ventricular contractions [PVCs] for definition of compensatory pause.) The configuration and the duration of the QRS complexes are normal.

Hemodynamic Implications
The PNC may cause decreased stroke volume because the ventricle does not have sufficient time to fill before the premature contraction. The radial pulse palpated following the PNC may be much fuller, owing to the extra ventricular volume, because the compensatory pause allows for extra ventricular fill time.

Treatment
No treatment is necessary unless the PNCs are related to digitalis toxicity. In this case, digoxin is withheld until the digoxin level is again within the therapeutic range.

Ventricular Arrhythmias

Ventricular arrhythmias originate from foci located somewhere in the ventricles. Ventricular pacemakers are erratic, slow, and undependable. An effective cardiac output is rarely maintained, and a life-threatening situation is created. Ventricular arrhythmias constitute an emergency. Immediate intervention and conversion of the arrhythmia to a rhythm that produces effective circulation is essential. The goal of long-term maintenance therapy is the prevention of the arrhythmia and sudden cardiac death.[31,32]

PREMATURE VENTRICULAR CONTRACTIONS

Definition and Cause
The most common of all arrhythmias, the premature ventricular contraction (PVC) is a premature beat arising from an ectopic focus in the ventricle.[17,21,26,29] Occur-

ring occasionally in the majority of the normal population, PVCs may be precipitated by anxiety, tobacco use, alcohol, or caffeine consumption. PVCs are the arrhythmia seen most often after MI.

Any condition resulting in ischemia of the myocardium (myocardial infarction, CAD, CHF) may cause PVCs. Hypokalemia, cardiomyopathy, and myocardial irritation from ventricular catheters, such as pacemaker leads or monitoring lines, may also precipitate PVCs.

ECG Appearance

The ECG may appear normal except for the premature beats (Fig. 8 29). Depolarization begins in the ventricle and follows an abnormal pathway that results in a tall and wide QRS complex (greater than 0.12 second). Such a complex is said to be bizarre. In most instances, the PVC does not conduct retrograde through the atrium to the SA node. The sinus mechanism is not interrupted and the PP interval including the PVC is double the normal sinus-induced PP interval. Because the PVC occurs early in the cycle, there is a longer-than-normal pause between the PVC and the next sinus beat. This is a compensatory pause. The sinus impulse that immediately follows the PVC is not conducted because of the ventricular refractory period induced by the PVC. Most often, the sinus mechanism is not interrupted, and the next impulse is initiated, from the SA node, at the regular interval in the existing sinus rhythm. If the PVC is conducted backward and interrupts the sinus mechanism, the sinus mechanism resets and a compensatory pause does not appear.[18,22] The T wave is opposite in deflection to the R wave of the PVC. PVCs that occur close to the vulnerable period of the preceding T wave are of concern because they may fall on the T wave and precipitate ventricular fibrillation (the R-on-T phenomenon).

Hemodynamic Implications

Occasional PVCs have minimal consequences. Increasingly frequent or multifocal PVCs suggest an increasingly irritable ventricle with potential for the development of life-threatening ventricular arrhythmias.

Patterns of PVCs

PVCs often occur in ratios to normal sinus beats. Bigeminy (Fig. 8–30) is a PVC coupled with each sinus beat. Trigeminy is a PVC every third beat. Quadrigeminy is a PVC every fourth beat, and a couplet (Fig. 8–31) is two PVCs occurring together.

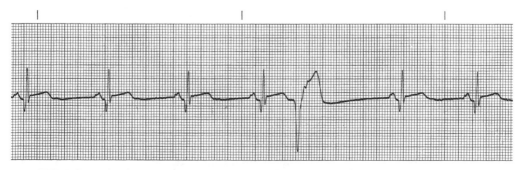

FIGURE 8–29. Normal sinus rhythm with unifocal premature ventricular contractions.

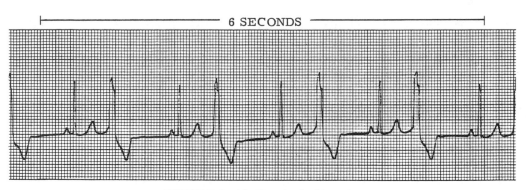

FIGURE 8–30. Ventricular bigeminy.

Treatment

Occasional PVCs in the individual with a healthy heart do not require treatment. Recently, treatment of occasional PVCs has decreased because of the severe side effects associated with many of the antiarrhythmics.[22] Removal of the irritant or treatment of the underlying cause are the initial interventions. Further treatment is based on the hemodynamic consequences of the PVCs. A symptomatic individual may complain of feeling "skipped beats" or fluttering sensations in the chest or throat. Rest and oxygen therapy may eliminate the arrhythmia. In the acute care setting, intravenous lidocaine may be administered when PVCs, couplets, or multifocal PVCs occur at rates of greater than 6 per minute (a standard point for intervention). Lidocaine slows conduction in the ventricles and Purkinje system. It also reduces automaticity in the ventricles and accelerates repolarization.[28] In the cardiac rehabilitation setting, some individuals may have chronic PVCs that do or do not change with exercise and do not require treatment even at rates greater than six PVCs per minute. Others may experience an expected increase in PVCs during some phase of their exercise or recovery period. In such individuals, the exercise prescription should include specific parameters delineating the circumstances under which the individual's exercise should be terminated and appropriate treatment initiated. When necessary, treatment of chronic PVCs is typi-

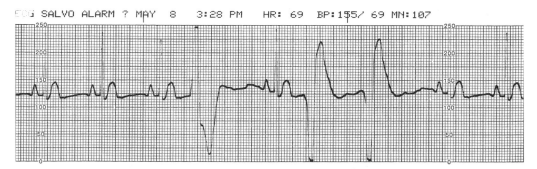

FIGURE 8–31. Premature ventricular contractions: single PVC, then couplet. Note the compensatory pause. The RR interval containing the PVC is two times the RR interval between sinus beats.

cally accomplished with procainamide or other antiarrhythmic medications such as amiodarone, quinidine, propranolol, tocainamide, or mexiletine. Treatment of any underlying cause is continued concomitantly.

VENTRICULAR TACHYCARDIA

Definition and Cause

Three or more PVCs, occurring sequentially at a rate of 150 to 200 bpm, constitute a run of VT. The PVCs may be of the same or varied configuration, indicating multiple foci. VT is usually the result of an irritable, ischemic ventricle and is due to ischemic coronary heart disease or acute MI. Frequent episodes of VT may also occur in the presence of a ventricular aneurysm. Unifocal VT is often related to an irritable focus at the border of a scar from a previous MI. Polymorphic VT is thought to be related to ongoing severe myocardial ischemia or to be the proarrhythmic effect of an antiarrhythmic drug.[26,27,32,33] In the healthy heart, VT may occur paroxysmally, produce no symptoms, and convert spontaneously to an effective cardiac rhythm. Sustained VT is life-threatening because an effective cardiac output is not maintained. As the ventricle becomes increasingly ischemic, VT degenerates to ventricular fibrillation. This progression of arrhythmias is believed to be responsible for sudden cardiac death unrelated to myocardial infarction and for many deaths after MI.

ECG Appearance

The QRS is wide, bizarre, and usually of high amplitude (Fig. 8–32). There are usually no identifiable P waves, and the RR intervals are usually regular. It is very important to differentiate VT from SVT so that the appropriate treatment may be initiated without hesitation.

Hemodynamic Implications

Coronary artery blood flow is estimated to decrease 60 percent in VT owing to ineffective cardiac output from a rapidly contracting ventricle.[4,19,32] Syncopal episodes occur. (If the patient remains alert with no signs of decreased cardiac output, the arrhythmias may actually be supraventricular, a rhythm that may also begin paroxysmally and have large, regular QRS complex. However, some patients do experience repeated episodes of ventricular tachycardia that are hemodynamically well tolerated.[34]

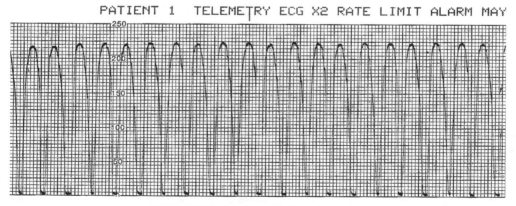

FIGURE 8–32. Ventricular tachycardia.

Treatment

Once the rhythm has been identified, treatment should begin immediately and without hesitation. Synchronized electrical cardioversion is the treatment of choice, with addition of lidocaine, procainamide, or amiodarone to prevent reoccurrence of VT and restore NSR. Bretylium may also be used. The correction of magnesium and potassium deficits is warranted in the successful treatment of VT.[22,26] In the acute care setting, persistent VT, secondary to myocardial ischemia, may also be treated with intra-aortic balloon counterpulsation.

When VT occurs spontaneously, unrelated to an acute myocardial infarction, an electrophysiologic study (EPS) is necessary to evaluate the arrhythmia and to determine the most effective treatment, if treatment is indicated.

Prophylactic drug therapy in patients with recurrent VT is highly individualized. Currently no single agent appears to stand out in its effectiveness. Amiodarone, encainide, and flecainide are some of the most commonly used antiarrhythmic agents. These and others have limited effectiveness and most have a high incidence of significant side effects, many of which are related to the central nervous system. Proarrhythmia, the worsening or new appearance of ventricular tachycardia or ventricular fibrillation, is seen in 10 to 20 percent of individuals taking these drugs.[21,27] Further study is required to determine whether magnesium replacement alone can be effective in eliminating or even preventing atrial and ventricular ectopy.[24]

Antiarrhythmic therapy can be evaluated by means of EP studies or 24-hour ambulatory ECGs. The ambulatory ECGs are an effective, noninvasive means of evaluating the effectiveness of antiarrhythmics during activities of daily living.[21]

The Food and Drug Administration (FDA) has approved an automatic implantable cardioverter defibrillator for use in patients who have chronic intractable VT or fibrillation that cannot be controlled by drug therapy. When tachycardia or fibrillation is sensed by the implanted pulse generator, it sends an electrical shock to the heart. This very-low-voltage shock depolarizes the entire myocardium and allows the sinus node to regain control of the rhythm.

The presence of a ventricular aneurysm or a scar from a previous MI may be suspect when there are frequent episodes of uniform VT.[26] Documented by cardiac catheterization with left ventricular angiography and EPS, the myocardium at the border of the aneurysm is often the site for ectopic foci. Recurrent VT, unrelieved by drugs, may be controlled by surgical resection of the aneurysm and the tissue at its border.[21,35] Another technique, catheter radiofrequency ablation of the ectopic focus, guided by electrophysiologic mapping, appears to be successful in eliminating intractable arrhythmias while maintaining a lower mortality rate than surgical resection.[21,27,36,37]

VENTRICULAR FIBRILLATION

Definition and Cause

VF is chaotic activity of the ventricle originating when multiple foci in the ischemic ventricle fire simultaneously. Because of electrical disorganization, the ventricles do not contract as a unit. There is absolutely no effective cardiac output or coronary perfusion. VF is associated with severe myocardial ischemia; it may follow an ongoing episode of VT or may be precipitated by a drug overdose (digitalis, procainamide, potassium chloride, and others), anesthesia, electrical shock, or cardiac surgery. This is a life-threatening arrhythmia that usually results in clinical death if not treated within 4 minutes.

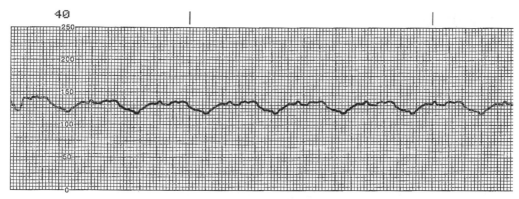

FIGURE 8-33. Ventricular fibrillation.

ECG Appearance

There are no recognizable P waves, QRS complexes, or T waves. The erratic wave forms vary in size and may initially be unrecognizable waves of large amplitude (coarse VF) that quickly decrease in amplitude (fine VF) as myocardial death occurs. A flat baseline (asystole) indicates absolute electrical silence and death (Figs. 8-33 and 8-34).

Hemodynamic Implications

There is no systemic or coronary circulation. Clinical death occurs within 4 minutes.

Treatment

Defibrillation with 200 to 400 watt-seconds is done immediately. If unavailable or ineffective, cardiopulmonary resuscitation must be initiated immediately, according to basic life support or advanced cardiac life support guidelines.[38] Bretylium, lidocaine, epinephrine, magnesium, and many other drugs may be used during the resuscitation efforts to treat arrhythmias, hypoxia, acidosis, and hypokalemia.

If resuscitation efforts are successful, an antiarrhythmic agent should be started to prevent recurrence of the ventricular arrhythmia.[22] EP studies may be used to evaluate the origin of the arrhythmia and identify effective drug therapy to prevent the recurrence of VT and VF.[32]

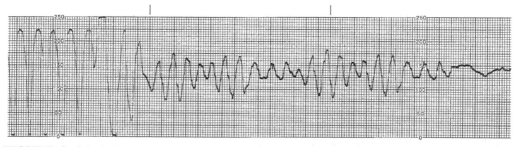

FIGURE 8-34. Progression of ventricular arrhythmias. Note that the rhythm rapidly changes from VT to coarse VF and then to fine VF.

Heart Blocks

Heart blocks are anatomic or functional interruptions in the normal conduction of an impulse through the heart's conductive pathways. This text briefly describes some of the more common blocks.

SINOATRIAL BLOCK

Definition and Cause

In sinoatrial node block (SA node block), the impulse is discharged from the SA node, but for some reason the impulse is unable to reach the surrounding atrial tissue. Although SA block is most frequently the result of drug therapy (digitalis or quinidine), it may occur in CAD.

ECG Appearance

The appearance of all waves is normal. There is an occasional or frequent interruption in the rhythm in which one or more cardiac cycles are missed. The rhythm is the same before and after the pause. If the pause is prolonged, an ectopic focus may fire. The sinus node usually continues to function as the pacemaker.

Hemodynamic Implications

There are hemodynamic implications only if the pause is prolonged. Prolonged pauses may be associated with bradycardia and signs of decreased cardiac output.

Treatment

Treatment is not necessary unless bradycardia is profound and the individual becomes symptomatic. Atropine, epinephrine, or isoproterenol may be administered to increase the heart rate if bradycardia occurs. Medications should be withdrawn if the block is the result of drug therapy.

Atrioventricular Blocks

Atrioventricular conduction blocks (AV blocks) are abnormal delays or failure of conduction through the AV node or bundle of His. The electrical impulse arises normally from the SA node and depolarizes the atria, but, on reaching the AV node or bundle of His, the conduction is slowed to greater than 0.20 second or completely blocked. The block may be a result of CAD, rheumatic heart disease, or MI. Therapy with quinidine, digitalis, and/or procainamide may also delay AV conduction. Treatment is based on the symptomatology the patient demonstrates and on the etiology of the block.

FIRST–DEGREE AV BLOCK

Definition and Cause

In first-degree AV block, all impulses arise normally from the SA node. The impulse is, however, slowed for greater than 0.20 second at the AV node or bundle of His and is then conducted to the ventricle. The delay may be as great as 0.8 second and usually remains constant. First-degree AV block may be seen in healthy individuals, especially in those with increased vagal tone such as well-conditioned athletes.[14,39] It may also be caused by congenital heart disease, rheumatic fever, or acute inferior MI, or seen as a complication of coronary artery bypass surgery. It is also caused by drug toxicity including digitalis, calcium channel blockers, beta blockers, quinidine, or procainamide.[14,30]

ECG Appearance

The configuration of all waves is normal. The PR interval is, however, prolonged (Fig. 8–35).

Hemodynamic Implications

There are no hemodynamic implications. First-degree AV block must be observed for progression to further block, especially when there is an acute onset.

Treatment

Correction of first-degree block requires treatment of the underlying cause. If it is related to drug therapy, dosages may be adjusted or the drug discontinued when the benefits of treatment are offset by the complication of heart block. Atropine may be given intravenously if there is significant bradycardia and the PR interval is greater than 0.26 second.

SECOND-DEGREE ATRIOVENTRICULAR BLOCK MOBITZ TYPE I (WENCKEBACH)

Definition and Cause

In the Wenckebach phenomenon, there is a repeated pattern of progressively lengthening PR intervals until finally an atrial impulse is completely blocked at the AV node. The dropped beats may appear regularly or sporadically. Inferior wall MI, cardiac surgery, electrolyte imbalance, or digoxin, quinidine, or procainamide therapy may precipitate this unusual transient arrhythmia. Wenckebach phenomenon usually appears suddenly but rarely progresses to complete heart block.[14]

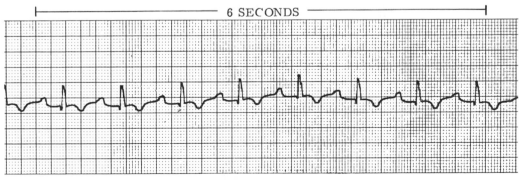

FIGURE 8–35. Normal sinus rhythm with first-degree AV block. (Note the PR interval, 0.28 second.)

ECG Appearance

The heart rate is usually slow because of a block in the AV node, but there is regular P wave activity. The PR interval is progressively lengthened until the P wave is completely blocked and there is no ventricular complex (Fig. 8–36). It is a cyclical phenomenon.[39] The degree of AV block is expressed in a ratio of P waves to QRS complexes (i.e., 4:3 indicates that every fourth P wave is not conducted).

Hemodynamic Implications

The Wenckebach rhythm is fairly well tolerated unless profound bradycardia, a rate less than 40 bpm, results. If bradycardia is profound and the cardiac output is inadequate, the individual exhibits signs of decreased cardiac output (cold, clammy skin, syncope, low blood pressure).

Treatment

Treatment is necessary only if the heart rate is slow and the individual exhibits symptoms of low cardiac output. Atropine may be used to increase the heart rate if the PR intervals exceeds 0.26 second or symptomatic bradycardia develops.[40] Medications that slow AV conduction (digoxin, quinidine, calcium channel blockers, and procainamide) may be withheld. In rare instances, an artificial pacemaker may be necessary to establish a rate consistent with an adequate cardiac output.

SECOND-DEGREE ATRIOVENTRICULAR BLOCK MOBITZ TYPE II

Definition and Cause

Mobitz type II block is rare. It is clinically very significant; it indicates disease in the distal conduction system and may occur as the result of a large anterior or anteroseptal MI, severe CAD, cardiomyopathy, or chronic degeneration of the conduction system. Second-degree AV block may also occur with digitalis toxicity or with propranolol or procainamide use. In Mobitz type II block, atrial impulses occur at a regular rate but are irregularly conducted to the ventricle. The P waves occur in a regular ratio to the QRS (i.e., 2:1 or 3:1). However, a progressive lengthening of the PR interval before the blocked P wave is absent. The site of the block is usually below the bundle of His and is a form of bilateral bundle branch block. This block usually progresses to complete heart block and therefore requires close observation and immediate therapeutic intervention.[22,39]

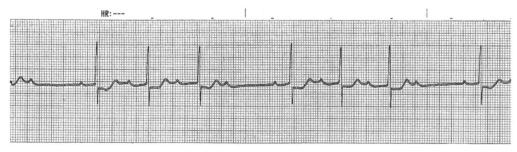

FIGURE 8–36. Second-degree AV block Mobitz type I (Wenckebach). (Note the progressively lengthening PR interval and then the absence of the QRS complex.)

ECG Appearance

The atrial rate is regular. P waves are normal in appearance and the PP interval is constant. The ventricular rate is slow and irregular. Conduction of the atrial impulse to the ventricle is intermittent. The PR interval is consistent (Fig. 8–37). The QRS complex may be normal in appearance but most often is wider than normal, with a bundle branch pattern, because of the level of the block.

Hemodynamic Implications

Symptoms experienced depend on the ventricular rate. When impulses are conducted from the atria to the ventricle, the normal atrioventricular sequence remains intact. If the ventricular rate is adequate, the individual will not experience symptoms of low cardiac output. This block is often progressive and symptoms of low cardiac output appear as the ventricular rate slows.

Treatment

The insertion of a permanent pacemaker and the withdrawal of medications that may increase AV conduction time are the treatment of choice. If the block is secondary to drug toxicity, the block will resolve within 96 hours of discontinuing the drug.[39] Atropine or isoproterenol may be administered initially for symptomatic bradycardia in an attempt to increase the conduction of impulses across the AV node. However, this usually has little effect because of the level of the block.[39]

COMPLETE HEART BLOCK

Definition and Cause

In complete or third-degree atrioventricular heart block, the atrial and ventricular rhythms are independent of one another and therefore the rhythm is termed AV dissociation. There is a failure of conduction of impulses from the atria to the ventricle. The block may be anywhere in the AV conduction system: the AV node, the bundle of His, or the bundle branches.[4,19,40] Any apparent sequence of the independent atrial and ventricular rhythms is coincidental. The atrial rate is faster than the ventricular rate and there is no fixed PR interval. An escape rhythm from the junctional or ventricular myocardium must take over as the pacemaker of the ventricle. The intrinsic ventricular

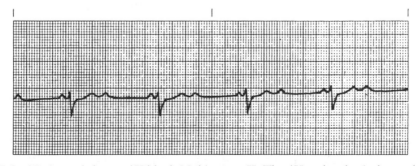

FIGURE 8–37. Second-degree AV block Mobitz type II. The AV node selectively conducts some betas while blocking others. Those that are not blocked are conducted through to the ventricles, although they may encounter a slight delay in the node. Once in the ventricles, conduction proceeds normally.

rate is 20 to 40 bpm. Complete heart block is usually seen as a complication of acute MI or severe angina in which sustained ischemia of the AV node has occurred. It may also be caused by some calcium channel blockers, beta-blockers, class I antiarrhythmics, and digitalis toxicity. Endocarditis, cardiomyopathy or degenerative diseases of the conduction system may result in complete heart block.

ECG Appearance
The atrial and ventricular rhythm appear as independent regular rhythms. The P wave is of normal configuration. The appearance of the QRS depends on the location of the ventricular pacemaker. The QRS is normal in appearance if the rate is controlled by a junctional focus; the lower the site of the escape focus, the wider and more bizarre the QRS complex. PP and RR intervals are regular. There is no relationship between the P and R waves. Ventricular irritability may be seen as a result of the slow heart rate and the resulting myocardial ischemia (Fig. 8–38).

Hemodynamic Implications
A slow heart rate, low cardiac output, and compromised coronary perfusion may result in acute CHF. Individuals may also experience syncope, which, when a result of complete heart block, is known as the Stokes-Adams syndrome. Although this rhythm may be well tolerated at rest in some individuals, symptoms may occur with exercise because of the inability of the ventricle to accelerate properly in response to activity.[19,22,41]

Treatment
Complete heart block is usually a life-threatening emergency because the ventricle is an unreliable pacemaker. However, some older individuals may be asymptomatic when the ventricular escape rhythm is 45 to 60 bpm, and they may tolerate it even with mild exertion.[22] Emergency treatment may include intravenous atropine or isoproterenol, or temporary transvenous or external pacing. Determination of the need for permanent pacing is based on the underlying cause of the block.

Bundle Branch Blocks

Bundle branch blocks (BBBs) are blocks in conduction along either the right or left bundle branch or both. (The term "bundle branches" refers to the major branches of

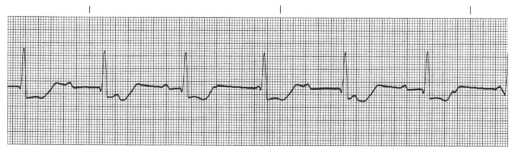

FIGURE 8–38. Complete heart block. (Note that the atrial and ventricular rates are independently occurring rhythms.)

the intraventricular conduction system.) A block in the bundle of His or bundle branches slows the depolarization of the ventricle because the impulse must travel retrograde to the "blocked" ventricle from the ventricle with the "normal" conduction pathway. The depolarization, now occurring at separate times, is represented on the ECG by two joined QRS complexes. The QRS is wider than 0.10 second with a notched configuration that represents two R waves: R and R′ (R prime). The tracing reflects the nonsimultaneous depolarization and is diagnostic of BBB. There is usually no serious impairment to conduction as long as one branch remains intact.[27] A 12-lead ECG is necessary for diagnosis. BBB is best seen in leads V_1 and V_6. BBBs are common complications of MI and are often precursors to complete heart block.[14,39,40]

RIGHT BUNDLE BRANCH BLOCK

Definition and Cause

Right bundle branch block (RBBB) is an anatomic or functional block in the right bundle branch that slows the depolarization and contraction of the right ventricle. Although seen in healthy hearts, RBBB is most frequently seen in anterior MI.

ECG Appearance

Atrial conduction is normal. The QRS is greater than 0.12 second and is notched (rSR′) in lead V_1. There are large S waves in leads I and V_6. The T wave is opposite in deflection to the QRS (Fig. 8–39).

Hemodynamic Implications

There are no hemodynamic implications. Despite delayed conduction, diastolic fill time and cardiac output remain normal.

Treatment

No treatment is necessary.

LEFT BUNDLE BRANCH BLOCK

Definition and Cause

Left bundle branch block (LBBB) is caused by a block in the left bundle branch that delays conduction and contraction of the left ventricle. LBBB occurs in ischemic heart disease, MI, valvular heart disease, and in other cases of serious heart disease. In some instances, LBBB may be rate-dependent (i.e., it appears only when a "critical

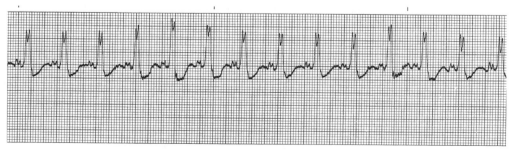

FIGURE 8–39. Right bundle branch block.

rate" is reached). The significance of this event is yet to be determined. The LBBB disappears immediately when the individual's heart rate falls below the critical rate and can be immediately reproduced by raising the heart rate to the critical level.

ECG Appearance
The rate and rhythm are normal, with a widened QRS, greater than 0.12 second, that appears notched in the left chest leads (V_5 and V_6) (Fig. 8–40).

Hemodynamic Implications
There are no complications.

Treatment
No treatment is necessary for the block itself.

ARTIFICIAL PACEMAKERS

An artificial pacemaker is an electronic device that can sense intrinsic electrical cardiac events and provide repetitive electrical stimuli to the heart muscle when they are absent. These stimuli, like the heart's natural pacemaker, allow the origination and conduction of an impulse through the heart. Artificial pacemakers have become increasingly more complex in the past 10 years. They are implanted minicomputers that store and analyze information and respond as they are programmed to a variety of cardiac conduction abnormalities. Today, approximately one million individuals have implanted pacemakers.[42]

The pacemaker coordinates sensed and paced cardiac events by means of an internal clock. Timing intervals between events determine how long the pacemaker waits following sensed or previously paced events before emitting a pacing stimulus.[43] Refractory periods, when the pacemaker is temporarily turned off for a set interval, prevent oversensing of other electrical activity.

Pacemakers are indicated in several cardiac rhythm abnormalities. Ninety percent of permanent pacemakers are implanted for sick sinus syndrome or AV node and His-Purkinje conduction disorders.[42,44,45] Other indications include symptomatic blocks distal to the bundle of His, overdrive suppression of SVT or VT that is resistant to drug therapy, and rate maintenance of both chambers to prevent tachyarrhythmias.

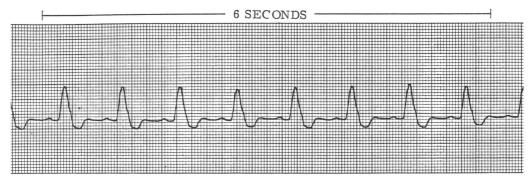

|← ─────────── 6 SECONDS ─────────── →|

FIGURE 8–40. Normal sinus rhythm with complete left bundle branch block (Lead I).

Temporary pacemakers are indicated as emergency treatment in virtually all symptomatic or hemodynamically compromising bradycardias and are often used prophylactically after MI or coronary artery bypass surgery.[26,43,45] Temporary pacing may be done transvenously or transcutaneously or via epicardial leads placed during open heart surgery. Temporary transvenous leads are positioned in the right ventricle from a right internal jugular or left subclavian approach. This is a very reliable method of temporary pacing. Transcutaneous pacing is a safe, fast, and generally effective method of pacing in emergency situations. Large pacing electrodes are placed over the cardiac apex and on the posterior chest wall between the scapulae. Although effective for short-term emergency pacing, it is very uncomfortable for the patient.

Specific guidelines for the use of pacemakers have been developed by the Joint American College of Cardiology/American Heart Association Task Force on Assessment of Cardiovascular Procedures.[45] As pacemakers become increasingly more complex in their functions and programmability, they also become increasingly expensive and more complex to use. The guidelines provide some direction for proper utilization and protection from overutilization.

Pacemaker Components

Pacemakers are composed of a pulse generator (a battery and electrical circuit) and a lead wire. The pulse generator initiates the electrical stimulus to the heart. It may also have a sensing mechanism with which it senses the individual's heartbeat.

Lithium iodide is the power source for essentially all permanent pacemaker generators that are implanted today. They have a life expectancy of 5 to 15 years. Nuclear-powered pacemakers, with a 20-to-40-year life expectancy, are no longer implanted because of safety, expense, and environmental issues.

With permanently implanted pacemakers, the pulse generator usually "fails" over a period of weeks to months. The symptoms exhibited depend on the patient's underlying rhythm. The failure of the battery is usually detected by a change in heart rate, either bradycardia or uncontrolled tachyarrhythmias and associated symptoms, or by pacemaker interrogation, which is done with a pacemaker-specific electronic programmer.

The lead is the conducting wire and electrode tip. It extends from the generator to the patient's heart and delivers the stimulus to the myocardium. The lead may be placed transvenously by threading it through the subclavian vein into the right atrium. When properly positioned, the electrode tip lies against the atrial or ventricular endocardium. It is held in place by a tine-like tip. If the pacemaker is placed during open heart surgery, the electrodes may be sutured directly to the epicardium.

Types of Pacemakers

Pacemakers are classified as either temporary or permanent and single- or dual-chamber. Temporary pacing, usually via the transvenous approach, is used when the arrhythmia is believed reversible, to evaluate the effects of a pacer-supported rhythm or as an emergency intervention until the permanent pacer can be inserted. Single-chamber pacing is that system which stimulates either the atria or ventricle. Usually it is the ventricle that is paced. Dual-chamber pacing stimulates both the atria and the ventricle. Both modes may be used temporarily or permanently.

Rate responsive permanent pacemakers modulate heart rate in response to body movements, respiratory rate, and blood temperature in individuals with chronotropic incompetence.[43,44]

Classification/NASPE Code

Pacemakers are classified according to five parameters: Chamber-paced, chamber-sensed, mode of response, programmable features, and special tachyarrythmia features. Each category designates a specific but standard function of the pacemaker.

"Chamber-paced" and "chamber-sensed" refer to the chamber of the heart in which the electrode lies (atrial, ventricular, or dual chamber). Chamber sensed depends on the presence and function of the sensing mechanism and in which one of the chambers this function occurs. (It may occur in both.) "Mode of pacing" refers to sensing function and how it relates to stimulus release. Programmable pacemakers have a variety of modes and specific functions that can be adjusted by external reprogramming. The letters describing this category are arranged in a hierarchy from absence of function to complex operation, with each higher level incorporating the functions of the previous levels. The letter "C" for communicating indicates that the pacemaker has telemetric capabilities. It may be capable of transmitting data about the pacemaker, the programmed features, past cardiac events, and the pacemaker's response to these events. Rate-responsive pacemakers modulate heart rate in response to at least one physiologic variable. Body movement, respiratory rate, and core blood temperature are examples of physiologic variables to which pacemakers may be programmed to respond. Special antitachycardia functions are available in some highly specialized pacemakers. This type of pacemaker is capable of one or more antitachycardia functions. Either a pacing stimulus, P, and/or a synchronized or unsynchronized shock, S, are emitted on detection of a tachyarrhythmia.[44]

To allow uniform description of pacemaker function, a five letter pacemaker code has been adopted by the North American Society of Pacing and Electrophysiology (NASPE), and this code is used universally. The first letter refers to the chamber pace. The second letter refers to the chamber sense and the third letter indicates how the pulse generator responds to the impulse. The fourth and fifth letters identify the programmability and the special tachyarrhythmia features of the pacemaker (see Table 8–3). The reader is referred to other sources for further details.[42–44,46]

Modes of Pacing

There are four pacing modes: fixed-rate or asynchronous, demand or inhibited, triggered or synchronous, and dual. Fixed-rate pacemakers fire continuously without regard to the patient's own rhythm. This preset firing may result in competition; that is, the ventricles may receive impulses simultaneously from both natural and artificial pacemakers, which compete for dominance. This competition may cause chaotic rhythm disturbances and is the primary disadvantage of fixed-rate pacemakers. Demand or inhibited pacemakers sense the inherent rhythm of the heart and do not discharge an impulse if the heart initiates its own impulse. The pacemaker fires only when needed.

Triggered or synchronous pacemakers pace constantly when there is no intrinsic

TABLE 8–3 NASPE Pacemaker Code

First letter Chamber-paced	O = None A = Atria V = Ventricle D = Dual (A + V)
Second letter Chamber-sensed	O = None A = Atria V = Ventricle D = Dual (A + V)
Third letter Mode of response	O = None T = Triggered I = Inhibited D = Dual (T + I)
Fourth letter Programmability and rate modulation	O = No adjustment possible P = Simple programmable M = Multiprogrammable C = Communicating R = Rate modulating
Fifth letter Antitachyarrhythmia function	O = None P = Pacing S = Shock D = Dual (P + S)

beat. When the pacemaker senses a ventricular depolarization owing to natural pacing, the pacemaker releases its impulse. Because the ventricle is already depolarized and refractory to another stimulus, the pacer impulse is ineffectual.

Dual-chamber pacemakers are capable of sensing and pacing both the atria and the ventricles. This enables each atrial contraction, whether spontaneous or paced, to be followed at a preset interval with a ventricular contraction. These are AV-sequential pacemakers. Their primary advantage is that they preserve the normal sequence of cardiac events. The atrial contribution to ventricular filling is maintained. Dual-chamber pacemakers are more versatile than single-chamber units. AV-sequential pacemakers may be reprogrammed to either single-chamber (atrial or ventricular) or dual-chamber function as needed.

Pacemakers are programmed when they are implanted to meet the current needs of the individual. After implantation, pacemaker functions may be adjusted or reprogrammed by means of an external, pacemaker-specific, electronic programmer.

Electrocardiogram Appearance

On the ECG, the pacemaker impulse is recorded as a spike immediately preceding the depolarization of the atria and/or ventricles (Figs. 8–41 and 8–42). The spike may be of varying amplitude. It is instantaneous and has no real duration. In some instances a 12-lead ECG may be required to detect the pacing spike because it is very small, but most are easily visible. When a pacemaker is stimulating adequately, each pacing spike produces a cardiac response. If the electrode is in the atria, each spike should produce a P wave. If the electrode is in the ventricles, each spike should pro-

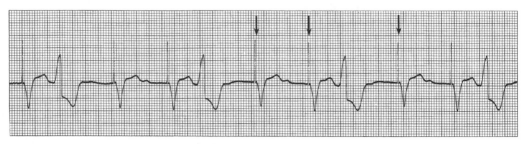

FIGURE 8–41. Ventricular pacemaker rhythm. (Note the spike preceding each ventricular complex. The ventricular complex is wide and bizarre because the impulse is initiated in the ventricle.)

duce a QRS complex. The pacemaker is then said to be in capture. When a pacing spike fails to produce a response, the pacemaker is said to be out of capture. Frequent causes of failure to capture are a loss of contact between the electrode and the chamber wall, depletion of the power source, or a fracture in the electrode[45,47] (Fig. 8–43).

In appearance, the waves of the cardiac cycle differ from those of the individual's natural rhythm because the pacemaker impulses arise from a different site in the myocardium. Conduction does not follow normal pathways. In a ventricularly paced rhythm, the QRS is often wide and bizarre in appearance.

Occasionally, the patient's own intrinsic stimulus occurs at the same time as the pacemaker-generated stimulus. Both stimuli initiate depolarization of the ventricle at the same time from different directions and result in a shared or "fusion" beat appearing on the ECG. The QRS follows the pacing spike and is a distorted blend of the two contributing wave forms (Fig. 8–44).

Complications

Complications associated with pacemaker function include: local infection or hematoma formation at the lead or pulse generator insertion sites, arrhythmias from

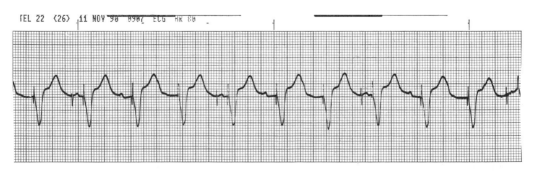

FIGURE 8–42. Atrioventricular pacemaker rhythm. (Note that the atrial pacing is intermittent. The individual's intrinsic P wave can be identified on those complexes that do not have an atrial pacing spike. Every QRS is paced.)

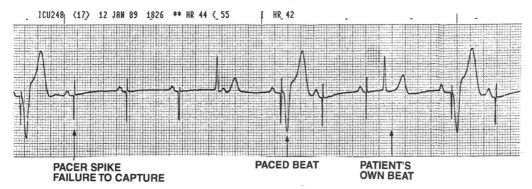

FIGURE 8-43. Failure to capture. (Note the pacing spikes that are not followed by any waveform.)

irritation of the ventricle, perforation of the right ventricle by the catheter, and loss of capture. The individual is treated symptomatically for each complication, with appropriate adjustments made to the pacemaker to ensure optimal functioning. Pacemakers may also be damaged or accidentally reprogrammed by defibrillation current. To minimize this risk, defibrillation paddles should always be placed at least 10 cm from the pulse generator.[43]

Response to Exercise

The response to exercise of an individual who has a pacemaker depends on the person's underlying cardiac disease, level of fitness before pacemaker placement, and degree of dependence on the pacemaker, as well as the type of pacemaker implanted. Individuals with normal SA node function and dual chamber pacers often have a "normal" cardiovascular response to exercise because they maintain the normal sequence of cardiac events. Those with ventricularly paced rhythms may not tolerate exercise as well because they may not have the benefit of the atrial kick (which contributes up to 30 percent of the cardiac output). Most individuals who are likely to exercise receive

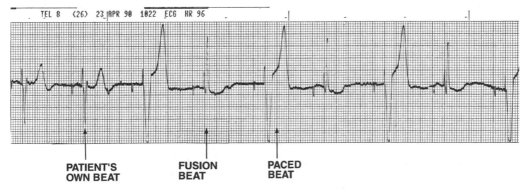

FIGURE 8-44. Fusion beat. (Note the unusual configuration of the fusion beat in comparison to the paced beats and the patient's intrinsic heartbeats.)

rate-responsive or rate-modulating pacemakers. Exercise testing can evaluate the appropriateness of the sensor response to the exercise intensity before the beginning of exercise training. Cardiac rehabilitation staff members must be familiar with the type and function of each individual's pacemaker. Pacemaker identification cards, carried by patients, provide information about the type and function of the implanted unit. Long-term follow-up is an important part of these individuals' ongoing health care.

Individuals with pacemakers should be taught to recognize such symptoms as shortness of breath and fatigue to determine their tolerance for exercise. With proper cardiac monitoring, exercise can be undertaken safely and confidently. It is possible for these individuals to achieve training effects and a relatively high level of fitness.[41,42,47] Even elderly and severely impaired individuals may be able to obtain a modest increase in work capacity that may help them maintain a higher level of independence.

ELECTROPHYSIOLOGIC STUDIES

An electrophysiologic (EP) study is an invasive technique used to detect and locate abnormalities in impulse origination and conduction in the heart. During a specialized cardiac catheterization procedure, electrode catheters are passed transvenously into the heart, and the electrical potential of specific areas of the heart can be observed and evaluated. Developed initially as a diagnostic tool, EP studies are now used for the diagnosis and treatment of many specific cardiac arrhythmias. The major indication for EP studies is ventricular arrhythmia unresponsive to routine drug therapy, especially in individuals who have experienced an episode of sudden cardiac death. Symptomatic supraventricular arrhythmias that are unresponsive to drug therapy and syncope of undetermined origin are also indications for EP evaluation.[17,22,27,32,48]

Diagnosis of a particular arrhythmia is made by observing the arrhythmia via intracardiac ECG or by electrically stimulating the heart and attempting to deliberately induce the specific arrhythmia. Under carefully controlled conditions, the arrhythmia is observed and then promptly terminated by transvenous pacing or electrical cardioversion. This allows the physician to observe potentially lethal tachyarrhythmias to determine the effectiveness of current treatment or determine what other therapies may be necessary. Drug therapies may be adjusted on the basis of repeat EP studies. If the particular arrhythmia cannot be reinduced following the initiation of a particular drug, the antiarrhythmic drug is effective. If it is ineffective, other drug therapies may be tested in this manner; if effective, it appears to correlate well with long-term prognosis for the individual in regard to that arrhythmia.[21,31] EP studies have allowed a much more rapid selection process of effective antiarrhythmics in individuals with recurrent life-threatening arrhythmias.[21,22]

EP studies may be used for direct treatment of cardiac arrhythmias by mapping ventricular conduction so that surgical resection or catheter radiofrequency ablation of an ectopic focus may be performed. EP studies are also used to predict the efficacy of an antiarrhythmic device or pacemaker.

The major drawbacks are the risks inherent to cardiac catheterization and the psychologic impact of repeat studies should they become necessary.

IMPLANTABLE CARDIOVERTER-DEFIBRILLATOR

The implantable cardioverter-defibrillator (ICD) is a battery-powered electrical device implanted to detect and correct life-threatening ventricular arrhythmias. Used in conjunction with appropriate antiarrhythmic drugs, the ICD monitors the heart through epicardial or transvenous leads and discharges an R-wave synchronized shock up to 33 joules when it senses VT or VF.[31] The generator is implanted in the abdominal wall and connected to sensing electrodes and patches attached to the epicardial surface of the heart or transvenous electrodes that are passed via the left subclavian vein into the right ventricular apex. With the transvenous electrodes, a single patch electrode for defibrillation may be implanted in the left midaxillary region. Single-therapy devices are able to monitor rate only or rate and QRS morphology, and deliver a shock sufficient to convert the arrhythmia to normal sinus rhythm. Tiered-therapy devices deliver multiple or tiered therapies: antitachycardia pacing (fast-pacing); single-chamber, ventricular-demand pacing for bradycardia (slow-pacing); and cardioversion and defibrillation shocks for life-threatening tachyarrhythmias.

An ICD is indicated in individuals who have survived an episode of sudden cardiac death unrelated to myocardial infarction and who have no inducible arrhythmia during EPS and those who have experienced recurrent tachyarrhythmias that are inducible during EPS but refractory to drug therapy.[42,49,50,51] ICDs may take up to 25 seconds to detect a tachyarrhythmia and deliver therapy. Individuals will be aware of the shock from the ICD, although they may or may not be aware of the VT or VF. They will describe it as a sharp kick in the chest or a brief electrical shock. Others touching the person during the therapy may feel a slight tingling sensation, but it is harmless.[42,50,52] If the cardiac rehabilitation specialist witnesses a shock, it is important to immediately assess the individual, including vital signs and the symptoms experienced before and after the shock. If the individual is symptomatic, it is important to identify the current rhythm. Any arrhythmia will require treatment. Individuals whose rhythm fails to convert after a maximum number of shocks from the ICD will require external defibrillation followed by cardiopulmonary resuscitation (CPR), if necessary. No treatment is indicated if the individual does not have symptoms and there is no arrhythmia. The ICD has worked effectively. A physician should re-evaluate the individual with an ICD if he or she experiences a change in the number of shocks in a day or if symptoms persist. Regular follow-up care is essential for these individuals.

The ICD has been well tolerated and has significantly decreased the mortality rate from recurrent cardiac arrest in this high-risk population to approximately 1.8 percent in the first year. Its safety record represents a promising approach to the management of individuals at particularly high risk for recurrent lethal arrhythmias.[52] About 40,000 ICDs are now implanted nationally.[44]

Individuals with ICDs can benefit significantly from cardiac rehabilitation, but it is important for both the individual and the cardiac rehabilitation specialist to be well aware of the patient's exercise tolerance evaluation, indicating any exercise-induced arrhythmias, and to be aware of the individual's tachycardia rate detection level (the rate at which the ICD is activated). It is recommended that the target heart rate be 20 to 30 bpm below the rate detection level.[11] This is an adequate safety margin so that the individual may exercise safely and confidently. The overall goal is to provide protection from SCD while allowing the individual to maximize his or her activity level.

ELECTROCARDIOGRAM CHANGES SEEN WITH EXERCISE

Individuals with healthy hearts demonstrate several expected and insignificant ECG changes during exercise (Table 8–4). Most notable is the significant tachycardia

TABLE 8–4 ECG Changes during Exercise*

Healthy Individual†	Individual with CAD‡
1. Slight increase in amplitude of P wave	1. Appearance of a BBB at a "critical heart rate"
2. Shortening of PR interval	2. Recurrent or multifocal PVCs during exercise and/or recovery
3. Slight shift to right of QRS axis	3. VT (three or more consecutive ventricular beats)
4. ST-segment depression of less than 1 mm	
5. Decreased amplitude of the T wave	
6. Single or rare PVCs during exercise and recovery	4. Appearance of bradyarrhythmias/ tachyarrhythmias—rapid rate abruptly slowing or vice versa, not related to exercise
7. Single or rare PJCs or PACs	5. ST-segment depression/elevation of greater than 1 mm, 0.08 second after the J point
	6. Bradycardia in response to exercise
	7. Tachycardia that results in a HR greater than the individual's upper limit
	8. Increase in frequency or severity of any arrhythmia the individual is known to have

*Decreases in the resting heart rate and the submaximal heart rate are observed in both groups with physical conditioning.
†All these ECG changes are normal in response to exercise.
‡Occurrence of any one of these changes should result in cessation of exercise and thorough evaluation of the ECG change and related symptoms.

that occurs with moderate to heavy physical exertion accompanied by a rapid return to the pre-exercise heart rate following cessation of the exercise (during recovery). The healthy individual may experience single or rare premature atrial, junctional, or ventricular contractions during exercise. These arrhythmias are without hemodynamic consequences.[11,54] Individuals with CAD should demonstrate the same changes during exercise, but at a much lower level of exercise. Beneficial ECG changes and a lower heart rate (at rest and during submaximal exercise) that occur as a result of physical conditioning are demonstrated by both healthy individuals and those with CAD. Individuals with CAD also develop the ability to engage in more vigorous activity before reaching their ischemic threshold (training effect). Individuals who have undergone cardiac transplants pose a challenge to the cardiac rehabilitation professional. Because of the lack of direct sympathetic innervation their heart rate rises more slowly and peaks at a lower rate than the rate of the normal heart.[40,55]

Abnormal ECG responses observed during exercise reflect an imbalance between myocardial oxygen supply and demand. Usually they are either exertional arrhythmias or alterations in the ST segment and T wave (see Table 8–2).[5,10] Exertional arrhythmias occur during both exercise and the recovery period. They are significant in their relationship to an individual's cardiac output. If the arrhythmia causes inadequate cardiac output, it may induce syncope, angina, or CHF. Alterations in the ST segment and T wave (see Fig. 8–5) fall into three categories: horizontal, downsloping, and upsloping. ST-segment depression or elevation of 1 mm or greater measured at 0.08 second from the J point indicates ischemia of the myocardium. It is an abnormal response to exercise. When exercise in cardiac rehabilitation is monitored, this parameter should be assessed carefully in relation to other clinical symptoms to determine intervention. There is little or no agreement concerning the significance of the varying shapes of both the ST segment and T wave that occur with exercise.[5]

Many pathophysiologic conditions, including anemia, hypoxemia, and ventricular aneurysm, as well as cardioactive drugs, cause the same ST segment and T wave changes commonly induced by exercise. In determining the significance of ST-segment depression during exercise, it is important not only to observe and evaluate the associated symptoms but also to observe and evaluate how quickly the individual's ECG returns to normal on cessation of the exercise. Table 8–4 lists other abnormal ECG changes that may be observed. For all these abnormalities and any other new and potentially significant clinical symptoms reported by the patient, including fatigue, chest discomfort, dizziness, and palpitations, exercise should be terminated. Observation of the arrhythmia and assessment of the patient, including vital signs and objective and subjective symptoms, should be done immediately and appropriate treatment should be instituted. If the situation is non-emergent, the individual should remain at the cardiac rehabilitation site under observation until symptoms have completely abated. The patient should be instructed to seek prompt evaluation by a physician. Information regarding the episode should be forwarded to the physician by the cardiac rehabilitation staff. Appropriate results from the physician's evaluation should be forwarded to the cardiac rehabilitation staff before the individual exercises again. In addition, new arrhythmias or other new symptoms observed before exercise should always be evaluated before the person is permitted to exercise. Exercise is contraindicated in any patient found to be in complete heart block or demonstrating CHF symptoms. Such individuals should seek immediate medical attention.

DRUG EFFECTS ON THE ELECTROCARDIOGRAM

Drugs that affect the heart rate may have some effect on the ECG pattern. Cardiac glycosides, antiarrhythmics, and beta-blockers all have varying effects on the cardiac cycle. Digitalis has the greatest potential for causing profound ECG changes.[6] Beta-blockers, in particular, may cause bradycardia. They may produce heart rates in the range of 40 to 50 bpm. Although these drugs do cause bradycardia, the linear relationship between increased exertion and increased heart rate remains.[11,55]

Digitalis preparations and calcium ion antagonists increase AV conduction time. The most frequently observed sign of digitalis toxicity is AV block. Digitalis may also produce sagging in the ST segment (Fig. 8–45) and shortening of the Q-T interval

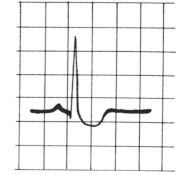

FIGURE 8–45. Digitalis effect. Note the rounded sagging appearance of the ST segment. (From Brunner, LS and Suddarth, DS: Textbook of Medical Surgical Nursing, ed 5. JB Lippincott, Philadelphia, 1984, p. 571, with permission.)

(measured from the Q wave through the T wave). In digitalis toxicity, arrhythmias of all types (atrial, junctional, and ventricular) have been documented[1] (Table 8–5).

Quinidine and procainamide may prolong the AV conduction time and cause a prolonged P-R interval. A wide QRS complex and a wide, notched T wave or even an inverted T may also be seen. In toxicity, patients frequently demonstrate an AV block, widening of the QRS (to as much as one and a half normal duration), or ventricular arrhythmias.[27]

Diuretics that cause hypokalemia may cause the development of arrhythmias, particularly PVCs.

Drugs used in the treatment of concurrent illnesses may also cause changes in the ECG. Phenothiazines (e.g., promethazine hydrochloride [Phenergan] chlorpromazine hydrochloride [Thorazine]) and tricyclic antidepressants (e.g., amitriptyline hydrochloride [Elavil], doxepin hydrochloride [Sinequan]) cause T-wave changes, PR and QT prolongation, conduction disorders, and supraventricular and ventricular arrhythmias.[4,27] MAO inhibitors can also induce arrhythmias.[6] It is therefore important to keep current records of patients' complete medical and pharmacologic regimens. Patients should be encouraged repeatedly to keep the cardiac rehabilitation team aware of any changes in their medications, as changes could have a dramatic effect on their exercise prescription and their response to exercise.[11,55]

TABLE 8–5 Effects of Selected Drugs on the ECG

Drug	ECG Effect
Digitalis	1. Shortens ventricular activation time 2. Increases AV conduction time 3. Shortens QT interval 4. Depresses ST segments and makes them sag 5. In large doses: Decreases T wave amplitude Prolongs PR interval Sinus bradycardia, PACs, PVCs, and bigeminy Multiple conduction abnormalities 6. Toxicity: AV block
Quinidine and procainamide	1. Prolonged PR interval 2. Wide QRS complex; lengthened QT interval 3. Depressed, widened or notched T wave 4. Toxicity: SA or AV block Ventricular arrhythmias Up to 50% increase in QRS duration
Phenothiazines (Phenergan, Thorazine)	1. Nonspecific T wave changes 2. Decreased T wave amplitude 3. Intraventricular conduction disturbances 4. Supraventricular and ventricular arrhythmias
Tricyclic antidepressants (Elavil, Sinequan)	1. T wave changes 2. PR interval, QT interval, and QRS complex prolongation 3. Conduction disturbances 4. Supraventricular and ventricular arrhythmias

SUMMARY

Information regarding the significance of ECGs in the diagnosis and treatment of cardiac pathology was presented. The individual wave forms were identified and related to the heart's corresponding electrical and muscular activity. Lead placements for proper ECG recording at rest and during exercise were identified and illustrated.

In addition, the basic concepts of rate, rhythm, and wave form configuration for the interpretation of ECGs most commonly encountered in a cardiac rehabilitation setting were presented. Arrhythmias, abnormalities in initiation and/or conduction of the heart beat, were described, with sample electrocardiographic strips for the purpose of illustration. Information outlining each arrhythmia's specific etiology, hemodynamic implication, and treatment was included for common arrhythmias and conduction blocks. Brief discussions of pacemakers, electrophysiologic studies, ICD, and the effects of drug therapy on the ECG concluded the chapter.

Review questions and ECG rhythm strips in workbook fashion are given after the references to provide an opportunity for evaluation of basic arrhythmia identification skills.

REFERENCES

1. Gilmore, SB and Woods SL: Electrocardiography and vectorcardiography. In: Woods, SL et al (eds): Cardiac Nursing, ed 3. Lippincott, Philadelphia, 1995, p 290.
2. Goldman, MJ: Principles of Clinical Electrocardiography, ed 12. Large Medical Publications, Los Altos, Calif, 1986.
3. The normal electrocardiogram. In: Guyton, AC and Hall, JE: Textbook of Medical Physiology, ed 9. Saunders, Philadelphia, 1996, p 129.
4. Menzel, LK and White, JM: Electrocardiogram interpretation. In Colchesy, JM et al (eds): Critical Care Nursing, ed 2, Saunders, Philadelphia, 1996, p 127.
5. Ritchle, DE. Exercise and Activity. In: Woods, SL, et al (eds): Cardiac Nursing, ed 3. Lippincott, Philadelphia, 1995, p 708.
6. Hartley, LH: Exercise for cardiac patients, long term maintenance. Cardiol Clin 11:270, 1993.
7. Dubin, D: Rapid Interpretation of EKGs, ed 4. Cover Publishing Co, Tampa, 1988.
8. Brannon, FJ: Experiments and Instrumentation in Exercise Physiology. Kendall-Hunt, Dubuque, Iowa, 1978.
9. Sumner, SM and Grau, PA: Guidelines for running a 12-lead EKG. Nursing '85 15:12, 1985.
10. Vinsant, MO and Spence, MI: Common Sense Approach to Coronary Care, ed 5. Mosby, St Louis, 1989.
11. Wenger, NK: Rehabilitation of the patient with coronary heart disease. In: Schlant, RC and Alexander, RW (eds): Hurst's The Heart—Arteries and Veins, ed 8. McGraw-Hill, New York, 1994, Vol 2, p 1223.
12. Fisch, C: Electrocardiography and vectorcardiography. In: Braunwald, E (ed): Heart Disease: A Textbook of Cardiovascular Medicine, ed 4. Saunders, Philadelphia, 1992, p 116.
13. Purcell, JA and Haynes, L: Using the ECG to detect MI. Am J Nurs 84:5, 1984.
14. O'Donnell, L: Complications of MI, beyond the acute stage. Am J Nurs 96(9): 25, 1996.
15. Marriott, HJL: Practical Electrocardiography, ed 8. Williams & Wilkins, Baltimore, 1988.
16. Conover, M: Understanding Electrocardiography: Arrhythmias and the 12-Lead Electrocardiogram, ed 6. Mosby Year Book, St. Louis, 1992.
17. Zipes, DP and Jalife, J: Cardiac Electrophysiology from Cell to Bedside. Saunders, Philadelphia, 1990.
18. Lipman, BS, Dunn, M, and Massic, E: Clinical Electrocardiography, ed 8. Year Book Medical Publishers, Chicago, 1989.
19. Myersburg, RJ, Kessler, KM, and Castellanos, A: Recognition, clinical assessment and management of arrhythmias and conduction disturbances. In: Schlant, RC and Alexander, RW (eds): Hurst's The Heart—Arteries and Veins, ed 8. McGraw-Hill, New York, 1994, Vol 1, p 705.
20. Woods, SL: Electrocardiography and vectorcardiography. In Woods, SL et al (eds): Cardiac Nursing, ed 3. Lippincott, Philadelphia, 1995, p 290.
21. Cardiac arrhythmias. In: Cheitlin, MD, Sokolow, M, and McIlroy, MB: Clinical Cardiology, ed 6. Appleton & Lange, Norwalk, Conn, 1993, p 512.
22. Hastillo, A and Hess, ML: Diagnosis and treatment of cardiac arrhythmias. In: Ayers, SM et al (eds): Textbook of Critical Care, ed 3. Saunders, Philadelphia, 1995, p 502.
23. Creswell, LL et al: Hazards of postoperative atrial arrhythmias. Ann Thorac Surg 56:539, 1993.

24. McCoy, AK: A new standard-creating an algorithm for atrial dysrhythmias. Am J Nurs (suppl) 84(11):27, 1994.
25. McKenry, LM, and Salerno, E: Pharmacology in Nursing, ed 16. Mosby, St. Louis, 1986.
26. Clyne, CA and Kimmelstiel, CD: Clinical management of cardiac arrhythmias in the coronary care unit. In: Rippe, JM et al (eds): Intensive Care Medicine, ed 3. Little Brown Co., Boston, 1996, Vol 1, p 532.
27. Zipes, DP: Management of cardiac arrhythmias; pharmacological, electrical and surgical technique. In: Braunwald, E (ed): Heart Disease: A Textbook of Cardiovascular Medicine, ed 4. Saunders, Philadelphia, 1992, p 628.
28. Stahl, L: How to manage common arrhythmias in medical patients. Am J Nurs 95(3):36, 1995.
29. Jacobson, C: Arrhythmias and conduction defects. In: Woods, SL et al (eds): Cardiac Nursing, ed 3. Lippincott, Philadelphia, 1995, p 321.
30. Loeb, S (ed): Cardiovascular Disorders in Disease. Springhouse Corporation, Springhouse, PA, 1993, p 572.
31. Lehman, MH and Steinman, RT: Preventing sudden cardiac death. Postgrad Med 82:7, 1989.
32. Marchlinski, FE: VT: Clinical presentation, course and therapy. In: Zipes, DP and Jalife, J: Cardiac Electrophysiology from Cell to Beside. Saunders, Philadelphia, 1990, p 756.
33. Antiarrhythmic drugs. In Tierney, LM, McPhee, S, and Papadakis, A (eds): Current Medical Diagnosis and Treatment, ed 35. Appleton & Lange, Stamford, Conn, 1996, p 344.
34. Bardy, GH and Olson, WH: Clinical characteristics of spontaneous-onset sustained VT and VF in survivors of cardiac arrest. In: Zipes, DP and Jalife, J: Cardiac Electrophysiology from Cell to Bedside, Saunders, Philadelphia, 1990, p 778.
35. Cox, J: Surgical Treatment of Cardiac Arrhythmias. In: Schlant, RC and Alexander, RW (eds): Hurst's The Heart—Arteries and Veins, ed 8, McGraw-Hill, New York, 1994, p 863.
36. Saksena, S et al: Clinical investigation of antiarrhythmic devices: A statement for health care professionals from a joint task force of the North American Society of Pacing and Electrophysiology, the American College of Cardiology, the American Heart Association and Working Groups on Arrhythmias and Cardiac Pacing of the European Society of Cardiology. Pacing and Clinical Electrophysiology 18(4 PT 1):637, 1995.
37. Scheinman, MM: Treatment of cardiac arrhythmias with catheter ablative technique. In: Schlant, RC and Alexander, RW (eds): Hurst's The Heart—Arteries and Veins, ed 8. McGraw-Hill, New York, 1994, p 859.
38. American Heart Association: Guidelines for cardiopulmonary resuscitation and emergency cardiac care, part III: Advanced cardiac life support. JAMA 268:2199, 1992.
39. Lewandowski, DM and Jacobson, C: AV blocks: Are you up to date? Am J Nurs 95(12):27, 1995.
40. Erikson, BA: Dysrhythmias. In: Kinney, MR and Packa, DR (eds): Andreoli's Comprehensive Cardiac Care, ed 8. CV Mosby, St. Louis, 1996, p 86.
41. Superko, HR: Effects of cardiac rehabilitation on permanently paced patients with third degree heart block. Journal of Cardiac Rehabilitation 3:561, 1983.
42. Stephenson, N and Combs, WJ: Artificial cardiac pacemakers and implantable cardioverter defibrillators. In: Kinney, MR and Packa, DR: Andreoli's Comprehensive Cardiac Care, ed 8. Mosby, St. Louis, p 220.
43. Belz, MK, Wood, MA, and Ellenbogen, KA: Pacemakers and implantable cardioverter defibrillator in the intensive care setting. In: Ayers, SM et al (eds): Textbook of Critical Care, ed 3. Saunders, Philadelphia, 1995, p 513.
44. Jones, MC: Pacemakers. In: Clochesy, JM et al (eds): Critical Care Nursing, ed 2. Saunders, Philadelphia, 1996, p 167.
45. Dreifus, LS et al: Guidelines for implantation of cardiac pacemakers and antiarrhythmia devices. J Am Coll Cardiol 18:10, 1991.
46. Bernstein, AD et al: The NASPE/BPEG generic pacemaker code for antibradyarrhythmia and adaptive rate pacing and antitachyarrhythmia devices. Pacing and Clinical Electrophysiology 10:794, 1987.
47. Tamarisk, NK: Enhancing activity levels with permanent cardiac pacemakers. Heart Lung 17(1):6, 1988.
48. Akhtar, M: Technique of electrophysiological testing. In: Schlant, RC and Alexander, RW: Hurst's The Heart—Arteries and Veins, ed 8. McGraw-Hill, New York, 1994, p 881.
49. Cooper, DK, Valladeres, BK, and Futterman, LG: Care of the patient with the automatic implantable cardioverter-defibrillator: A guide to nurses. Heart Lung 87(1):640, 1987.
50. Collins, MA: Implantable cardioverter defibrillator. Am J Nurs 94:34, 1994.
51. Ayers, SM: Cardiovascular. In: Ayers, SM: Textbook of Critical Care, ed 3. Saunders, Philadelphia, 1995, p 448.
52. Callans, DJ and Josephson, ME: Future developments in implantable cardioverter defibrillators: The optimal device. Prog Cardiovasc Dis 36(3):227, 1993.
53. Brooks, R et al: The automatic implantable cardioverter defibrillator: Early development, current utilization and future directions. In: Braunwald, E (ed): Heart Disease Update. Saunders, Philadelphia, 1990, p 193.
54. Dehn, MM: Rehabilitation of the cardiac patient: The effects of exercise. Am J Nurs 80:5, 1980.
55. Miller, NH: Cardiac rehabilitation: Management of the patient after MI. In: Kinney, MR and Packa, DR: Andreoli's Comprehensive Cardiac Care, ed 8. Mosby, St. Louis, 1996, p 402.

CHAPTER 8 REVIEW QUESTIONS

Instructions: Briefly answer the following questions as they apply to electrocardiography. (Answers follow.)

1. ECG interpretation is based on _____ , _____ , _____ , and _____ .

2. _____ is the hallmark ECG sign of myocardial ischemia.

3. Disturbances in cardiac rhythm (cardiac arrhythmias) are caused by abnormalities in either _____ or _____ or both.

4. The _____ , the "natural pacemaker of the heart," fires intrinsically at a rate of _____ times per minute.

5. _____ leads and _____ leads make up the 12 standard ECG leads. _____ is often used as a single monitoring lead during exercise.

6. Match the wave or waves of the ECG in Figure 8–46 that are described by one of the following definitions or phrases.

   a. _____ ventricular depolarization

   b. _____ the cardiac cycle

   c. _____ absolute and relative refractory period

   d. _____ ventricular repolarization

   e. _____ atrial depolarization

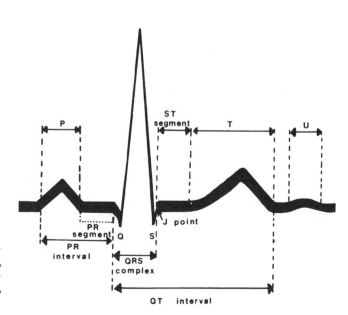

FIGURE 8–46. ECG wave configuration. (From Underhill, SL, et al: Cardiac Nursing. JB Lippincott, Philadelphia, 1983, p. 204, with permission.)

7. Identify the most common heart blocks.
   a.
   b.
   c.
   d.
   e.

8. All are characteristics of NSR except:
   a. The rhythm is essentially regular.
   b. The impulse arises from the sinoatrial node at a rate of 60 to 100 bpm.
   c. The appearance of the QRS complexes is variable.
   d. The rate may decrease slightly with deep inspiration and increase with expiration.

9. In individuals with coronary artery disease and angina, sinus tachycardia:
   a. increases myocardial oxygen demand
   b. may significantly decrease coronary artery perfusion because of the decrease in the duration of diastole
   c. may result in an anginal episode if the underlying cause is not identified and treated to decrease the heart rate
   d. all of the above.

10. Regularly occurring premature ventricular contractions (PVCs) may be identified

    as _____ when a PVC is coupled with every normal beat and

    as _____ when the PVC occurs every third beat.

11. Briefly explain the mechanism by which the heart meets the increased oxygen demand of exercise.

    How does this differ in the individual with atherosclerosis?

12. Sinus bradycardia:
    a. may be well tolerated
    b. is often seen in individuals who are physically fit and in many individuals during sleep
    c. may be profound (less than 40 bpm) and lead to signs and symptoms of low cardiac output
    d. may be seen in individuals on digoxin therapy
    e. all of the above

13. Identify the average duration of the:

    a. P wave _____

    b. PR interval _____

    c. QRS complex _____

    d. ST segment _____

    e. T wave _____

14. When an abnormal ECG change is detected and persists or increases in frequency with exercise, the health professional should do all of the following except:
    a. terminate the exercise with the appropriate monitored cool-down period
    b. check and record the individual's vital signs and associated symptoms
    c. allow the individual to resume exercise as soon as the abnormality disappears
    d. notify the client's physician of the ECG change
    e. caution the client against exercise until the ECG change is evaluated
    f. none of the above

15. All of the following are normal ECG changes seen with exercise except:
    a. depression of the ST segment of less than 1 mm
    b. tachycardia
    c. recurrent and/or multifocal PVCs during exercise or in the recovery phase
    d. decreased amplitude of T wave

16. An anatomic or functional interruption to conduction of an impulse through the normal conductive pathway is:
    a. atrial fibrillation
    b. heart block
    c. heart failure
    d. ventricular muscle depolarization

17. Identify four characteristics of PVCs.
    a.
    b.
    c.
    d.

18. Premature ventricular contractions may be precipitated by:
    a.
    b.
    c.

19. Briefly describe why arrhythmias, arising in the ventricles (other than occasional PVCs) require immediate treatment.

20. Atrial flutter is characterized by all of the following except:
    a. Ventricular response may be irregular or regular and stated in a ratio of atrial to ventricular activity.
    b. The atrial activity has a saw-toothed configuration on ECG and is known as "F" or flutter waves.
    c. There is an abnormal configuration to the QRS waves

21. List the categories of cardiac drugs that most commonly affect the ECG and give their effects.
    a.
    b.
    c.
    d.

22. Atrial arrhythmias:
   a. include atrial fibrillation, atrial flutter, and premature atrial contractions as the most common
   b. arise from ectopic foci in the atria
   c. have P waves of abnormal or various configurations, or there may be an absence of identifiable P waves
   d. may have normal QRS configurations
   e. all of the above

23. Why is it essential to maintain up-to-date medication profiles on all patients in a cardiac rehabilitation program?

24. What is the biggest advantage of atrioventricular sequential pacemakers?

25. How is a pacemaker detected on ECG?

26. What are the two indications for an implantable cardioverter-defibrillator?

27. For an individual with an ICD, explain the margin of safety between the target heart rate for an exercise session and the rate detection level of the ICD.

ANSWERS TO REVIEW QUESTIONS

1. Rate, rhythm, regularity, and the individual wave configurations
2. ST-segment depression/elevation of greater than 1 mm occurring 0.08 second after the J point
3. Automaticity, conduction
4. Sinoatrial node, 60 to 100
5. Six limb, six chest, modified chest lead V5 (CMV5)
6. a. QRS complex
   b. the entire PQRST complex
   c. ST segment and T wave
   d. T wave
   e. P wave
7. a. sinoatrial node block (SA node block)
   b. first-degree AV block (Mobitz I)
   c. second-degree AV block (Mobitz II)
   d. complete heart block
   e. bundle branch block
8. C is the correct answer
9. D is the correct answer
10. bigeminy, trigeminy (in that order)
11. Because the heart is extremely efficient in extracting oxygen from the blood at normal rates, the healthy heart meets increased oxygen demand brought on by exercise by increasing the heart rate (and consequently, increasing the coronary artery blood flow) and through dilation of the coronary arteries.

    In CAD there are changes in the vessel walls that inhibit dilation, and therefore the increase in heart rate is the only mechanism that increases oxygen supply to the myocardium during exercise.

12. E is the correct answer.
13. a. P wave: 0.08 to 0.12 second
    b. PR interval: less than 0.20 second
    c. QRS: 0.06 to 0.12 second
    d. ST segment: 0.12 second
    e. T wave: 0.16 second
14. C is the correct answer.
15. C is the correct answer.
16. B is the correct answer.
17. Any four of these answers:
    a. QRS is prolonged owing to the abnormal pathway of myocardial conduction and depolarization.
    b. A compensatory pause follows the PVC.
    c. Often occurs in the cool-down or recovery phase following exercise.

   d. If untreated, may degenerate into life-threatening arrhythmias of ventricular tachycardia or ventricular fibrillation.
   e. The T wave is opposite in deflection to the R wave of the PVC.

18. Premature ventricular contractions may be precipitated by any three of these answers:
    a. caffeine
    b. alcohol
    c. anxiety
    d. tobacco
    e. any ischemia-producing event

19. With the exception of occasional PVCs, arrhythmias that have their origin in the ventricles are life-threatening because the ventricular pacemakers are undependable, and chaotic rhythms may result in a cardiac output that may be well below what is necessary to meet the body's metabolic demands.

20. C is the correct answer.

21. a. Cardiac glycosides. Effect: Increased AV conduction time; sagging ST segment; shortened Q-T interval.
    b. Beta blockers. Effect: Bradycardia at rest; slower heart rate than may be predicted with exercise.
    c. Calcium antagonists. Effect: Increased AV conduction time; slowing of heart rate.
    d. Antiarrhythmics. Effect: Varies with the drug and the arrhythmia it is being used to treat.

22. E is the correct answer.

23. Different medications have various effects on patients when they exercise and may cause some complications or ECG changes. Knowledge of patients' medication profile allows for more appropriate interpretation of a change in the ECG or a new symptom brought on by exertion.

24. The atrioventricular pacemaker mimics the normal conduction system of the heart, the atria, and ventricle pump in sequence. The atrial kick is maintained.

25. The properly functioning pacemaker is detected by the appearance of a spike (a deflection with no duration) just before the atrial and/or the ventricular depolarization wave.

26. a. Individuals who have survived an episode of SCD, unrelated to an MI, and who have no inducible arrhythmia during EP studies
    b. Individuals who have experienced recurrent tachyarrhythmias that are inducible during EP studies but are refractory to drug therapy.

27. The individual's target heart rate should be set 20 to 30 beats below the rate detection level of the ICD (the rate at which the ICD is activated).

RHYTHM STRIP REVIEW

Interpret each of the following rhythm strips by answering the following questions:

1. What is the rate?
2. What is the rhythm? regular or irregular?
3. Are there P waves?
4. What is the QRS duration?
5. By evaluating the P-R interval, what is the relationship between the P waves and the QRS complexes?

   (Answers follow.)

RHYTHM STRIP REVIEW NOTES

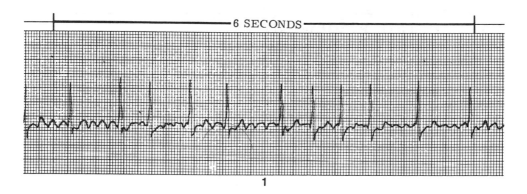

6 SECONDS

1

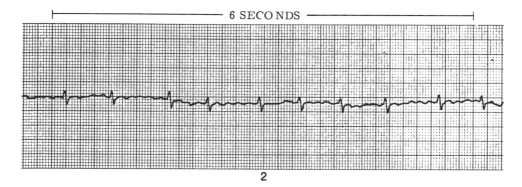

6 SECONDS

2

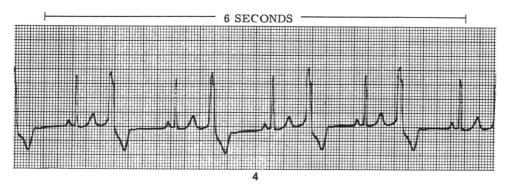

3

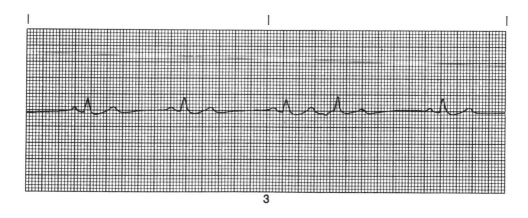

6 SECONDS

4

RHYTHM STRIP REVIEW NOTES

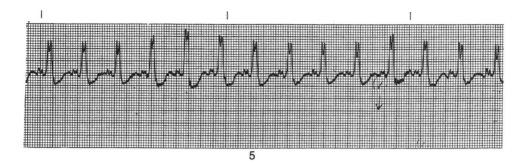

5

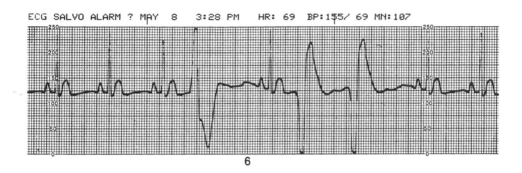

ECG SALVO ALARM ? MAY 8 3:28 PM HR: 69 BP:155/ 69 MN:107

6

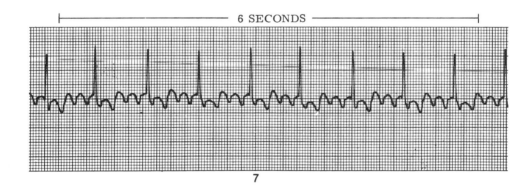

6 SECONDS

7

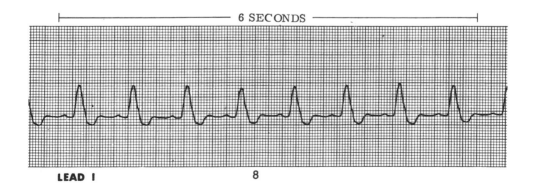

6 SECONDS

LEAD I 8

RHYTHM STRIP REVIEW NOTES

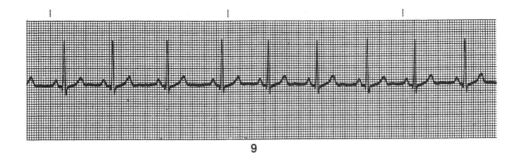

9

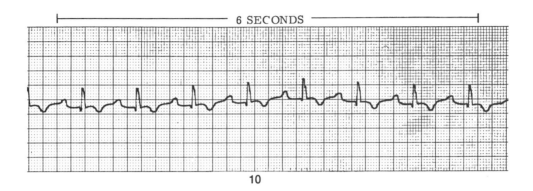

10

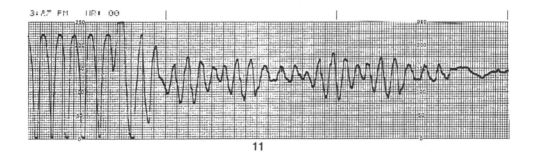

11

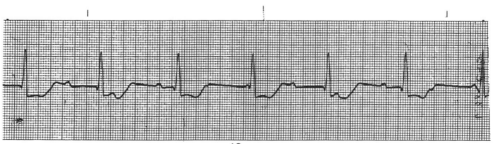

12

RHYTHM STRIP REVIEW NOTES

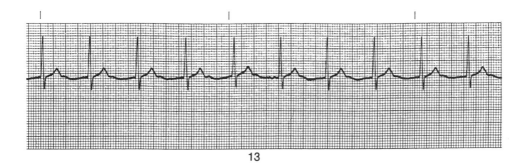

13

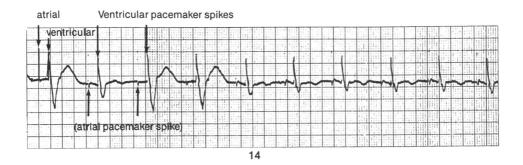

atrial   Ventricular pacemaker spikes

ventricular

(atrial pacemaker spike)

14

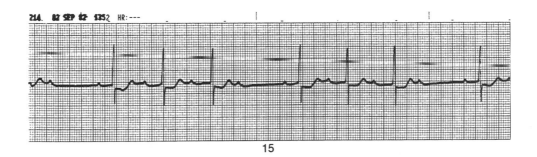

15

PATIENT 1   TELEMETRY ECG X2 RATE LIMIT ALARM MAY

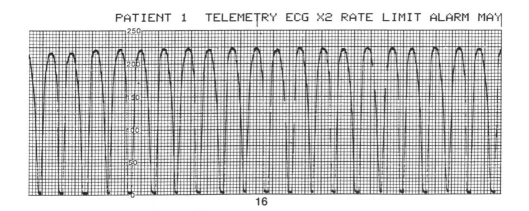

16

RHYTHM STRIP REVIEW NOTES

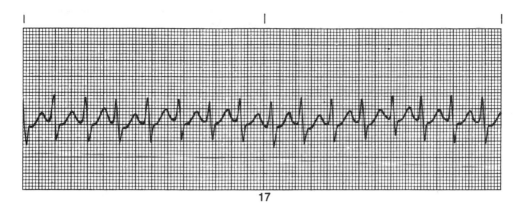

17

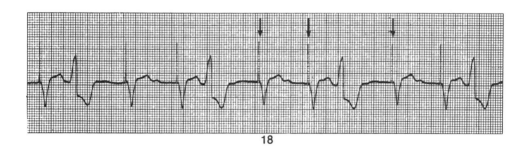

18

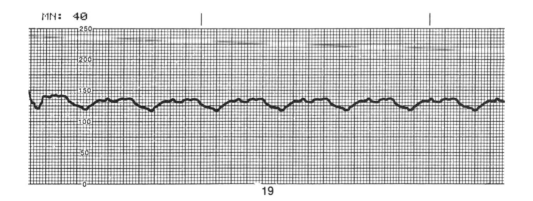

19

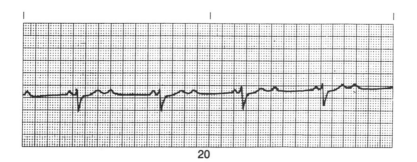

20

RHYTHM STRIP REVIEW ANSWERS

1. Atrial fibrillation with rapid ventricular response
2. Atrial fibrillation with controlled ventricular response
3. Sinus bradycardia with one premature nodal contraction
4. Ventricular bigeminy
5. Normal sinus rhythm with right bundle branch block (RBBB)
6. Normal sinus rhythm with unifocal premature ventricular contractions
7. Atrial flutter
8. Normal sinus rhythm with left bundle branch block (LBBB)
9. Normal sinus rhythm
10. Normal sinus rhythm with first-degree atrioventricular (AV) block
11. Progression of ventricular arrhythmias. Ventricular tachycardia degenerates to course ventricular fibrillation and then fine ventricular fibrillation
12. Complete heart block or third degree heart block
13. Junctional rhythm
14. Atrioventricular sequentially paced rhythm
15. Second-degree AV block, type I (Wenckebach)
16. Ventricular tachycardia
17. Supraventricular tachycardia (SVT)
18. Ventricular paced rhythm
19. Ventricular fibrillation
20. Second-degree AV block, type II

CHAPTER 9

Assessment of the Cardiac Patient

Many patients referred to outpatient cardiac programs are likely to have undergone some sort of assessment procedure(s) by their referring physicians to determine medical status, risk stratification, and monitoring requirements during exercise and as a basis for formulating the exercise prescription. Many of these tests are of a technical nature and the team of specialists responsible for providing outpatient cardiac rehabilitation services may not participate in these assessments. Although this chapter briefly addresses more technologic tests such as radionuclide imaging, echocardiography, and coronary angiography, the primary focus is to describe the various assessment techniques and procedures that are likely to be performed by the cardiac rehabilitation team responsible for Phases II and III cardiac rehabilitation.

INFORMATION REGARDING PATIENT MEDICAL STATUS

Before scheduling individual assessments, information regarding a patient's medical status must be obtained. This information comes from the patient and the referring physician.

Information Provided by the Patient

Specific forms have been developed to obtain information from, as well as to provide information for, the patient. Usually, these forms are mailed to the prospective rehabilitation patient after he or she has made the initial request for information. Although the packet of application forms can be expensive to mail, properly completed forms in advance of laboratory assessment at the rehabilitation site can save considerable time for the rehabilitation staff. Five separate forms should be included in the patient program application packet: the patient information letter, the medical history questionnaire, an insurance form, a medical release authorization form, and an instruction sheet for the graded exercise test (GXT). Examples of these forms are found in Appendix A.

249

The primary purpose of the patient information letter is to inform the prospective patient of the appropriate entry procedures, including the accurate completion of the enclosed forms, the information to be supplied by the referring physician, and the scheduling of the laboratory assessment. Information regarding the cost of the program and insurance reimbursement may also be included.

The medical history and risk factor analysis forms included in the packet of patient application forms should be reviewed for accuracy in a later interview. The interview is an essential part of the assessment process and is conducted by the rehabilitation personnel. The assessment procedures essentially begin with the interview.

There are many ways to administer a medical history. Medical histories may be self-administered by the patient, computer-administered, obtained through interviews by physicians or the rehabilitation staff, or obtained by a combination of these methods.

Although the cardiovascular history (including symptoms and medications) is the most significant part of the medical history for cardiac patients, the medical history should also include information pertaining to other major systems of the body. It can be divided into three categories: past history, family history, and present symptoms. Information regarding allergies, medications, injuries, operations, and hospitalizations should also be reviewed and documented.[1-3]

Information regarding the patient's quality of life (QOL) should be included as part of the comprehensive medical history. This information should include an evaluation of physical function status, previous exercise history, occupational activities, job satisfaction, social activities, hobbies, relationships with family and friends, sense of self-reliance, sexual adjustment, mood, and general satisfaction with life. These assessments may be divided into three domains: (1) physical status and functional abilities; (2) psychological status and well-being; and (3) social interactions and role functions.[3]

Information Provided by the Referring Physician

The medical evaluation by the referring physician will probably include a medical history; a physical examination; and evaluation of blood pressure, serum cholesterol, lipoprotein levels, additional blood components (e.g., hematocrit, electrolytes, etc.), and pulmonary function.[1,2] The referring physician's form must be completed and returned to the rehabilitation staff before initiation of treatment or further evaluation. It would also be prudent to obtain the physician's signature on STAT and PRN emergency orders along with the prescription for cardiac rehabilitation (Appendix B).

If a GXT has not been previously performed, once the aforementioned information is obtained from the patient and the referring physician, the patient may be scheduled for a GXT at the cardiac rehabilitation center. Because measurements of body composition are usually obtained by the rehabilitation staff, assessment of body composition and the GXT are addressed in this chapter. Assessments of risk factors and psychosocial status will be discussed in Chapter 13.

ASSESSMENT AT THE CARDIAC REHABILITATION CENTER

When a patient comes to the rehabilitation center for a scheduled assessment, he or she is interviewed and the medical history and risk factor appraisal forms are confirmed for accuracy. At this time, the patient signs the informed consent and release forms before the conduction of any further assessment.

Informed Consent

Specific policies for the protection of the legal rights and safety of patients must be developed. Obtaining informed consent ensures preservation of the patient's rights and documents his or her voluntary assumption of risk. Informed consent is a method of communication between a qualified health care provider, informing the patient of the intent to test or treat, and a patient, indicating an understanding of the procedures to be performed. It also provides for the patient to give permission freely, allowing the rehabilitation staff to perform specified medical procedures. It therefore requires that the patient be informed of the purpose, nature, risks, and benefits of the procedure(s). The informed consent must also contain a statement indicating that the patient must not withhold information, that the patient has been given an opportunity to ask questions, and that those questions have been answered to his or her satisfaction. A statement as to availability of emergency equipment and personnel qualified to handle emergency situations should also be included. The informed consent forms should be developed through careful study of national and local practices and adopted for use by the rehabilitation staff only after approval by the medical supervisor and appropriate legal advisors.[1-6] An example of informed consent for the GXT and cardiac rehabilitation can be found in Appendix C. After all preliminary forms and procedures have been completed, exercise evaluation of the patient may begin.

Graded Exercise Test

All patients wishing to enter a cardiac rehabilitation program should be evaluated for exercise tolerance before beginning the program. This evaluation is not always in the form of a GXT, and the referring physician must decide the mode and extent of evaluation necessary for providing the rehabilitation staff with exercise guidelines for each patient. However, many GXTs are being performed in the referring physician's office or at the rehabilitation site, and it is quite common for the rehabilitation clinicians to participate in the administration of the GXT under the supervision of a physician.[2,3] Conditions that preclude a patient from exercise testing are listed in Table 9–1.

The Electrocardiogram. Equipment basic to obtaining electrocardiographic (ECG) data include a cardiograph with multilead capabilities and a monitor to continuously view the ECG. Although individual preferences vary, most practitioners require a 12-lead ECG at rest (supine, sitting, and standing), during and following the completion of the GXT. Some experts feel that the standard 12-lead system is impractical in emergency situations because the electrodes covering the chest impede defibrillation procedures. As a result, a modified lead $V_5(CMV_5)$ is frequently used, and it has been reported to be 98 percent accurate in detecting cardiac problems during exercise testing[2,7] (see Chapter 8).

Some practitioners feel that the 12-lead ECG recordings are not necessary at all times during exercise testing and prefer to use a variety of ECG leads.[2] Assuming that

TABLE 9–1 Contraindications to Exercise Testing

Absolute Contraindications

1. Recent significant change in the resting ECG suggesting infarction or other acute cardiac event
2. Recent complicated myocardial infarction
3. Unstable angina
4. Uncontrolled ventricular arrhythmia
5. Uncontrolled atrial arrhythmia that compromises cardiac function
6. Third degree AV block without pacemaker
7. Acute congestive heart failure
8. Severe aortic stenosis
9. Suspected or known dissecting aneurysm
10. Thrombophlebitis or intracardiac thrombi
11. Active or suspected myocarditis or pericarditis
12. Recent systemic or pulmonary embolus
13. Acute infections
14. Significant emotional distress (psychosis)

Relative Contraindications

1. Resting diastolic blood pressure >115 mm Hg or resting systolic blood pressure >200 mm Hg
2. Moderate valvular heart disease
3. Known electrolyte abnormalities (hypokalemia, hypomagnesemia)
4. Fixed-rate pacemaker (rarely used)
5. Frequent or complex ventricular ectopy
6. Ventricular aneurysm
7. Uncontrolled metabolic disease (e.g., diabetes, thyrotoxicosis, or myxedema)
8. Chronic infectious disease (e.g., mononucleosis, hepatitis, AIDS)
9. Neuromuscular, musculoskeletal, or rheumatoid disorders that are exacerbated by exercise
10. Advanced or complicated pregnancy

Source: From ACSM Guidelines for Exercise Testing and Prescription ed 5. Williams & Wilkins, Baltimore, 1995, p. 42, with permission.

the electrocardiograph has the capability, an example of one procedure for obtaining ECGs might be[3]:

Pre-exercise (minimum of 5 minutes):	12-lead ECG in supine position
	12-lead ECG in sitting position (usually with cycle ergometer)
	12-lead ECG in standing position
Exercise (usually 9–12 minutes)	3-lead (II, aVF, V_5) during last 10 seconds of each minute or 12-lead at end of each stage of test
Postexercise (usually 6 minutes):	12-lead at end of each minute of cool-down (if given) and/or recovery (patient supine position)

When necessary, 12 leads and/or rhythm strips can be obtained, or individual leads can be selected for recording. In addition to obtaining ECGs during the GXT, frequent blood pressure measurements are also obtained and recorded. Blood pressures and ratings of perceived exertion (see Chapter 11) are usually obtained at rest while the patient is in the supine, sitting, and standing positions, during the last minute of each stage of the GXT, immediately following the completion of the GXT and every 2 or 3 minutes during cool-down and recovery.

Recording the Electrocardiogram. Even when the practitioner has followed proper procedures for patient preparation in applying the electrodes, quality ECG recordings during exercise are more difficult to obtain than those at rest. ECG tracings can be of poor quality because of AC interference, static electricity, or other forms of electromagnetic radiation. Patients wearing nylon or other synthetic clothing can create static electricity, which interferes with quality ECG tracings. For this reason, before the GXT, the patient should be asked to wear cotton clothing. Additional reasons for poor ECG tracings include loose electrodes, movement artifact, poor patient preparation, and large amounts of fatty tissue present at electrode sites. Methods for checking electrode leads when poor tracings are being obtained are outlined in Table 9–2.

MODALITIES FOR THE GXT

Before discharge from the hospital, a low-level exercise test should be administered. The exercise test begins at a low intensity and is often terminated:

1. At a heart rate of 120 to 130 beats per minute
2. At 70 percent of age-predicted maximum heart rate
3. To a termination point of 5 to 6 metabolic equivalents
4. To a symptom-limited end point[8,9]

If no exercise test has been performed before hospital discharge, it is desirable to perform a symptom-limited test (SL-GXT) within 3 to 4 weeks following the cardiac event. The results of the SL-GXT are used as the basis for the exercise prescription.[10,11] To re-evaluate the exercise prescription, exercise testing should be performed after the initial 6 weeks of rehabilitation training and at least yearly thereafter.[12] Regardless of the frequency of administering the GXT, exercise modalities that produce a volume load on the left ventricle (dynamic exercise) are preferred to those that create a pressure load (static activity).[2,13] The modalities available that provide dynamic exercise for graded exercise testing include steps, escalators, ladder mills, treadmills, and cycle ergometers. The most common modalities utilized for the exercise test are the treadmill, the bicycle, and the arm ergometer.[13,14] Each modality has advantages and disadvantages, and the personnel responsible for deciding which modality to use must do so in accordance with the specific needs of the patient.

The treadmill has become the first choice among the three testing modalities.

TABLE 9–2 Troubleshooting Poor
ECG Tracings

Troublesome ECG Lead	Electrode and Lead-Wire Check
II and III	LL
I and II	RA
I and III	LA
I, II, and III	RL
aVR, aVL, aVF	I, II, III (as above)
V_1, V_2, V_3, etc.	V_1, V_2, V_3, etc.

Walking on a treadmill requires little skill, is a more accurate predictor of $\dot{V}O_2$max, and uses more leg muscles, thus reducing leg fatigue, which is one of the most common reasons for premature test termination. The main disadvantages of the treadmill are its expense, the inability to test persons with balance problems, the difficulty in obtaining good ECG tracings, and the difficulty in determining accurate blood pressure measurements due to treadmill noise and patient movement. Newer treadmills have attempted to solve these problems by minimizing the treadmill noise and increasing the accuracy of electronic sphygmomanometers. However, blood pressure measurements obtained with automated, electronic sphygmomanometers have not been satisfactory and the standard procedure requiring the test administrator to hold the stethoscope over the brachial artery is the preferred method for blood pressure measurement.[13,14]

Use of the bicycle ergometer for testing is particularly attractive because of its relatively low cost and ease of calibration. It is also the modality of choice when testing patients with poor balance, poor vision (e.g., diabetics), or limited range of motion or pain in the joints of the lower extremities (e.g., arthritics). Blood pressure measurements are more accurate during bicycle tests, and ECG recordings are usually good because upper body movement is minimal when compared with other modalities. It should be noted that some patients find the bicycle seat uncomfortable and have difficulty keeping their feet on the pedals or maintaining a regular pace. In addition, localized muscle (quadriceps) fatigue may prevent maximal testing of the cardiovascular system.[3,14]

For patients who cannot perform leg exercise, arm ergometry is used as the GXT modality. Although arm ergometry is used in patients with vascular, orthopedic, or neurologic conditions, the results are not equivalent to those obtained during leg exercise testing and, whenever possible, leg exercise should be used.

MEASUREMENT OF OXYGEN UPTAKE

Data gathered from the GXT are usually reported in terms of metabolic equivalents (METs). One MET is the amount of oxygen consumed at rest and equals the uptake of approximately 3.5 milliliters of oxygen per kilogram of body weight per minute.[15] Thus, MET levels (multiples of resting $\dot{V}O_2$) attained during maximal exercise testing are determined by dividing the estimated $\dot{V}O_2$ max achieved during the test by the resting $\dot{V}O_2$ (3.5 mL/kg per min). Fortunately, various experiments of actual $\dot{V}O_2$max measurements have been conducted and tables of MET equivalents have been devised to save time and cost and to avoid errors in computing the actual METs achieved.

A maximal GXT is generally defined in terms of a specific end-point target heart rate (heart rate and $\dot{V}O_2$ max are linearly related and are based on the patient's age; see Chapter 4). This is usually referred to as the age-adjusted maximum heart rate (AAMHR), and can be estimated by subtracting the individual's age from 220. In most cases, tests that do not elicit a heart rate equal to 100 percent of the AAMHR are considered to be submaximal. However, use of the AAMHR method to predict maximal heart rates is inherently inaccurate because of the wide variation in actual maximal heart rates. In addition, some medications lower the heart rate and thereby render the AAMHR inaccurate as a predictor of maximal effort. Therefore the clinician must remember that the AAMHR procedure should be used only as a guideline when predicting maximal responses to a GXT. Most clinicians currently use the Borg scale of perceived exertion (see Chapter 11) as a more accurate indicator of maximal effort and basis for test termination.[16,17] For the cardiac patient or otherwise physically impaired individual, the GXT end point may be based on symptoms such as the onset of angina, ECG changes, and dysrhythmias. Therefore, the classification of the GXT as maximal or submaximal is determined not by heart rate, but by the onset of symptoms (SL-GXT) and the MET level achieved at the end point of the SL-GXT is considered the maximal capacity for that individual and can be used for the purpose of exercise prescription. The heart rate at which the maximal MET level was achieved should also be noted and used in the formulation of the exercise prescription (see Chapter 11).

It should be noted that gas-exchange techniques that give direct measurements of oxygen uptake are currently used in exercise physiology laboratories primarily for research purposes. Direct measurements of oxygen uptake have not been used to a great extent in the clinic setting during the GXT. If performed correctly and by appropriately trained personnel, direct measurements of oxygen uptake are more accurate than procedures that estimate $\dot{V}O_2$max. Direct measurement of oxygen utilization involves measuring the volume of air exhaled and determining the difference in the amount of oxygen in inspired air compared with the amount of oxygen in the air expired by the patient. Oxygen uptake is the result of the cardiac output and the arteriovenous oxygen difference (see Chapter 4). Direct measurement of oxygen uptake provides an accurate assessment of the anaerobic threshold, an important clinical consideration because it determines a patient's limitations at submaximal levels. However, use of gas-exchange techniques is costly and time-consuming and causes discomfort to the patient. For these reasons, it remains a common practice to estimate the oxygen consumed during the GXT rather than measure it directly.[16–19]

BLOOD PRESSURE RESPONSE DURING GXT

Before and during the GXT, blood pressure measurements as well as ECGs must be recorded frequently. Because the available automated devices for taking blood pressures have not been found to be reliable in the detection of exertional hypotension, blood pressure should be measured using a standard stethoscope and sphygmomanometer.[16,18] Systolic and diastolic blood pressures (SBP, DBP) should be recorded during the 5-minute rest period before the beginning of the GXT. Blood pressures are to be recorded in the supine, sitting (if ergometer is the mode for testing), and standing positions. During the GXT, SBP and DBP should be recorded during the last minute of each stage (usually every 3 minutes) and more frequently if warranted. During the recovery phase (at least 6 minutes), blood pressures are measured immediately after the termination of the GXT (patient in upright position), and every 1 to 2 minutes during the 6-minute recovery period or longer if warranted. If a cool-down is given, blood pressures are measured during cool-down and then during either the sitting or supine recovery period. Many decisions as to when to obtain blood pressure measurements, rating of perceived exertion, ECGs, etc. will be dictated by the individual patient response. The information presented in this text is to be used as guidelines for decision making by the clinicians responsible for the care of the patient.

During the exercise test, the normal response for the systolic blood pressure is to rise with increasing workloads. A decrease in SBP of 20 mm Hg or failure of the SBP to rise with increasing workloads is reason for test termination and can be one cause for an SL-GXT. An excessive rise in the systolic blood pressure (250 mm Hg) and/or the diastolic blood pressure (120 mm Hg) is also cause for test termination. Following exercise, systolic blood pressure is elevated in the immediate upright and supine positions and should gradually return to normal during recovery.[3,18]

RATE-PRESSURE PRODUCT (DOUBLE PRODUCT)

The rate-pressure product (RPP) is the product of the heart rate and the systolic blood pressure. It is usually a five-digit figure, the last two digits of which are dropped. The product is an excellent indicator of aerobic conditioning because the RPP decreases for a given workload as the patient becomes more conditioned. Cardiac and deconditioned subjects generally have higher RPPs for a given workload than physically trained individuals. The RPP relates well to measured myocardial oxygen consumption, and it is possible to precipitate a patient's angina repeatedly at the same RPP when a standardized workload or exercise test is performed. The RPP illustrates the importance of considering both heart rate and blood pressure responses when writing an appropriate exercise prescription.[17,20]

TEST PROTOCOLS

Regardless of the modality selected for the GXT, a variety of standard protocols are available for the clinician's use. This text presents the most commonly used protocols; personnel responsible for administration of the GXT should keep in mind that standard protocols may have to be adapted for individuals with low functional capacity, orthopedic limitations, and other medical problems.

One aspect of the GXT that is not well addressed in some standard protocols is that of adequate warm-up at the beginning of the GXT and provisions for a cool-down when the test has been terminated. The clinician responsible for protocol selection will need to make the decision whether or not to include a warm-up and a cool-down as part of the regular test protocol. Protocols that have been chosen for clinical testing as well as those chosen to determine functional capacity may include a low-intensity warm-up, 8 to 12 minutes of continuous exercise, and an appropriate cool-down period.[3,6] Some test protocols begin at such a low level that adequate warm-up is an inherent part of the test. Most protocols do not specifically state what the cool-down should be and the decision for providing a cool-down period will have to be made by the person administering the test in accordance with the purpose of the test and the patient's physiologic responses to the test. Some practitioners feel that there should be no cool-down period and that the patient should be placed in the supine position immediately following completion of the GXT.[16]

Treadmill Tests

Despite its limitations, the Bruce treadmill protocol (Table 9–3) remains the test of choice for most physicians because of its ease of administration and economy of time.

TABLE 9–3 Bruce Treadmill Protocol

Stage	Speed, *mph*	Grade, %	Time, *min*	METs
1	1.7	10	3	5
2	2.5	12	3	7
3	3.4	14	3	10
4	4.2	16	3	13
5	5.0	18	3	16
6	5.5	20	3	19
7	6.0	22	3	22

Source: From Computer Assisted Exercise System. Marquette Electronics, Milwaukee, 1980, with permission.

TABLE 9–4 Adapted Bruce Treadmill Protocol

Stage	Speed, *mph*	Grade, %	Time, *min*	METs
1	1.7	0	3	2
2	1.7	5	3	3
3	1.7	10	3	5
4	2.5	12	3	7
5	3.4	14	3	10
6	4.2	16	3	13
7	5.0	18	3	16
8	5.5	20	3	19
9	6.0	22	3	22

Source: From Computer Assisted Exercise System. Marquette Electronics, Milwaukee, 1980, with permission.

In many cases, however, it may be too strenuous to use with the cardiac or otherwise deconditioned patient. Because of the large and uneven MET increments (2 to 3 METs of work every 3 minutes) in the Bruce protocol, it is not recommended for use by some clinicians because it tends to overestimate exercise capacity.[2,6,13] In such cases, the physician may choose the adapted Bruce treadmill protocol (Table 9–4), which provides two low-level initial stages that allow a warm-up period for the patient. Because of its constant speed (2 or 3.3 mph) and gradual increase in treadmill grade of 1 percent each minute, the Balke-Ware protocol is preferred by many clinicians.[6,13] The current trend in exercise protocols is to individualize the test according to each patient's capability.[3,13]

Bicycle Ergometer Tests

The bicycle ergometer GXTs are usually performed at a pedaling rate of 50 rpm, but the resistance to pedaling usually increases every 3 or 6 minutes. A number of ergometers are currently used for conducting GXTs and some workloads are set in kiloponds, others in kilogram meters per minute, and still others in watts. These variances create some difficulty in standardizing tests and, although interpolations will probably have to be made, Tables 9–5 and 9–6 should help in converting test data into MET levels achieved. An example of a bicycle ergometer protocol for multistage testing is

TABLE 9–5 Conversion of Work Load in Kiloponds (KP) to METs for Bicycle Ergometry

Body Weight (lb)	Workloads (KP*)								
	0.5	1	1.5	2	2.5	3	3.5	4	5
110	3.6	5.1	6.9	8.6	10.3	12.0	13.7	15.4	16.3
132	3.3	4.3	5.7	7.1	8.6	10.0	11.4	12.9	14.0
154	3.1	3.7	4.9	6.1	7.3	8.6	9.8	11.0	13.5
176	3.0	3.2	4.3	5.4	6.4	7.5	8.6	9.6	11.0
198	2.9	2.9	3.8	4.8	5.7	6.7	7.6	8.6	10.0
220	2.8	2.6	3.4	4.3	5.1	6.0	6.9	7.7	9.2

*0.5 KP = 150 kg/min = 25 watts
 1.0 KP = 300 kg/min = 50 watts
 1.5 KP = 450 kg/min = 75 watts, etc.
Source: Adapted from American College of Sports Medicine,[23] p. 299.

TABLE 9–6 Oxygen Requirements of Bicycle Ergometric Workloads

				Workload							
Watts		25	50	75	100	125	150	175	200	250	300
kg/min		150	300	450	600	750	900	1050	1200	1500	1800
Total Oxygen Used		600	900	1200	1500	1800	2100	2400	2700	3300	3900
kcal/min		3.0	4.5	6.0	7.5	9.0	10.5	12.0	13.5	16.5	19.5
Body Weight											
(lb)	(kg)	*Oxygen Used (ml/kg/min of body weight)*									
88	40	15.0	22.5	30.0	37.5	45.0	52.5	60.0	67.5	82.5	97.5
110	50	12.0	18.0	24.0	30.0	36.0	42.0	48.0	54.0	66.0	78.9
132	60	10.0	15.0	20.0	25.0	30.0	35.0	40.0	45.0	55.0	65.0
154	70	8.5	13.0	17.0	21.5	25.5	30.0	34.5	38.5	47.0	55.5
176	80	7.5	11.0	15.0	19.0	22.5	26.0	30.0	34.0	41.0	49.0
198	90	6.7	10.0	13.3	16.7	20.0	23.3	26.7	30.0	36.7	43.3
220	100	6.0	9.0	12.0	15.0	18.0	21.0	24.0	27.0	33.0	39.0
242	110	5.5	8.0	11.0	13.5	16.5	19.0	22.0	24.5	30.0	35.5
264	120	5.0	7.5	10.0	12.5	15.0	17.5	20.0	22.5	27.5	32.5

Source: From Ellestad,[27] p. 161, with permission.

TABLE 9–7 A Protocol for Multistage GXT
Utilizing the Bicycle Ergometer

Stage	Speed, *rpm*	Workload	Time, *min*
Warm-up	50	0	2–3
1	50	.5 KP	2–3
2	50	1.0 KP	2–3
3	50	1.5 KP	2–3
4	50	2.0 KP	2–3
5	50	2.5 KP	2–3
6	50	3.0 KP	2–3
7	50	3.5 KP	2–3
8	50	4.0 KP	2–3
Cool-down	50	0	3–6

Source: Adapted from Guidelines for Exercise Testing and Prescription, ed 4. Lea & Febiger, Philadelphia, 1991, p 62, with permission.

given in Table 9–7. The bicycle test protocol used by the YMCA[21] and the Astrand-Rhyming[22] bicycle tests are additional protocols that are commonly used for the GXT.

Arm Ergometry GXT

An arm ergometer is commonly used as the mode for the GXT in patients who have peripheral vascular disease (PVD) or musculoskeletal, neuromuscular, or other disorders that prevent their being tested on the treadmill or with the bicycle ergometer. The test may be performed in the seated or standing position and the test protocol is usually continuous. The stages are usually 2 minutes in length with the workload increasing by 0.5 KP (25 watts or 150 kg/m/min) for each 2-minute stage. Some patients may be able to perform better if the test is a discontinuous one that allows for 1 to 2 minutes of rest between the 2-minute exercise stages. As with other testing protocols, arm ergometry tests need to be individualized as opposed to following a standard protocol.[18,23]

Ramping Tests

A recent protocol suggested for individualizing the GXT is that of ramping. The ramping method may be used with the treadmill, bicycle, and arm ergometer. Ramping tests are characterized by being progressive and having even increases in speed, grade, and workload. Small, even, and more frequent work increments are preferable to larger, uneven, and less frequent increases. Each test is individualized for each patient and the protocol needs to be adapted so that a test duration of 8 to 12 minutes can be achieved. To assist in the prediction of workloads for each patient, the patient can be questioned regarding his or her usual activities that have known MET levels. This inquiry into activity level can occur during the pre-GXT interview or may be included as part of the Patient Program Application Forms (Appendix A). The Duke Activity Status Index[25] questionnaire (Table 9–8) has been found helpful in predicting oxygen uptake and can assist the clinician in selecting the appropriate test protocol for each patient. Standard GXT protocols need to be adapted to accommodate each patient and are to be used as guidelines and not as exact testing procedures.[6,13,16,24]

TABLE 9–8 The Duke Activity Status Index[25]

Activity: Can you. . . .	Weight
Take care of yourself (eat, dress, bathe, and use the toilet)?	2.75
Walk indoors, such as around your house?	1.75
Walk a block or two on level ground?	2.75
Climb a flight of stairs or walk up a hill?	5.50
Run a short distance?	8.00
Do light work around the house, like dusting or washing dishes?	2.70
Do moderate work around the house, like vacuuming, sweeping floors, or carrying in groceries?	3.50
Do heavy work around the house, like scrubbing floors or lifting or moving heavy furniture?	8.00
Do yard work, like raking leaves, weeding, or pushing a power mower?	4.50
Have sexual relations?	5.25
Participate in moderate recreational activities, like golf, bowling, dancing, doubles tennis, or throwing a basketball or football?	6.00
Participate in strenuous sports, like swimming, singles tennis, football, basketball, or skiing?	7.50

The Duke Activity Status Index (DASI) = the sum of the weights for "yes" replies. Oxygen uptake $(\dot{V}O_2) = (0.43 \times DASI) + 9.6$.

TEST AND EXERCISE TERMINATION

The guidelines for test and exercise therapy termination should be in accord with the particular situation and must be developed by the personnel in charge of the rehabilitation program. Some indications for exercise and test termination are given in Table 9–9.

TABLE 9–9 Indications for Test and Exercise Therapy Termination

1. Acute MI or suspicion of MI
2. Onset of moderate to severe angina
3. Drop in SBP with increasing workload accompanied by signs or symptoms or drop below resting pressure
4. Serious arrhythmias (e.g., second- or third-degree A-V block, sustained ventricular tachycardia or increasing PVCs, atrial fibrillation with fast ventricular response)
5. Signs of poor perfusion, including pallor, cyanosis, or cold and clammy skin
6. Unusual or severe shortness of breath
7. CNS symptoms, including ataxia, vertigo, visual or gait problems, or confusion
8. ECG changes from baseline greater than 2 mm horizontal or downsloping ST-segment depression or elevation (except in aVR)
9. Leg cramps or intermittent claudication (grade 3 on 4 point scale)
10. Hypertensive response (SBP > 260 mm Hg: DBP > 115 mm Hg)
11. Exercise-induced bundle branch block that cannot be distinguished from ventricular tachycardia
12. Technical inability to monitor the ECG
13. Patient's request

Source: Adapted from American College of Sports Medicine: ACSM's Guidelines for Exercise Testing and Prescription, ed. 5. Williams & Wilkins, Baltimore, 1995, p. 97.

INTERPRETATION OF GXT RESULTS

Interpretation of test results and their application to exercise therapy requires knowledge of physiology, pathophysiology, and exercise and should always be supervised by the medical director. The end point for test termination may be related to the patient's age and to the point at which symptoms such as angina, dyspnea, dysrhythmias, adverse blood pressure responses, and the like occur. Occasionally patients may be too unstable to participate in exercise therapy. If so, the decision must be made on an individual basis and in consideration of the medical and legal consequences.

The results of the GXT enable the therapist to classify a patient according to functional capacity and the MET level achieved on the GXT can be estimated from Figure 9–1. The functional classification is helpful in predicting subsequent cardiac events and determining prognosis for survival, and it assists in the determination of maintenance levels for cardiac exercise therapy. Classification also aids in advising patients about recreational and occupational activities. If a patient performs less than 5 METs on the GXT, the prognosis for that patient is poor.[16]

To interpret the results of a GXT correctly, the clinician must also be aware of the specificity and sensitivity of the test. An exercise test that is interpreted as abnormal in a person who does not have coronary artery disease (CAD) is called a false-positive test: conversely, a test interpreted as normal in a person who is found to have CAD is called false-negative. Test specificity refers to the percent of people without CAD who have a negative GXT and therefore correctly identifies persons without CAD (a true-

Functional class	Clinical status	O_2 cost ml/kg/min	Met$_s$	Bicycle ergometer	Bruce 3 min stages mph/%gr	Kattus mph/%gr	Balke-Ware % grade at 3.3 mph (1-min stages)	Ellestad 3/2/3 min stages mph/%gr	USAF-SAM mph/%gr	"Slow" USAF-SAM mph/%gr	McHenry mph/%gr	Stanford % grade at 3 mph	Stanford % grade at 2 mph	Met$_s$
Normal and I	Healthy, dependent on age, activity	56.0	16	1 watt = 6 KPDS	5.0 / 18			6 / 15						16
		52.5	15	For 70 KG body weight KPDS 1500			26		3.3 / 25					15
		49.0	14			4 / 22	25	5 / 15						14
		45.5	13		4.2 / 16		24 / 23		3.3 / 20		3.3 / 21			13
		42.0	12	1350		4 / 18	22 / 21				3.3 / 18	22.5		12
	Sedentary healthy	38.5	11	1200		4 / 14	20 / 19 / 18	5 / 10	3.3 / 15		3.3 / 15	20.0		11
		35.0	10	1050			17			2 / 25		17.5		10
		31.5	9	900	3.4 / 14		16 / 15			2 / 20		15.0		9
		28.0	8			4 / 10	14 / 13	4 / 10	3.3 / 10		3.3 / 12	12.5		8
	Limited	24.5	7	750	2.5 / 12	3 / 10	12 / 11	3 / 10		2 / 15		10.0	17.5	7
II		21.0	6	600			10		3.3 / 5	2 / 10	3.3 / 9	7.5	14	6
	Symptomatic	17.5	5	450	1.7 / 10	2 / 10	9 / 8 / 7	1.7 / 10			3.3 / 6	5.0	10.5	5
		14.0	4	300			6		3.3 / 0	2 / 5		2.5	7	4
III		10.5	3		1.7 / 5		5 / 4				2.0 / 3	0.0	3.5	3
		7.0	2	150	1.7 / 0		3 / 2		2.0 / 0	2 / 0				2
IV		3.5	1				1							1

FIGURE 9–1. Estimated ventilatory oxygen cost per stage for most of the commonly used treadmill protocols. (From Froehlicher, VF, Myers, J, Follansbee, WP, Labovitz, AJ: Exercise and the Heart, ed 3. Mosby-Year Book, St. Louis, 1993, p. 17, with permission.)

TABLE 9–10 Conditions Contributing
to False-Positive Tests

---

1. Resting repolarization abnormalities (e.g., LBBB)
2. Cardiac hypertrophy
3. Accelerated conduction defects (e.g., Wolff-Parkinson-White syndrome)
4. Digitalis
5. Nonischemic cardiomyopathy
6. Hypokalemia
7. Mitral valve prolapse
8. Vasoregulatory abnormalities
9. Pericardial disorders
10. Technical or observer error
11. Coronary spasm in the absence of significant CAD
12. Anemia
13. Female gender

Source: From ACSM's Guidelines for Exercise Testing and Prescription, ed 5. Williams & Wilkins, Baltimore, 1995, p. 142, with permission.

negative test). Test sensitivity refers to the percent of patients tested who have CAD and who have an abnormal GXT (a true-positive test). Test specificity is reduced by false-positive tests and test sensitivity is reduced by false-negative tests. If 100 people who are free of CAD are tested and 90 percent of those tested have a normal GXT and 10 percent have an abnormal GXT (false-positive), the test specificity is 90 percent for prediction of CAD. If 100 persons with CAD are tested and 90 percent of those tested have a positive test and 10 percent have a negative (false-negative) test, the sensitivity of the test is 90 percent for prediction of CAD. The specificity of the GXT has been found to be 79 percent and GXT sensitivity is reported to be 68 percent. The predictive value of the GXT indicates whether or not the test correctly identifies persons with CAD and those without it (true-positive and true-negative tests). Interpretation of GXT results is strongly influenced by an individual's age, sex, risk factors, MET level achieved, rate-pressure product, and symptoms. Interpretation of the GXT must reflect a consideration of these factors.[18] Tables 9–10 and 9–11 list conditions that contribute to increased incidence of false-positive and false-negative tests. To assist the clinician in decisions as to when to terminate the GXT and to provide examples of test interpretation, see the case histories presented at the end of this chapter.

TABLE 9–11 Conditions Contributing to False-Negative Tests

---

1. Failure to reach an ischemic threshold
2. Monitoring an insufficient number of leads to detect ECG changes
3. Failure to recognize non-ECG signs and symptoms that may be associated with underlying disease (e.g., hypotension)
4. Angiographically significant disease compensated by collateral circulation
5. Musculoskeletal limitations to exercise preceding cardiac abnormalities
6. Technical or observer error

Source: From ACSM's Guidelines for Exercise Testing and Prescription, ed 5. Williams & Wilkins, Baltimore, 1995, p. 141, with permission.

EMERGENCY PROCEDURES, MEDICATIONS, AND BASIC EQUIPMENT

Written emergency procedures should be established and signed by the appropriate medical personnel. Equipment and medications for emergencies must be available during all testing and exercise sessions. An example of emergency procedures and a list of standard emergency medications and equipment[26] is given in Appendix D. Emergency procedures must be constantly updated to keep pace with changes in technology and research in emergency medicine. Because situations and the laws that govern them are unique, personnel in charge of rehabilitation programs would be prudent to have a carefully documented plan for dealing with emergency situations. The plan should include specific instructions for the administration of basic and advanced life support, the periodic review of emergency procedures, and a plan for emergency drills for all members of the cardiac rehabilitation staff. All plans should be approved by the appropriate medical and legal advisors. The safety of patients involved in rehabilitation programs is the highest priority.

Additional Physical Assessments

In addition to the GXT, various additional physical measurements are also important in assessing the patient. These assessments may be performed on a separate visit to the rehabilitation center either before or after the administration of the GXT, or on the same day as the GXT is performed. These measurements can be performed quickly and, with the exception of pulmonary function, do not require extensive or expensive equipment. The information provided by the assessments is useful in planning, evaluation, and motivational aspects of the program. Usually they are obtained at the rehabilitation center by any member(s) of the trained rehabilitation staff, such as a nurse, exercise specialist, and/or laboratory technician. Although most of the procedures are simple, adequate time and training must be provided to ensure that the measurements are properly taken. These measurements may include a pulmonary function test, height, body weight, body girth measurements, and percentage of body fat (estimated by skinfolds and anthropometric measurements). They may also include various measurements for strength and range of joint motion, although measures of strength are usually not taken until the patient has been in the cardiorespiratory rehabilitation program for 4 to 6 weeks.[28]

Pulmonary Function Testing

Pulmonary function testing is indicated for the cardiac patient primarily to determine:

1. The presence of lung disease or abnormal lung function
2. The extent of the abnormality, if one exists
3. The disabling effect of the abnormality
4. The appropriate exercise prescription for the patient with abnormal lung function.[1,29]

For information on pulmonary assessment, see Chapter 10.

Height

Accurate height is desirable for utilizing height-weight charts and for use in various formulas for the prediction of percentage of body fat or metabolic equivalents. Use of a stadiometer is recommended for measurement (Fig. 9–2). The patient should re-move both shoes and socks before measurement and stand with his or her back to the measuring device with feet together and arms relaxed at the sides of the body. The eyes should be directed straight ahead and the measuring square should be adjusted to rest lightly on the scalp. The measurement should be recorded to the nearest quarter-inch or centimeter.

Body Weight

For obtaining body weight, a standard balance scale is preferred to a spring-balance or digital scale because it is more easily calibrated. All weighings on the same patient should be performed with the same scale. The scale should be checked in the zero position before each weighing, the balance should be returned to zero after each weighing, and the scale should be recalibrated periodically. The patient can be weighed at the same time that the height measurement is obtained. Weight recorded during the patient's participation in the rehabilitation program may be measured with or without socks and shoes as long as the measurement technique is consistent.

Percentage Body Fat

Body composition can be divided into two components: lean body mass and body fat. The lean body mass encompasses all the body's nonfat tissues including the skeleton, water, muscle, connective tissue, organ tissues, and teeth. The body fat

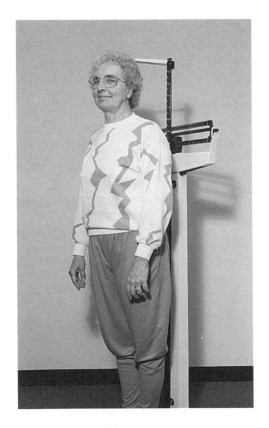

FIGURE 9–2. Use of the stadiometer to measure height. (Courtesy of Bio-Energitks Rehabilitation, Prospect, PA.)

component includes both the essential and nonessential lipid stores. Essential fat includes fat that is a part of organs and tissues such as nerves, brain, heart, lungs, liver, and mammary glands.[30] The storage of nonessential fat is primarily within the adipose tissue depots.

There are many ways in which to measure body composition and several new technologies have been developed and found reliable but not valid. These technologies include the use of dual energy x-ray absorptiometry (DXA), near-infrared (NIR) interactance devices, and bioelectrical impedance analysis (BIA).[30-36] These technologies need to be researched further, are costly, and hence are not recommended for general use to measure body composition in a cardiac rehabilitation program. Other technologies that can be used to determine body composition include radiography, ultrasound, nuclear magnetic resonance, and potassium-40 count. These technologies not only are expensive, but for various reasons are not recommended for general assessment of body composition.[30]

Hydrostatic weighing (HW) has been the standard against which other measures of predicting body composition have been compared. HW techniques are largely reserved for research in human performance laboratories, and their use in cardiac rehabilitation settings is usually not practical because of equipment expense, time and space constraints, discomfort of total head submersion, and the amount of time required to complete the assessment.[23,37,38]

Skinfold Assessment

The most accurate, cost-effective, and practical technique for predicting percentage of body fat is that of measuring skinfold thickness. The skinfold equations are derived by using multiple regressions that predict the percentage of body fat from the measurements of various skinfold sites.[23,37,38] The skinfold method of assessing body composition has the potential for error if the clinician taking the measurements lacks the proper training and experience. In obtaining the skinfold measurement, a fold of skin and subcutaneous tissue is pinched between the thumb and forefinger and lifted firmly away from the underlying muscle. (Active contraction of the muscle in the skinfold site before measurement helps the clinician to discriminate between the muscle and the subcutaneous tissue.) The fold should be held between the finger and thumb and the skinfold caliper should be applied perpendicular to the fold and approximately 1 centimeter from the thumb and forefinger (in the center of the fold, not near the base or apex). The caliper should be released to allow full tension to be applied to the skinfold, but the thumb and forefinger should not be released (Fig. 9–3).[37]

Depending on the regression equation being used for estimation of body fat, measurements should be recorded to the nearest 0.5 or 1.0 centimeter. A minimum of two measurements per site are recommended and all skinfold measurements should be taken on the right side of the body.[37]

Tables 9–12 and 9–13 provide an estimation for the prediction of percentage body fat from the sum of three skinfold measurements for men and women, respectively.[39] The three skinfold sites and instructions for measurement of men are as follows:

1. Triceps skinfold. Measure at the midpoint between the acromion and the olecranon process on the posterior aspect of the upper arm. Pinch the skinfold in the vertical plane with the arm relaxed and extended (see Fig. 9–3).
2. Chest skinfold. Measure between the anterior axillary line and the nipple on a diagonal fold, ⅔ distance to the nipple.

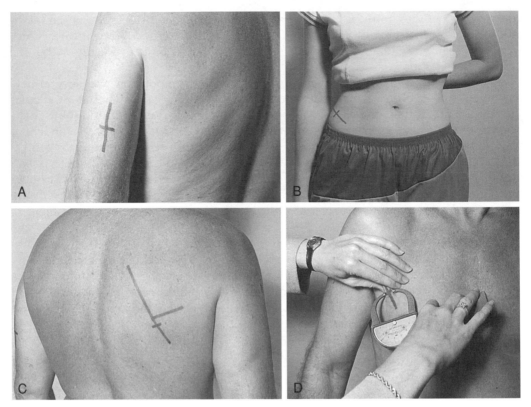

FIGURE 9-3. Lange skinfold calipers and location of skinfold measurement sites. (Courtesy of Bio-Energitks Rehabilitation, Prospect, PA.)

3. Subscapular skinfold. Measure on a diagonal line from the vertebral border of the scapula to within 1 to 2 cm from the inferior angle of the scapula.

The measurements for women are as follows:

1. Triceps skinfold. Measure the same as for men.
2. Abdominal skinfold. Measure approximately 2 cm laterally from the umbilicus in a vertical plane.
3. Suprailiac skinfold. Measure a diagonal fold above the iliac crest at the anterior axillary line.

Body Mass Index

The body mass index (BMI) is a simple assessment that is calculated by dividing body weight in kilograms by height in meters squared (kg/m^2). An alternate method that gives the same result is to multiply body weight in pounds by 700 and divide the result by the height in inches squared.[23,37,40] Recent research indicates that obesity-related health problems begin to increase when the BMI is greater than 25 and morbid obesity occurs when the BMI is greater than 40.[23,40]

TABLE 9–12 Percent Fat Estimate for Men: Sum of Triceps, Chest, and Subscapular Skinfolds

Sum of Skinfolds (mm)	*Age to Last Year*								
	Under 22	23–27	28–32	33–37	38–42	43–47	48–52	53–57	Over 57
8–10	1.5	2.0	2.5	3.1	3.6	4.1	4.6	5.1	5.6
11–13	3.0	3.5	4.0	4.5	5.1	5.6	6.1	6.6	7.1
14–16	4.5	5.0	5.5	6.0	6.5	7.0	7.6	8.1	8.6
17–19	5.9	6.4	6.9	7.4	8.0	8.5	9.0	9.5	10.0
20–22	7.3	7.8	8.3	8.8	9.4	9.9	10.4	10.9	11.4
23–25	8.6	9.2	9.7	10.2	10.7	11.2	11.8	12.3	12.8
26–28	10.0	10.5	11.0	11.5	12.1	12.6	13.1	13.6	14.2
29–31	11.2	11.8	12.3	12.8	13.4	13.9	14.4	14.9	15.5
32–34	12.5	13.0	13.5	14.1	14.6	15.1	15.7	16.2	16.7
35–37	13.7	14.2	14.8	15.3	15.8	16.4	16.9	17.4	18.0
38–40	14.9	15.4	15.9	16.5	17.0	17.6	18.1	18.6	19.2
41–43	16.0	16.6	17.1	17.6	18.2	18.7	19.3	19.8	20.3
44–46	17.1	17.7	18.2	18.7	19.3	19.8	20.4	20.9	21.5
47–49	18.2	18.7	19.3	19.8	20.4	20.9	21.4	22.0	22.5
50–52	19.2	19.7	20.3	20.8	21.4	21.9	22.5	23.0	23.6
53–55	20.2	20.7	21.3	21.8	22.4	22.9	23.5	24.0	24.6
56–58	21.1	21.7	22.2	22.8	23.3	23.9	24.4	25.0	25.5
59–61	22.0	22.6	23.1	23.7	24.2	24.8	25.3	25.9	26.5
62–64	22.9	23.4	24.0	24.5	25.1	25.7	26.2	26.8	27.3
65–67	23.7	24.3	24.8	25.4	25.9	26.5	27.1	27.6	28.2
68–70	24.5	25.0	25.6	26.2	26.7	27.3	27.8	28.4	29.0
71–73	25.2	25.8	26.3	26.9	27.5	28.0	28.6	29.1	29.7
74–76	25.9	26.5	27.0	27.6	28.2	28.7	29.3	29.9	30.4
77–79	26.6	27.1	27.7	28.2	28.8	29.4	29.9	30.5	31.1
80–82	27.2	27.7	28.3	28.8	29.4	30.0	30.6	31.1	31.7
83–85	27.7	28.3	28.8	29.4	30.0	30.5	31.1	31.7	32.3
86–88	28.2	28.8	29.4	29.9	30.5	31.1	31.6	32.2	32.8
89–91	28.7	29.3	29.8	30.4	31.0	31.5	32.1	32.7	33.3
92–94	29.1	29.7	30.3	30.8	31.4	32.0	32.6	33.1	33.4
95–97	29.5	30.1	30.6	31.2	31.8	32.4	32.9	33.5	34.1
98–100	29.8	30.4	31.0	31.6	32.1	32.7	33.3	33.9	34.4
101–103	30.1	30.7	31.3	31.8	32.4	33.0	33.6	34.1	34.7
104–106	30.4	30.9	31.5	32.1	32.7	33.2	33.8	34.4	35.0
107–109	30.6	31.1	31.7	32.3	32.9	33.4	34.0	34.6	35.2
110–112	30.7	31.3	31.9	32.4	33.0	33.6	34.2	34.7	35.3
113–115	30.8	31.4	32.0	32.5	33.1	33.7	34.3	34.9	35.4
116–118	30.9	31.5	32.0	32.6	33.2	33.8	34.3	34.9	35.5

Source: From Jackson, AS and Pollock, ML: Practical assessment of body composition. Phys Sportsmed 13(5):87, 1985, with permission of McGraw-Hill

TABLE 9–13 Percent Fat Estimate for Women: Sum of Triceps, Abdomen, and Suprailiac Skinfolds

Sum of Skinfolds (mm)	18–22	23–27	28–32	33–37	38–42	43–47	48–52	53–57	Over 57
8–12	8.8	9.0	9.2	9.4	9.5	9.7	9.9	10.1	10.3
13–17	10.8	10.9	11.1	11.3	11.5	11.7	11.8	12.0	12.2
18–22	12.6	12.8	13.0	13.2	13.4	13.5	13.7	13.9	14.1
23–27	14.5	14.6	14.8	15.0	15.2	15.4	15.6	15.7	15.9
28–32	16.2	16.4	16.6	16.8	17.0	17.1	17.3	17.5	17.7
33–37	17.9	18.1	18.3	18.5	18.7	18.9	19.0	19.2	19.4
38–42	19.6	19.8	20.0	20.2	20.3	20.5	20.7	20.9	21.1
43–47	21.2	21.4	21.6	21.8	21.9	22.1	22.3	22.5	22.7
48–52	22.8	22.9	23.1	23.3	23.5	23.7	23.8	24.0	24.2
53–57	24.2	24.4	24.6	24.8	25.0	25.2	25.3	25.5	25.7
58–62	25.7	25.9	26.0	26.2	26.4	26.6	26.8	27.0	27.1
63–67	27.1	27.2	27.4	27.6	27.8	28.0	28.2	28.3	28.5
68–72	28.4	28.6	28.7	28.9	29.1	29.3	29.5	29.7	29.8
73–77	29.6	29.8	30.0	30.2	30.4	30.6	30.7	30.9	31.1
78–82	30.9	31.0	31.2	31.4	31.6	31.8	31.9	32.1	32.3
83–87	32.0	32.2	32.4	32.6	32.7	32.9	33.1	33.3	33.5
88–92	33.1	33.3	33.5	33.7	33.8	34.0	34.2	34.4	34.6
93–97	34.1	34.3	34.5	34.7	34.9	35.1	35.2	35.4	35.6
98–102	35.1	35.3	35.5	35.7	35.9	36.0	36.2	36.4	36.6
103–107	36.1	36.2	36.4	36.6	36.8	37.0	37.2	37.3	37.5
108–112	36.9	37.1	37.3	37.5	37.7	37.9	38.0	38.2	38.4
113–117	37.8	37.9	38.1	38.3	39.2	39.4	39.6	39.8	40.0
118–122	38.5	38.7	38.9	39.1	39.4	39.6	39.8	40.0	40.7
123–127	39.2	39.4	39.6	39.8	40.0	40.1	40.3	40.5	41.3
128–132	39.9	40.1	40.2	40.4	40.6	40.8	41.0	41.2	41.9
133–137	40.5	40.7	40.8	41.0	41.2	41.4	41.6	41.7	41.9
138–142	41.0	41.2	41.4	41.6	41.7	41.9	42.1	42.3	42.5
143–147	41.5	41.7	41.9	42.0	42.2	42.4	42.6	42.8	43.0
148–152	41.9	42.1	42.3	42.8	42.6	42.8	43.0	43.2	43.4
153–157	42.3	42.5	42.6	42.8	43.0	43.2	43.4	43.6	43.7
158–162	42.6	42.8	43.0	43.1	43.3	43.5	43.7	43.9	44.1
163–167	42.9	43.0	43.2	43.4	43.6	43.8	44.0	44.1	44.3
168–172	43.1	43.2	43.4	43.6	43.8	44.0	44.2	44.3	44.5
173–177	43.2	43.4	43.6	43.8	43.9	44.1	44.3	44.5	44.7
178–182	43.3	43.5	43.7	43.8	44.0	44.2	44.4	44.6	44.8

Source: From Jackson, AS and Pollock, ML: Practical assessment of body composition. Phys Sportsmed 13(5):87, 1985, with permission of McGraw-Hill

Waist-to-Hip Ratio

The waist-to-hip ratio (WHR), independent of BMI, has been found to be associated with high central obesity (fat concentrated in the abdominal region), mortality, and chronic metabolic disease, especially in older men and women. High WHR correlates with coronary risk factors such as hypertension, hyperglycemia, lower levels of high-density lipoproteins (HDL) and elevated levels of total cholesterol, low-density lipoprotein (LDL), and apolipoprotein B.[37,41-44]

The WHR is a simple method to indicate upper and lower body distribution of fat. Upper body fat (android, central, male) occurs when the distribution of excess body fat is primarily in the back and abdominal regions. Lower body fat (gynoid, gluteal-femoral, peripheral, female) is the deposition of fat primarily in the buttocks, hips, and thighs. Individuals with more central fat, especially in the abdominal region, are at greater risk for CAD and premature death.[23,37,41-44]

Measurement of WHR is inexpensive, economical of time, and requires only a tape measure to measure the hip and waist circumferences. The waist (abdominal) circumference is measured at the natural waist, which is the smallest circumference below the rib cage above the umbilicus. If the natural waist is not easily determined, measure at the level of the umbilicus with the patient's abdomen relaxed. The hip circumference is measured at the largest circumference of the posterior protrusion of the buttocks. To determine the WHR, divide the waist circumference by the hip circumference. It is desirable for the WHR to be 0.90 or less for men and 0.80 or less for women. A WHR of 0.95 or greater for men and 0.85 or greater for women increases the risk for disease.[37]

Assessment of Functional Outcomes

For accreditation, good record keeping that indicates patient outcomes is necessary for evaluation of rehabilitation programs. Records that can show positive changes in the behavior, function, and well-being of patients will be able to show that the programs are effective. Functional status is frequently measured by the MET level achieved on the GXT and the measurements obtained of blood pressures, RPE, RPP, ECG changes, and symptoms.

Measurements of body composition by means of skinfolds, BMI, and WHR are also convenient and valid indicators of risk for CAD. Outcome data should be collected under identical circumstances at the beginning of the program, on discharge from the program, and within 1 year following program entry. These data are necessary to show the cost-effectiveness and patient benefits of cardiac rehabilitation.[3,45]

RADIONUCLIDE IMAGING, ECHOCARDIOGRAPHY, AND CORONARY ANGIOGRAPHY

Because of its availability, lower cost, and yield of clinically useful information, the exercise stress test is an important tool in the diagnosis of CAD. However, advances in cardiovascular testing technology have added noninvasive radionuclide imaging techniques and echocardiography (with exercise or pharmacologic stress) to the invasive procedure, coronary angiography, for the diagnosis of CAD. This discussion of the technologic advances for diagnosis of CAD is not intended to be fully descriptive as to procedures for administering the various tests. Rather, it serves to give a brief overview to provide the clinician with basic information important to the understanding of diagnostic procedures and their results.[46–56]

Radionuclide Imaging

Radionuclide imaging is an area of nuclear cardiology concerned with the assessment of myocardial perfusion and ventricular function. Because imaging can be used with pharmacologic as well as exercise stress, it is possible to evaluate patients who are unable to exercise.[46,48–51]

MYOCARDIAL PERFUSION IMAGING

Myocardial perfusion imaging is performed with exercise testing or with intravenous infusion of pharmacologic coronary artery dilating agents such as dipyridamole (Persantine) or adenosine. Perfusion imaging is useful in the diagnosis and evaluation of ischemic heart disease, myocardial scarring, myocardial infarction, risk stratifications of patients after recent myocardial infarction (MI), evaluation of a patient with prior revascularization, and similar diagnostic and prognostic procedures.[48,51]

Although various radioactive tracers have been used in radionuclide perfusion imaging, thallium-201 is still the most common agent used for perfusion scanning.[48,50,55] If thallium scanning is used with an exercise stress test, the test is usually performed on a bicycle ergometer or a treadmill. Before the beginning of the exercise test, an intravenous line is begun so that when the patient is at, or near, maximal exertion, the thallium can be injected. To circulate the thallium tracer, the patient continues the exercise test for another minute following injection. The patient is then placed in a supine position under a scintillation camera, which is used for radioactive emissions detection. When the camera is interfaced with a computer system, the images that are produced are two-dimensional planar scintigrams, which show perfusion of the myocardium.[51] Scans are usually taken within 10 minutes following the exercise test and again in 3 to 4 hours.[48,52,55] The distribution of thallium-201 is proportional to myocardial blood flow and in absence of CAD, distribution of thallium-201 is fairly homogenous. In patients with CAD, at peak exercise, thallium-201 is underperfused and there is a reduction in the accumulation of thallium-201 in the myocardial cells.[50] Additional scans are taken 3 to 4 hours after the initial imaging to assess for redistribution of thallium. The presence of thallium redistribution ("filling in" of defects that were noted on the immediate postexercise images) indicates that transient ischemia was present at the time of the initial injection of thallium.[55]

Other methods used to assess myocardial perfusion include positron emission tomography (PET) and single-photon emission computerized tomography (SPECT). The radioactive marker used during the PET scan is 18F-fluorodeoxyglucose (FDG). Delayed thallium-201 perfusion scans (performed 8 to 72 hours after initial thallium perfusion following exercise) or repeat imaging (performed after a second injection of thallium) have been shown to produce results that are similar to PET imaging with less cost.[55] Myocardial imaging via SPECT gives a three-dimensional scan of the distribution of a radionuclide compared with the conventional two-dimensional, planar scan obtained during perfusion evaluation via thallium-201. The newer radionuclide technetium-99m (Tc-99m)-based agents, sestamibi and teboroxime, are currently being utilized and studied during procedures to assess myocardial perfusion.[48,50,51] The advantages and disadvantages of the newer technologies have not been fully investigated, and myocardial perfusion imaging via thallium-201 with conventional planar scanning currently remains the commonly performed procedure.[51,53,55]

ASSESSMENT OF VENTRICULAR FUNCTION

Assessment of ventricular function employs a technique known as "blood pool imaging." In this procedure, the patient is injected intravenously with a radioactive tracer during rest, exercise, or other intervention and a scintillation camera is placed over the patient's chest to detect the radionuclide. A picture is then created that shows how the blood is pumped through the heart, and evaluations of left and right ejection fractions, ventricular volumes, cardiac output, diastolic filling rates, and regional wall motion abnormalities can be determined. If blood pool imaging is to be performed during exercise, the cycle ergometer is usually the preferred mode. The patient exercises on the ergometer in the supine, upright, or semi-upright position and the camera is positioned to obtain a 45° left anterior oblique image. The workload on the ergometer increases every 3 minutes to peak performance and measurements of the ejection fraction and regional wall motion at rest and during exercise are compared. Two methods can be used for blood pool imaging, the equilibrium method and the first-pass method.[50,51,55]

Equilibrium Method. So that imaging can be performed over an extended period of time, the equilibrium or "gated" method of blood pool imaging requires stable blood cell labeling. To accomplish this, nonradioactive stannous pyrophosphate is injected intravenously into the patient and, 20 to 30 minutes later, the radionuclide Tc-99m is injected.[51,55] Images of ventricular function are obtained during several hundred cardiac cycles, and by using sophisticated computer techniques a multigated radionuclide cineangiogram (MUGA) is generated. Scans can be performed as often as necessary for 4 to 6 hours after injection of the tracer.[51,53,55]

First-pass Method. The first-pass method does not require blood cell labeling because the scans are obtained during the "first pass" of the radionuclide through the myocardial circulation. The radioactive tracer used for the images is a bolus injection of Tc-99m and ventricular activity is recorded with a scintillation camera. The first-pass method is likely to provide a more accurate assessment of right ventricular function than does the MUGA scan. Visual and quantitative evaluation of regional wall motion is probably more accurate with the equilibrium (MUGA) method. Recent advances in technology allow acquisition of first-pass imaging data during treadmill testing, as well as the conventional cycle ergometry evaluations. The equilibrium and the first-pass methods give ejection fraction results that compare favorably with those obtained via cardiac catherization, with less risk to the patient.[50,51,55]

PHARMACOLOGIC STRESS PERFUSION IMAGING

Because the coronary blood flow is greatest during high-flow rates and nonhomogeneity of perfusion is more easily seen after peak exercise, stress thallium imaging is usually performed after an exercise stress test. However, many patients are unable to exercise effectively because of medications or physical limitations such as peripheral vascular disease, orthopedic problems, severe obstructive pulmonary disease, and severe diabetes mellitus. Elderly patients or those in poor physical condition may also be unable to effectively exercise. As a result of the need to assess patients who are unable to exercise, pharmacologic stress tests were developed.[16,48–51,55] Pharmacologic agents used for assessing patients unable to exercise can be classified into two groups: (1) agents that produce coronary vasodilatation such as dipyridamole and adenosine and (2) agents that produce ischemia by increasing myocardial oxygen demand (dobutamine).[48,49,51,55]

Dipyridamole (Persantine) increases endogenous levels of adenosine with consequent increases in myocardial blood flow caused by a decrease in arteriolar vascular resistance throughout the heart. Following injection of dipyridamole, coronary vascular beds supplied by normal, healthy coronary arteries show an increase in blood flow. Vascular beds supplied by an artery in which stenosis exists show smaller changes in resistance to flow, and there are smaller increases in blood flow. This reduction in blood flow is caused by the already-reduced coronary resistance in a stenotic vessel to maintain a normal level of flow at rest. The differences in blood flow between various regions of the heart can be detected by the thallium-201 perfusion imaging techniques previously discussed.[49–51,55] The pharmacologic stress test using dipyridamole infusion with thallium-201 is performed in the fasting state (4 to 6 hours). Dipyridamole is administered during a 4-minute intravenous infusion and reaches its peak effect in 7 to 8 minutes. Thallium-201 is injected within 5 minutes after dipyridamole and initial images are obtained within 10 minutes after thallium injection. Delayed images are obtained 3 to 4 hours later to evaluate for redistribution. If the patient is able to exercise, handgrip exercises, low-level treadmill (or similar activity), and cycling in combination with dipyridamole infusion increase the peak level of coronary blood flow and can be performed after administration of dipyridamole.[51,55] Dipyridamole perfusion imaging has been found to give results comparable to those of conventional exercise-thallium imaging. In addition to its role in myocardial perfusion evaluation in patients who are not able to exercise to near-peak performance, intravenous dipyridamole perfusion imaging has prognostic value in patients who have peripheral vascular disease or have had a recent MI.[51,55]

Adenosine is a naturally occurring agent and a powerful coronary vasodilator that decreases coronary vascular resistance and increases coronary flow. It is formed both intracellularly and extracellularly and is also administered intravenously in pharmacologic stress testing. During the test, infusion of adenosine occurs in 4 to 6 minutes and the duration of the effect of adenosine lasts 1 to 2 minutes. Because of the extremely short half-life of adenosine, thallium must be administered 1½ to 2 minutes before infusion of adenosine has been completed. Adenosine-thallium imaging has not been studied as extensively as dipyridamole-thallium imaging, but the results from adenosine scintigraphy appear to be similar to those obtained from conventional exercise scanning and dipyridamole imaging.[51,55]

Dobutamine is a pharmacologic agent that has been used to diagnose and assess for the presence of CAD in a patient who is unable to exercise effectively. In patients who have bronchospastic disease and for whom dipyridamole or adenosine infusion is contraindicated, dobutamine is particularly useful. Dobutamine, unlike dipyridamole, increases the heart rate, blood pressure, and myocardial contractility, which results in an increase in myocardial oxygen demand and may precipitate ischemia. Although dobutamine thallium-201 imaging might be effective for perfusion imaging testing, it seems to be more effective in inducing regional myocardial dysfunction and is more commonly used in conjunction with echocardiography. More research is necessary to determine the role of stress imaging using dobutamine infusion as the pharmacologic agent, but the use of dobutamine will be addressed again in the next section of this chapter in the discussion of echocardiography.[49–51,55]

Echocardiography

Echocardiography is an evaluation technique that provides images of the anatomy, structural defects, and blood flow of the heart with the use of ultrasonography, which does not necessitate the use of radioactive tracers. Ultrasonography may be used in different modes including M-mode, two-dimensional spectral, and color-flow Doppler. The common techniques for evaluation of the heart are the transthoracic and transesophageal echocardiograms. In transthoracic echocardiography, the probe, or transducer, is placed on the surface of the chest, while the transesophageal technique requires the transducer to be placed in the patient's esophagus. (The latter technique is used in patients in whom transthoracic echocardiogram images may be comprised by obesity, pulmonary disease, chest wall deformities, and so forth.) Regardless of the ultrasonographic mode or technique used, all forms are included in the general term "echocardiography." A more detailed discussion of each is beyond the scope of this text.[47,53,55]

In addition to information about the anatomy of the heart, the valves, and various diseases, echocardiography can provide information about overall ventricular function, abnormalities in wall motion and thickening, and blood flow through the cardiovascular system. It is also used to detect regional myocardial ischemia.[47,53,55]

Echocardiography can be performed at rest, during or following exercise, and with a pharmacologic stress-inducing agent. When it is used during exercise testing, the preferred exercise mode is either the bicycle ergometer or the treadmill. Because it is not feasible to perform the echocardiographic examination in an upright walking patient, if the treadmill is used, the echocardiographic images are obtained immediately before and immediately after a standard exercise stress protocol. If the bicycle ergometer is the mode of exercise stress, imaging can be obtained at the end of each stage of exercise testing. The most common pharmacologic agents used for echocardiographic stress testing are dipyridamole and dobutamine.[48,51,55]

Before the beginning of the exercise test, echocardiographic images are taken of the patient's heart at rest. The patient then begins a standard exercise stress test protocol (with ECG) and images are taken at the end of each exercise stage (bicycle ergometer) or immediately following the completion of the exercise test (treadmill). Like any standard exercise stress test, the test is terminated if symptoms develop or when the patient reaches peak exercise. Using one of several available computer programs, the images obtained at rest and during or after exercise are then compared for differences in wall motion quality, calculation of ejection fraction, detection of CHD, assessing the prognosis of patients who have had myocardial infarction and those with revascularizations, and for the evaluation of several additional anatomic and functional features.[48,51,55] The results from exercise stress echocardiography compare positively with those obtained by radionuclide techniques, and exercise echocardiography has some distinct advantages over radionuclide imaging: it is less expensive; it does not use radioactive tracers, the equipment is small and easily portable, and it is extremely versatile. Stress echocardiography is also diagnostically useful in patients, especially women, who have high occurrences of false-positive electrocardiographic stress tests.[51]

Because it permits continuous monitoring of left ventricular function, echocardiography is well suited for use in pharmacologic stress testing. Intravenous infusions of dipyridamole or dobutamine are the most commonly used agents that induce the "stress." Dipyridamole is usually infused as a fixed dose and scanning is performed throughout the infusion. Dobutamine stress echocardiography involves incremental infusions in 3-minute stages. In each case, the patient's ECG and blood pressure are continuously monitored simultaneously with echocardiographic imaging. Unlike dipyridamole, dobutamine increases the myocardial oxygen demand by increasing heart rate, blood pressure and myocardial contractility. This effect of dobutamine may evoke ischemia in patients with CAD and, in the presence of coronary stenosis, dobutamine has been found to be more effective than dipyridamole in inducing regional myocardial dysfunction for similar coronary lesions.[49–51,55] More research is needed to assess the use of dobutamine infusion in echocardiography, as serious side effects have been reported.[56,57]

Coronary Angiography

Coronary angiography uses a catheter inserted into an artery, vein, or both, and ultimately into the heart to obtain information as to the presence and/or extent of atherosclerotic CAD or other disease and defects. Usually one of three methods for right and left heart catheterization are utilized:

1. Entry of a catheter through the femoral vein into the right side of the heart and entry of a catheter through the femoral artery into the ascending aorta and left ventricle
2. Catheterization of the right and left sides of the heart by entry through the brachial vein and artery
3. Catheterization of the right heart through the femoral vein followed by passage of a small needle across the intra-atrial septum into the left atrium and insertion of a catheter into the left ventricle.[50]

As the catheters are carefully advanced toward and into the heart and coronary arteries, their progress is guided by the use of a fluoroscope.[52] Injections of a contrast material is then made through the catheters and x-rays are obtained to study the circulation in the major coronary vessels and their branches.[50,54] Thus, the angiogram produces x-ray pictures of the heart that are used to "map" the coronary circulation, detect obstructions, assess the pumping action of the heart, detect valvular and congenital defects, obtain pressure measurements important in determination of vascular resistance, and detect common disorders such as vasospasm and other structural abnormalities. The most common use for coronary angiography is to identify stenosis in the coronary arteries that may dictate the need for further medical intervention including coronary artery bypass grafting (CABG) and percutaneous transluminal angioplasty (PTCA). Angiography is an invasive procedure that involves greater risk than the previously discussed noninvasive procedures. Those at greater risk during the angiographic procedures include those with a left main coronary artery stenosis greater than 50 percent, those with unstable angina and low functional capacity, and those with congestive heart failure (CHF) and advanced age. Major complications that can result from angiography include MI and resultant death, cerebral vascular accidents, arterial access problem, and major rhythm disturbances.[50,54]

GRADED EXERCISE TEST CASE HISTORIES

The GXT performed by the cardiac rehabilitation personnel may be used to determine functional capacity or diagnose disease. The information gained from the GXT is generally used to formulate exercise prescriptions, to assess functional changes at discharge from the program, and in follow-up procedures.[3] An often difficult decision for the inexperienced clinician is that of determining precisely when the GXT is of adequate duration for exercise prescription purposes to warrant test termination. The case histories presented in this section may provide some insight into this decision-making process, because they illustrate that test termination most often is a result of factors other than those attributed to age-related maximum heart rates. It should be noted that Borg's revised scale[58] is used to determine RPE.

CASE STUDIES*

CASE STUDY 1

The patient is a 57-year-old woman with a history of CAD and coronary artery bypass grafts (CABG) and angina. Her medications are Persantine and Synthroid; her body fat is 32 percent; and her age-adjusted maximum heart rate (AAMHR) is 163 bpm. Table 9–14 summarizes the results of her GXT.

TABLE 9–14 GXT Data for Case Study 1

Age: 57   Sex: F   AAMHR: 163 bpm   70% AAMHR: 114 bpm
Brief History: CAD, CABG, angina
Medications: Persantine, Synthroid
Resting ECG: Slight ST-T flattening, no PVCs or other dysrhythmias
Resting HR: 65 bpm   Resting BP: 128/84
Protocol: Adapted Bruce Treadmill

Stage	HR (bpm)	BP (3-min)	METs	RPE (rev)	Comments and Reason for Termination
1	80			1	
	82			2	
	80 . . . . . 146/84		2	2	Dyspnea (level 1)
2	84			2	
	84			3	
	86 . . . . . 150/86		3	3	Dyspnea (level 1)
3	96			3	
	92			3	
	96 . . . . . 158/86		5	4	Dyspnea (level 2)
4	112			4	
	118			5	Dyspnea (level 3), fatigue,
	118 . . . . . 168/86		7	7	ECG showed 2 mm ST/T sagging.

End-point HR: 118 bpm   End-point BP: 168/86   RPP: 198   RPE: 7
Conclusion: A mildly positive treadmill test with no dysrhythmias: heart rate and blood pressure responses were good. The test was terminated at the end of stage 4 (7 METs), which was considered adequate for prescription purposes. Risk: Intermediate.

*Case studies are courtesy of Bio-Energetiks Rehabilitation, Prospect, PA.

TABLE 9–15 GXT Data for Case Study 2

Age: 60   Sex: F   AAMHR: 160 bpm   70% AAMHR: 112 bpm
Brief History: CAD, angina, MI
Medications: Inderal, Lanoxin, Lasix, Isordil
Resting ECG: ST-T depression of 1 mm, no dysrhythmias
Resting HR: 52 bpm   Resting BP: 140/80
Protocol: Adapted Bruce Treadmill

Stage	HR (bpm)	BP (3-min)	METs	RPE (rev)	Comments and Reason for Termination
1	63			1	
	68			2	
	68 . . . . . 140/88		2	2	
2	72			3	
	74			3	
	75 . . . . . 168/88		3	4	
3	80			6	
	82 . . . . . 176/90		~4	8	Throat dryness, chest pain and burning (level 3).

End-point HR: 82 bpm   End-point BP: 176/90   RPP: 144   RPE: 8
Conclusion: The test was terminated after 2 minutes into Stage 3 (~4 METs) due to chest pain (level 3) and is positive for angina. The ST-T changes are mild and difficult to interpret because the patient is taking Lanoxin. Blood pressure responses were fairly normal although somewhat hypertensive in view of the low workload the patient was able to achieve. Risk: Intermediate.

TABLE 9–16 GXT Data for Case Study 3

Age: 81   Sex: M   AAMHR: 139 bpm   70% AAMHR: 97 bpm
Brief History: ASHD, MI, arthritis (knees), pacemaker implant
Medications: Pronestyl, Lanoxin, Cardizem, Dyazide, Transderm-Nitro 10, Clinoril
Resting ECG: Frequent pacer beats, ST-T sagging 1½ mm
Resting HR: 74 bpm   Resting BP: 110/70
Protocol: Adapted Bruce Treadmill

Stage	HR (bpm)	BP (3-min)	METs	RPE (rev)	Comments and Reason for Termination
1	84			5	
	84			1	
	82 . . . . . 112/70		2	1	
2	86			2	
	86			2	
	88 . . . . . 120/70		3	3	
3	88			3	
	86			4	
	88 . . . . . 124/72		5	4	
	90			5	
4	92			5	Dyspnea (level 3), fatigue,
	92 . . . . . 132/78		7	6	T-wave inversion noted.

End-point HR: 92 bpm   End-point BP: 132/78   RPP: 121   RPE: 6
Conclusion: T waves inverted during last stage, indicating possible ischemia, but since there were no symptoms, most likely due to old MI or post-pacemaker activity— difficult to interpret due to meds. Risk: Intermediate.

CASE STUDY 2

The patient is a 60-year-old woman with a history of CAD, angina, and MI. Her medications are Inderal, Lanoxin, Lasix and Isordil; her body fat is 28 percent, and her AAMHR is 160 bpm. Table 9–15 gives a summary of her GXT.

CASE STUDY 3

The patient is an 81-year-old man with a history of ASHD, MI, hypertension, arthritis, and a pacemaker implant. His body fat is 28 percent; his AAMHR is 139; and his medications are Pronestyl, Lanoxin, Cardizem, Dyazide, Clinoril, and Transderm-Nitro 10. Table 9–16 summarizes the results of his GXT.

CASE STUDY 4

The patient is a 52-year-old man whose body fat is estimated to be 38 percent. He is a smoker with a history of hypertension and pacemaker implant. His medications are Quinidine, Minipress, and hydrochlorothiazide. Table 9–17 summarizes the results of his GXT.

TABLE 9–17 GXT Data for Case Study 4

Age: 52   Sex: M   AAMHR: 168 bpm   70% AAMHR: 118 bpm

Brief History:	Hypertension, pacemaker implant, obesity, smoker
Medications:	Quinidine, Minipress, hydrochlorothiazide
Resting ECG:	Pacer spikes with occasional PVCs (less than 10/min), 1 episode of coupling noted.

Resting HR: 72 bpm   Resting BP: 120/80
Protocol: Adapted Bruce Treadmill

Stage	HR (bpm)	BP (3-min)	METs	RPE (rev)	Comments and Reason for Termination
1	82			1	2 episodes of coupling,
	85			2	frequent PVCs, bigeminy,
	82	140/82	2	2	asymptomatic
2	85			2	1 episode of coupling,
	86			3	occasional PVCs,
	86		3	3	asymptomatic
3	86	140/90		4	1 episode of coupling,
	90			4	occasional PVCs,
	96	140/92	5	5	asymptomatic
4	102			6	
	102			6	Dyspnea (level 3+),
	102	142/92	7	7	Leg fatigue

End-point HR: 102 bpm   End-point BP: 142/92   RPP: 144   RPE: 7
Conclusion: Frequent ventricular coupling and episodes of bigeminy that decreased in frequency during Stages 3 and 4. Pacer firings were intermittent with no ST-T changes noted. GXT was negative for angina, and positive for ventricular dysrhythmia. MET level attained was 7. Risk: Intermediate to High.

TABLE 9-18 GXT Data for Case Study 5

Age: 70   Sex: F   AAMHR: 150 bpm   70% AAMHR: 105 bpm
Brief History: Hypertension, obesity, arthritis (knees, wrists, spine)
Medications: Hydrochlorothiazide, Aldomet
Resting ECG: Normal
Resting HR: 62 bpm   Resting BP: 146/92
Protocol: Ramping (Bicycle Ergometer)

Stage	Workload	HR (bpm)	BP (3-min)	METs	RPE (rev)	Comments and Reason for Termination
1	.5 KP	88			3	Headache with pounding
		95			5	sensation. GXT terminated
		114	220/136	<2	7	due to severe hypertensive response to exercise.

End-point HR: 113 bpm   End-point BP: 220/136   RPP: 248   RPE: 7
Conclusion: Severe hypertensive response to exercise, severely deconditioned. No dysrhythmias or chest pain noted. Negative test for ischemia to level tested (<2 METs). Risk: Intermediate to High because of age, poor functional capacity, and severe hypertensive response to a very low workload.

CASE STUDY 5

The patient is a 70-year-old woman with an estimated body fat of 44 percent. She is hypertensive, obese, and arthritic, and her medications are hydrochlorothiazide and Aldomet. Because of the limitations imposed by her arthritis, she is being tested on a bicycle ergometer. A summary of her GXT is shown in Table 9-18.

CASE STUDY 6

The patient is a 73-year-old man with a history of hypertension, COPD, arthritis, and cancer (CA) of the colon. His body fat is estimated to be 30 percent; his medications are Procainamide, Ativan, Ecotrin, and Tylenol; he is a smoker. The results of his GXT are shown in Table 9-19.

CASE STUDY 7

The patient is a 52-year-old man with a history of CAD, MI, and hypertension. His body fat is estimated to be 25 percent, and his medications are Corgard and Procainamide. Because the patient had previously been involved in a cardiac rehabilitation program, the Bruce protocol seemed appropriate for his GXT. The results of his GXT are shown in Table 9-20.

CASE STUDY 8

The patient is a 50-year-old man with a history of an MI, CAD, CABG (triple vessel), peripheral vascular disease (PVD), and hyperlipidemia. His body fat is estimated to be 20 percent, and his medications are Cardizem, Isordil, and Trans-

TABLE 9–19 GXT Data for Case Study 6

Age: 73   Sex: M   AAMHR: 147 bpm   70% AAMHR: 103 bpm
Brief History: Hypertension, COPD, arthritis, CA, colostomy, hyperlipidemia, smoker
Medications: Procainamide, Ativan, Ecotrin, Tylenol
Resting ECG: Normal
Resting HR: 76 bpm   Resting BP: 148/92
Protocol: Adapted Bruce Treadmill

Stage	HR (bpm)	BP (3-min)	METs	RPE (rev)	Comments and Reason for Termination
1	98			.5	
	98			.5	
	98	194/98	2	1	
2	102			1	
	106			2	Slight dyspnea (level 1)
	112	206/104	3	3	
3	114			4	Moderate hypertensive
	116			6	response, dyspnea (level 3),
	122	220/106	5	7	fatigue

End-point HR: 122 bpm   End-point BP: 220/106   RPP: 268   RPE: 7
Conclusion: No dysrhythmias noted during GXT but PACs were seen on recovery. ST-T depression (1 mm) in leads II, III, and aVF indicate a mildly positive GXT suggesting possible right coronary artery disease. A moderate hypertensive response to level tested (7 METs). Risk: Intermediate to High.

TABLE 9–20 GXT Data for Case Study 7

Age: 52   Sex: M   AAMHR: 169 bpm   70% AAMHR: 118 bpm
Brief History: CAD, MI, hypertension
Medications: Corgard, Procainamide
Resting ECG: Normal
Resting HR: 56 bpm   Resting BP: 126/86
Protocol: Bruce Treadmill

Stage	HR (bpm)	BP (3-min)	METs	RPE (rev)	Comments and Reason for Termination
1	76			1	
	76			1	
	80	148/90	5	2	
2	92			3	Frequent PVCs, bigeminy,
	110			5	one episode of coupling
	110	168/94	7	6	

End-point HR: 110 bpm   End-point BP: 168/94   RPP: 184   RPE: 6
Conclusion: At peak exercise (7 METs), PVCs increased in frequency with bigeminy and one episode of coupling. No ST-T changes were noted, but the GXT is considered positive for ischemia because of dysrhythmias. Risk: High.

TABLE 9–21 GXT Data for Case Study 8

Age: 50   Sex: M   AAMHR: 170 bpm   70% AAMHR: 119 bpm
Brief History: CAD, MI, CABG, PVD, hyperlipidemia
Medications: Cardizem, Isordil, Transderm-Nitro 5
Resting ECG: Baseline ST abnormalities with ST-T flattening in II, III, and aVF
Resting HR: 48 bpm
Protocol: Adapted Bruce Treadmill

Stage	HR (bpm)	BP (3-min)	METs	RPE (rev)	Comments and Reason for Termination
1	68			2	
	78			2	
	82	138/84	2	3	
2	84			3	Bilateral leg tightness and pain
	82			4	(level 1)
	84	146/90	3	5	
3	94			6	Leg pain (level 2), ST-T
	94			6	depression in V_5
	94	150/94	5	7	
4	98	156/98		9	Bilateral leg pain intense (3+), ST-T depression: 3 mm

End-point HR: 98 bpm   End-point BP: 156/98   RPP: 152   RPE: 9
Conclusion: Positive GXT for ischemia; 3 mm depression noted in V_5. No angina occurred, but the test was positive for claudication. PVCs and occasional bigeminy during cool-down and recovery. Risk: High.

TABLE 9–22 GXT Data for Case Study 9

Age: 55   SEX: F   AAMHR: 165 bpm   70% AAMHR: 116 bpm
Brief History: MVP, atypical angina, possible coronary artery spasms, hypertension, hyperlipidemia
Medications: Inderal, hydrochlorothiazide
Resting ECG: ST flattening
Resting HR: 62 bpm   Resting BP: 150/86
Protocol: Adapted Bruce Treadmill

Stage	HR (bpm)	BP (3-min)	METs	RPE (rev)	Comments and Reason for Termination
1	110			1	Some ST depression apparent
	110			1	
	110	140/88	2	1	
2	112			2	ST depression, patient
	114			2	complained of chest pain
	114	142/90	3	3	
3	114			4	Chest pain increasing, ST
	116			5	depression
	116	158/92	5	5	
4	130			7	Severe chest pain radiating
	136			8	into arms and neck (level
	142	164/94	7	9	3+)

End-point HR: 142 bpm   End-point BP: 164/94   RPP: 232   RPE: 9
Conclusion: Positive GXT for angina and for ischemia, although it may be a false-positive for CAD due to MVP. METs achieved: 7; ST-T depression of 3 mm. Recommend thallium GXT for further evaluation. Risk: High.

derm-Nitro 5. Table 9–21 shows the results of his GXT.

CASE STUDY 9

The patient is a 55-year-old woman with a history of mitral valve prolapse (MVP), atypical angina, possible coronary artery spasms, hypertension, and hyperlipidemia. Her body fat is estimated to be 18 percent, and her medications are Inderal and hydrochlorothiazide. Table 9–22 shows the results of her GXT.

The case studies provide examples of responses to GXTs. In each case, the reason for test termination should be clear to the reader. Test termination guidelines are given in Table 9–9 and in Chapters 7 and 8.

SUMMARY

The procedures commonly followed to evaluate patients with cardiovascular disease have been reviewed. The prudent clinician should be initially concerned with evaluating the medical status of a prospective patient through the comprehensive medical history. The information should include personal, medical, and family health histories; lifestyle health habits; and results from the most recent physical examination by the patient's physician.

Results of laboratory evaluations give valuable information about the medical status of a patient. Those of particular significance include blood test results, pulmonary function testing, and ECGs. Information gathered through assessments such as body weight, percent body fat, body mass index, and waist-to-hip ratio is also valuable to the understanding of the medical status of a patient.

Before administration of the exercise evaluation, GXT, several forms must be read, completed, and (in some cases) signed by the patient. A primary concern for the clinician is the informed consent form, which should be devised with the aid of legal counsel and signed by each patient before a GXT or exercise program is undertaken.

The evaluation of cardiorespiratory capacity through the GXT has value, not only for diagnosis of ischemic heart disease and similar disorders, but also for formulating exercise prescriptions. Although the clinician may administer the GXT using a treadmill, a bicycle, or an arm ergometer, the mode of choice in most cases is the treadmill. Rather than a single-level test, a graded test such as the adapted Bruce or a ramping test is preferred. However, the most commonly administered treadmill test is the Bruce protocol.

The clinician administering the GXT should be alert for such patient symptoms as angina, dyspnea, and ECG changes that indicate the test should be terminated. Equipment and medications to be used in case of emergency must be available during all testing and exercise sessions.

Advances in cardiovascular testing technology have added noninvasive radionuclide imaging techniques and echocardiography to an invasive procedure, coronary angiography, for the diagnosis of CAD. Radionuclide imaging gives valuable information about myocardial perfusion and ventricular function. Echocardiography is an evaluation technique that provides images of the anatomy, structural defects, and blood flow of the heart with the use of ultrasonography and does not necessitate the use of radioactive tracers. Radionuclide imaging and echocardiography can be used with pharmacologic as well as exercise stress.

Coronary angiography is an invasive procedure using a catheter inserted into an artery, a vein, or both, and ultimately into the heart to obtain information as to the presence and/or extent of atherosclerotic CAD or other disease and defects. Because coronary angiography is an invasive procedure, it involves greater risk to the patient than radionuclide imaging and echocardiography. Coronary angiography is necessary before revascularization techniques such as CABG and PTCA.

Finally, this chapter includes case studies that illustrate outcome data to be obtained from the GXT, including heart rates, blood pressures, MET level achieved, ratings of perceived exertion, and rate-pressure products. Criteria indicating cause for test termination have also been included.

REFERENCES

1. American College of Sports Medicine: ACSM's Guidelines for Exercise Testing and Prescription, ed 5. Williams & Wilkins, Baltimore, 1995, pp 29–48.
2. Fletcher, GF et al: AHA medical/scientific statement: exercise standards. Circulation 82(6):2286–2322, 1990.
3. American Association of Cardiovascular and Pulmonary Rehabilitation: Guidelines for Cardiac Rehabilitation Programs, ed 2. Human Kinetics, Champaign, 1995, pp 29–59.
4. Herbert, WG and Herbert, DL: Legal considerations. In: Pollock, ML and Schmidt, DH (eds): Heart Disease and Rehabilitation, ed 3. Human Kinetics, Champaign, 1995, pp 433–444.
5. Herbert, DL and Herbert, WG: Medicolegal aspects of rehabilitation of the coronary patient. In: Wenger, NK and Hellerstein, HK (eds): Rehabilitation of the Coronary Patient, ed 3. Churchill Livingstone, New York, 1992, pp 567–580.
6. McKirnan, MD and Froelicher, VF: General principles of exercise testing. In: Skinner, JS (ed): Exercise Testing and Exercise Prescription for Special Cases, ed 2. Lea & Febiger, Philadelphia, 1993, pp 3–27.
7. Vinsant, MO and Spence, MI: Commonsense Approach to Coronary Care, ed 5. Mosby, St. Louis, 1989.
8. Wenger, NK: In-hospital exercise rehabilitation after myocardial infarction and myocardial revascularization: physiologic basis, methodology, and results. In: Wenger, NK and Hellerstein, HD (eds): Rehabilitation of the Coronary Patient, ed 3. Churchill Livingstone, New York, 1992, pp 351–363.
9. Squires, RW et al: Cardiovascular rehabilitation: status, 1990. Mayo Clin Proc 65:731–755, 1990.
10. Comoss, PM: Standards for cardiac rehabilitation programs and practice. In: Pollock, ML and Schmidt, DH (eds): Heart Disease and Rehabilitation, ed 3. Human Kinetics, Champaign, 1995, pp 287–306.
11. Hamm, LF and Leon, AS: Exercise training for the coronary patient. In: Wenger, NK and Hellerstein, HK (eds): Rehabilitation of the Coronary Patient, ed 3. Churchill Livingstone, New York, 1992, pp 367–402.
12. Balady, GJ et al: AHA medical/scientific statement: cardiac rehabilitation programs. Circulation 90(3):1602–1610, 1994.
13. Froelicher, VF, et al: Exercise and the Heart, ed 3. Mosby-Year Book, St. Louis, 1993, pp 10–31.
14. Wasserman, K et al: Principles of Exercise Testing and Interpretation, ed 2. Lea & Febiger, Philadelphia, 1994, pp 95–111.
15. Thomas, CL (ed): Taber's Cyclopedic Medical Dictionary, ed 17. FA Davis, Philadelphia, 1993.
16. Froelicher, VF and Umann, TM: Exercise testing: clinical applications. In: Pollock, ML and Schmidt, DH (eds): Heart Disease and Rehabilitation, ed 3. Human Kinetics, Champaign, 1995, pp 57–80.
17. Kavanagh, T: Cardiac rehabilitation. In: Goldberg, L and Elliot, DL (eds). FA Davis Company, Philadelphia, 1994, pp 48–75.
18. American College of Sports Medicine: op cit, pp 86–149.
19. Froehlicher, VF, Myers, J, Follansbee, WP, et al: Exercise and the Heart. Mosby-Year Book, St. Louis, 1993, pp 32–47.
20. Froehlicher et al: op cit, pp 71–98.
21. Golding, L, Myers, C, and Sinning, W: The Y's Way to Physical Fitness, ed 3. Human Kinetics, Champaign, 1989.
22. Astrand, PO and Rodahl, K: Textbook of Work Physiology, ed 3. McGraw-Hill, New York, 1986, p 376.
23. American College of Sports Medicine: Guidelines for Exercise Testing and Prescription, ed 4. Lea & Febiger, Philadelphia, 1991, pp 53–72.
24. Myers, J et al: Individualized ramp treadmill. Chest 101:236s–241s, 1992.
25. Hlatky, MA et al: A brief self-administered questionnaire to determine functional capacity (the Duke Activity Status Index). Am J Cardiol 64:651–654, 1989.
26. American Heart Association: Textbook of Advanced Cardiac Life Support. American Heart Association, Dallas, 1994.
27. Ellestad, MH: Stress Testing: Principles and Practice, ed 3. FA Davis, Philadelphia, 1986, p 161.
28. American College of Sports Medicine: op cit, p 189.

29. Humberstone, N: Respiratory therapy and treatment. In: Irwin, S and Tecklin, JS (eds): Cardiopulmonary Physical Therapy, ed 2. Mosby, St. Louis, 1990, p 283.
30. Gettman, LR: Fitness testing. In: ACSM's Resource Manual for Guidelines for Exercise Testing and Prescription, ed 2. Lea & Febiger, Philadelphia, 1993, pp 229–246.
31. Cassady, SL et al: Validity of near infrared body composition analysis in children and adolescents. Med Sci Sports Exerc 25(10):1185–1191, 1993.
32. Clark, RR, Kuta, JM, and Sullivan, JC: Prediction of percent body fat in adult males using dual energy x-ray absorptiometry, skinfolds and hydrostatic weighing. Med Sci Sports Exerc 25(4):528–535, 1993.
33. Douphrate, DI et al: Evaluation of three near-infrared instruments for body composition assessment in an aged cardiac patient population. J Cardpulm Rehabil 14(6):399–405, 1994.
34. Kohrt, WM: Body composition by DXA: tried and true? Med Sci Sports Exerc 27(10):1349–1353, 1995.
35. Van Loan, MD, et al: Evaluation of body composition by dual energy x-ray absorptiometry and two different software packages. Med Sci Sports Exerc 27(4):587–591, 1995.
36. U.S. Department of Health and Human Services: Bioelectrical Impedance Analysis in Body Composition Measurement. NIH Technology Assessment Statement, Dec 12, 1994, pp 1–35.
37. Verrill, D et al: Recommended guidelines for body composition assessment in cardiac rehabilitation. J Cardpulm Rehabil 14(2):104–121, 1994.
38. Organ, LW, Eklund, AD, and Ledbetter, JD: An automated real time underwater weighing system. Med Sci Sports Exerc 26(3):383–391, 1994.
39. Jackson, JS and Pollock, ML: Practical assessment of body composition. The Physician and Sportsmedicine 13(5):76–90, 1985.
40. Harvard Women's Health Watch: The new weight guidelines. Harvard Medical School 3(3):1, 1995.
41. Ades, PA, Ross, SJ, and Poehlman, ET: Body composition-coronary risk factor interactions in older female coronary patients. J Cardpulm Rehabil 15(5):352, 1995.
42. Alexander, JK: Obesity and the cardiovascular system. In: Schlant, RC and Alexander, RW (eds): Hurst's The Heart, ed 8. McGraw-Hill, New York, 1995, pp 297–300.
43. Leon, AS: Scientific rationale for preventive practices in atherosclerotic and hypertensive cardiovascular disease. In: Pollock, ML and Schmidt, DH (eds): Rehabilitation of the Coronary Patient, ed 3. Human Kinetics, Champaign, 1995, pp 115–146.
44. Smith, CR: Fat distribution linked to mortality risk. The Physician and Sportsmedicine 21(5):40, 1993.
45. Hall, LK and Gettman, LR: Policies and procedures in P&R programs. In: ACSM's Resource Manual for Guidelines for Exercise Testing and Prescription, ed 2. Lea & Febiger, Philadelphia, 1993, pp 562–569.
46. American College of Sports Medicine: op cit, pp 101–102.
47. Armstrong, WF: Exercise and other stress echocardiography. In: Wenger, NK and Hellerstein, HK (eds): Rehabilitation of the Coronary Patient, ed. 3. Churchill Livingstone, New York, 1992, pp 183–190.
48. Beller, GA: Radionuclide-based exercise testing. In: Wenger, NK and Hellerstein, HK (eds). Rehabilitation of the Coronary Patient, ed. 3. Churchill Livingstone, New York, 1992, pp 171–189.
49. Beller, GA: Pharmacologic stress imaging. JAMA 265(5):633–638, 1991.
50. Franklin, BA et al: Additional diagnostic tests: Special populations. In: ACSM's Resource Guidelines for Exercise Testing and Prescription, ed 2. Lea & Febiger, Philadelphia, 1993, pp 285–308.
51. Froehlicher, VF, Follansbee, WP, Myers, J, and Labovitz, AJ: op cit, pp 252–322.
52. Hillegass, EA: Cardiac tests and procedures. In: Hillegass, EA and Sadowsky, SH (eds): Essentials of Cardiopulmonary Physical Therapy, Saunders, Philadelphia, 1994, pp 327–353.
53. Lee, RW and Ewy, GA: Diagnostic procedures for patients with coronary heart disease. In: Wenger, NK and Hellerstein, HK (eds): Rehabilitation of the Coronary Patient, ed 3. Churchill Livingstone, New York, 1992, pp 231–255.
54. Morrison, DA and Crowley, ST: Coronary angiography and interventional techniques in the management of patients with coronary artery disease. In: Pollock, ML and Schmidt, DH (eds): Heart Disease and Rehabilitation, ed 3. Human Kinetics, Champaign, 1995, pp 95–104.
55. Schmidt, DH, Port, SC, and Gal, RA. Nuclear cardiology and echocardiography: noninvasive tests for diagnosing patients with coronary artery disease. In: Pollock, ML and Schmidt, DH (eds). Heart Disease and Rehabilitation, ed 3. Human Kinetics, Champaign, 1995, pp 81–94.
56. Williams, BR: Imaging techniques: radionuclide testing, PET, MRI. In: Wenger, NK and Hellerstein, HK (eds): Rehabilitation of the Coronary Patient. Churchill Livingstone, New York, 1992, pp 249–255.
57. Picano, E et al: Safety and tolerability of dobutamine-atropine stress echocardiography: A prospective, multicentre study. The Lancet 344:1190–1192, 1994.
58. Borg, GV: Psychophysical bases of perceived exertion. Med Sci Sports Exerc 14:377–387, 1982.

CHAPTER **10**

Pulmonary Assessment

The assessment of a patient's pulmonary status has four purposes applicable to pulmonary rehabilitation:

1. To evaluate the appropriateness of the patient's participation in a pulmonary rehabilitation program.
2. To determine the therapeutic measures most appropriate to the participant's treatment program.
3. To monitor the participant's physiologic response to exercise
4. To appropriately progress the participant's treatment program over a period of time.

Achieving these stated purposes necessitates an ongoing assessment throughout the entire rehabilitative process. The initial assessments of patients with pulmonary disease allow careful and appropriate selection of pulmonary rehabilitation candidates. Patients must be evaluated to verify the need for pulmonary rehabilitation and to predict those who will benefit within the given structure of the program.

An appropriate individualized rehabilitation treatment program can be formulated only after a comprehensive pulmonary evaluation has been performed. A pulmonary rehabilitation treatment program must be tailored to the individual's dysfunctions and his or her perceived needs. Mutually acceptable and realistic goals must be agreed on by the patient and the pulmonary rehabilitation staff.

Once the treatment program has been devised, the patient must be frequently assessed during the course of therapy. An evaluation of the participant's performance during each session makes it possible for the treatment program to reflect alterations in medical strategies, daily fluctuations in ability, and improvement in function. The success and safety of each rehabilitation session can be assured if the participant is continually assessed.

Exercise progression can be appropriately determined on the basis of an assessment of the participant's abilities to perform his or her exercise sessions. When heart rates plateau at lower levels and/or perceived exertion rates fall below the prescribed level during similar exercise intensity, exercise may be progressed. (This principle of exercise progression assumes that all other parameters are within safe and acceptable ranges.)

Optimal care is continually formulated, and the overall success of the treatment program can be ensured only by an ongoing assessment of the patient.

Assessment takes many forms. Information is obtained through the patient interview and physical examination, which includes observation, inspection, palpation, and auscultation. Information is also received from the referring physician and chart reviews regarding test results and interpretations, including laboratory values, chest x-rays, pulmonary function tests, arterial blood gas analyses, and electrocardiograms (ECGs). Graded exercise tests are not always performed in a diagnostic work-up for chronic lung disease, but they are necessary before admission to a pulmonary rehabilitation program.

PATIENT INTERVIEW

A patient interview should begin with the "chief complaint," the patient's *perception* of why pulmonary rehabilitation is being sought. Commonly, the chief complaint centers around a loss of function. Participants differ in the type and degree of activity loss that motivates them to seek pulmonary rehabilitation. Identifying the chief complaint is the beginning of goal setting in the rehabilitation process.[1] Loss of activity should be translated into a measurable, achievable goal.

A medical history contains pertinent pulmonary symptoms specific to that patient: cough, sputum production, wheezing, and shortness of breath. By requesting the patient to relate his or her medical history, knowledge of the patient's disease processes can be evaluated. A medical history also addresses occupational, social, medication, and family histories.

Cough history is an important assessment when interviewing a patient with pulmonary disease. Participants often minimize the extent of cough and sputum production. This may not be a conscious deception of minimizing symptoms but instead may be a result of the insidious onset of coughing that has become so incorporated in the patient's life that he or she is not aware of its frequency. It can be helpful to ask for such specific information as: Do you cough? Do you cough more in the morning upon arising from bed? Do you produce sputum? If so, what is the amount.[2]

Participants are asked to relate episodes of shortness of breath and wheezing by answering such questions as: How often do these episodes occur? When was the onset of these symptoms? Is there anything that either precipitates the occurrence or helps to alleviate the intensity of these symptoms? This information is necessary to devise an appropriate individualized pulmonary rehabilitation program.

An occupational history for patients with pulmonary disease provides information regarding exposures to toxins and irritants.[3] Inquiring about their *present* occupations will provide information on exposures that may put them at risk for hypersensitive occupational asthma. A *past* occupational history will contain information on exposure to hazardous materials that may cause a more chronic type of occupational lung disease. Asbestosis, silicosis, beryliosis, and many other occupational lung diseases have long latency periods between exposure to the toxin and the beginning of symptomatology.[4]

Social habits, such as smoking, alcohol consumption, and recreational or habitual drug use, should be documented. Each of the aforementioned has pulmonary implications.

Smoking history should be calculated in pack-years. Total pack-years are equal to the number of packs smoked per day times the number of years smoked. A patient who smoked three packs per day for 10 years has a 30-pack-year history, as does a patient who smoked one pack per day for 30 years. The greater the pack-year history (especially over 60 pack-years), the more likely it is that the patient will have a smoking-related illness.[2]

An admission of excessive alcohol consumption may be difficult to obtain. Inquiring about extreme behaviors may make it easier for patients to be honest about the amount of alcohol they consume. For example, the interviewer might ask, "Do you ever drink two to three cases of beer a day?"[5] Excessive alcohol consumption allows patients to harbor opportunistic pulmonary infections, and special precautions may need to be considered with this population.

Drug use of any sort involves health risks. Drugs that are smoked, such as marijuana and crack cocaine, deliver toxins directly to the lungs. The most common acute complication of these toxins is pulmonary edema.[2]

Knowing that cigarette smoking, excessive alcohol consumption, and drug usage are objectional health behaviors, patients may tend to minimize and understate the extent of consumption and use. A nonjudgmental atmosphere will assist accurate information gathering. If there is a question of accuracy, the family may have to be consulted.

A medication history is necessary to alert the clinician to the need for special considerations when prescribing exercise. For example, a patient who has been maintained on long-term steroids for pulmonary bronchospasm is at risk for osteoporosis.[7] The resulting potential for fractures may necessitate a low-impact mode of exercise.

A patient's family history is also important. An environment of passive smoke may add to a pulmonary dysfunction,[8] and there may be a familial propensity for bronchospasm.[9] There are also pulmonary diseases that are genetic in origin, such as immotile cilia or alpha-antitrypsin deficiency.[10]

Finally, a patient's family/home environment should be assessed. What are the psychosocial issues surrounding the patient and his or her family? What is the housing situation? What are the patient's responsibilities within the family? What types of support systems are presently in place for this patient?

PHYSICAL EXAMINATION

Vital Signs

Vital signs are taken for diagnostic purposes and are measured before the onset of exercise at each pulmonary rehabilitation session. Some of the vital signs and their significance are addressed in the following discussion.

Temperature elevation above normal (98.6°F or 37°C) commonly indicates an infection. Although the pulmonary system is a probable site for infection in patients with pulmonary disease, nonpulmonary infections can also be devastating to such patients.

Resting heart rate values may be elevated in the patient with pulmonary disease as a result of bronchodilator drug therapy.[11] Heart rates may also be elevated in the presence of infection. If arrhythmias are suspected, heart rate should be determined by ECG tracings.

Respiratory rate and the character of ventilation should be closely evaluated. The normal resting respiration rate is 12 to 18 breaths per minute. Respiratory rates may be elevated in patients with pulmonary dysfunction in an attempt to maintain as near normal a Paco$_2$ value as possible. Breathing patterns can be described by the rhythm and amplitude of the respiratory cycle. Patients may have an increase in the rate and/or depth of their breathing patterns, but rhythms are not usually altered. Changes in rate and character of ventilation can occur in the normal population for a variety of reasons including exercise, altitude changes, and drawing attention to a person's respiratory pattern. The evaluator, therefore, must conceal the assessment of respiratory rate from the client. One way to ensure an accurate measurement is to count the respirations while the patient assumes that the heart rate is being assessed.

An individual's height should be measured because there is a direct relation between height and lung volumes. A stadiometer is recommended for this measurement (see Chapter 9 for the procedure).

Weight should be measured on a standard balance scale, and each evaluation of weight should be performed on the same scale (Chapter 9 explains this procedure). Weight gains should be interpreted as a possible decrease in activity and/or a decrease in cardiac function. An unexplained weight loss may be a sign of carcinoma.

Resting blood pressure measurements average from 90/60 to 120/90 mm Hg. Resting arterial blood pressures exceeding 160/95 mm Hg are considered to be hypertensive.[12] Blood pressures vary with age, drug therapy, stress, level of fitness, and pathologic conditions. Blood pressure may be elevated in a patient with pulmonary disease during an infection. Pulsus paradoxus, an exaggerated decrease of 10 mm Hg or greater in the systolic blood pressure during inspiration, may be present in patients with severe airway obstruction.

Observation, Inspection, and Palpation

By observing the neck and shoulders of a patient with pulmonary disease, the clinician can determine the extent of use of the accessory muscles of ventilation. The severity of respiratory distress might well be judged by accessory muscle use at rest and the presence of paradoxic breathing.[13] Jugular venous distention (JVD) can also be discerned by observing the neck. JVD is a sign consistent with right ventricular failure from pulmonary disease (cor pulmonale).[14] Another sign of right ventricular failure is peripheral edema.

A normal configuration of the thorax is important for proper ventilation. By observing and measuring the thorax, one can assess anteroposterior (AP) and lateral dimensions of the thorax. Any change in the normal configuration (AP to lateral ratio of 2:1) indicates structural abnormalities within the rib cage. Emphysema causes destruction of the lung parenchyma that results in an increase in the AP diameter and a narrowing of the ratio (1:1). Because of hyperinflation of the lungs, the chest appears rounder and is therefore referred to as a "barrel chest." The subcostal angle (the angle formed anteriorly by the borders of the costocartilage) is normally approximately 90°. Alterations in this angle often reflect a change in the underlying lung parenchyma.

The chest should appear symmetric at rest. During inhalation and exhalation, both sides of the thorax should have equal lateral movement. By placing his or her hands over the anterior base of the lungs and aligning the thumbs over the costochondral borders, the clinician can grossly assess symmetry during ventilatory maneuvers. Placement of the clinician's hands over the posterior bases of the lungs, with the thumbs parallel to the vertebral column, further enhances assessment of chest symmetry (Fig. 10–1).

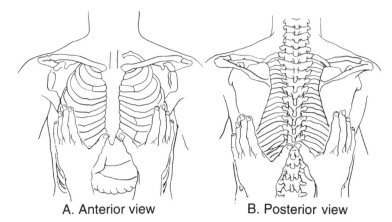

A. Anterior view   B. Posterior view

FIGURE 10–1. Placement of the clinician's hands to assess the symmetrical movement of the patient's thorax. (Adapted from Rothstein, JM, Roy, SH, and Wolf, SL: The Rehabilitation Specialist's Handbook, ed. 2. FA Davis, Philadelphia, 1998, pp. 494–495, with permission.)

On observation of the skin and the nail beds, two characteristics of pulmonary disease can be seen. The first, cyanosis, is a bluish discoloration of the skin that indicates hypoxemia.[14] Common sites for observing cyanosis are the perioral and periorbital sites and the fingernail and toenail beds. The second observation, digital clubbing of the fingers and toes, is an increase in the angle created by the distal phalynx and the point at which the nail exits from the digit. The tip of the digit becomes bulbous. The condition is often associated with chronic hypoxia[14] (Fig. 10–2).

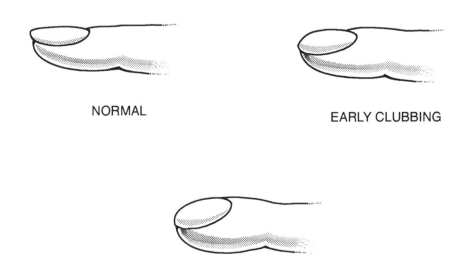

NORMAL   EARLY CLUBBING

ADVANCED CLUBBING

FIGURE 10–2. The progression of digital clubbing of the finger. (From Bell, C, et al: Home Care and Rehabilitation in Respiratory Medicine. JB Lippincott, Philadelphia, 1984, with permission.)

To assist their breathing, patients with chronic pulmonary disease may assume postures that structurally elevate and/or stabilize the shoulder girdle (Fig. 10–3). The thoracic attachments of the pectoralis major and minor and the serratus anterior can be used to expand the thorax and become muscles of inspiration.[15] With elevation and stabilization of the shoulder girdle, the thorax is already in the position to assist with inspiration. Some of the postures that assist in breathing are sitting with hands clasping the edge of the chair or bed, elbows locked and the shoulder girdle elevated; standing while bending slightly forward and leaning on locked elbows on a window sill; and standing while leaning backward against a wall with hands on knees and locked elbows. Observing the posture that a patient assumes at rest and during exercise will help in assessment of the severity of lung dysfunction.

Auscultation of the Lungs

Auscultation involves listening to air as it enters and exits the lungs. A stethoscope is placed firmly on the patient's thorax over the lung tissue. The patient is asked

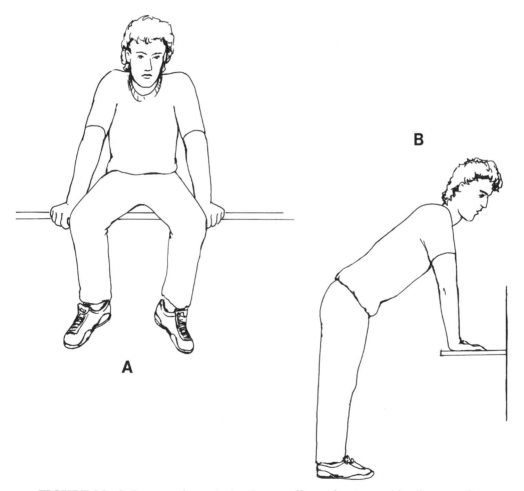

FIGURE 10–3. Postures that assist inspiratory efforts of patients with pulmonary disease.

to inhale fully through an open mouth and then to exhale quietly.[16] The clinician should listen for breath sounds over the anterior, lateral, and posterior chest wall. Breath sounds occurring on the right thorax should be compared with those on the left at comparable levels. A general auscultatory examination (Fig. 10–4) provides an over-all assessment of the patient's breath sounds without risk of the patient tiring or hyperventilating. After the patient takes a brief rest, a more specific auscultatory examination in an area where abnormalities were heard can commence.

Inhalation and the beginning of exhalation normally emit a soft rustling sound. The end of exhalation is silent. This characteristic of a normal breath sound is termed "vesicular." It should be noted that, on listening over various portions of the thorax, different intensities are normally heard. The bases of the lungs are quieter than the apices. A loud breath sound can be found over the right anterior upper thorax. When a louder, more hollow, and echoing sound occupies a larger portion of the ventilatory cycle, the breath sounds are referred to as "bronchial." Bronchial breath sounds can normally be heard over the trachea during quiet breathing. When the breath sounds are very quiet and barely audible, they are termed "diminished." With those three terms—vesicular, bronchial, and diminished—the listener can describe the intensity of the breath sound[17] (Fig. 10–5).

In addition to the normal and abnormal quality of the breath sound, there may be other sounds and vibrations—adventitious sounds—that can be heard during auscultation. They are superimposed on the already-described intensity of the breath sound. According to the American College of Chest Physicians and the American Thoracic Society, there are two types of adventitious sounds: crackles and wheezes.[18] Crackles, formerly termed "rales," are thought to occur when previously closed small airways and alveoli are rapidly reopened.[19] Patients with such problems as atelectasis, which is the collapse of alveoli, present with crackles over the collapsed area.[20] As the patient inhales deeply, some of the airways open and the characteristic crackling is heard. In

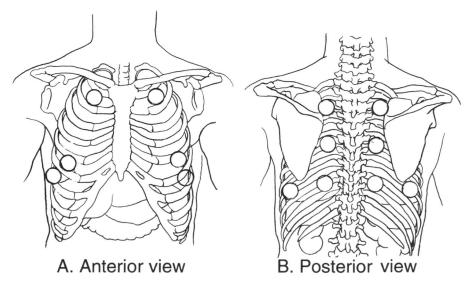

A. Anterior view   B. Posterior view

FIGURE 10–4. Anterior, lateral, and posterior auscultation sites. (Adapted from Rothstein, JM, Roy, SH, and Wolf, SL: The Rehabilitation Specialist's Handbook, ed. 2. FA Davis, Philadelphia, 1998, pp. 494–495, with permission.)

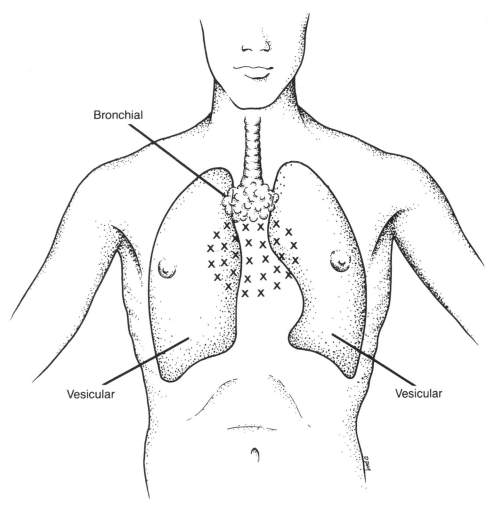

FIGURE 10–5. Normal auscultatory findings over different aspects of the thorax. (From Rothstein, JM, Roy, SH, and Wolf, SL: The Rehabilitation Specialist's Handbook, ed. 2. FA Davis, Philadelphia, 1998, p. 499, with permission.)

pulmonary edema, the fluid in the lung parenchyma may cause the small airways to close. Crackles can be heard on inhalation in a patient with pulmonary edema. The same is true of pneumonia, bronchiectasis, and other secretion-producing pulmonary pathologies.[21] Crackles are also heard in such restrictive pulmonary diseases as pulmonary fibrosis.[22]

Wheezes, on the other hand, are more musical in nature. They can be likened to blowing up a balloon and then pulling on its neck to produce a whistling sound as the balloon deflates. It is the decreased size of the neck of the balloon that produces the wheeze, and that is true within the lung also. Anything that can decrease the size of the lumen of the airway creates a wheezing sound. Asthma, with its bronchoconstriction, bronchial mucosal edema, and increased secretion production, typically produces a wheeze. Tumor growth into the lumen of an airway, an aspirated foreign body lodged in an airway, or excessive secretions can also produce a wheezing sound.[13] Under normal conditions, the size of the airway lumen increases during inspiration and decreases during expiration. Mild wheezing occurs at the end of expiration when the airway is the most narrow and the obstruction would further reduce the diameter of the airway. As wheezing worsens, it takes up more and more of the expiratory phase of breathing, and severe wheezing affects both inspiration and expiration.

There is not always agreement among practitioners on the subjective findings of auscultation. Reliability of auscultation has been found to be best when practitioners are asked to identify wheezing,[23] but there is less agreement when practitioners report the intensity of breath sounds and the presence of crackles.[23] The use of a recording device, phonopneumography, to make the assessment of breath sounds more objective is being investigated.

LABORATORY TESTS

Various laboratory studies should be performed to help in an evaluation of the appropriateness of a participant for pulmonary rehabilitation. They include chest x-rays (CXR), pulmonary function tests (PFT), graded exercise tests (GXT), arterial blood gas analysis (ABG), oxygen saturation measurements (SaO_2), and ECGs. The following discussion focuses on the use of ABG, SaO_2, and the ECG as they relate to an exercise-testing situation.

Radiographic Techniques

A CXR provides information pertaining to the bony thorax, the lungs, the heart, the structures of the hilum, the diaphragm, the interpleural space, and the soft tissues of the thorax.[25] As a diagnostic tool by itself, a CXR has limited capacities. Viewed in sequence, however, CXRs can show disease progression or resolution, and are helpful for monitoring disease processes. Correlating clinical data with radiographic findings can make a CXR very useful in diagnosing disorders of the pulmonary system.

Computer tomography (CT) of the lung provides a computer-generated cross-sectional picture of the thorax using the tomographic technique. Conventional CT takes cross-sectional pictures, or slices, every 10 millimeters. These views, seen sequentially, can differentiate various types of tissue (fat, calcification, tumor) making it useful in identifying some intrathoracic diseases better than a routine CXR. High-resolution CT uses slices that are 1 to 2 mm thick. These high-resolution images are useful in diagnosing interstitial fibrosis, bronchiectasis, and emphysema.[26] CT is not indicated for routine diagnostic use. However, if lung volume reduction surgery is being considered, CT can detect bullous disease and any inhomogeneity of emphysema.[27]

Magnetic resonance imaging (MRI) has limited indications for the thorax. MRI can provide images in multiple planes, making it advantageous for evaluating processes near the lung apex, the spine, and the thorocoabdominal junction.[26] The MRI may have an advantage over CT scan when evaluating the mediastinum.[28]

Pulmonary Function Tests

A PFT can assist in:

1. Establishing the diagnosis of lung disease
2. Documenting the extent of the abnormality
3. Determining the reversibility of the abnormality
4. Predicting the prognosis of a patient with pulmonary disease
5. Deciding on appropriate exercise-testing protocols

Five important pulmonary function measurements to be discussed are the forced vital capacity (FVC), the forced expiratory volume in 1 second (FEV_1), maximum minute ventilation ($\dot{V}Emax$), the forced expiratory flow rate over 25 to 75 percent of the FVC ($FEF_{25-75\%}$), and the diffusion capacity of the lung for carbon monoxide (DLCO). The measurements should be obtained with the patient in either the sitting or the standing position.[29] Maximal patient effort is needed to obtain reproducible values.[29] Measurements of volume or flow can be compared to normative values based on a patient's height, age, ethnicity, and gender. A comparison of a subject's PFT values over a period of time can demonstrate stability or progression of the disease.

VITAL CAPACITY

Vital capacity (VC) is the amount of air that can be exhaled following a maximal inspiratory effort. When the VC is forcibly and quickly exhaled, the maneuver is called a forced vital capacity (FVC). VC is recorded in liters, and may vary as much as 20 percent from the predicted normal values in healthy individuals. It may also vary somewhat from time to time in the same individual, depending on such factors as medical status, body position, bronchodilator therapy, and patient effort. It varies directly with height and indirectly with age. Normative values for VC are found in Tables 3–12 and 3–13 in Chapter 3. A VC less than 50 percent of the predicted value indicates severe respiratory impairment.[30]

FORCED EXPIRATORY VOLUME IN 1 SECOND

FEV_1 is the volume of gas expired during the first second of an FVC maneuver (Fig. 10–6). The FEV_1 is reported in liters per second, and it varies directly with height and indirectly with age. Because FEV_1 measures the volume of gas expired over time, it is a measurement of flow. Airway obstruction lengthens the exhalation time of a VC maneuver. By evaluating flow rates, the severity of airway obstruction can be determined. An individual whose FEV is less than 40 percent of predicted FEV is considered to have severe respiratory impairment.[30] Normative values for FEV_1 are found in Tables 3–16 and 3–17 in Chapter 3.

Expressing FEV_1 as a percent of FVC (calculated by $FEV_1/FVC \times 100$, but commonly written FEV_1/FVC) corrects for variations in height, age, sex, and alterations in VCs.[31] FEV_1 as it relates to FVC then becomes a more useful predictor of airway obstruction. For example, compare the results of pulmonary function tests in a healthy 50-year-old man whose height is 180 cm (6 ft) to those in a 60-year-old woman who is 160 cm (5 ft, 4 in). The man's FVC is predicted to be 4.8 liters, and his FEV_1 is 4.1 liters

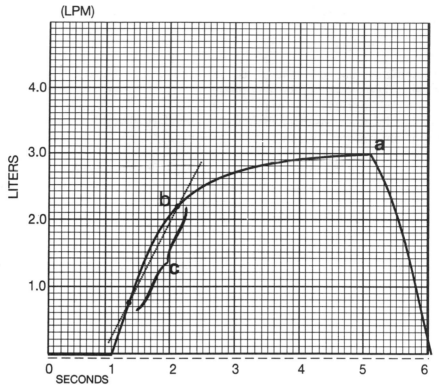

FIGURE 10-6. Values assessed with the forced vital capacity maneuver. *A*, The total volume of gas exhaled (FVC) is 3 liters. *B*, The volume of gas exhaled in the first second (FEV[1]) is 2.2 liters. The volume of gas exhaled in the first second expressed as a percentage of the total volume exhaled (FEV[1]/FVC) is 73%. *C*, The forced expiratory flow (FEF$_{25\%-75\%}$) is 1.77 liters per second.

per second. The woman's predicted values are an FVC of 2.79 liters and an FEV_1 of 2.40 liters per second. Although the two individuals have very different FVC values, 4.8 and 2.79 liters, and FEV_1 values, 4.1 and 2.4 liters per second, they are quite similar in the FEV_1/FVC percents, 84 and 86 percent. FEV_1/FVC is, in health, greater than 75 percent.[22] An FEV_1/FVC of less than 40 percent indicates a severe respiratory impairment.[32]

MAXIMUM VOLUNTARY VENTILATION AND MAXIMUM MINUTE EXPIRED VOLUME

The maximum voluntary ventilation (MVV) is the maximum amount of air that can be moved in 1 minute. It is measured as follows: The patient is asked to breathe as hard and as fast as possible for 15 seconds. The volume is recorded and multiplied by 4 to convert the findings to liters per minute. The maximum voluntary ventilation can also be predicted by multiplying the FEV_1 by 35.[33] Because the former method is so dependent on effort for an extended period of time, the latter method is often used, but an actual measurement is preferred.[34] The MVV is an indicator of the ventilatory limit of the pulmonary system, especially in patients with chronic obstructive pulmonary disease (COPD), and is useful in evaluating an exercise test.[35]

The minute expired volume ($\dot{V}E$) is the amount of air expired per minute. $\dot{V}E$max is the amount of air expired per minute at peak exercise. During an exercise test, healthy subjects do not achieve their ventilatory limit, even when exercising at or near their maximum heart rates. The $\dot{V}E$max in a healthy person is approximately 60 to 70 percent of the total MVV at maximal exercise ($\dot{V}E$max/MVV = 60 to 70 percent).[36] In contrast, a patient whose pulmonary system is compromised by obstructive disease will approach 100 percent of MVV before ever reaching the predicted maximum heart rate.[36]

FORCED EXPIRATORY FLOW

The $FEF_{25-75\%}$ reflects the amount of time required to exhale the middle half of a forced vital capacity maneuver. The volume attained during an FVC maneuver is divided into quarters. The first and last quarter are ignored, and the middle two quarters (half) of the volume are determined. That volume is then divided by the time it took to exhale it.[29] $FEF_{25-75\%}$ is recorded in liters per second. $FEF_{25-75\%}$ has a wide range of normal values, making it difficult to use as a screening tool. However, within subjects, a decrease in this value may detect the early stages of lung disease.[37] $FEF_{25-75\%}$ normally decreases with age. The test is also called the maximum midexpiratory flow rate (MMEFR).

DIFFUSION CAPACITY OF THE LUNGS FOR CARBON MONOXIDE

The D_{LCO} is an analysis of the ability to diffuse a single held breath of an inhaled gas from the pulmonary alveoli to the pulmonary capillary.[38] The subject is first asked to empty the lungs of all possible air, then inhale as deeply as possible a combination of carbon monoxide and helium, and hold that breath for 10 seconds. Finally, the gas is fully exhaled and analyzed for carbon monoxide content. The amount of carbon monoxide that crossed the alveolar capillary membrane is then determined. The normal diffusing capacity is approximately 25 milliliters per minute per mm Hg.[12]

Although the D_{LCO} test cannot be performed by simple spirometry, it is useful as a predictor of a subject's ability to oxygenate arterial blood during exercise. Patients whose D_{LCO} is greater than 55 percent of the normative value can be predicted to maintain their oxygenation during exercise.[39] Patients with COPD who are most likely to become hypoxic during exercise have D_{LCO} values less than 55 percent of predicted.[39] Studying younger patients with cystic fibrosis, Lebecque et al.[40] showed that a D_{LCO} greater than 80 percent was predictive of the ability to maintain oxygenation during exercise, whereas a patient with a D_{LCO} less than 65 percent of predicted D_{LCO} was likely to desaturate. The criterion for severe impairment is a D_{LCO} less than 40 percent of predicted D_{LCO}.[30,41]

EXERCISE TESTING IN PATIENTS WITH PULMONARY DISEASE

The evaluation of functional capacity is part of the assessment of a patient with pulmonary disease. A graded exercise test (GXT) can provide the objective information to document a patient's symptomatology and physical impairment. It can also provide the information necessary to prescribe safe exercise for the successful management of patients in a pulmonary rehabilitation program. Other uses of an exercise test are to document oxygen desaturation and changes in pulmonary function during exercise.

Physiologic Testing Parameters

PULMONARY FUNCTION TESTS

Before the exercise testing session, the pulmonary function tests previously mentioned in this chapter should be performed. The results of FEV_1 will help decide the appropriate protocol to use for the GXT. Maximum voluntary ventilation should be determined before the exercise test because it is one of the criteria for test termination (V̇Emax approaches MVV). The DLCO can help predict patients who may not oxygenate their blood adequately during exercise. After exercise, the PFTs are again administered to assess the effects of exercise on lung function. A reduction of 10 percent in either FEV_1 or $FEF_{25-75\%}$ is an indication of need for bronchodilator therapy.[42]

ARTERIAL BLOOD GAS ANALYSIS AND OXYGEN SATURATION

An ABG analysis provides the best method for determining arterial oxygenation and the adequacy of alveolar ventilation. Table 10–1 shows normal values obtained by an arterial blood gas sample. The recording of the partial pressure of oxygen (PaO_2) and the partial pressure of carbon dioxide ($PaCO_2$) can detect hypoxemia and hypercapnea during execise. During exercise, arterial blood gas samples are drawn from a catheter (which has been previously placed in the radial artery) every 1 to 1½ minutes. When analyzed, the ABG measurement provides information regarding the need for supplemental oxygen as well as information regarding anaerobic threshold and the ventilatory reserve.[43]

An estimate of PaO_2 can be made by using pulse oximetry, which measures the degree of saturation of hemoglobin with oxygen (SaO_2). Although there is not a one-to-one correlation between SaO_2 and PaO_2, according to the oxyhemoglobin dissociation curve, a relationship between the two values does exist. Changes in SaO_2 correlate closely with the changes in PaO_2 on the flat portions of the oxyhemoglobin desaturation curve, but when the SaO_2 falls to the steep slope of the curve, a small decrease in SaO_2 will produce a significant drop in PaO_2[44] (Fig. 10–7). Evaluating PaO_2 by arterial oxygen saturation is limited by the accuracy of the oximeter which has confidence limits of $\pm$ 4 to 5 percent.[42]

Measuring exhaled volumes of gas for carbon dioxide (CO_2) content can predict $PaCO_2$. However, the CO_2 levels of the expired air do not necessarily correspond accu-

TABLE 10–1 Normal Values
for Arterial Blood Gas
Sampling with the Subject
Breathing Room Air

FIO_2	0.21
PaO_2	95–100 mm Hg
$PaCO_2$	35–45 mm Hg
pH	7.35–7.45
HCO_3^-	24 mEq/m

FIO_2 = fraction of inspired oxygen, PaO_2 = partial pressure of oxygen, $PaCO_2$ = partial pressure of carbon dioxide, HCO_3^- = bicarbonate ion.

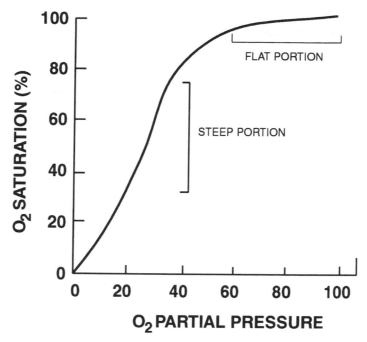

FIGURE 10–7. Oxyhemoglobin dissociation curve.

rately to the alveolar concentration of CO_2 or to the partial pressure of CO_2 in the blood.

Although ABG analysis is an invasive testing procedure, actual blood gas measurements are far more accurate than those made by using noninvasive procedures. On the other hand, oximetry is noninvasive and does provide a continuous stream of data. These features may be valuable in some clinical situations.

THE EXERCISE ELECTROCARDIOGRAM

The ECG gives a recording of the electrical activity of the cardiac conduction system. Electrocardiography is used to detect cardiac arrhythmias, conduction abnormalities, and cardiac ischemia. Before exercise, patients are prepared for 12-lead exercise ECG tracings. Electrode sites, methods for checking poor tracings, and suggestions for recordings and interpretations are given in Chapters 8 and 9.

BLOOD PRESSURE

During the GXT, blood pressure measurements must be recorded frequently. Measurements should be recorded in supine, sitting, and standing positions at rest, at 2-minute intervals during exercise, and during recovery from the test. During the exercise test, systolic blood pressure should rise with increasing workloads, and the diastolic pressure should remain about the same. The highest systolic blood pressure should be achieved at the maximal workload, but the test should be terminated if the systolic pressure reaches 250 mm Hg and/or the diastolic pressure is 110 mm Hg or greater. The test should also be terminated if the systolic or diastolic blood pressure falls more than 10 mm Hg with increasing exercise loads.

$\dot{V}O_2$max MEASUREMENT

Measurements of maximum oxygen consumption ($\dot{V}O_2$max) (see Chapter 4) are used to identify vocational and leisure activities that lie within or outside the bounds of a participant's ability. According to some estimates, a person can perform a job for up to 8 hours if the maximal workload of that job requires no more than 40 percent of the worker's $\dot{V}O_2$max.[45] Justification for return to work or for disability can be objectively judged by the use of $\dot{V}O_2$max. If $\dot{V}O_2$max is below 15 milliliters per kilogram per minute or fewer than 5 METs (see Chapter 9), the participant is considered to have a moderately impaired respiratory system[46] and to be physically impaired for practically all types of employment.[30]

Formulas are available to predict a participant's $\dot{V}O_2$max by using the amount of work accomplished on a specific exercise protocol (see Chapter 9). Actual $\dot{V}O_2$max determinations necessitate the use of headgear with a mouthpiece and a nose clip to collect the gas samples necessary to make the actual $\dot{V}O_2$max determination. Although the actual $\dot{V}O_2$max is a valuable measurement, the anxiety produced by the equipment may be so objectionable to some pulmonary patients that a less-than-maximal test will result and therefore an inaccurate $\dot{V}O_2$max will be obtained. Decisions about the need for actual $\dot{V}O_2$max values versus predicted values should be made on an individual basis.

Exercise-Testing Protocols

Exercise testing of the pulmonary patient is not usually diagnostic; it is used to document the amount of impairment caused by an already diagnosed condition. The purposes of an exercise test are to establish the functional capacity of a patient with pulmonary disease, evaluate the need for oxygen therapy during exercise, and prescribe appropriate exercise intensity.

A graded (gradually increasing intensity) exercise test should stress the patient to the point of limitation while vital signs are monitored to ensure the patient's safety. Numerous testing procedures are available to assess the functional abilities of patients with pulmonary disease. Protocols and equipment requirements for measuring functional ability range from the very simple 12-minute walk test (which requires only the ability to measure heart rate, blood pressure, time, and distance) to the more sophisticated treadmill and cycle protocols. The treadmill and cycle protocols may include any of the following measurements: $\dot{V}O_2$max, heart rate, electrocardiogram, blood pressure, respiratory rate, PaO_2, $PaCO_2$, pH, SaO_2, A-aO_2 difference, A-$\dot{V}O_2$ difference, respiratory quotient (R), dead space volume (VDS), and dead space to tidal volume ratio (VDS/VT).[47]

Testing protocols vary with the preference and training of the examiners, availability of equipment, and abilities of the patient population. See Table 10–2 for examples of protocols used in exercise-testing patients with pulmonary disease.

THE 12-MINUTE WALK

The 12-minute walk is a simple way to asses functional ability. The subject is asked to cover as much distance as possible in 12 minutes.[48] Because functional ability

TABLE 10–2 Protocols Used for Exercise-Testing the Patient with
Pulmonary Disease

Mode	Author	Protocol
Walk test	Cooper[48]	Ambulate as far as possible in 12 min
	Guyatt et al.[50]	Ambulate as far as possible in 6 min
Cycle test	Jones[53]	Begin with 100 kpm (17 W), increase 100 kpm every min
	Jones and Campbell[54]	Begin with 25 W, 15-W increase every min
	Berman and Sutton[55]	Begin with 100 kpm/min, increase 100 kpm/min every min or 50 kpm/min every min when FEV_1 less than 1 liter/s
	Mass. Respiratory Hospital[56]	Begin with 25 W, increase 10 W every 20 sec or 5 W every 20 sec when FEV_1 less than 1 liter/s
Treadmill tests	Naughton et al.[58]	2 mph constant 0 grade
		3.5% grade every 3 min
	Balke and Ware[59]	3.3 mph constant 0 grade
		3.5% grade every 2 min
	Mass. Respiratory Hospital[56]	1.5 mph constant 0 grade
		4% grade every 2 min
		2% grade every 2 min if FEV_1 is less than 1 liter/s

increases with training, the distance walked in 12 minutes also should increase. Performance of a 12-minute walk has been shown to correlate positively with FVC and $\dot{V}O_2$max as determined by cycle ergometry and treadmill tests.[48,49] When used for pretesting and post-testing, the 12-minute walk becomes an easy, inexpensive, and objective measurement of changes in ability. For pulmonary patients, the 12-minute walk may be modified to 6 minutes or sometimes 2 minutes.[50,51]

CYCLE ERGOMETER

Cycle ergometer protocols are advantageous for patients who lack agility, coordination, and/or balance. Because the person is seated, the test performed can be safer. Blood pressure measurements, arterial blood gas samples, and ECG tracings are easier to obtain during a cycle ergometer test because of the stability of the upper body during exercise. One major disadvantage of using a cycle ergometer protocol is that leg fatigue often causes test termination before the patient achieves maximal capability.[52]

There are a variety of testing protocols for cycle ergometers. Jones[53] uses a progression of 17 watts (W) every minute (speed is constant at 50 rpm). Another protocol suggested by Jones and Campbell begins with a workload of 25 W and increases by increments of 15 W every minute.[54]

According to the ability of each patient, an individualized protocol can be chosen for the exercise test session. Berman and Sutton[55] suggest increments of 100 kpm every minute with patients whose FEV_1 is greater than 1 liter per second. If the FEV_1 is found to be less than 1 liter per second, the increments are lowered to 50 kpm per minute.

Some cycle protocols do not achieve steady states; instead, they use a more "ramped" increase in workload. With pedal speed kept constant, the workload is increased every 20 seconds. Again, these decisions should be based on the ability of each patient. For example, if a patient has an FEV_1 of less than 1 liter per second, the protocol would increase the workload 5 W every 20 seconds. If the FEV_1 is greater than 1 liter per second, then the workload can be increased 10 W every 20 seconds.[56] (See Chapter 9 for additional ergometry tests.)

TREADMILL TESTING

Treadmill tests provide a more accurate functional assessment of the patient with pulmonary disease than does a cycle ergometer test. The number of protocols available for treadmill testing allow accommodation to a number of individual abilities. For example, a patient who may have difficulty walking faster than 2 mph will perform best when following the Naughton protocol.[57,58] A patient who is able to walk faster than 2 mph may be evaluated by the Balke test protocol.[37,59] A Bruce protocol is rarely indicated in exercise testing of pulmonary patients because the test is best suited for healthier patients capable of higher workloads.[60,61] Some patients cannot maintain speeds of 2 mph and require treadmill speeds of 1.5 mph or less.[56,61] Not all treadmills, however, can accommodate speeds below 2 mph. (Additional treadmill protocols can be found in Chapter 9.)

Test and Exercise Termination

The symptom-limited end point of an exercise test for patients with pulmonary disease is somewhat different from that already described for cardiac patients (Chapter 9). Criteria for stopping a pulmonary exercise test may include but not be limited to the following.[30,33,47]

1. Maximal shortness of breath
2. A fall in Pao_2 of more than 20 mm Hg or a Pao_2 less than 55 mm Hg
3. A rise in $Paco_2$ more than 10 mm Hg or a $Paco_2$ greater than 65 mm Hg
4. Cardiac ischemia or arrhythmias
5. Symptoms of fatigue
6. Increase in diastolic blood pressure readings of 20 mm Hg, systolic hypertension greater than 250 mm Hg, decrease in blood pressure with increasing workloads
7. Leg pain
8. Total fatigue
9. Signs of insufficient cardiac output
10. Reaching a ventilatory maximum

Interpretation of Graded Exercise Test Results

With assessment of functional abilities, an appropriate vocational assessment can be completed and documentation necessary for addressing disability provided.[45]

The need for supplemental oxygen is identified if a patient becomes hypoxic during the exercise test session. A decrease in PaO_2 of more than 20 mm Hg or a PaO_2 less than 55 mm Hg are indications for oxygen supplementation.[62] Guidelines for supplemental oxygen prescription should include a high flow rate with an FIO_2 of 24 to 27 percent and should be criterion-based, that is, sufficient to maintain an SaO_2 greater than 85 percent.

Pulmonary function tests administered before an exercise test and readministered after an exercise test will determine if exercise-induced bronchospasm is present.

For prescribing an exercise program based on the GXT, see Chapter 11. For emergency procedures, see Chapter 9.

PULMONARY TESTING CASE STUDIES

CASE STUDY 1

The patient is a 61-year-old woman with a diagnosis of COPD, asthma, and orthostatic hypotension. She has recently had a mastectomy. Medications are Tamoxatrin, imipramine, Ventolin MDI, Atrovent MDI, Ativan, and Slo-phyllin. Table 10–3 summarizes her exercise test.

CASE STUDY 2

The patient is a 77-year-old man with a diagnosis of COPD, asthma, chronic bronchitis, hypertension, and peptic ulcer disease. Medications are Beclovent MDI, Atrovent MDI, Robitussin, and Maxair MDI. Table 10–4 summarizes his exercise test.

CASE STUDY 3

The patient is a 69-year-old man with a diagnosis of COPD, pneumoconiosis (he is formerly a foundry worker—possible silicosis), HTN, CAD, MI (LVEF 43 percent), ulcers, L CVA, PVD, and gout. Medications are Lasix, ASA, diltiazem, Alipurinol, digoxin, Lanoxin, and NTG. Table 10–5 summarizes his exercise test.

CASE STUDY 4

The patient is a 73-year-old man with a diagnosis of COPD and glaucoma. Medications are Maxair MDI, Beclovent MDI, Atrovent MDI, prednisone, Dilantin, aminophylline, and Pilocar drops. Table 10–6 summarizes his exercise test.

TABLE 10–3 Raw Data—Case Study 1

Age: 61 Sex: F AAMHR: 159 Ht: 162.6 cm Wt: 56.4 kg
Smoking: 45 pack-years; quit 8 years ago
Occupation: Clerk, part-time
Resting ECG: Normal; Resting HR, 108; Resting BP, 130/70; Resting RR, 16
Resting PFTs: FVC, 1.77 liter (57%); FEV$_1$ 0.68 liter/s (28%); FEV$_1$/FVC, 38% MVV = 17.8 L/min
Protocol: Modified cycle

Time	Workload (W)	HR (bpm)	BP (mm Hg)	RR (br/min)	$\dot{V}_E$ (liter/min)	$\dot{V}_{O_2}$ (liter/min)	METs	ABG PaO$_2$/PaCO$_2$/pH
Rest	00.0	108	130/70	16			1.0	55/38/7.44
1:01	25.0	118		18.8	12.3	0.37	1.9	
2:01	40.0	120	136/82	19.1	16.1	0.51	2.6	41/44/7.36
2:14	45.0	123		23.4	16.8	0.55	2.8	

Reason for test termination: Leg fatigue
Exercise ECG: Normal

Max Values

	Actual	Predicted	Percent of Predicted
HR	123	159	78
V$_{O_2}$	0.6	1.3	44

Ventilatory Values

Actual $\dot{V}_{Emax}$	16.8
MVV	17.8
Predicted $\dot{V}_E$	23.8
$\dot{V}_{Emax}$ MVV	94%

Postexercise PFTs: FVC, 1.55 L (50%); FEV$_1$ 0.60, liter/s (25%); FEV$_1$/FVC, 39%

Comments: There was a significant bronchospastic response after exercise. Also there was decrease in oxygenation with exercise.
Interpretation: Submaximal exercise test. Moderately severe ventilatory (pre- and post-PFTs) and diffusion (ABGs) limitations.

TABLE 10–4 Raw Data—Case Study 2

Age: 77 Sex: M AAMHR: 143 Ht: 169 cm Wt: 82.3 kg
Smoking: 75 pack-years; quit 2 years ago
Occupation: Retired
Resting ECG: Normal; Resting HR, 61; Resting BP, 128/82; Resting RR, 18.6
Resting PFTs: FVC, 2.76 liter (72%); FEV$_1$, 1.55 liter/s (53%); FEV$_1$/FVC, 56% MVV 44.2 L/min
Protocol: Modified cycle

Time	Workload (W)	HR (bpm)	BP (mm Hg)	RR (br/min)	$\dot{V}_E$ (liter/min)	$\dot{V}_{O_2}$ (liter/min)	METs	ABG PaO$_2$/PaCO$_2$/pH	SaCO$_2$ %
Rest	00.0	61	128/82	18.6	8.9		1.0	71/34/7.40	94
1:00	25.0	74		19.0	13.8	0.49	1.7		92
2:03	55.0	84	170/86	21.3	20.4	0.83	2.9		90
3:01	85.0	94		21.7	25.4	0.98	3.4		90
4:00	115	111		25.5	32.3	1.20	4.2	57/45/7.33	87
4:30		123		29.7	39.3	1.31	4.5		87

Reason for test termination: Dyspnea
Exercise ECG: Normal

Max Values

	Actual	Predicted	Percent of Predicted
HR	123	146	87
V$_{O_2}$	1.3	1.6	80

Ventilatory Values

Actual $\dot{V}_{Emax}$	39.3
MVV	44.2
Predicted $\dot{V}_{Emax}$	54.3
$\dot{V}_{Emax}$ MVV	89%

Postexercise PFTs: FVC, 2.69 liter (70%); FEV$_1$, 1.70 liter/s (58%); FEV$_1$/FVC, 63%

Comments: There was a 10% improvement in FEV$_1$ postexercise. Oxygenation decreased during exercise, SaO$_2$ dropped to 87%.
Interpretation: Maximal test with moderately severe obstructive lung disease. Results indicate moderate ventilatory mechanical limitation with diffusion abnormality. No significant changes in ECG with exercise. Patient stopped exercise test because of pulmonary limitations.

TABLE 10-5 Raw Data—Case Study 3

Age: 69 Sex: M AAMHR: 151 Ht: 181 cm Wt: 66.8 kg
Smoking: 70 pack-years; quit 11 years ago
Occupation: Retired; former foundry worker
Resting ECG: 2–3 mm ST depression RHR, 84; RBP, 140/76; RRR, 13.1 br/min
Resting PFTs: FVC, 3.88 liter (82%); FEV$_1$, 1.61 liter/s (44%); FEV$_1$/FVC, 41% MVV = 36.9 L/min
Protocol: Treadmill

Time	Workload	HR (bpm)	BP (mm Hg)	RR (br/min)	V̇E (liter/min)	V̇O$_2$ (liter/min)	METs	ABG PaO$_2$/PaCO$_2$/pH	SaCO$_2$ %
Rest		84	140/76	13.1	12.8		1.0	72/29/7.39	96
1:01	1.5 mph 0% grade	90		16.7	21.0	0.52	2.2		92
2:02		90		20.0	25.4	0.63	2.7		90
2:45		96		23.4	30.8	0.73	3.1		87
3:17	1.5 mph 0% grade	89	190/84	22.8	31.0	0.70	3.0	57/45/7.33	87

Reason for test termination: Dyspnea and fatigue
Exercise ECG: No significant changes with exercise

Max Values	Actual	Predicted	Percent of Predicted
HR	96.0	152	63
V̇O$_2$	0.8	1.9	40

Ventilatory Values

Actual V̇Emax	31.0
MVV	36.9
Predicted V̇Emax	56.4
V̇Emax MVV	84%

Postexercise PFTs: FVC, 3.99 liter (84%); FEV$_1$, 1.59 liter/s (44%); FEV$_1$/FVC, 40%

Comments: Spirometry at rest showed moderately severe obstructive lung disease. There was no significant change postexercise.
Interpretation: Submaximal exercise test without reaching anaerobic threshold. Moderately severe gas exchange abnormality with diffusion-type limitations. Decrease in exercise heart rate at highest workload, indicating cardiac limitation or deconditioning. Suggest pulse oximetry on activity.

TABLE 10–6 Raw Data—Case Study 4

Age: 73 Sex: M AAMHR: 145 Ht: 178 cm Wt: 69.0 kg
Smoking: 50 pack-years; quit 3 years ago
Occupation: Retired, former truck driver
Resting ECG: PVCs, couplets twice; RHR, 93; RBP, 138/80; RRR, 22.5 br/min
Resting PFTs: FVC, 3.13 liter (71%); FEV_1 1.14 liter/s (34%); FEV_1/FVC, 36% MVV = 29.2 L/min
Protocol: Treadmill

Time	Workload		HR (bpm)	BP (mm Hg)	RR (br/min)	$\dot{V}_E$ (liter/min)	$\dot{V}_{O_2}$ (liter/min)	METs	ABG $PaO_2/PaCO_2$/pH
Rest			93	138/80	22.5	19.5		1.0	63/43/7.40
1:03	1.5 mph	0% grade	96		22.1	20.3	0.47	2.0	
2:01	1.5 mph	0% grade	98		19.7	22.0	0.61	2.5	52/45/7.40
3:01	1.5 mph	4% grade	114		23.2	24.6	0.68	2.8	44/47/7.38
4:01	1.5 mph	4% grade	113	190/84	26.4	28.5	0.78	3.2	42/50/7.36

Reason for test termination: Mouth and nose discomfort from mouthpiece and nose clip, some shortness of breath
Exercise ECG: Few PVCs seen; nonspecific ST-T-segment changes

Max Values	Actual	Predicted	Percent of Predicted
HR	114.0	148	72
$\dot{V}_{O_2}$	0.8	1.7	47

Ventilatory Values

Actual $\dot{V}_{Emax}$	28.5
MVV	29.2
Predicted $\dot{V}_{Emax}$	39.9
% Predicted $\dot{V}_{Emax}$/MVV	97%

Postexercise PFTs: FVC, 3.35 liter (76%); FEV_1, 1.21, liter/s (36%); FEV_1/FVC, 36%

Comments: Spirometry at rest showed severe degree of airflow obstruction. Significant drop in PaO_2 during exercise, $PaCO_2$ rose 7 mm Hg.
Interpretation: Submaximal exercise test because of pulmonary limitations and discomfort. Anaerobic threshold not reached. Heart rate reserve normal. Breathing reserve poor. Need for oxygen with exercise.

SUMMARY

Assessment of the patient with pulmonary disease is a continuous process. A thorough assessment allows the appropriate treatment program to be conceived, administered safely and effectively, and altered (either progressed or regressed) according to the patient's needs. The value of the ongoing nature of pulmonary assessment is discussed.

Pulmonary assessment includes the interview, the physical examination, and laboratory tests. Each area of assessment provides information that the clinician can use to tailor the treatment program to best suit the patient. It is of little benefit to develop a treatment program to which the patient either cannot or will not adhere.

The pulmonary assessment interview includes the chief complaint, that is, the patient's reason for seeking medical intervention, as well as medical, occupational, social, and family histories.

Physical examination includes observation of the patient's posture, breathing pattern (rate, rhythm, and use of accessory musculature), skin color and appearance of the distal extremities, and thoracic configuration. Palpation gives insight into symmetry and excursion of the thorax during the respiratory cycle. Auscultation allows the clinician to listen to the air movement within the thorax. Abnormal breath sounds (diminished or bronchial) and adventitious sounds (crackles and wheezes) will, if heard, alert the clinician to the site of the abnormality.

Laboratory tests, including pulmonary function tests, chest x-rays, and arterial blood gas analyses, are used to diagnose pulmonary disease and to monitor the progress of the disease process. An exercise tolerance test, although not usually performed as a diagnostic test, is used to determine exercise prescription, document symptoms and functional capacity, assess the need for supplemental oxygen, and justify job-related abilities or disabilities. Case studies illustrating exercise testing and termination criteria have been included.

REFERENCES

1. Payton, O, Nelson, C, and Ozer, M: Patient Participation in Program Planning. FA Davis, Philadelphia, 1990.
2. Hobson, L and Hammon, W: Chest assessment. In: Frownfelter, D (ed): Chest Physical Therapy and Pulmonary Rehabilitation, ed 3. Year Book Medical Publishers, Chicago, 1996.
3. Surveillance for respiratory hazards in the occupational setting: The official ATS statement. American Review of Respiratory Diseases 126:952–956, 1982.
4. Luce, J: Lung Diseases of Adults. American Lung Association, 1986.
5. Cohen-Cole, S: The Medical Interview: The Three Function Approach. Year Book Medical Publishers, Chicago, 1991.
6. Purtilo, R: Health Professional/Patient Interaction, ed 3. Saunders, Philadelphia, 1984.
7. Ciccone, C: Pharmacology in Rehabilitation. FA Davis, Philadelphia, 1990.
8. Fielding, J: Smoking effects and control, part 1. N Engl J Med 313(8):491–498, 1985.
9. Burki, N: Pulmonary Diseases. Medical Examination Publishing, New York, 1982.
10. Farzan, S: A Concise Handbook of Respiratory Diseases, ed 2. Reston Publishing, Reston, Va, 1985.
11. Zadai, C: Pulmonary pharmacology. In: T Malone (ed): Physical and Occupational Therapy: Drug Implications for Practice. Lippincott, Philadelphia, 1989, pp 97–119.
12. Price, S and Wilson, L: Pathophysiology: Clinical Concepts of Disease Processes, ed 2. McGraw-Hill, New York, 1982.
13. Gaskell, D and Webber, B: The Brompton Hospital Guide to Chest Physiotherapy, ed 4. Blackwell Scientific Publications, Oxford, England, 1980.
14. Bell, C et al: Home Care and Rehabilitation in Respiratory Medicine. Lippincott, Philadelphia, 1984.
15. Williams, P (ed): Gray's Anatomy, the anatomical basis of medicine and surgery, ed 38. Churchill Livingstone, New York, 1995.

16. Traver, G: Assessment of the Thorax and Lungs. Am J Nurs 73(3):466–471, 1973.
17. Murphy, R: Auscultation of the lung: Past lessons, future possibilities. Thorax 36:99–107, 1981.
18. Pulmonary terms and symbols: A report of the ACCP-ATS Joint Committee on Pulmonary Nomenclature. Chest 67:583–593, 1975.
19. Forgacs, P: Crackles and wheezes. Lancet 2:203–205, 1967.
20. Ploysongsang, Y and Schonfeld, S: Mechanism of the production of crackles after atelectasis during low volume breathing. American Review of Respiratory Diseases 126:413–415, 1982.
21. Loudon, R: The lung speaks out. American Review of Respiratory Diseases 126:411–412, 1982.
22. Harper, R: A Guide to Respiratory Care: Physiology and Clinical Applications. Lippincott, Philadelphia, 1981.
23. Holleman, D and Simel, D: Does the Clinical Examination Predict Airflow Limitation? JAMA 273(4):313–319, 1995.
24. Mahagnah, M and Favriely, N: Repeatability of Measurements of Normal Lung Sounds. Am J Respir Crit Care Med 149:477–481, 1994.
25. Downie, P (ed): Cash's Textbook of Chest, Heart and Vascular Disorders for Physiotherapists, ed 4. Lippincott, Philadelphia, 1987.
26. Weinberger, S: Recent advances in pulmonary medicine, first of two parts. N Engl J Med 328(19): 1389–1397, 1993.
27. McIvor, A and Chapman, K: Diagnosis of chronic obstructive pulmonary disease and differentiation from asthma. Current Opinion in Pulmonary Medicine 2:148–154, 1996.
28. Pugatch, R: Radiologic evaluation in chest malignancies: A review of imaging modalities. Chest 107(6): 294S–297S, 1995.
29. Cherniack, R: Pulmonary Function Testing. Saunders, Philadelphia, 1977.
30. American Thoracic Society: Evaluation of impairment secondary to respiratory disease. American Review of Respiratory Diseases 126:945–951, 1982.
31. Ruppel, G: Manual of Pulmonary Function Testing, ed 2. Mosby, St Louis, 1979.
32. Report of Snowbird Workshop on standardization of spirometry. American Review of Respiratory Diseases 119:831–838, 1979.
33. Ries, A: The role of exercise testing in pulmonary diagnosis. Clin Chest Med 8:81–89, 1987.
34. Dillard, T: Ventilatory limitations of exercise. Chest 92:195–196, 1987.
35. LoRusso, T et al: Reduction of max exercise capacity in obstructive and restrictive disease. Chest 104:1748–1754, 1993.
36. Weisman, I and Zeballos, R: An integrated approach to the interpretation of cardiopulmonary exercise testing. Clin Chest Med 15(2):421–445, 1994.
37. Guenter, C and Welch, M: Pulmonary Medicine, ed 2. JB Lippincott, Philadelphia, 1982.
38. Jones, R and Mead, F: A theoretical and experimental analysis of anomalies in the estimation of pulmonary diffusing capacity by single breath holding method. Quarterly Journal of Experimental Physiology 46:131–143, 1961.
39. Owens, G et al: The diffusing capacity as a predictor of arterial oxygen desaturation during exercise in patients with chronic obstructive pulmonary disease. N Engl J Med 310:1218–1221, 1984.
40. Lebecque, P et al: Diffusion capacity and oxygen desaturation effects on exercise in patients with cystic fibrosis. Chest 91:693–697, 1987.
41. Epler, G, Saber, F, and Guensler, E: Determination of severe impairment (disability) in interstitial lung disease. American Review of Respiratory Diseases 121:647–659, 1980.
42. O'Ryan, J and Burns, D: Pulmonary Rehabilitation from Hospital to Home. Year Book Medical Publishers, Chicago, 1984.
43. Reis, A: Position paper of the American Association of Cardiovascular and Pulmonary Rehabilitation. Scientific basis for pulmonary rehabilitation. J Cardpulm Rehabil 10:418–441, 1990.
44. Guyton, A: Textbook of Medical Physiology, ed 9. Saunders, Philadelphia, 1996.
45. Hodgkin, J, Zorn, E, and Connors, G: Pulmonary Rehabilitation. Guidelines to Success. Butterworth Publishers, Boston, 1984.
46. Ostiguy, G: Summary of task force report on occupational respiratory diseases. Can Med Assoc J 121: 414–421, 1979.
47. Zadai, C: Rehabilitation of the patient with chronic obstructive pulmonary disease. In: Irwin, S and Tecklin, J (eds): Cardiopulmonary Physical Therapy. Mosby, St. Louis, 1985.
48. Cooper, K: A means of assessing maximal oxygen intake: Correlation between field and treadmill walking. JAMA 203:201–204, 1968.
49. McGavin, C, Gupta, S, and McHardy, G: Twelve minute walking test for assessing disability in chronic bronchitis. BMJ 1:822, 1976.
50. Guyatt, G, Berman, L, and Townsend, M: Long-term outcome after respiratory rehabilitation. Can Med Assoc J 137:1089–1095, 1987.
51. Butland, R et al: Two, six and twelve minute walking tests in respiratory disease. BMJ 284:1007–1008, 1982.
52. American College of Sports Medicine: Guidelines for Exercise Testing and Prescription, ed 4. Lea & Febiger, Philadelphia, 1991.

53. Jones, N: Exercise testing in pulmonary evaluation: Rationale, methods and the normal respiratory response to exercise. N Engl J Med 293:541–544, 1975.
54. Carter, R et al: Exercise gas exchange in patients with moderate severe to severe chronic obstructive pulmonary disease. J Cardpulm Rehab 9(6):243–248, 1989.
55. Berman, L and Sutton, J: Exercise for the pulmonary patient. J Cardpulm Rehab 6(2):55–59, 1986.
56. Massachusetts Respiratory Hospital, Exercise Testing Protocol, Braintree, Mass.
57. Bell, C: Exercise Stress Testing and Physical Conditioning Program in Pulmonary Rehabilitation Medical Manual, University of Nebraska Medical Center, pp 50–91, 1977.
58. Naughton, J, Balke, B, and Poarch, R: Modified work capacity studies in individuals with and without coronary artery disease. J Sports Med 4:208–212, 1964.
59. Balke, B and Ware, R: An experimental study of physical fitness of Air Force personnel. US Armed Forces Med J 10:675–688, 1959.
60. Bruce, R: Methods of exercise testing: Step test, bicycle, treadmill, and isometrics. Am J Cardiol 33:715–720, 1974.
61. Ellestad, M: Stress Testing: Principles and Practice, ed 3. FA Davis, Philadelphia, 1986.
62. Wilson, P, Bell, C, and Norton, A: Rehabilitation of the Heart and Lungs. Beckman Instruments, Fullerton, Calif, 1980.

CHAPTER 11

The Exercise Prescription

An individualized plan should be formulated for each patient who enters the rehabilitation program. The specific plan designed for each patient by the rehabilitation staff is devised from the patient's medical history, prognosis, and functional capacity and should reflect the patient's individual needs, goals, and anticipated outcomes.[1,2] Although the comprehensive rehabilitation program includes several facets designed to provide interventions for restoring functional capacity, reducing risk factors, and promoting positive psychosocial behavioral changes that lead to maintenance of health and social independence,[3,4] this chapter focuses on factors to be considered in formulation of the exercise prescription for outpatient cardiac rehabilitation.

Because of the increasing amount of research reporting the beneficial effects of cardiac rehabilitation on secondary prevention of coronary artery disease (CAD), exercise training has become widely recognized as an important component in developing rehabilitation interventions for patients with coronary artery disease.[5-16] Secondary prevention programs have been shown to be effective for patients with other types of coronary heart disease (CHD) including those recovering from coronary artery bypass graft surgery (CABG), myocardial infarction (MI), valve replacement, pacemaker implantation, percutaneous transluminal coronary angioplasty (PTCA), and cardiac transplantation, as well as for patients with left ventricular dysfunction and congestive heart failure (CHF).[4,5,9,11,16-19]

The major goals of cardiac rehabilitation are to limit the negative physiologic and psychologic effects of cardiac illness, reduce the risk of sudden death, control cardiac symptoms, stabilize or reverse the atherosclerotic disease, and enhance the patient's psychosocial and vocational status.[3,4,9,16-18,20-25] These goals are accomplished through exercise training to improve functional capacity, education for risk factor modification, and counseling.[2,3,26]

Largely because of the success of cardiac rehabilitation in returning patients with cardiac disease to a better quality of life, patients with chronic obstructive pulmonary disease (COPD) are being referred to rehabilitation programs in increasing numbers. Rehabilitation programs for patients with COPD provide a valuable adjunct to medical therapy in helping to control the symptoms of lung disease and to improve functional capacity so that patients may achieve the highest possible level of independent function. A primary goal of pulmonary rehabilitation is to attempt to reverse a patient's disability from the disease rather than reverse a progressive disease process.[27]

The major goals of cardiac and pulmonary (cardiopulmonary) rehabilitation programs are quite similar in that their objectives are to restore patients with cardiopulmonary diseases to their optimal physiologic, psychologic, social, and vocational status.[3,4,16,26,27] Although there are some differences in exercise prescription for cardiac and pulmonary patients, the basic guidelines for each group remain so similar that the two are presented in a broad, general manner directed toward "cardiopulmonary" rehabilitation, with more specific discussions included as needed. The case studies presented in this chapter are, of course, specific to cardiac and pulmonary patients.

To write a comprehensive exercise prescription for a patient with cardiopulmonary disease, the clinician must:

1. Demonstrate an understanding of the physiologic factors that are essential to the attainment of normal cardiopulmonary function and physical fitness.
2. Identify through evaluative procedures the status of an individual with regard to those factors.
3. Recognize and skillfully apply the training principles necessary for physiologic adaptation to improve the functional status of impaired patients and assist patients in maintaining normalized function once it has been attained.

The clinician who prescribes exercise for cardiopulmonary patients must consider the patient's age, gender, clinical status, related medical problems, habitual physical activity, and musculoskeletal integrity. The information obtained from symptom-limited graded exercise tests (SL-GXT) (see Chapters 9 and 10) will be the most useful tool to establish guidelines for exercise training for patients with known or suspected cardiopulmonary disease. Identification and definition of the physiologic and clinical basis for the prescription of exercise in cardiopulmonary patients are presented in this chapter. The exercise prescription will vary with the individual's development or recurrence of disease, and, for safety and functional improvement, may need to be readjusted periodically. Examples of exercise prescriptions using case histories from Chapters 9 and 10 have been included in this chapter so that the knowledge of training principles can be integrated with the information obtained from the evaluation procedures. The formulation of the exercise prescription is scientifically based, individualized, and presented to illustrate the process of writing an exercise prescription in a clear, practical manner. The cardiopulmonary rehabilitation staff should view the development of exercise prescriptions as an art as well as a science[28] and should be prepared to modify exercise prescriptions in accordance with the responses and adaptations of individual patients.

The major factors essential to the attainment and maintenance of optimal functional capacity through exercise training are improved cardiorespiratory endurance, body composition, muscular strength and endurance, and flexibility (range of joint motion). The development of each factor requires a specific training technique. To be effective, training methods designed to improve cardiorespiratory endurance must differ from those used to improve strength or flexibility. This variance in training methods illustrates the principle of "specificity of training,"[20,30] and rehabilitation clinicians must understand and be competent in the application of this principle to patient exercise prescriptions. Although training is specific and training programs differ, inherent in each well-designed program are principles related to the mode, intensity, duration, frequency, and rate of progression of the exercise. All these factors are essential to the exercise prescription, but the highest priority must be placed on the development of cardiorespiratory endurance, which appears to be most beneficial in the primary and secondary prevention of CHD.[2,16,28,29] The following discussion of principles of exercise prescription is included to illustrate the role each factor plays in cardiopulmonary exercise therapy.

RISK STRATIFICATION

Increasing numbers of patients with severe CHD and other diseases are being referred for comprehensive rehabilitation. This inclusion of exercise therapy as an adjunct to traditional medical treatment has necessitated the addition of risk stratification to the rehabilitation process.[2,31,32] The levels of risk are outlined in Table 11–1. An assessment of the clinical course, the extent of myocardial damage, left ventricular function, presence or absence of residual myocardial ischemia, ventricular arrhythmias, and other test results are used as guidelines for risk stratification. A careful evaluation of these factors is needed to appropriately assess the patient's prognosis for reinfarction, cardiac arrest, or heart failure, and to determine his or her functional capacity.[2,31,32] The mode, intensity, duration of medical supervision, and frequency of continuous electrocardiographic monitoring should be guided by the level of risk, be it low, moderate, or high, in which the patient is stratified. Risk assessment can be used to de-

TABLE 11–1 Guidelines for Risk Stratification of Patients
with Cardiac Disease

Risk Level	Characteristics
Low	No significant left ventricular dysfunction (i.e., ejection fraction ≥50%)
	No resting or exercised-induced myocardial ischemia manifested as angina and/or ST-segment displacement
	No resting or exercise-induced complex arrhythmias
	Uncomplicated MI, CABG, PTCA, or athrectomy
	Functional capacity ≥6 METs on GXT 3 or more weeks after clinical event
Intermediate	Mild to moderately depressed left ventricular function (ejection fraction 31%–49%)
	Functional capacity <5–6 METs on GXT 3 or more weeks after clinical event
	Failure to comply with exercise intensity prescription
	Exercise-induced myocardial ischemia (1–2 mm ST-segment depression) or reversible ischemic defects (echocardiography or nuclear radiography)
High	Severely depressed left ventricular function (ejection fraction ≤30%)
	Complex ventricular arrhythmias at rest or appearing or increasing with exercise
	Decrease in systolic blood pressure of >15 mm Hg during exercise or failure to rise with increasing workloads
	Survivor of sudden cardiac death
	Myocardial infarction complicated by CHF, cardiogenic shock, and/or complex ventricular arrhythmias
	Severe coronary artery disease and marked exercise induced myocardial ischemia (>2 mm ST-segment depression)

Source: Guidelines for Cardiac Rehabilitation Programs (p 14) by American Association of Cardiovascular and Pulmonary Rehabilitation, 1995, Human Kinetics, Champaign, with permission.

termine if more extensive cardiac evaluations are necessary, if cardiac rehabilitation, surgical, or other medical treatments are indicated, and the nature of the medical supervision to be provided for exercise training. In addition to assessing the patient's functional status and overall prognosis for a cardiac event, the objective of risk stratification identifies patients who need a formal, monitored exercise-based rehabilitation program. Risk stratification usually occurs before or soon after patient entry into the cardiac rehabilitation program.[2,26,32] Additional information on risk stratification will be discussed in Chapter 12 as it pertains to the exercise session, the degree of medical supervision, and the frequency of continuous ECG monitoring. The risk stratification of a patient is to be used as a guide in the medical management of the patient, including the nature and timing of the rehabilitation program.

Determination of Pulmonary Impairment

The status of a patient with pulmonary disease can be classified by the degree of impairment of the pulmonary system. Although the results of a physical examination determine the degree of dyspnea, frequency of cough, amount of sputum, number of pack-years in a smoker, findings on auscultation, results of chest x-rays, and extent of occupational exposure, the results of pulmonary function testing are the most important criteria for documenting the degree of pulmonary impairment. Table 11-2 presents the criteria developed by the Social Security Administration, the American Thoracic Society, and the American Medical Society.[33] In the 1995 statement by the American Thoracic Society, a staging of chronic obstructive pulmonary disease was proposed that included not only pulmonary function test results but also arterial blood gas values, the impact on quality of life, and the predicted amount of health care expenditure.[34] Table 11-3 presents this new staging of disability.

The degree of pulmonary impairment is used to alert the rehabilitation staff to the individual needs of a patient with pulmonary disease. For example, participants with mild pulmonary impairment may maintain their levels of oxygenation during exercise, whereas patients with a moderate or severe degree of impairment have been shown to decrease, increase, or maintain their oxygenation during exercise.[27] The amount of pulmonary impairment also is considered when prescribing exercise intensity.[35-37] (See the section on intensity of exercise in this chapter.)

TABLE 11-2 Pulmonary Function Test Criteria for the
Determination of Degree of Pulmonary Impairment*

Test	Normal (%)	Mildly Impaired (%)	Moderately Impaired (%)	Severely Impaired (%)
VC	80	60–79	51–59	50 or less
FEV_1	80	60–79	41–59	40 or less
FEV_1/FVC	75	60–74	41–59	40 or less
DLCO	80	60–79	41–59	40 or less

*Values reported are given in units of percent of predicted.
Source: Adapted from the American Thoracic Society,[33] with permission.

TABLE 11–3 Categorization of Patients with Chronic Obstructive
Pulmonary Disease Based on the American Thoracic Standards of
Definitions, Epidemiology, Pathophysiology Diagnosis, and Staging

	Stage I	Stage II	Stage III
Patients, n	Majority	Minority	Minority
FEV$_1$	>50% predicted	35 to 49% predicted	<35% predicted
ABG values	Not hypoxemic	ABG eval necessary	ABG eval necessary
Impact on quality of life	Minimal	Significant	Profound
Per capital health care $	Modest	Large	Large
Primary physician	Generalist	Specialist	Specialist

Source: Joughlin and Digenio,[39] with permission.

CARDIORESPIRATORY ENDURANCE

No single exercise can promote improvement in all factors identified as major contributors to functional capacity and physical fitness. A complete exercise prescription for the patient with cardiopulmonary disease, therefore, includes exercises to effect changes in all parameters. However, throughout this discussion the importance of one factor, cardiorespiratory endurance, is emphasized for the maintenance of health and the rehabilitation of individuals with cardiorespiratory disease. In writing an exercise prescription, no other component demands more specialized knowledge than cardiorespiratory endurance. The key purpose of the exercise prescription is to increase or maintain functional capacity.

Although health care providers are among those who strongly advocate exercise for health maintenance as well as for augmentation of their patients' rehabilitation or treatment, not all of them receive formal training in exercise physiology. Many are unfamiliar with cardiorespiratory training principles and methodologies. Therefore, exercise prescription tends to be rather vague and often "canned" (not individualized). As in all types of training, to be most effective, the cardiovascular exercise prescription must be specific about the intensity, duration, frequency, and mode of exercise performed and must be individualized for each patient.

Intensity of Exercise

There is an intensity or level of aerobic exercise that is necessary to improve cardiorespiratory endurance. Although intensity and duration are separate entities and will be discussed separately, it is difficult to discuss intensity without mentioning duration because of the interaction between the two. Prescribing exercise intensity for all adults—those who have cardiac or pulmonary problems or those who are apparently healthy—is the most challenging task in designing the exercise program because individualization and appropriate monitoring are required to ensure that the maximum prescribed intensity is not exceeded. The intensity of exercise is usually expressed in relative terms as a percent of functional capacity or a percentage of age-adjusted maximum heart rate (AAMHR).[28] By using the data derived from the laboratory and clinical assessment (see Chapter 9 and 10), the clinician can begin to formulate the exercise intensity portion of the rehabilitative exercise program. Table 11–4 outlines the data often used in developing the exercise prescription.

TABLE 11–4 Data Obtained from the Exercise Test to Be Used in
the Development of an Exercise Prescription

Subjective

  Angina pectoris
  Dyspnea
  Fatigue—weakness
  Leg discomfort
  Dizziness

Objective

  Physical examination
    Breath sounds
    Peripheral pulses
    Precordial examination for dyskinetic areas, murmurs, and gallops (before and after exercise)
    Blood pressure response
    Pulmonary function test results (before and after exercise)
    Heart rate response
    General appearance
    Oximetry/arterial blood gas results
  Physical performance
    Time on treadmill/cycle
    Maximum workload (watts, kg-m per minute, kp-m per minute)
    Rate of perceived exertion
    Rate pressure product (max HR × max systolic BP)
  Electrocardiogram
    Repolarization changes—ST segment and J point
    Rate response
    Dysrhythmias
    Conduction abnormalities—atrioventricular and ventricular
  Cardiorespiratory/metabolic measurements (limited availability)
    Anaerobic threshold (AT)
    Carbon dioxide output ($\dot{V}CO_2$)
    Gas exchange ratio (R)
    Minute ventilation ($\dot{V}E$)
    Oxygen uptake ($\dot{V}O_2$)
    Respiratory quotient (RQ)

Source: Adapted from Mikolich, JR and Fletcher, GF: The exercise prescription. In Fletcher, GF (ed): Exercise and the Practice of Medicine, ed 2. Futura Publishing Company, Mount Kisco, NY, 1988, p. 82, with permission.

Three techniques are commonly used to prescribe and monitor exercise intensity: heart rate, metabolic energy expenditure ($\dot{V}O_2$ or metabolic equivalents [METs]), and rating of perceived exertion (RPE).[2,5,6,9,11,19,28,38–42]

HEART RATE

During dynamic exercise involving large muscle groups, a relatively linear relationship exists between heart rate and oxygen uptake. There are several widely used methods for establishing target heart rate (THR) and target heart rate range (THRR) for apparently healthy adults, as well as for patients with cardiac and pulmonary disease.[28]

There are three commonly used methods for determining THR and THRR for the exercise prescription: (1) the heart rate reserve method or Karvonen formula; (2) percentage of maximal heart rate achieved on the GXT; and (3) resting heart rate plus 20 to 30 bpm.[2,5,28,40-44] A fourth method for establishing THRR and THR that will be briefly presented is to plot the relationship between heart rate (HR) and $\dot{V}O_2$.

The heart rate reserve, Karvonen formula,[43] is calculated by taking a percentage (usually 40 to 85 percent) of the difference between the resting heart rate (in the seated position) and the maximal achieved heart rate on a graded exercise test (GXT) and adding that value to the resting heart rate. Table 11–5 illustrates the calculation of the THRR using the Karvonen method.

The THRR is used to define safety guidelines for exercise intensity during the exercise session. Individuals with low levels of functional capacity should probably begin their exercise regimes at 40 to 50 percent of heart rate reserve.[28] To ensure a cardiorespiratory endurance training effect, the THR for a specific patient defines the most appropriate HR within the prescribed THRR. For most individuals, the training intensity would be approximately 60 percent of heart rate reserve.[41] For pulmonary patients with mild to moderate impairment, the recommended THR should be calculated by using a minimum of 50 to 60 percent of the maximum functional capacity.[45] Patients with moderate to severe pulmonary impairment reach their maximum voluntary ventilations (MVVs), equal to $\dot{V}Emax$, before the cardiovascular maximums are approached. For these patients, exercise intensities that approach their maximum ventilatory limits or the upper end of the THRR can be used. Fluctuations of approximately 10 percent normally occur in a patient's exercise HR during a single exercise session.

A second method to calculate THRR is to use a fixed percentage of the maximum heart rate (MHR) attained on the GXT. Generally the percentage used to calculate the THR is between 55 and 90 percent.[2,28] This method to determine THRR is easier to calculate than the Karvonen method and a number of clinicians prefer its use. It has been reported that a THR of 75 percent MHR correlates with the heart rate at ventilatory (anaerobic) threshold (VT) and, in absence of direct measurement of VT, can be used as a guide to determine THR in patients with cardiac disease.[39] Cardiac rehabilitation programs using the percentage of MHR attained on the GXT for determining exercise intensity have been reported to use an average of 65 percent.[42] In cases in which patients enter rehabilitation with a symptom-limited GXT (SL-GXT), the HR at which the SL-GXT was terminated becomes the "maximum" HR for that subject. The maximum

TABLE 11–5 Heart Rate Reserve or
Karvonen[43] Method for Determining Target
Heart Rate Range

Given:	Lower Limit	Upper Limit
Maximum HR	140	140
Resting HR	−70	−70
Heart rate reserve	70	70
Desired intensity	×.40	×.85
(40–85% HR range)	—	—
	28	59.5
Add resting HR	+70	+70.0
Target HR range	98	129 beat/min

HR attained on the SL-GXT is then used in formulas for calculation of THR and THRR. If no SL-GXT or GXT has been given, the age-adjusted maximum heart rate (AAMHR) may be used in the formulas for calculating THR and THRR. The AAMHR may be estimated by simply subtracting the patient's age from 220. The major problems with estimating HRmax arise from individual differences and medications that may alter expected resting and maximum heart rates.

The third method commonly used to establish the exercise training THR is to simply take the patient's resting heart rate and add 20 to 30 bpm to that value. This is the simplest of the three methods that have been presented and is often used when no GXT or SL-GXT has been performed and the patient has been referred for cardiac rehabilitation.[42]

A fourth method used to establish patient THRs and THRRs is to plot the heart rate against measured $\dot{V}O_2$max. Because this method requires an accurate measurement of $\dot{V}O_2$max, it is not practical to use in situations where direct measurements of $\dot{V}O_2$max are not obtained. Estimations of $\dot{V}O_2$max can be obtained from maximal MET levels achieved on a GXT or an SL-GXT. THRRs by this method are usually calculated between 50 and 85 percent of $\dot{V}O_2$max achieved or estimated.[2,28]

METABOLIC ENERGY EXPENDITURE

Some clinicians prefer to prescribe exercise intensity by using activities that require a percent of maximal METs achieved during the evaluation process. Usually the activities chosen for prescription by this method correspond to 40 to 85 percent of maximal METs achieved during evaluation.[46,47] Table 11–6 provides a list of activities and their average exercise intensities in METs.

As with any method of exercise prescription, in the beginning phases of rehabilitation, the exercise intensity should be prescribed at the lower end of the target range, in this case, near 40 percent of maximal METs. It is a prudent practice, when prescribing exercise by METs, to also monitor HRs by telemetry (in early rehabilitation) and/or palpation (in later stages) of rehabilitation. Adding HR monitoring to prescriptions by METs ensures that maximal safe exercise will not be exceeded, especially in situations that naturally cause increases in HRs (e.g., hot, humid environment) and in the rate-pressure product (RPP) (see Chapter 9).

The prescription of exercise intensity in METs should be adjusted as cardiorespiratory endurance increases, but the THRR should remain relatively the same. As training adaptation occurs, increases in workload will be necessary to maintain the workload at the prescribed MET level, even though the THRR will not change appreciably.

RATING OF PERCEIVED EXERTION

As patients become familiar with the "feeling" associated with exercise at the appropriate target level, the need for an objective measurement (e.g., monitoring HR) decreases. At that point the "perceived exertion" provides a subjective means of monitoring exercise intensity.[48] Borg's Rating of Perceived Exertion (RPE) Scale[49,50] (Table 11–7) is used by the patient with cardiac disease to rate the intensity of an exercise activity. A rating of 12 to 13 (somewhat hard) on the 20-point scale corresponds to approximately 60 percent of the HR range, whereas a rating of 16 (hard) corresponds to 85 percent. If the 10-point scale were used, these ratings would be between 4 and 6.[51] Adding a zero to each number of the 20-point scale indicates at what heart rate the pa-

TABLE 11–6 Cardiorespiratory–Endurance–Promoting Potential of Various Activities

Intensity (70-kg Person)	Endurance-Promoting	Occupational	Recreational
1½–2 METs 4–7 mL/kg/min 2–2½ kcal/min	Too low in energy level	Desk work, driving auto, electric calculating machine operation, light housework, polishing furniture, washing clothes	Standing, strolling (1 mph), flying, motorcycling, playing cards, sewing, knitting
2–3 METs 7–11 mL/kg/min 2½–4 kcal/min	Too low in energy level unless capacity is very low	Auto repair, radio and television repair, janitorial work, bartending, riding lawnmower, light woodworking	Level walking (2 mph), level bicycling (5 mph), billiards, bowling, skeet shooting, shuffleboard, powerboat driving, golfing with power cart, canoeing, horseback riding at a walk
3–4 METs 11–14 mL/kg/min 4–5 kcal/min	Yes, if continuous and if target heart rate is reached	Bricklaying, plastering, pushing wheelbarrow (100-lb load), machine assembly, welding (moderate load), cleaning windows, mopping floors, vacuuming, pushing light power mower	Walking (3 mph), bicycling (6 mph), horseshoe pitching, volleyball (6-person, noncompetitive), golfing (pulling bag cart), archery, sailing, (handling) small boat, fly fishing (standing in waders), horseback riding (trotting), badminton (social doubles)
4–5 METs 14–18 mL/kg/min	Recreational activities promote endurance. Occupational activities must be continuous, lasting longer than 2 min	Painting, masonry, paperhanging, light carpentry, scrubbing floors, raking leaves, hoeing	Walking (3½ mph), bicycling (8 mph), table tennis, golfing (carrying clubs), dancing (foxtrot), badminton (singles), tennis (doubles), many calisthenics, ballet
5–6 METs 18–21 mL/kg/min	Yes	Digging garden, shoveling light earth	Walking (4 mph), bicycling (10 mph), canoeing (4 mph), horseback riding (posting to trotting), stream fishing (walking in light current in waders), ice or roller skating (9 mph)
6–7 METs 21–25 mL/kg/min 7–8 kcal/min	Yes	Shoveling 10 times/min (4½ kg or 10 lb), splitting wood, snow shoveling, hand lawnmowing	Walking (5 mph), bicycling (11 mph), competitive badminton, tennis (singles), folk and square dancing, light downhill skiing, ski touring (2½ mph), water skiing, swimming (20 yards/min)

Continued

317

TABLE 11–6 Cardiorespiratory–Endurance–Promoting Potential of Various Activities (*Continued*)

Intensity (70-kg Person)	Endurance-Promoting	Occupational	Recreational
7–8 METs 25–28 mL/kg/min 8–10 kcal/min	Yes	Digging ditches, carrying 36 kg or 80 lb, sawing hardwood	Jogging (5 mph), bicycling (12 mph), horseback riding (gallop), vigorous downhill skiing, basketball, mountain climbing, ice hockey, canoeing (5 mph), touch football, paddleball
8–9 METs 28–32 mL/kg/min 10–11 kcal/min	Yes	Shoveling 10 times/min (5½ kg or 14 lb)	Running (5½ mph), bicycling (13 mph), ski touring (4 mph), squash (social), handball (social), fencing, basketball (vigorous), swimming (30 yards/min), rope skipping
10+ METs 32+ mL/kg/min 11+ kcal/min	Yes	Shoveling 10 times/min (7½ kg or 16 lb)	Running (6 mph = 10 METs, 7 mph = 11½ METs, 8 mph = 13½ METs, 9 mph = 15 METs, 10 mph = 17 METs), ski touring (5 mph), handball (competitive), squash (competitive), swimming (greater than 40 yards/min)

Source: Fox, SM, Naughton, JP, and Gorman, PA: Physical activity and cardiovascular health. Part 3. The exercise prescription: Frequency and type of activity. Modern Concepts in Cardiovascular Disease 41:25–30, 1972, pp 26–27, by permission of the American Heart Association.

TABLE 11-7 Borg's Rating of Perceived
Exertion Scale and the Revised 10-Grade Scale

20-Point RPE	10-Point Rating Scale
6	0 Nothing at all
7 Very, very light	0.5 Very, very weak (just noticeable)
8	1 Very weak
9 Very light	2 Weak (light)
10	3 Moderate
11 Fairly light	4 Somewhat strong
12	5 Strong (heavy)
13 Somewhat hard	6
14	7 Very strong
15 Hard	8
16	9
17 Very hard	10 Very, very strong (almost maximum)
18	
19 Very, very hard	Maximal

Source: Adapted from Borg, GV. Psychophysical bases of perceived exertion. Med Sci Sports Exerc 14:377–387, 1982, © by the American College of Sports Medicine, with permission.

tient is performing the exercise. For example, the Borg rating of 13 has been reported to correspond to a heart rate of 130 bpm.[2] Borg's RPE scale may be particularly useful when evaluating patients on beta-blocking or some calcium channel blocking medications and when supervising patients in atrial fibrillation. It is also a useful adjunct to the GXT and provides valuable information as to how the patient is tolerating the exercise test. It provides information during the exercise session that the clinician can use to evaluate and alter, if necessary, the exercise prescription.

Patients with pulmonary disease can use a similar scale by rating their perceived shortness of breath (Table 11-8). Because such patients often have poor ventilatory reserves but adequate HR reserves, the use of a scale or perceived shortness of breath becomes helpful for monitoring exercise intensity by subjective means. Ratings of between 4 and 6—mildly short of breath to moderately short of breath—define the

TABLE 11-8 Subjective Definitions for a 10-Point
Perceived Shortness of Breath Scale

Rate of Perceived Exertion/Shortness of Breath	
1 Rest	Not short of breath
2 Minimal activity	Minimally short of breath
3 Very light activity	Slightly short of breath
4 Light activity	Mildly short of breath
5 Somewhat hard activity	Mildly to moderately short of breath
6 Hard activity	Moderately short of breath
7	Moderately to severely short of breath
8 Very hard activity	Severely short of breath
9	Breathing is not in control
10 Very, very hard activity	Maximally short of breath

Source: Adapted from Pulmonary Rehabilitation Program, Massachusetts Respiratory Hospital, Braintree, MA.

range in which patients generally work. Patients with pulmonary disease do not tend to deny their shortness of breath as patients with cardiac disease may deny perceived exertion. These patients, being aware of their inability to recover rapidly from shortness of breath, tend to exaggerate their perception of shortness of breath so as not to exceed their abilities. With training, a patient's perception of shortness of breath may change because of an increase in physiologic training, an increase in motivation to exercise, and/or a desensitization to dyspnea. As those changes in training occur, exercise progression requires higher workloads to achieve the same RPE rating.

For the patient with pulmonary disease, exercise targets and exercise progression during training should be based on symptoms of shortness of breath and fatigue more than on HRs or fixed work levels.[27,52,53] Clinicians usually prefer to prescribe exercise for patients with both cardiac and pulmonary disease by using a combination of prescription by HR and the RPE or shortness of breath. When prescribing exercise, the therapist should express the desired intensity as a range because during exercise the patient usually shows fluctuations from prescribed THRs or METs of about 10 percent. It should also be emphasized that maximum aerobic capacity can be increased by either increasing the intensity of the activity or extending the duration of the exercise session. For persons with low functional capacities, extending the duration of the exercise session at a low intensity over a period of weeks is safer than increasing the intensity of the activity.[5]

ADDITIONAL CONSIDERATIONS

Additional considerations in prescribing the intensity of exercise should include such factors as age, gender, blood pressure response, and orthopedic limitations. Those factors are discussed in Chapters 4 and 12. Table 11–9 summarizes the relationships among the various methods used to prescribe exercise intensity.

Duration of Exercise

Each cardiorespiratory (CR) session should consist of a 10- to 15-minute warm-up period, a CR training period of 20 to 60 minutes of aerobic activity, and a 5- to 15-

TABLE 11–9 Classification of Intensity of Exercise
Based on 30 to 60 Minutes of Endurance Training

Relative Intensity			
HRmax (%)	$\dot{V}o_2$ max or HRmax reserve (%)	RPE (20–point scale)	Intensity
35	30	10	Very light
35–59	30–49	10–11	Light
60–79	50–74	12–13	Moderate
80–89	75–84	14–16	Heavy
90	85	16	Very heavy

HRmax, maximum heart rate; $\dot{V}o_2$ max, maximum oxygen uptake; RPE, rate of perceived exertion.
Source: From Pollock and Wilmore,[54] p. 105, with permission.

minute cool-down period. During the 20 to 60 minutes of CR exercise, the HR should be maintained, as nearly as possible, at the target level and within the THRR.[2,28]

In the initial stages of cardiac rehabilitation, the duration of the CR exercise session is more likely to be 15 to 20 minutes in length. Some patients will not be able to perform 15 to 20 minutes of CR activity and will need to have shorter, more frequent exercise sessions. As each individual progresses, the length of the CR session can gradually increase until the desired goal for each patient is attained. Generally, no increase in intensity of CR activity is recommended until the patient can perform 20 to 30 minutes of continuous aerobic exercise.[28] Because there is a relationship between the intensity and the duration of activity, and CR improvement is dependent on the total energy expended during any single bout of activity, current policy is to prescribe CR exercise at moderate levels (lower intensities—longer duration) rather that at more intense levels (higher intensities—shorter duration). This moderate approach to exercise prescription for the cardiac patient reduces musculoskeletal injury and decreases cardiac risk.[28,55] As the functional capacity of the patient improves, the exercise prescription should be adjusted accordingly. Functional capacity is improved by increasing the intensity and/or duration of the CR activity. The average duration for the exercise session has been reported to be approximately 45 minutes.[42]

The length of time the patient remains in Phases II and III cardiac rehabilitation depends on such factors as reimbursement, risk stratification, individual achievement of goals, and a number of other considerations. The current average duration for outpatient cardiac programs that do not risk-stratify their patients is 12 weeks.[42] In programs that risk-stratify their patients, low-risk patients were reported to be in the cardiac rehabilitation program from approximately 2 to 9 weeks; intermediate-risk patients for 4 to 12 weeks; and high-risk patients continued in outpatient cardiac rehabilitation for an average of 7 to 13 weeks. The average duration of the cardiac rehabilitation program for each category was 5.6 weeks for low-risk patients, 7.8 weeks for intermediate-risk patients, and 10 weeks for high-risk patients.[42]

It is difficult to predict the length of time a patient will remain in the Phase II and Phase III outpatient programs. Patients should be progressed to Phase III only when they are determined to be clinically stable, can demonstrate independence in performing self-monitoring techniques (especially during their physical activities), and no longer require intensive ECG monitoring.[19,56]

Frequency of Exercise

Frequency of exercise refers to the number of exercise sessions in which a patient engages per day and/or per week. Depending on individual functional capacities, frequency of CR exercise may vary from several short exercise sessions per day to three to five bouts per week. In patients whose functional capacities are less than 3 METs, short sessions of 5 minutes (more or less) performed several times a day may be prescribed. Generally, patients with functional capacities greater than 5 METs should exercise three to five times per week.[2,28]

Exercise Prescription Progression

The rate of progressing patients from light CR activities (lower functional capacities) to more difficult CR activities (requiring higher functional capacities) usually involves three stages: (1) the initial conditioning stage, (2) the improvement stage, and (3) the maintenance stage.[28] Of course, rate of exercise progression depends on such factors as age, functional capacity, health status, compliance, and various individual needs and considerations. During the various stages of progression and conditioning, patient goals and expected outcomes should be established by the patient and the exercise clinician.

INITIAL CONDITIONING STAGE

One goal that is especially important in the early stages of initial conditioning is to ensure that each exercise session is undertaken at low levels of intensity and duration. Taking this approach will help to avoid muscle soreness and musculoskeletal or other injury that is likely to result if the exercise sessions are undertaken at higher levels of intensity and/or duration. During the first few weeks of the initial conditioning stage, HRs should be monitored frequently so that patients exercise fairly close to their THRs (which should be prescribed at the lower end of their THRRs). Whether patients need to exercise by interspersing activity of short duration with periods of rest will depend on individual needs and abilities, but the duration of the total activity performed usually lasts 12 to 15 minutes, gradually progressing to 20 minutes.[28] The role of the clinician in prescribing activity for patients at the appropriate intensity and duration is extremely important because the clinician must be able to adjust the exercise prescription to meet individual needs. Although there is considerable variation among patients, usually the initial conditioning stage lasts from 4 to 6 weeks.[28]

During the first week of pulmonary rehabilitation, this initial phase is used to ensure safety with exercise and to train the patient to achieve the appropriate intensity of exercise. This time also teaches the patient to tolerate the sensation of breathlessness with exercise.[57] Because dyspnea has always been the point at which patients cease activity, teaching patients to maintain a level of activity while being short of breath requires time.

IMPROVEMENT STAGE

The improvement stage may last from 4 to 5 months.[28] It is during this stage that the intensity and duration of the exercise sessions are gradually increased so that the patient is exercising within the THRR and within his or her functional capacities (40 to 85 percent of $\dot{V}o_2$ max.) Durations of aerobic activity also are gradually increased (every 2 or 3 weeks) so that patients are exercising for at least 20 to 30 minutes per exercise session as the end of the improvement stage approaches. It is especially important for older patients and/or those with disease to begin this stage with intermittent activity (if necessary) and progress gradually to activity that is continuous. The duration of the exercise session should be increased before the intensity is increased, but, where feasible, the patient should attempt to exercise in the upper portion of the THRR.[28]

MAINTENANCE STAGE

Most patients require approximately 6 months of exercise training to reach the maintenance stage of conditioning. Usually this stage involves continuing the exercise routine that was acquired at the end of the improvement stage. To maintain fitness levels, the exercise sessions must be continued on a regular basis.

Mode of Aerobic Exercise

The rules of specificity of training apply to CR endurance, and the clinician must prescribe the activities that are most useful in improving functional capacity. Generally, any physical activity that is rhythmic, can be sustained for prolonged periods of time, and uses large muscle groups can be classified as an aerobic activity. High-impact activities (e.g., running and jumping) are not generally recommended for promoting CR endurance because of the increased risk of injury inherent in their use. Low-impact and/or non-weight-bearing activities have a lower incidence of injury and are generally recommended for cardiopulmonary patients.

Because it is necessary to maintain an appropriate intensity of exercise, activities that are particularly useful for improving functional capacity include walking, jogging (perhaps), riding stationary bicycles, and arm-leg cycle ergometers.[2,28] With patients using the arm cycle ergometer, the THR should be approximately 10 bpm lower than THR calculated from GXT data.[2]

One meta-analysis of several studies[58] investigated the roles that intensity, duration, frequency, and mode of activity play in improving functional capacity through central and peripheral physiologic changes. The data indicated that the intensity of the exercise prescription was more important than duration, frequency, or mode in eliciting positive central adaptations, provided the exercise was performed at an intensity of at least 80 percent of $\dot{V}O_2$max. Peripheral adaptations to aerobic training appeared to be a more significant factor in improving functional capacity when the exercise was performed at an intensity below 80 percent of $\dot{V}O_2$max. For most cardiopulmonary patients, exercising at a functional capacity of 80 percent of $\dot{V}O_2$max is unrealistic and unsafe and should be prescribed with caution. No doubt the future will provide more study of the relationships of intensity, frequency, duration, and mode of aerobic activity as they apply to improving functional capacity.[58]

Although the majority of cardiopulmonary rehabilitation programs use lower-extremity exercise as the mainstay, there is growing evidence that upper-extremity exercise is useful, especially in the patient with pulmonary disease. Many patients with COPD have a very limited endurance for arm exercise.[59] It is not surprising, then, that patients with COPD report dyspnea induced by upper-extremity activity. Activities that require the arms to be unsupported or overhead, such as many activities of daily living, are the most difficult to accomplish.[60,61] Patients with pulmonary disease tolerate upper-extremity exercise quite poorly, perhaps because these muscles are being used as accessory muscles for respiration.[62] Upper-extremity exercise training has been shown to reduce ventilatory demand in patients with COPD.[63] Because of specificity of training, an increase in upper extremity endurance does not necessarily translate into a decrease in dyspnea during activities of daily living.[64] The mode of exercise chosen should be compatible with the desired outcome.

Body Composition

Various factors have important roles in the development of obesity or overweight. Genetic, hormonal, metabolic, and behavioral variables contribute to the development of obesity, but the main reason for increased body fat in individuals is believed to be an imbalance between energy input (caloric intake) and energy output (energy expenditure). Recent evidence, however, indicates that obesity and overweight may not result from overeating but from eating a diet with a high fat-to-carbohydrate ratio and sedentary lifestyles.[65-70] Recent research also indicates that fat deposited primarily in the trunk and abdominal area (central obesity, see Chapter 9) seems to be associated with a higher risk for the development of hypertension, diabetes, and CAD.[28]

Although considerable variations exist among individuals in their responses to weight loss regimens and body composition changes, generally programs developed for managing body weight should include some type of CR endurance training. The benefits of CR endurance training in helping to control body weight include increased caloric expenditure, a decrease in body fat, and a possible increase in lean body weight. To be effective in helping control excess body fat, the CR activity should use a minimum of 300 kcal per exercise session for a minimum of three times per week or 200 kcal per exercise session performed for a minimum of four times per week.[28] The following formula (based on the MET level of the activity) has been devised to assist the clinician with estimating the caloric expenditure during an exercise session.[28]

$$\text{METs} \times 3.5 \times \text{body weight in kg}/200 = \text{kcal/min}$$

Using CR exercise in combination with reduction of daily caloric intake should provide a weekly maximum weight loss of approximately 1 kg (2.2 lb). Additional guidelines that have been reported to be effective and should be considered in providing diet therapy for overweight patients include:[66-72]

1. Generally, do not restrict caloric intake to less than 1200 kcal per day.
2. Provide an exercise regime that provides an expenditure of approximately 300 kcal per session.
3. Allow for a gradual weight loss of approximately 1 kg (2.2 lb) per week.
4. Gradually reduce the amount of fat and increase the amount of complex carbohydrates and fiber consumed.
5. Include behavioral techniques to help manage eating and exercise behaviors.
6. Include participation in peer and social support groups.
7. Include regular counseling during the rehabilitation program as well as regular follow-up contact.

Patients with pulmonary disease may present with an ideal body weight, overweight, or more frequently, underweight. The incidence of malnutrition varies with the severity of the disease and between 40 and 50 percent of all hospitalized patients with COPD have been reported to be malnourished.[73] Malnutrition promotes muscle wasting, which also affects the respiratory muscles. Anthropometric measurement, rather than total body weight, can be used to estimate lean body mass and ensure that appropriate nutritional intervention is provided. Improved nutritional status should help to improve the patient's state of health, respiratory muscle function, and overall sense of well-being.[74]

Muscular Strength and Endurance

Two components of total physical fitness—muscular strength and muscular endurance—are usually discussed together because the acquisition of one (strength) usually causes improvement in the other (endurance), and vice versa. Both are acquired through adhering to the overload principle, which, simply stated, means that, to improve, an individual must increase the intensity, duration, and perhaps the frequency of the activity. If the goal is to maximize strength gains, an individual must increase the resistance (intensity) and decrease the number of repetitions (frequency) per exercise bout. Maximal gains in muscular endurance are acquired through an increase in repetitions and a decrease in resistance.[75]

A second principle that is important in the acquisition of strength and/or endurance is that of specificity of training: strength and/or endurance improvement is gained only in the muscle groups actively involved in the resistance training. Effects of training (improvement) are also specific to the range of motion through which the resistance is moved or lifted. For best results, the resistance activity should be performed through the full range of motion.[75]

Until recently, the feasibility of including resistance training in cardiopulmonary rehabilitation was controversial. Currently, research indicates that resistance training can be safe for selected cardiopulmonary patients, especially when the activity is of low intensity, is progressed fairly slowly, and is properly monitored.[76,77]

It is recommended that most patients do not begin a resistance training program until they have participated in a CR exercise program for at least 4 to 6 weeks.[26] Additional criteria to be used for patient entrance into a resistance training program include functional capacity of at least 5 to 6 METs, no evidence of ischemic ECG changes during the GXT, fairly normal blood pressure responses to activity, and absence of uncontrolled arrhythmias. Patients with unstable angina, uncontrolled hypertension, congestive heart failure (CHF), poor left ventricular function (LVF), uncontrolled arrhythmias, or severe valvular disease are usually excluded from resistance training.[2,75,77,78]

The rehabilitation clinicians must supervise patients involved in the resistance training program. Heart rates and blood pressures must be monitored and evidence of patient activity evoking the Valsalva maneuver (straining to lift a weight) should be avoided.[2,75,79] Patients who have had recent surgery should not engage in activities that cause pressure on the sternum.[2]

To initiate a resistance training program that will result in positive changes in patient strength and endurance, and for patient outcome assessment, several methods have been used for baseline evaluation of strength:

1. One repetition maximum (1-RM)—the amount of weight that can be lifted through the full range of motion once without holding the breath
2. 90 percent of 1-RM—the amount of weight that can be lifted through the full range of motion 2 or 3 times without holding the breath
3. Isokinetic testing—determining muscular strength at varying rates of muscular contraction.[77,79]

Because greater hemodynamic responses are seen when patients perform resistance training close to 1-RM, rather than assessing patients for initial strength performance, some clinicians prefer to start the patient at a very low resistance and increase the weight as tolerated.[77,79] Once the initial baseline for strength has been established, the resistance program should include from 8 to 10 exercises involving large muscle groups in the upper and lower body. Although performing resistance exercises for 8 to 15 repetitions at 40, 60, and 80 percent of 1-RM has been reported to be safe for patients with cardiac disease, greater hemodynamic responses were found to occur as the resistance increased. Rate pressure products (RPP—Chapter 9) were found to increase significantly at 60 to 80 percent compared with resistance training at 40 percent of 1-RM.[79] It appears that performance of 12 to 15 repetitions of 40 percent of 1-RM using 8 to 10 different exercises is safe for most patients with cardiac disease and it is recommended that resistance training be individualized for each patient and should not exceed 85 percent of 1-RM.[79] A minimum of one set of 12 to 15 repetitions for each exercise is recommended, to be completed 2 or 3 times a week.[2,79] The intensity of each activity may be gradually increased when the patient can lift the resistance 12 to 15 times with undue stress.[2] Table 11–10 presents the resistance training guidelines recommended for patients with cardiac disease who are candidates for a resistance training program.

Flexibility

Flexibility, or range of motion in a joint, is necessary for normal bodily movement. This component of total physical fitness is important to include in the rehabilitative

TABLE 11–10 **Weight Training Guidelines for Low-Risk Cardiac Patients**

- To prevent soreness and injury, initially choose a weight that will allow the performance of 12 to 15 repetitions comfortably, corresponding to approximately 30%–50% of the maximum weight load that can be lifted in one repetition. (Note: Selected stable, aerobically trained cardiac patients may eventually use loads corresponding to a more traditional program of weight training [i.e., 60%–80% of 1 RM])
- Perform one to three sets of each exercise.
- Avoid straining. Ratings of perceived exertion (6–20 scale) should not exceed fairly light to somewhat hard during lifting.
- Exhale (blow out) during the exertion phase of the lift. For example, exhale when pushing a weight stack overhead and inhale when lowering it.
- Increase weight loads by 5 to 10 lb when 12 to 15 repetitions can be comfortably accomplished.
- Raise weights with slow, controlled movements; emphasize complete extension of the limbs when lifting.
- Exercise large muscle groups before small muscle groups. Include devices (exercises) for the upper and lower extremities.
- Weight-train at least two to three times per week.
- Loosely hold hand grips when possible; sustained, tight gripping may evoke an excessive blood pressure response to lifting.
- Stop exercise in the event of warning signs or symptoms, especially dizziness, arrhythmias, unusual shortness of breath, and/or angina pectoris.
- Allow minimal rest periods between exercises (e.g., 30–60 sec) to maximize muscular endurance and aerobic training benefits.

Source: From *Guidelines for Cardiac Rehabilitation Programs* (p. 11) by American Association of Cardiovascular and Pulmonary Rehabilitation, 1991, Champaign, IL: Human Kinetics. Copyright 1991 by American Association of Cardiovascular and Pulmonary Rehabilitation. Reprinted by permission.

process, especially for the older adult who may lack flexibility and consequently may have difficulty in performing activities of daily living. When including flexibility exercises in the rehabilitation program, particular attention should be given to the range of motion in the lower back and posterior thigh, since "stiffness" in that region is often associated with chronic low back pain. Flexibility activities should also be prescribed for the upper and lower trunk, neck, hips, and muscles in the lower legs.[28] Examples of flexibility activities are given in Appendix E.

Stretching activities are usually performed as part of the warm-up preceding aerobic activity as well as during the cool-down following its completion. Flexibility exercises should be performed slowly and progression to greater ranges of motion should be gradual. Generally, the recommended procedure to follow in prescribing flexibility exercise is to perform a slow controlled movement followed by a static stretch that is "held" for 10 to 30 seconds. Each flexibility activity should be repeated three to five times, and the flexibility regime should be performed at least three times per week. During the execution of the flexibility exercises, the range of motion should not be so great as to cause pain.[28,80,81]

EXERCISE AND OXYGEN THERAPY

Supplemental oxygen improves the mortality and morbidity in hypoxemic patients with COPD.[82] The physiologic goals of oxygen therapy are to reverse or prevent tissue hypoxia. The long-term benefits of supplemental oxygen for patients who are hypoxemic only during exercise remains unknown because there have not been any reports that hypoxemia only during exercise causes any long-term ill effects.[34] Therefore the rationale for using supplemental oxygen during exercise sessions would be to prevent the immediate effects of hypoxemia, for example cardiac ischemia or rhythm disturbances,[83] or dyspnea,[84] and to increase exercise tolerance.[85] Nixon and co-workers[86] reported that supplemental oxygen minimized oxygen desaturation during the exercise session and enabled patients to exercise with a lower ventilatory and cardiovascular demand. Other authors also have reported an increase in exercise tolerance with the use of supplemental oxygen.[85,87,88]

Supplemental oxygen to decrease arterial hypoxemia during exercise becomes warranted when the SaO_2 dips below 88 percent saturation, PaO_2 dips below 55 mm Hg, or the PaO_2 drops more than 20 mm Hg during exercise.[27,34] Arterial blood gases should be monitored during the graded exercise test to document changes in PaO_2 during exercise (see Chapter 10). Pulse oximetry can evaluate a patient's arterial oxygen saturation during an exercise test or during the session, since it is a noninvasive procedure.

Supplemental oxygen is prescribed by the attending physician. Oxygen therapy should be based on the patient's diagnosis, age, amount of hypoxemia during different living conditions; at rest, during exercise, and during sleep.[34] A usual prescription may include a variety of liter flow rates according to the patient's activity level. Oxygen flow rate during exercise, when minute ventilation is higher than at rest, may have to be increased to provide an FiO_2 that will maintain the PaO_2 above 55 mm Hg or the SaO_2 above 85 percent.[34,82,89] Flow rates may have to be readjusted when the patient is at rest or sleeping.[82] The necessary liter flow may dictate the probability of the oxygen source.

Supplemental oxygen can be provided in a variety of ways. The most common device used during rehabilitation sessions is the nasal cannula, using either liquid O_2 or compressed gas in a portable canister. More recent advances in oxygen delivery are transtracheal O_2, reservoir cannulas, and inspiratory phased oxygen delivery (Oxymizer). Because none of the oxygen is "wasted" when these latter methods of oxygen delivery are used, lower liter flows and therefore longer durations from the portable oxygen source are possible.[90]

By transtracheal administration, oxygen is delivered directly into the trachea through an opening in the neck. The method has been shown to use only 50 percent as much oxygen as the nasal cannula delivery system.[91] Other benefits from transtracheal oxygen are improved cosmesis, increased comfort, and improved compliance.[92] There are also disadvantages to the use of transtracheal oxygen that must be considered. Surgical emphysema, catheter fracture, local infection, catheter dislodgement, and mucus plugging have been reported.[91,93] Exercise studies using transtracheal oxygen demonstrate that exercise performance is enhanced with his method of oxygen delivery as compared with more traditional methods, although the mechanisms for the improvement are not readily apparent.[94]

Reservoir cannulas store oxygen in a collecting chamber within the nasal cannula tubing or in the transtracheal oxygen pendent. During inhalation, the breath is drawn from this chamber, or reservoir, of oxygen. During exhalation, the chamber refills. The reservoir cannulas have been shown to be 2 to 4 times more efficient in the use of oxygen than continuous flow methods.[95] The reservoir is larger than the continuous flow cannula, making the disadvantage of cosmesis a consideration for some patients.

Inspiratory phased delivery of oxygen, or demand oxygen delivery system (DODS), uses a reservoir attached to the apparatus of oxygen delivery. Inhalation removes oxygen from the reservoir during high inspiratory flow rates, as in early inspiration, but not during expiration. This method of oxygen delivery is more efficient than the nasal cannula delivery system: less oxygen is wasted.[90] It has been reported that DODS during exercise used only one-seventh the amount of oxygen as compared with the more traditional oxygen delivery system.[96]

FORMULATING THE EXERCISE PRESCRIPTION (CASE STUDIES)*

The information presented in this chapter should provide guidelines for writing exercise prescriptions for cardiopulmonary patients with cardiopulmonary disease. Tables 11–11 to 11–20 illustrate the use of intensity, duration, frequency, and mode of activity as they apply to the prescription of comprehensive programs for rehabilitating cardiopulmonary patients. The examples presented integrate the information obtained from the assessment (Chapter 9 and 10), and case studies 1, 5, 7, and 8 from Chapter 9 have been included to show exercise prescriptions for four patients with cardiovascular disease. Case studies 1, 2, 3, and 4 from Chapter 10 have been included to illustrate prescriptions for the pulmonary patient. The exercise prescriptions presented in Table 11–11 to 11–15 and 11–16 to 11–20 are the initial exercise prescriptions that were written after the assessment and before initiating exercise therapy. Progressions and exercise prescription adjustments will be presented in Chapter 12.

Text continued on page 339.

---

*Case studies 11–1 through 11–15 are courtesy of Bio-Energetiks Rehabilitation, Prospect, Pa.

**TABLE 11–11 Sample Exercise Prescription Form
for the Cardiac Patient**

Name _____ F   M   Age ____   Date _____

Ht (in) _____   Wt. (lb) _____

Dx: _____

Meds: _____

Comments: _____

GXT Data: Date Performed _/_/_   Where _____

Rest HR _____   Protocol _____

Max HR _____   Max METs _____

Max BP _____   RPE (10-Pt. Scale) _____

Re-evaluation scheduled _/_/_

C-R Rx:

Functional Capacity (METs) = 40% to 85% of Max METs

= .40 to .85 × _____

THRR (Heart Rate Reserve) bpm = (Max HR − Rest HR)(40% to 85%) + (Rest HR)

= (_____ − _____)(40% to 85%) + (_____)

= _____ bpm

Mode of Exercise _____ Bike _____ Row _____ Walk _____ Walk/Jog

Length of session: _____ Frequency: _____

Comments: _____

_____

_____

Flexibility Rx: _____

_____

Muscular S & End Rx: _____

_____

% Body Fat   Desirable M <20 %

                              F <30 %

Body Wt _____ lb   Body Mass Index (BMI) _____

_____ kg   Desirable BMI M & F   20–24.9

TABLE 11–12 Exercise Prescription for Case Study 1, Chapter 9

Name   Case Study 1   (F)   M   Age   57   Date _____

Ht (in)   59   Wt. (lb)   149.5

Dx: CAD, CABG, Angina

Meds: Persantine, Synthroid

Comments: ST-T sagging—2 mm at Max HR GXT & Dyspnea, Fatigue

GXT Data: Date Performed   3/19/96   Where   X Clinic

     Rest HR   65   Protocol   Adapted Bruce TM

     Max HR   118   Max METs   7

     Max BP   168/86   RPE (10-Pt. Scale)   7

     Re-evaluation scheduled   6/25/96

C-R Rx:

   Functional Capacity (METs) = 40% to 85% of Max METs

$$= .40 \text{ to } .85 \times \underline{\quad 7 \quad}$$

$$= 2.8 \text{ to } \sim 6 \text{ METS}$$

   THRR (Heart Rate Reserve) bpm = (Max HR − Rest HR)(40% to 85%) + (Rest HR)

$$= (\quad 118 \quad - \quad 65 \quad)(.40 \text{ to } .85) + (\quad 65 \quad)$$

$$= \sim 86 \text{ bpm to } 110 \text{ bpm}$$

   Mode of Exercise   X   Bike   Row   X   Walk   Walk/Jog

   Length of session: 20–30 min.   Frequency: 2–3/wk

Comments: Initial HR determined from lower end of HRR = ~86 bpm

RPP = 198

Flexibility Rx: Begin with flex for calf, hamstring, quads, hip flexors. Hold 10 sec, progress to 30 sec. Add shoulder, trunk, neck and back exercise. 3 ×s/wk prior to Ex. 1 ×/day at home.

Muscular S & End Rx: N/A. Begin when patient able

% Body Fat   32%   Desirable M   <20   %

                                    F   <30   %

Body Wt   149.5   lb   Body Mass Index (BMI)   30.063

         68   kg   Desirable BMI M & F   20–24.9

Referred also for nutrition education and weight reduction. Although classified as Intermediate risk, suggest continuously monitoring at first, followed by intermittent, progressing to self.

TABLE 11–13 Exercise Prescription for Case Study 5, Chapter 9

| Name | Case Study 5 | (F) | M | Age | 70 | Date | |

| | | Ht (in) | 59 | | Wt. (lb) | 180 |

Dx: Hypertension, Obesity, Arthritis (knees, wrists, spine)

Meds: Hydrochlorothiazide, Aldomet

Comments: Severe hypertensive response to exercise, Max BP 220/136, severely deconditioned, orthopedic limitations.

GXT Data: Date Performed 2/7/96 Where Clinic X

    Rest HR 62 Protocol Ramping-Bike

    Max HR 113 Max METs ~2

    Max BP 220/136 RPE (10-Pt. Scale) 7

    Re-evaluation scheduled 5/22/96

C-R Rx:

    Functional Capacity (METs) = 40% to 85% of Max METs

$$= .40 \text{ to } .85 \times \underline{\quad \sim 2 \quad}$$

$$= .80 \text{ to } 1.7 \text{ METS}$$

    THRR (Heart Rate Reserve) bpm = (Max HR − Rest HR)(40% to 85%) + (Rest HR)

$$= (\underline{\quad 113 \quad} - \underline{\quad 62 \quad})(.40 \text{ to } .85) + (\underline{\quad 62 \quad})$$

$$= \sim 83 \text{ bpm to } 105 \text{ bpm}$$

Mode of Exercise   X   Bike   Row   Walk   Walk/Jog

    (no arms on Schwinn Airdyne until adapt. occurs)

Length of session: 20–30 min.   Frequency: 3 ×s/wk

Comments: Patient limited by BP response and deconditioning. Intermittent CR exercise initially with 2–3 min of exercise and 1–2 min of rest. Progress to continuous activity as tolerated. RPP = 248.

Flexibility Rx: General program with emphasis on joints; 3 ×s/day

Muscular S & End Rx: Mild strength and endurance program when BP controlled.

| % Body Fat | 44% | Desirable | M | <20 % |
| | | | F | <30 % |

| Body Wt | 180 | lb | Body Mass Index (BMI) | 36.196 |
| | 82 | kg | Desirable BMI M & F | 20–24.9 |

Patient referred for nutrition education and weight reduction. BMI, low functional capacity, BP response, and age indicate she is Intermediate to High risk. Continuously monitor, progress to intermittent and to self-monitoring as indicated.

TABLE 11–14 Exercise Prescription for Case Study 7, Chapter 9

Name	Case Study 7		F (M) Age 51	Date

Ht (in)   74   Wt. (lb)   238

Dx: CAD, MI, Hypertension, Arrhythmias

Meds: Corgard, Procainamide

Comments: Mild hypertensive response to exercise on GXT, PVCs, Coupling (1), Bigeminy at Max HR

GXT Data: Date Performed   1/24/96   Where   Clinic X

    Rest HR   56   Protocol   Bruce TM

    Max HR   110   Max METs   7

    Max BP   168/94   RPE (10-Pt. Scale)   6

    Re-evaluation scheduled   4/25/96

C-R Rx:

Functional Capacity (METs) = 40% to 85% of Max METs

$$= .40 \text{ to } .85 \times \underline{\quad 7 \quad}$$

$$= 2.8 \text{ to } 5.5 \text{ METs}$$

THRR (Heart Rate Reserve) bpm = (Max HR − Rest HR)(40% to 85%) + (Rest HR)

$$= (\quad 110 \quad - \quad 56 \quad)(.40 \text{ to } .85) + (\quad 56 \quad)$$

$$= \sim 78 \text{ bpm to } 102 \text{ bpm}$$

Mode of Exercise	X	Bike		Row	X	Walk		Walk/Jog

Length of Session: 20–30 min.   Frequency: 3 ×s/wk

Comments: Patient referred to physician for medication change to stabilize arrhythmia prior to exercise therapy. RPP = 184

Flexibility Rx: Flex for calf, hamstring, quads, hip, 3 ×s/week prior to therapy, 1 ×/day at home, progress from 10 to 30 sec. Add shoulders, trunk, and neck as indicated.

Muscular S & E Rx: N/A at this time. Add later, if stabilized.

% Body Fat   25%   Desirable M   <20   %

                                  F   <30   %

Body Wt   238   lb   Body Mass Index (BMI)   30.424

       108   kg   Desirable BMI M & F   20–24.9

Referred for nutrition education and weight reduction. Referred to physician for medication change to stabilize arrhythmias. Since he is stratified as High risk, monitor continuously, progress to intermittent and to self-monitoring as indicated.

TABLE 11–15 Exercise Prescription for Case Study 8, Chapter 9

Name	Case Study 8	F Ⓜ	Age	50	Date

Ht (in) ___69___ Wt. (lb) ___160___

Dx: CAD, MI, CABG, Hyperlipidemia, PVD

Meds: Cardizem, Isordil, Transderm 5

Comments: Mild hypertensive response to exercise on GXT, ST-T depression of 3 mm in V_5 at Max HR, Bilateral leg claudication at 3 METs, PVCs, Bigeminy during cool-down and recovery.

GXT Data: Date Performed ___2/6/96___ Where ___Clinic X___

Rest HR	48	Protocol	Bruce TM
Max HR	98	Max METs	5
Max BP	156/98	RPE (10-Pt. Scale)	9

Re-evaluation scheduled ___5/8/96___

C-R Rx:

Functional Capacity (METs) = 40% to 85% of Max METs

= .40 to .85 × ___5___

= 2.0 to 4.25 METS

THRR (Heart Rate Reserve) bpm = (Max HR − Rest HR)(40% to 85%) + (Rest HR)

= (__98__ − __48__)(.40 to .85) + (__48__)

= 68 to 91 bpm

Mode of Exercise	X	Bike		Row	X	Walk		Walk/Jog

Length of session: ___20 to 60 min.___ Frequency: ___3 ×s/wk___

Comments: Subjective gradation of pain (3+) at Max HR. May need longer cool-down. RPP = 152.

Flexibility Rx: Stretching for calves, hamstrings, quads, hips, 3 ×s/week prior to exercise therapy and daily at home on alternate days.

Muscular S & End Rx: N/A Begin when patient can tolerate.

% Body Fat	20%	Desirable M	<20 %
		F	<30 %

Body Wt	160	lb	Body Mass Index (BMI)	23.524
	73	kg	Desirable BMI M & F	20–24.9

Referred for lipid-lowering nutritional plan and nutrition education. Since the patient is stratified as High risk, continuously monitor, progress to intermittent and to self-monitoring as indicated. Initially will need 2 to 3 min. of rest between exercise bouts, progress to continuous activity as tolerated.

TABLE 11–16 Sample Pulmonary Exercise Prescription Form

Exercise Rx

Name _____   F   M   Age _____   Date _____

           Pack-years _____   Ht. (in) _____   Wt. (lb) _____

Dx: _____

Meds: _____

Comments: _____

_____

GXT Data: Date Performed ___/___/___   Where: _____

          Rest HR _____   Protocol: _____

          Max HR _____   Max METs: _____

          Re-evaluation scheduled ___/___/___

PFT Interpretation: _____

_____

C-R Rx:
   Functional Capacity (METs) = 40% to 85% of Max METs

$$= .40 \text{ to } .85 \times \underline{\hspace{2cm}}$$

$$= \underline{\hspace{2cm}} \text{ METs}$$

   THRR (bpm) = (Max HR − Rest HR)(.40% to .85%) + (Rest HR)

$$= \underline{\hspace{2cm}} \text{ bpm}$$

   RPE (10-point scale)   = _____

   Type of Exercise _____ Bike _____ Row _____ Walk _____ Walk/Jog

           _____ Stairs _____ Arm ergometry

_____

_____

   Length of session: _____   Frequency: _____

   Comments: _____

_____

Flexibility Rx: _____

_____

Monitoring and Oxygen Needs:

Telemetry _____   Oximetry _____

Supplementary oxygen _____

Comments: _____

_____

TABLE 11–17 Exercise Prescription for Case Study 1, Chapter 10

Exercise Rx

Name <u>Case Study 1, Chapter 10</u> (F) M Age <u>61</u> Date _____

Pack-years <u>45</u> Ht. (in) <u>65</u> Wt. (lb) <u>124</u>

Dx: COPD, Asthma, Orthostatic hypotension, S/P Mastectomy

Meds: Tamoxatrin, imipramine, Ventolin MDI, Atrovent MDI, Slo-phyllin, Ativan

Comments: ECG normal before and after exercise. Quit smoking 8 years ago. Termination: Leg
fatigue

GXT Data: Date Performed <u>4/5/95</u> Where: <u>Clinic X</u>

Rest HR <u>108 bpm</u> Protocol: <u>Modified cycle</u>

Max HR <u>123 bpm</u> Max METs: <u>2.8</u>

Re-evaluation scheduled _____

PFT Interpretation: <u>Bronchospastic response to exercise moderately severe mechanical and</u>
diffusion limitations

C-R Rx:

Functional Capacity (METs) = 40% to 85% of Max METs

= .40 to .85 × <u>2.8</u>

= 1.1 to 2.4 METs

THRR (bpm) = (Max HR − Rest HR)(.40 to .85) + (Rest HR)

= <u>114–121</u> bpm

RPE (10-point scale) = <u>4 to 5</u>

Type of Exercise <u>X</u> Bike _____ Row <u>X</u> Walk _____ Walk/Jog

_____ Stairs <u>X</u> Arm ergometry

Circuit program: 10-min walk, 5-min bike (20 watts), 5 minutes arm
ergometer, RPE not to exceed 5

Length of session: <u>20 min of total</u> Frequency: <u>4–5 ×/wk</u>

Comments: Suggest Ventolin and Atrovent MDIs prior to exercise rest periods as needed. 16
stairs needed to home, work on pacing, not ex program yet.

Flexibility Rx: General flexibility exercises with emphasis on head, neck, and shoulders.

Muscular strength and endurance Rx: Not applicable at this time. If METs increase, consider light
weights later.

Monitoring and Oxygen Needs:

Telemetry _____ Oximetry <u>X</u>

Supplementary oxygen <u>3 liters</u>

Comments: Dropped PaO_2 during exercise. Oximetry eval with 3 liters of oxygen with exercise.
Keep sats above 88%

TABLE 11–18 Exercise Prescription for Case Study 2, Chapter 10

Exercise Rx

Name   Case Study 2, Chapter 10   F   Ⓜ   Age   77   Date _____

Pack-years   75   Ht. (in)   67.6   Wt. (lb)   180

Dx: COPD, Asthma, Chronic bronchitis, HTN, Peptic ulcers

Meds: Atrovent MDI, Beclovent MDI, Max Air, Robitussin

Comments: No significant ECG changes, termination due to dyspnea. Quit smoking 2 years ago

GXT Data: Date Performed   6/12/91   Where: Clinic X

Rest HR   61   Protocol: Modified cycle

Max HR   123   Max METs: 4.5

Re-evaluation scheduled _____

PFT Interpretation: Moderately severe obstruction. Moderate ventilatory mechanical and diffusion limitations

C-R Rx:
    Functional Capacity (METs) = 40% to 85% of Max METs

$$= .40 \text{ to } .85 \times \quad 4.5$$

$$= 1.8 \text{ to } 3.8 \text{ METs}$$

   THRR (bpm) = (Max HR − Rest HR)(.40 to .85) + (Rest HR)

$$= 85 - 114 \text{ bpm}$$

RPE (10-point scale)   =   4 to 5

Type of Exercise   X   Bike _____ Row   X   Walk _____ Walk/Jog

_____ Stairs   X   Arm ergometry

Cycle 60 to 80 watts for 10 minutes, walking 10 minutes. Arm ergometry for 5 minutes at 25 watts

Length of session: 25 min   Frequency: 3 ×/wk

   Comments: Intersperse rest periods only if needed during each stage of circuit. Rest between modes as needed.

Flexibility Rx: General flexibility program with attention to low back

Monitoring and Oxygen Needs:

Telemetry _____   Oximetry _____

Supplementary oxygen Supplemental O_2 to keep sats above 88%

Comments: Pao_2 57 with sats at 87% at 4.5 METs. Dyspnea correlated well with decreased sats.

TABLE 11–19 Exercise Prescription for Case Study 3, Chapter 10

Exercise Rx

Name   Case Study 3, Chapter 10   F   (M)   Age   69   Date _____

Pack-years   70   Ht. (in)   72.4   Wt. (lb)   147

Dx: COPD, Pneumoconiosis, HTN, CAD, S/P MI, L CVA, PVD, Gout, Ulcers

Meds: Lasix, ASA, diltiazem, Alipurinol, digoxin, Lanoxin, NTG

Comments: ST seg depression pre- and post-exercise. HR is disproportionately increased indicating cardiac limitation. Smokefree 11 years. Termination: Dyspnea and fatigue.

GXT Data: Date Performed   5/11/95   Where: _____

Rest HR   84   Protocol: Modified treadmill

Max HR   96   Max METs: 3.1

Re-evaluation scheduled   / /

PFT Interpretation: Moderately severe obstructive disease, no change with exercise.

C-R Rx:

Functional Capacity (METs) = 40% to 85% of Max METs

= .40 to .85 × __3.1__

= 1.2 to 2.6 METs

THRR (bpm) = (Max HR − Rest HR)(.40 to .85) + (Rest HR)

= 88–94 bpm

RPE (10-point scale)   =   4

Type of Exercise   X   Bike _____ Row   X   Walk _____ Walk/Jog

_____ Stairs   X   Arm ergometry

Cycle 50 rpm no resistance 2 sets of 3 min each with rests 1–2 minutes.

Walking 3–5 minutes with 1–2 min rests

Length of session: 12–15 min ex, 4–8 min rest   Frequency: 4–5 ×/wk

Comments: Intersperse rest periods as needed. No upper extremity work as yet. Progression: 15 min continuous exercise.

Flexibility Rx: General flexibility, special attention to L upper and lower extremity

Monitoring and Oxygen Needs:

Telemetry   X   Oximetry   X

Supplementary oxygen Needed during ex session to maintain $SaO_2 \geq 88\%$

Comments: Decreased O_2 sats to 87% and increased heart rate with low-level exercise. Suggest telemetry and oximetry during exercise session, SaO_2 to stay above 88%.

TABLE 11-20 Exercise Prescription for Case Study 4, Chapter 10

Exercise Rx

Name _____Case Study 4, Chapter 10_____   F (M)   Age __73__   Date _____

_____ Pack-years ___50___   Ht. (in) __71.5__   Wt. (lb) ___152___

Dx: COPD, Glaucoma

Meds: Beclovent MDI, Max Air MDI, Atrovent MDI, prednisone, Dilantin, aminophylline,

Pilocar drops

Comments: Few PVCs, nonspecific ST-T changes. Smokefree 3 years. Termination: Nose/mouth

discomfort, some dyspnea.

GXT Data: Date Performed ___4/5/95___   Where: _____Clinic X_____

Rest HR _____93_____   Protocol: _____Treadmill_____

Max HR _____114_____   Max METs: _____3.2_____

Re-evaluation scheduled _____

PFT Interpretation: Severe airflow obstruction. No change pre- and post-exercise test

C-R Rx:
   Functional Capacity (METs) = 40% to 85% of Max METs

                    = .40 to .85 × ___3.2___

                    = 1.3 to 2.7 METs

   THRR (bpm) = (Max HR − Rest HR)(.40 to .85) + (Rest HR)

                    = 101–111 bpm

   RPE (10-point scale)   = __4 to 5__

   Type of Exercise _____ Bike _____ Row __X__ Walk _____ Walk/Jog

          __X__ Stairs __X__ Arm ergometry

          Never been on a bike. Lives on 3rd floor walk-up walking 5 min, 1–2 min rest.

          Stairs 2–3 min within THRR

   Length of session: 3 sets walk _____ Frequency: 4–5 ×/wk

   Comments: Keep within THRR during 5-min walk, progress to 15 min continuous walking.

Consider arm erg as progression

Flexibility Rx: General flexibility, begin with LE and low back, add UEs as progression occurs.

Monitoring and Oxygen Needs:

Telemetry _____ Oximetry __X__

Supplementary oxygen _____3 liters_____

Comments: Heart rate reserve adequate, breathing reserve poor. PaO_2 drop to 42, $PaCO_2$ up to 50.

Keep sats above 88%.

SUMMARY

Guidelines for writing exercise prescriptions for patients with cardiopulmonary disease have been presented. Training principles associated with the development of each of the components of a comprehensive rehabilitation program (cardiorespiratory endurance, percent body fat, muscular strength and endurance, and flexibility) have been included. The principles of intensity, duration, frequency, and mode of activity have been described and interpreted as they relate to the improvement in functional capacity and normalization of daily activities so that patients may lead more productive lives. Examples of exercise prescriptions, four case histories of patients with cardiovascular disease, and four case histories of patients with pulmonary disease have been included. These case studies should assist students and clinicians in the application of the guidelines presented for writing comprehensive exercise prescriptions.

REFERENCES

1. Hall, LK and Gettman, LR: Policies and procedures in P & R programs. In: ACSM's Resource Manual for Guidelines for Exercise Testing and Prescription, ed 2. Lea & Febiger, Philadelphia, 1993, pp 562–569.
2. Pollock, ML, Welsch, MA, and Graves, JE: Exercise prescription for cardiac rehabilitation. In: Pollock, ML and Schmidt, DH (eds): Heart Disease and Rehabilitation, ed 3. Human Kinetics, Champaign, 1995, pp 243–276.
3. American Association of Cardiovascular and Pulmonary Rehabilitation: Guidelines for Cardiac Rehabilitation Programs, ed 2. Human Kinetics, Champaign, 1995, pp 87–95.
4. Balady, GJ et al: Cardiac rehabilitation programs: a statement for healthcare professionals from the American Heart Association. Circulation 90(3):1602–1610, 1994.
5. American College of Sports Medicine: Position stand—Exercise for patients with coronary artery disease. Med Sci Sports Exerc 26(3):i–v, 1994.
6. Butler, RM and Rogers, FJ: Exercise in healthy individuals. In: Goldberg, L and Elliot, DL (eds): Exercise for Prevention and Treatment of Illness. FA Davis, Philadelphia, 1994, pp 3–23.
7. Fletcher, GF et al. AHA medical/scientific statement: Exercise standards. Circulation 82(6):2286–2322, 1990.
8. Hambrecht, R et al: Various intensities of leisure time physical activity in patients with coronary artery disease: Effects on cardiorespiratory fitness and progression of coronary atherosclerotic lesions. J Am Coll Cardiol 22:468–477, 1993.
9. Hamm, LF and Leon, AS: Exercise training for the coronary patient. In: Wenger, NK and Hellerstein, HK (eds): Rehabilitation of the Coronary Patient, ed 3. Churchill Livingstone, New York, 1992, pp 367–402.
10. Hedback, B, Perk, J, and Woodlin, P: Long-term reduction of cardiac mortality after myocardial infarction: 10-year results of a comprehensive rehabilitation program. Eur Heart J 14:831–835, 1993.
11. Kavanagh, T: Cardiac rehabilitation. In: Goldberg, L and Elliot, DL (eds): Exercise for Prevention and Treatment of Illness. FA Davis, Philadelphia, 1994, pp 48–74.
12. LaFontaine, T and Roitman, J: Life style changes can prevent or reverse the progression of atherosclerosis. J Cardpulm Rehabil 12(3):159–162, 1992.
13. Morris, JN: Exercise in the prevention of coronary heart disease: Today's best buy in public health. Med Sci Sports Exerc 26(7):807–814, 1994.
14. Paffenbarger, RS et al: Changes in physical activity and other lifeway patterns influencing longevity. Med Sci Sports Exerc 26(7):857–865, 1994.
15. Rodriguez, BL et al: Physical activity and 23-year incidence of coronary heart disease morbidity and mortality among middle-aged men. Circulation 89(6):2540–2545, 1994.
16. Wenger, NK et al: Cardiac Rehabilitation as Secondary Prevention. Clinical Practice Guideline. Quick Reference Guide for Clinicians, No. 17. Rockville, MD: U.S. Department of Health and Human Services. Public Health Service, Agency for Health Care Policy and Research and National Heart, Lung, and Blood Institute. AHCPR Pub. No. 96-0673, October, 1995.
17. Ben-Ari, E et al: Return to work after successful coronary angioplasty—Comparison between a comprehensive rehabilitation program and patients receiving usual care. J Cardpulm Rehabil 12(1):20–24, 1992.
18. Hare, DL et al: Cardiac rehabilitation based on group light exercise and discussion. J Cardpulm Rehabil 15(3)186–192, 1995.
19. Temes, WC: Cardiac rehabilitation. In: Hillegass, EA and Sadowsky, HS (eds). Essentials of Cardiopulmonary Physical Therapy. Saunders, Philadelphia, 1994, pp 633–675.

20. Bar, FW et al: Cardiac rehabilitation contributes to the restoration of leisure and social activities after myocardial infarction. J Cardpulm Rehabil 12(2):117–125, 1992.
21. Friedman, DB: Exercise and the Heart. Southwestern Medical Center, University of Texas, Dec 9, 1993, p 13.
22. Oldridge, NB: Universal access and insurance coverage: Missing pieces. J Cardpulm Rehabil 15(1):9–13, 1995.
23. Sherman, C: Sudden death during exercise. The Physician and Sportsmedicine 21(9):93–102, 1993.
24. Sherman, C: Reversing heart disease. The Physician and Sportsmedicine 22(1):91–95, 1994.
25. Thompson, PD: Athletes, athletics, and sudden cardiac death. Med Sci Sports Exerc 25(9):981–984, 1993.
26. American College of Sports Medicine: ACSM's Guidelines for Exercise Testing and Prescription, ed 5. Williams & Wilkins, Baltimore, 1995, pp 177–193.
27. Ries, AL: Position paper of the American Association of Cardiovascular and Pulmonary Rehabilitation: Scientific basis of pulmonary rehabilitation. J Cardpulm Rehabil 10:418–441, 1990.
28. American College of Sports Medicine: op cit, pp 153–176.
29. DeVries, HA and Housh, TJ: Physiology of Exercise, ed 5. Brown & Benchmark, Dubuque, 1994, pp 311–333.
30. McArdle, WD, Katch, FI, and Katch, VL: Essentials of Exercise Physiology. Lea & Febiger, Philadelphia, 1994, pp 345–369.
31. American Association of Cardiovascular and Pulmonary Rehabilitation. Guidelines for Cardiac Rehabilitation Programs, ed 2. Human Kinetics, Champaign, 1995, pp 7–25.
32. American College of Sports Medicine: op cit, pp 12–26.
33. American Thoracic Society: Evaluation of impairment/disability secondary to respiratory disorders. American Review of Respiratory Diseases 133:1205–1209, 1986.
34. American Thoracic Society: Definitions, epidemiology, pathophysiology, diagnosis and staging. Am J Respir Crit Care Med 152:S78–121, 1995.
35. Reis, A: Endurance exercise training at maximal targets in patients with chronic obstructive pulmonary disease. J Cardpulm Rehabil 7:594–601, 1987.
36. Carter, R et al: Exercise conditioning in the rehabilitation of patients with chronic obstructive pulmonary disease. Arch Phys Med Rehabil 69:118–121, 1988.
37. Punzal, P et al: Maximum intensity exercise training in patients with chronic obstructive pulmonary disease. Chest 100:618–623, 1991.
38. Gordon, NF and Scott, CB. Exercise intensity prescription in cardiovascular disease. J Cardpulm Rehabil 15(3):193–196, 1995.
39. Joughlin, HM and Digenio, AG: Calculation of exercise prescription using different formulae: Which method provides the best alternative to ventilatory threshold measurement? J Cardpulm Rehabil 14(5):345, 1994.
40. Londeree, BR et al: %$\dot{V}O_2$max versus %HRmax regressions for six modes of exercise. Med Sci Sports Exerc 27(3):458–461, 1995.
41. Swain, DP et al: Target heart rates for the development of cardiorespiratory fitness. Med Sci Sports Exerc 26(1):112–116, 1994.
42. Winslow, A et al: Exercise prescription for cardiac patients: A national survey of outpatient cardiac rehabilitation programs (CRPs). J Cardpulm Rehabil 15(5):358, 1995.
43. Karvonen, M, Kentala, K, and Mustala, O: The effects of training on heart rate: A longitudinal study. Annales Medicinae Experimentalis et Biologiae Fenniae 35:307, 1957.
44. Stamford, Bryant: Tracking your heart rate for fitness. The Physician and Sportsmedicine 21(3):227–228, 1993.
45. Hodgkins, J: Prognosis in chronic obstructive pulmonary disease. Clin Chest Med 11(3):555–569, 1990.
46. Fox, SM, Naughton, JP, and Gorman, PA: Physical activity and cardiovascular health. Modern Concepts in Cardiovascular Disease 41:25–30, 1972, pp 26–27.
47. American College of Sports Medicine: Guidelines for Exercise Testing and Prescription, ed 4. Lea & Febiger, Philadelphia, 1991, p. 102.
48. Borg, GV and Linderholm, H: Perceived exertion and pulse rate during graded exercise in various groups. Acta Med Scand (suppl) 472:194–206, 1967.
49. Borg, GV: Perceived exertion: A note on history and methods. Med Sci Sports Exerc 5:90–93, 1973.
50. Borg, GV: Psychophysical bases of perceived exertion. Med Sci Sports Exerc 14:377–387, 1982.
51. American College of Sports Medicine: op cit, 1991, p. 70.
52. Belman, M: Exercise conditioning in chronic obstructive pulmonary disease. Clin Chest Med 7(4):585–596, 1986.
53. Reis, A: The importance of exercise in pulmonary rehabilitation. Clin Chest Med 15:327–337, 1994.
54. Pollock, ML and Wilmore, JH: Exercise in Health and Disease: Evaluation and Prescription for Prevention and Rehabilitation, ed 2. Saunders, Orlando, 1990.
55. Franklin, BA et al: Exercise and cardiac complications. The Physician and Sportsmedicine 22(2):56–68, 1994.
56. American Association of Cardiovascular and Pulmonary Rehabilitation. op cit, pp 1–25.

57. Patessio, A, Ioli, F, and Donner, C: Exercise prescription. In: Casaburi, R and Petty, T. (eds): Principles and Practice of Pulmonary Rehabilitation, Saunders, Philadelphia, 1993.
58. LeMura, LM, von Duvillard, SP, and Bacharach, DW. Central versus peripheral adaptations for the enhancement of functional capacity in cardiac patients. A meta-analytic review. J Cardpulm Rehabil 10:217–223, 1990.
59. Celli, B, Rassulo, J, and Make, B: Dyssynchronous breathing during arm but not leg exercise in patients with chronic airflow obstruction. N Engl J Med 314:1485–1490, 1986.
60. Astrand, I, Guhuray, A, and Wahren, J: Circulatory response to arm exercise with different arm positions. J Appl Physiol 25:528–532, 1968.
61. Criner, G and Celli, B: Effect of unsupported arm exercise on ventilatory muscle recruitment in patients with chronic airflow obstruction. Am Rev Respir Dis 138:856–861, 1988.
62. Casaburi, R: Therapeutic modalities in pulmonary rehabilitation. In: Casaburi, R and Petty, T (eds): Principles and Practice of Pulmonary Rehabilitation, Saunders, Philadelphia, 1993.
63. Casaburi, R et al: Reductions in exercise lactic acidosis and ventilation as a result of exercise training in patients with obstructive lung disease. American Review of Respiratory Diseases 143:9–18, 1991.
64. Reis, A, Ellis, B, and Hawkins, R. Upper extremity exercise training in chronic obstructive pulmonary disease. Chest 93:688–692, 1988.
65. American Association of Cardiovascular and Pulmonary Rehabilitation. Round Table: The primary prevention of coronary artery disease. J Cardpulm Rehabil 14(2):79–86, 1994.
66. LaFontaine, T. The role of lipid management by diet and exercise in the progression, stabilization and regression of coronary artery atherosclerosis. J Cardpulm Rehabil 15(4):262–268, 1995.
67. Miller, WC: Introduction: Obesity, diet composition, energy expenditure and treatment of the obese patient. Med Sci Sports Exerc 23:273–274, 1991.
68. Miller, WC: Diet composition, energy intake, and nutritional status in relation to obesity in men and women. Med Sci Sports Exerc 23:280–284, 1991.
69. Schuler, G et al: Regular physical exercise and low-fat diet: Effects on progression of coronary artery disease. Circulation 86(1):1–11, 1992.
70. Shephard, RJ: Physical activity and reduction of health risks: How far are the benefits independent of fat loss? J Sports Med Phys Fitness 34(1):91–98, 1994.
71. American College of Sports Medicine: op cit, pp 206–219.
72. Perri, MG: Confronting the maintenance problem in the treatment of obesity. J Cardpulm Rehabil 13(3):164–166, 1993.
73. Hunter, A, Carey, M, and Larsh, H: The nutritional status of patients with chronic obstructive pulmonary disease. American Review of Respiratory Diseases 124:376–381, 1981.
74. Mancino, J, Donahoe, M, and Rogers, R: Nutritional assessment and therapy. In: Casaburi, R and Petty, T (eds): Principles and Practice of Pulmonary Rehabilitation. Saunders, Philadelphia, 1993.
75. Graves, JE et al: Specificity of limited range of motion variable resistance training. Med Sci Sports Exerc 21:84–89, 1989.
76. Franklin, BA et al: Resistance training in cardiac rehabilitation. J Cardiopulm Rehabil 11:99–107, 1991.
77. Stewart, KJ: Resistive training effects on strength and cardiovascular endurance in cardiac and coronary prone patients. Med Sci Sports Exerc 21:678–682, 1989.
78. American Association of Cardiovascular and Pulmonary Rehabilitation: op cit, pp 27–56.
79. Kelemen, MH: Resistive training safety and assessment guidelines for cardiac and coronary prone patients. Med Sci Sports Exerc 21:675–677, 1989.
80. Stralow, CR, Ball, TE, and Looney, M. Acute cardiovascular responses of patients with coronary disease to dynamic variable resistance exercise of different intensities. J Cardpulm Rehabil 13(4):255–263, 1993.
81. Stamford, B: A stretching primer. The Physician and Sportsmedicine 22(9):85–86, 1994.
82. Tiep, B: Long term home oxygen therapy. Clin Chest Med 11:505–521, 1990.
83. Cox, N et al: Exercise and training in patients with chronic obstructive lung disease. Sports Med 6:180–192, 1988.
84. Liker, E, Karnick, A, and Lerner, L: Portable oxygen in chronic obstructive lung disease with hypoxemia and cor pulmonale. Chest 68:236, 1975.
85. Zack, M and Palange, A: Oxygen supplemented exercise of ventilatory and non-ventilatory muscles in pulmonary rehabilitation. Chest 88:669–675, 1985.
86. Nixon, P et al: Oxygen supplementation during exercise in cystic fibrosis. Am Rev Respir Dis 142:807–811, 1990.
87. Bradley, B et al: Oxygen assisted exercise in chronic obstructive lung disease: The effect on exercise capacity and arterial blood gas tensions. Am Rev Respir Dis 118:239–243, 1978.
88. Davidson, A et al: Supplemental oxygen and exercise ability in chronic obstructive airway disease. Thorax 43:965–971, 1988.
89. Hodgkin, J: Pulmonary rehabilitation: Structure, components and benefits. J Cardpulm Rehabil 11:423–434, 1991.
90. Stewart, A and Howard, P: Devices for low flow O_2 administration. Eur Respir J 3:812–817, 1990.
91. Russi, E et al: Experiences with long term transtracheal oxygen therapy (abstract). Schweiz Rundsch Med Prax 79:850–853, 1990.

92. Tiep, B et al: Pulsed nasal and transtracheal oxygen delivery. Chest 97(2):364–368, 1990.
93. Walsh, D and Govan, J: Long term continuous domiciliary oxygen therapy by transtracheal catheter. Thorax 45(6):478–481, 1990.
94. Wesmiller, S et al: Exercise tolerance during nasal cannula and transtracheal oxygen delivery. Am Rev Respir Dis 14:789–791, 1990.
95. Soffer, M et al: Conservation of oxygen supply using a reservoir nasal cannula in hypoxemic patients at rest and during exercise. Chest 89:806–810, 1985.
96. Tiep, B et al: Demand oxygen delivery during exercise. Chest 91:15–20, 1987.

CHAPTER 12

The Exercise Therapy Session

CANDIDATES FOR REHABILITATION

Patients may be referred for cardiopulmonary exercise therapy after interpretation of their clinical data previously obtained via invasive and noninvasive testing procedures. Important results of the clinical evaluations are to determine:

1. Whether a patient is likely to benefit from exercise training
2. The patient's ability to return to employment
3. The success of current medical management
4. The amount of supervision and/or monitoring needed during the exercise session

Patient goals and expected outcomes are also determined as a result of the clinical evaluation, past history, the nature of the disease, and the patient's personal objectives.[1]

Patients with Cardiac Disease

Comprehensive cardiac rehabilitation programs provide services including medical evaluation, prescribed exercise, risk factor modification, education, counseling, and behavioral interventions. These services are designed to improve the physiologic and psychologic effects of cardiac disease, reduce the risk of sudden death or reinfarction, stabilize or reverse the atherosclerotic process, and enhance the patient's psychosocial and vocational status.[2]

Following completion of the clinical evaluation, cardiac patients are "stratified" according to their degree of risk for acute cardiovascular complications during exercise and their general prognosis (see Chapter 11, Table 11–1, for guidelines for risk stratification of cardiac patients).[3] Particularly important in determining the prognosis of a patient following a cardiovascular event is the type and severity of the disease, the extent of left ventricular dysfunction, the arrhythmic potential of the cardiac tissue, and exercise-induced ischemia as evidenced by significant ST-depression, angina, or both.[4,5] Some patients with cardiac disease are considered too unstable (too high risk) to benefit from exercise therapy and are excluded from exercise programs.[3] Table 12–1

TABLE 12–1 Absolute
Contraindications to Exercise Training

Unstable angina
Uncontrolled congestive heart failure
Dysrhythmias compromising hemodynamic status
Uncontrolled hypertension
Acute myocarditis
Severe valvular stenosis
Hypertrophic cardiomyopathy
Acute pulmonary embolism or deep venous thrombosis

Source: From Balady, GJ and Weiner, DA: Risk stratification in
cardiac rehabilitation. J Cardpulm Rehabil 11(1):39–45, 1991,
with permission.

summarizes the conditions that preclude a patient from being referred for exercise
training.

Major reasons for risk stratification include establishing the prognosis a patient is
likely to have, predicting the risk of further major events, and determining the patient's chance for survival, especially during the first year following an acute myocardial infarction (AMI) or coronary artery bypass graft surgery (CABG). Patients found
to be at low risk following AMI or CABG have a first-year mortality of 2 percent compared with a 10 to 25 percent mortality in moderate-risk patients. High-risk individuals' first-year mortality rates exceed 25 percent.[6]

Risk stratification is also important in providing the rehabilitation team with information necessary for patient management during the rehabilitative process and is used
in the decision-making process to determine which patients should be continuously
monitored during the exercise session.[7] Patients who are at intermediate and high risk
usually require a longer, more closely monitored, supervised exercise program than
those who are determined to be at low risk.[8] Table 12–2 presents guidelines to be used
in determining which patients should probably be continuously monitored.[9] Phase II

TABLE 12–2 Characteristics of Patients Most Likely to Benefit
from Continuous Electrocardiographic Monitoring
during Cardiac Rehabilitation

Severely depressed left ventricular function (ejection fraction less than 30%)
Resting complex ventricular arrhythmia
Ventricular arrhythmias that appear or increase with exercise
Survival of sudden cardiac death
Survival of myocardial infarction complicated by congestive heart failure, cardiogenic shock, and/or
    serious ventricular arrhythmias
Severe coronary artery disease and marked exercise-induced ischemia (ST depression greater than 2
    mm)
Inability to self-monitor heart rate (physical or intellectual impairment)

Source: Reprinted with permission from Parmley, WW: Position report on cardiac rehabilitation: Recommendations of the American College of Cardiology. (Journal of the American College of Cardiology 7(2):453,
1986.)

cardiac rehabilitation is generally characterized by intensive ECG monitoring and supervision and Phase III usually begins when the patient does not need continuous or frequent intermittent ECG monitoring.[4] The length of time a patient may remain in Phase II and/or Phase III is quite variable and dependent upon a number of factors including individual need for ECG monitoring and level of clinical supervision required.[10] (See Chapter 1 for more description of Phase II and Phase III cardiac rehabilitation.)

An additional benefit of risk stratification is to determine the amount of supervision (staff-to-patient ratio) recommended for individual patients during the exercise training sessions. The recommended staff-to-patient ratio for Phase II cardiac rehabilitation is one staff member to supervise each five patients and a second person who should be immediately available in case of emergency. The staff-to-patient ratio for Phase III is 1:15. At least one person with current Advanced Cardiac Life Support (ACLS) certification and medical and legal authority to provide such care is required to be present during supervised exercise sessions for high- and intermediate-risk patients.[10-13]

Patients with Pulmonary Disease

Patients with chronic obstructive pulmonary disease (COPD) can be grouped according to their degree of impairment, which may allow predictions of benefits of a pulmonary rehabilitation program. (See Tables 10–2 and 10–3 for classification of COPD.)

Patients with mild pulmonary disease (stage I) may not recognize their diseases. The impact of the disease process on their physical abilities is minimal and it does not correlate with diminished ability to perform most jobs.[14,15] Patients may not see the need to be an active participant in a pulmonary rehabilitation program, and would therefore not benefit from the program.

Moderate to moderately severe impairment (stage II) has a significant impact on the patient's physical functioning. There is a diminished ability to meet the physical demands of many jobs. Patients with moderate to moderately severe disease usually experience dyspnea on physical exertion and may show signs of exercise hypoxemia, ischemic heart disease, ventricular arrhythmias, and cor pulmonale. Enrolling in a pulmonary rehabilitation program could allow patients with this category of disease to become more functional and less dyspneic with exertion and perhaps to return to gainful employment.

Severe pulmonary impairment (stage III) has a profound impact on the patient's physical abilities, usually precludes gainful employment, and usually reflects total disability.[15] Pulmonary impairment of this severity results in a lack of adequate lung function reserve. Lung function may be too limited to allow a significant benefit from a pulmonary rehabilitation program.[16]

The patients most likely to benefit from a pulmonary rehabilitation program, then, are those who:

1. Have moderate to moderately severe pulmonary disease
2. Are stable on current medical management for their diseases
3. Have minimal disease in other organ systems

4. Are willing to learn about their disease
5. Are motivated to participate in an exercise program

Motivation seems to be the most important of all the factors.[16]

Patients with restrictive pulmonary disease and/or with mixed restrictive and obstructive diseases may also benefit from a pulmonary rehabilitation program. Pulmonary rehabilitation is not appropriate for some patients, especially those with such diseases as terminal lung cancer or acute respiratory failure.

Once a patient has been referred for cardiopulmonary rehabilitation, the rehabilitation team must provide a comprehensive program involving weight control, nutrition counseling, smoking cessation, social and psychological support, and, of course, the exercise program. The goal is to return the patient to a productive lifestyle and to prevent or reverse (when possible) the progression of the disease process.[17]

This chapter will present the principles discussed in Chapter 11, The Exercise Prescription, and gives examples of exercise prescription and progressions as they apply to cardiopulmonary rehabilitation. Case studies will be presented to illustrate the events that transpire during the exercise session. A discussion of patients with special needs in exercise training also will be briefly discussed.

COMPONENTS OF THE EXERCISE SESSION

Each exercise session usually includes a 5- to 15-minute warm-up, a cardiorespiratory (CR) exercise period of 20 to 60 minutes, a 5- to 15-minute cool-down, and perhaps some resistance training activities. The warm-up and cool-down periods are important components of the exercise session because cardiovascular complications during the exercise session are more likely to occur during these periods.[18]

Warm-up

The warm-up period may include flexibility exercises and should always include low-intensity CR activities performed below target heart rate (THR) levels and below the exercising rate of perceived exertion (RPE). The goal is to gradually elevate the heart rate (HR) from the resting level to just below the THR within the 5- to 15-minute warm-up period. Activities selected for the CR warm-up phase may be the same as those used for the CR endurance training, but performed at a lower intensity and HR. Longer warm-up and cool-down periods may be needed for older and/or deconditioned patients, but a 5-minute warm-up consisting of low-level CR activities is considered a minimal amount of warm-up before CR endurance training.[8,19-21]

Cardiorespiratory Endurance Training

The CR endurance training period should follow the warm-up phase. To produce the desired CR adaptations (increased functional capacity and so on), the goal of the CR endurance training period is for patients to perform 20 to 60 minutes of continuous aerobic activity. However, as indicated in Chapter 11, this is the goal, and especially in the early stages of CR conditioning, patients may not be able to perform continuous activity. It is fairly common for patients to initiate their CR programs by using discontinuous activity which includes frequent rest periods. No one part of the exercise prescription is more challenging to the clinician than that of prescribing the appropriate CR activity. It should be emphasized that, until the patient can perform 20 to 30 minutes of continuous aerobic exercise, it is best to increase the duration of the activity before the intensity of the CR activity is increased.[22] To avoid musculoskeletal injury and to decrease cardiac risk, moderate levels of CR activity (lower intensities, longer duration) rather than more intense levels (higher intensities, shorter duration) should be prescribed.[22,23] As functional capacity increases and physiologic adaptation improves, the exercise prescription should be adjusted accordingly (see Chapter 11).

Cool-down

The CR endurance training period should be followed by a 5- to 15-minute cool-down period. Abrupt cessation of exercise may cause pooling of blood in the extremities. As a result of peripheral pooling, the brain, heart, or intestines may have insufficient blood supplies and such symptoms as vertigo, syncope, palpitations, or nausea may occur. Cardiac arrhythmias are sometimes precipitated following CR exercise, and a cool-down seems to be beneficial in preventing the potentially lethal irregularities that may result from increased catecholamine levels in the blood that are caused by exercise.[8,22] Exercises similar to those used for the warm-up and/or CR endurance training period are appropriate, but should be performed at lower intensities. The heart rate should return to near-resting levels before the patient is considered to be cooled down.

Resistive Exercises

As stated in Chapter 11, resistive exercise may be appropriate for cardiopulmonary patients provided it is undertaken with caution. When it is so prescribed, it is usually performed after the cool-down period that follows the CR endurance training. Blood pressures should be monitored before, during, and after the resistive training period because the rate-pressure product (RPP) increases, largely because of increases in systolic blood pressure. The resistive part of the rehabilitation process is usually prescribed after a patient has been aerobically conditioned for at least 4 to 6 weeks.[10] The intensity begins gradually (usually at 30 to 40 percent of maximal effort) and progresses gradually until the patient can perform one to three sets of 12 to 15 repetitions. The resistance may be gradually increased to 60 percent of one maximal effort, but the decision to do so is based on each individual's responses to resistive training.[19,24,25]

CASE STUDIES

To enhance the clinician's decision-making skills with regard to progressions in and modification of the exercise prescription, this section includes case studies that describe a 12-week course of treatment for two patients with cardiovascular disease and case studies that describe an 8-week course of treatment for two patients with pulmonary disease. Each case study includes the initial exercise prescription and rationale as well as a summary of the data obtained during the exercise training sessions that justify change in the exercise prescription. In this way, the developmental progression of the training sessions, as well as many of the factors that enter into the decision-making process for writing and adjusting an exercise prescription, can be more easily understood. It should be emphasized that, regardless of the length of time a patient may be in Phase II or Phase III cardiac rehabilitation (i.e., the patient progresses from Phase II to Phase III, to Phase IV), the physiologic adaptations to the exercise prescription follow a certain pattern that is unique to each patient. Discharge from Phase III to a home or community-based Phase IV (maintenance) cardiac rehabilitation program should occur when the patient is stable, is able to self-monitor exercise activity, and can maintain the outcomes achieved in Phases II and III. Progression of the cardiac patient to Phase IV may take 6 months or longer (see Chapters 1 and 11).[22,26–28]

CASE STUDY 5, CHAPTER 9*

This section describes the rehabilitative treatment for the patient in Case Study 5, Chapter 9. An initial exercise prescription written for this patient is given in Table 12–3. The prescription is based on the results of her GXT (see Table 9–18) and the information obtained from her completed preliminary forms and interview.

Although this 70-year-old hypertensive woman does not have coronary artery disease, certain features of her medical history and response to the GXT have special significance: namely, her age, arthritic condition (which limits her orthopedically), severe hypertensive response to exercise, and extremely deconditioned state (less than 2 METs on the GXT), which resulted in a stratification of intermediate to high risk.

Her CR training heart rate was determined after careful consideration of her functional capacity, her target heart rate range (THRR), and her rating of perceived exertion (RPE) (see Table 12–3 for the exercise prescription for this patient). Because her functional capacity was approximately 2 METs, her HRmax was 113 bpm, and her BP response was 220/136 mm Hg, the THRR was calculated to be 83 to 105 bpm (Karvonen method).[29] When considering the rapid rise in both systolic and diastolic BP (to 220/136 mm Hg) in 3 minutes at an extremely low exercise intensity, it was considered dangerous for her to exercise at an HR above the lower end of her THRR. Therefore, her initial THR was determined to be around 83 bpm, and because she was extremely deconditioned, her CR training began with intermittent training. The duration of the CR training was adjusted by gradually reducing the number and length of rest periods between the intermittent bouts of exercise.

Because of her hypertensive response to exercise, her BP was monitored at regular intervals during the CR exercise session, and because her BP response was another indicator of the intensity of her CR exercise, the BP, not her HR, seemed to be her limiting factor. Remember that a diastolic BP of 120 mm Hg is one criterion for exercise termination (see Chapter 9).

The bicycle ergometer was the initial mode of choice for CR training for this patient. Because of her arthritic condition and her obesity, it was important to reduce the pressure on her weight-bearing joints. In addition, lower initial workloads and smaller workload increments were prescribed to avoid injury and to allow for improvement in her deconditioned state. The Schwinn Airdyne bicycle

*Case study courtesy of Bio-Energetiks Rehabilitation, Prospect, PA.

TABLE 12–3 Exercise Prescription for Case Study 5, Chapter 9

Name _____ Case Study 5 _____ Ⓕ M Age _70_ Date _____

Ht. (in.) _59_ Wt. (lb) _180_

Dx: Hypertension, Obesity, Arthritis (knees, wrists, spine)

Meds: Hydrochlorothiazide, Aldomet

Comments: Severe hypertensive response to exercise, Max BP 220/136, severely deconditioned, orthopedic limitations.

GXT Data: Date Performed _2/7/96_ Where _____ Clinic X _____

Rest HR _62_ Protocol _Ramping-Bike_

Max HR _113_ Max METs _~2_

Max BP _220/136_ RPE (10-pt. scale) _7_

Re-evaluation scheduled _5/22/96_

C-R Rx:

Functional Capacity (METs) = 40% to 85% of Max METs

$$= .40 \text{ to } .85 \times \underline{\quad \sim 2 \quad}$$

$$= \underline{.80 \text{ to } 1.7 \text{ METS}}$$

THRR (Heart Rate Reserve) bpm = (Max HR − Rest HR)(40% to 85%) + (Rest HR)

$$= (\underline{\quad 113 \quad} - \underline{\quad 62 \quad})(.40 \text{ to } .85) + (\underline{\quad 62 \quad})$$

$$= \underline{\sim 83 \text{ bpm to } 105 \text{ bpm}}$$

Mode of Exercise _X_ Bike _____ Row _____ Walk _____ Walk/Jog

(no arms on Schwinn Airdyne until adapt. occurs)

Length of session: _20–30 min_ Frequency: _3 ×s/wk_

Comments: Patient limited by BP response and deconditioning. Intermittent CR exercise initially with 2–3 min of exercise and 1–2 min of rest. Progress to continuous activity as tolerated. RPP = 248.

Flexibility Rx: General program with emphasis on joints; 3 ×s/day

Muscular S & End Rx: _Mild strength and endurance program when BP controlled._

% Body Fat _44%_ Desirable M _<20_ %

F _<30_ %

Body Wt _180_ lb Body Mass Index (BMI) _36.196_

_82_ kg Desirable BMI M & F _20–24.9_

Patient referred for nutrition education and weight reduction. BMI, low functional capacity, BP response, and age indicate she is Intermediate to High risk. Continuously monitor, progress to intermittent and to self-monitoring as indicated.

---

was used, but the patient was initially instructed not to use her arms to maintain her workload. The workload performed on the ergometer during each exercise bout was carefully recorded. When weight loss, orthopedic conditions, and functional capacity permitted, walking was added to her CR training program (see week 10 on Table 12–4).

TABLE 12-4 Summary of a 12-Week Cardiovascular Exercise Program for Case Study 5, Chapter 9

Date	Rest HR	Rest BP	TARGET HR	W-UP	CR Work Type-Min*	C-R HR	Laps Wkload	Cool-Down HR	Cool-Down BP	Wt. lb	Comments — BPs, Arrhythmias, Med. Changes, Symptoms, etc.
WEEK 1	66	162/92	83	76	B-3, R-2	80	0.5 KP	78	160/90	180	B1st BP—170/103 Exercise terminated p 3rd bike due to hypertensive response to ex.
					B-3, R-3	82	0.5 KP				B2nd BP—172/106 Pt. re-referred for BP control
					B-3, R-3	86	0.5 KP				B3rd BP—180/112 9' CRE_x Intermittent 10 minute cool-down
					B-3, Terminate						
WEEK 2	52	152/84	78	68	B-2, R-2	72	0.5 KP	60	148/82	178	Medication change: Tenormin Lower Target HR Good tolerance
					B-2, R-2	76	0.5 KP				B2nd BP—160/86 B4th BP—168/90 10' CRE_x Intermittent
					B-2, R-2	78	0.5 KP				10' cool-down
					B-2, R-2	75	0.5 KP				
					B-2, R-2	78	0.5 KP				
WEEK 3	52	140/78	78	66	B-3, R-1	70	0.5 KP	58	138/76	176	Good tolerance, below THR 8' cool-down
					B-3, R-1	70	0.5 KP				B2nd BP—156/82 B4th BP—154/80 12' CRE_x Intermittent
					B-3, R-1	70	0.5 KP				
					B-3, R-1	70	0.5 KP				
WEEK 4	50	152/74	78	68	B-5, R-1	78	0.6 KP	56	142/74	173	Good tolerance, on target
					B-5, R-1	72	0.6 KP				B2nd BP—148/76 B4th BP—144/74 20' CRE_x Intermittent
					B-5, R-1	78	0.6 KP				8' cool-down
					B-5, R-1	78	0.6 KP				

WEEK	Pre (RPE / BP)	Pre (HR / min)	Mode	HR	Resistance	Max HR	Post (RPE / BP)	CR	Tolerance
WEEK 5	48 / 130/82	78 / 60	B-5	78	0.6–.7 KP	172	60 / 132/78	B3rd BP—132/80 20' CR Continuous	Good tolerance 6' cool-down
			B-5	73	0.6–.7 KP				
			B-5	78	0.6–.7 KP				
			B-5	78	0.6–.7 KP				
WEEK 6	50 / 136/74	78 / 66	B-5	72	0.7 KP	170	54 / 132/72	B3rd BP—130/76 25' CR Continuous	Good tolerance 6' cool-down
			B-5	72	0.7 KP				
			B-5	73	0.7 KP				
			B-5	72	0.7 KP				
			B-5	78	0.7 KP				
WEEK 7	50 / 130/74	78 / 66	B-5	78	0.8 KP	168	58 / 128/72	BPs prn 30' CR Continuous	Good tolerance 6' cool-down
			B-5	76	0.8 KP				
			B-5	78	0.8 KP				
			B-5	76	0.8 KP				
			B-5	78	0.8 KP				
			B-5	78	0.8 KP				
WEEK 8	48 / 130/68	78 / 66	B-5	78	0.8–.9 KP	165	54 / 128/74	BPs prn 30' CR Continuous	Good tolerance 5' cool-down
			B-5	78	0.8–.9 KP				
			B-5	78	0.8–.9 KP				
			B-5	76	0.8–.9 KP				
			B-5	78	0.8–.9 KP				
			B-5	78	0.8–.9 KP				
WEEK 9	48 / 128/70	78 / 66	B-5	76	1.0 KP	163	50 / 110/70	BPs prn 30' CR Continuous	Good tolerance 5' cool-down
			B-5	76	1.0 KP				
			B-5	78	1.0 KP				
			B-5	76	1.0 KP				
			B-5	76	1.0 KP				
			B-5	76	1.0 KP				

Continued

TABLE 12–4 Summary of a 12-Week Cardiovascular Exercise Program for Case Study 5, Chapter 9 (*Continued*)

Date	Rest		HR		C-R Training			Cool-Down		Wt.	Comments
	HR	*BP*	TARGET	*W-UP*	*CR Work Type-Min**	*C-R HR*	*Laps Wkload*	*HR*	*BP*	*lb*	*BPs, Arrhythmias, Med. Changes, Symptoms, etc.*
WEEK 10	48	128/72	78	64	B-5	76	1.0 KP	50	114/70	160	BPs prn
					W-5	78	5 Laps				30' CR Continuous
					B-5	76	1.0 KP				Add walk to CR Ex.
					B-5	78	5 Laps				Good tolerance
					W-5	78	1.0 KP				5' cool-down
					B-5	76	5 Laps				
WEEK 11	50	118/74	78	66	B-5	76	1.1 KP	48	110/70	158	BPs prn
					W-5	76	6 Laps				30' CR Continuous
					B-5	76	1.1 KP				Increase Walking to ½ of Cr Ex
					W-5	78	6 Laps				Good tolerance
					B-5	76	1.1 KP				5' cool-down
					W-5	78	6 Laps				
WEEK 12	50	114/72	78	68	W-5	76	7 Laps	48	110/68	156	BPs prn
					B-10	76	1.2 KP				30' CR Continuous
					W-5	76	7 Laps				↑Length of CR bouts
					B-10	76	1.2 KP				Good tolerance
											5' cool-down

*B = Bike; W = Walk; R = Rest.
Re-evaluation

Because of her deconditioned state, the patient initially required shorter-than-average warm-up and cool-down periods. Her muscular weakness did not allow her to exercise continuously, and her cycling was limited to bouts of 2 or 3 minutes of exercise followed by 1 or 2 minutes of rest. Intermittent exercise was progressed to continuous when the patient could tolerate it. In Table 12–4, it can be seen that the patient in Case Study 5 was able to tolerate 20 minutes of continuous CR activity after 4 weeks of exercise training. The patient was not encouraged to perform CR exercise at home until her BP response was under control (after week 3, see Table 12–4).

The flexibility program for this patient emphasized range-of-motion exercises for her arthritic joints. Most stretching exercises were initially performed in positions in which her weight was supported (e.g., sitting). She was encouraged to perform her flexibility exercises daily, at home. As her functional capacity improved, she was able to modify her flexibility activities so that they could be performed in nonseated positions when appropriate.

Mild muscular strength and endurance exercises were prescribed for this patient after she could complete 20 minutes of continuous CR activity (week 5). During her strength and endurance exercises, her BP responses were initially evaluated during each exercise. As her functional capacity improved, she was able to complete her muscular strength and endurance activities without the need to constantly monitor her BP.

The patient's medical problems were compounded by her obesity and she was referred for nutritional counseling (Chapter 13). Fortunately, she was neither diabetic nor hyperlipidemic and was able to tolerate a general meal plan of reduced calories.

Table 12–4 summarizes the cardiorespiratory exercise program for the patient in Case Study 5. Note that the patient was initially unable to tolerate CR bouts of 3 minutes and was referred to her physician regarding her continuation in the program. An example of a re-referral form is in Appendix B. Her physician changed her blood pressure medication to Tenormin and she was advised to continue in the exercise program. Tenormin, a beta-blocking medication, reduced her resting heart rate from 66 bpm to approximately 50 bpm. Although general guidelines regarding the effect of a beta-blocking agent on heart rate are available, the actual effect is difficult to predict because it is influenced by dosage and individual patient response. A practical approach to changing the THR was used. The patient was exercised at the same workload as before the medication change and a THRR was established based on the response. The patient's HR response to the same workload was approximately 8 to 10 bpm lower as a result of the beta-blocking medication. Thus, her new THRR was determined to be 73 to 95 bpm.

As the patient improved in her exercise tolerance, the need for frequent BP measurements during exercise declined. BP was not measured during exercise after week 6 of CR training. Her flexibility and muscular strength training were also adjusted at this time. Her improved recovery from CR exercise resulted in a decrease in the time needed for her cool-down period.

The patient's compliance with her weight-reducing regimen was demonstrated by a weight loss of 24 lb over the 12-week period. Her weight loss enhanced her CR training response and enabled her to tolerate more walking exercise and longer bouts of continuous cycling.

CASE STUDY 8, CHAPTER 9*

This section describes the course of rehabilitative treatment for the patient in Case Study 8, Chapter 9. The initial exercise prescription written for this patient is shown in Table 12–5. The prescription is based on the results of his GXT (see Chapter 9, Table 9–21) and the information gathered from his completed preliminary forms and interview.

Aspects of this 50-year-old male cardiac patient's history that have particular significance in relation to the patient's exercise prescription include a hypertensive response to exercise, ST depression of 3 mm in V_5 (with no angina), bilateral leg claudication (pain level 1 at 3 METs and level 3+ at 5 METs), and ventricular arrhythmias that occurred during the cool-down and recovery periods. His risk stratification was high, and he was classified as a high-risk patient with cardiac disease who was continuously telemetry-monitored during the first 4 weeks of the exercise sessions. He then progressed to intermittent ECG monitoring.

In formulating his training THR, both the functional capacity (METs) achieved on his GXT and the Karvonen formula[29] were considered. The MET level achieved on the GXT was 5 METs, and the maximal HR he achieved on his GXT was 98 bpm. Considering that his blood pressure was 156/98 mm Hg at the maximal HR he achieved on the GXT (98 bpm), and that he experienced claudication and ST depression, the initial exercise prescription was written at the lower end of his THRR, that is 68 bpm (Table 12–5).

As well as continuously monitoring the ECG of this patient, the blood pressure response to exercise was monitored at regular intervals as needed. The bicycle ergometer and treadmill (or other means of walking) were selected as the primary modes for exercise in CR training because alternate bouts of walking and cycling should minimize his leg pain. (If the Schwinn Airdyne or similar ergometer is used, the patient should be instructed, initially, to refrain from using the arms to maintain the workload because to do so may increase the BP response to exercise.) As the functional capacity of the patient in Case Study 8 improved, he was allowed to use his arms in the CR activity. Workload performed on the bicycle and the walking distance covered per exercise bout were carefully recorded to give the patient and staff objective feedback as to the intensity of his exercise. Accurate recording of the data makes it easier to identify the point at which training adaptations occur. Educating the patient regarding training adaptations and linking the adaptations to changes in daily exercise data help to motivate the patient to comply with the training regime.

Initially, to prevent ventricular irritability, this patient required longer than average warm-up and cool-down periods. Also, his pain tolerance did not permit continuous exercise, and his walking and cycling bouts were limited to 2 to 3 minutes of exercise followed by 1 or 2 minutes of rest. Intermittent exercise was progressed to continuous exercise as he was able to tolerate, which occurred after week 2 of his program (Table 12–6). The progression from intermittent to continuous CR exercise was accomplished by gradually decreasing the rest period and increasing the length of each CR bout. The length of the total CR training period (excluding warm-up and cool-down) was gradually increased from an initial 12 minutes to 45 minutes over a period of 12 weeks. In addition to his scheduled

*Case study courtesy of Bio-Energetiks Rehabilitation, Prospect, PA.

TABLE 12-5 Exercise Prescription for Case Study 8, Chapter 9

Name ___Case Study 8___ F (M) Age __50__ Date _____

Ht. (in.) __69__ Wt. (lb) __160__

Dx: CAD, MI, CABG, Hyperlipidemia, PVD

Meds: Cardizem, Isordil, Transderm 5

Comments: Mild hypertensive response on GXT, ST-T depression of 3 mm in V_5 at Max

HR, Bilateral leg claudication at 3 METs, PVCs, Bigeminy during cool-down and

recovery.

GXT Data: Date Performed __2/6/96__ Where ___Clinic X___

Rest HR __48__ Protocol ___Bruce TM___

Max HR __98__ Max METs ___5___

Max BP __156/98__ RPE (10-pt. scale) ___9___

Re-evaluation scheduled __5/8/96__

C-R Rx:

Functional Capacity (METs) = 40% to 85% of Max METs

= .40 to .85 × __5__

= 2.0 to 4.25 METS

THRR (Heart Rate Reserve) bpm = (Max HR − Rest HR)(40% to 85%) + (Rest HR)

= (__98__ − __48__)(.40 to .85) + (__48__)

= 68 to 91 bpm

Mode of Exercise __X__ Bike _____ Row __X__ Walk _____ Walk/Jog

Length of session: __20 to 60 min__ Frequency: __3 ×s/wk__

Comments: Subjective gradation of pain (3+) at Max HR. May need longer cool-down. RPP = 152.

Flexibility Rx: Stretching for calves, hamstrings, quads, hips, 3 ×s/week prior to exercise therapy

and daily at home on alternate days.

Muscular S & End Rx: N/A Begin when patient can tolerate.

% Body Fat __20%__   Desirable M __<20__ %

    F __<30__ %

Body Wt __160__ lb   Body Mass Index (BMI) ___23.524___

       __73__ kg   Desirable BMI M & F ___20-24.9___

Referred for lipid-lowering nutritional plan and nutrition education. Since the patient is stratified as High risk, continuously monitor, progress to intermittent and to self-monitoring as indicated. Initially, will need 2 to 3 min of rest between exercise bouts, progress to continuous activity as tolerated.

---

therapy three times per week on alternate days, the patient was encouraged to exercise at home.

The flexibility program for this patient emphasized the musculature and joints of the legs and hips. Stretching was performed before and after CR training and he was monitored periodically to make sure that, while stretching, no strain-

Text continued on page 359

TABLE 12–6 Summary of a 12-Week Cardiac Exercise Program for Case Study 8, Chapter 9

Date	Rest		HR TARGET		C-R Training			Cool-Down		Wt.	Comments
	HR	*BP*	*TARGET*	*W-UP*	*C-R Work Type-Min**	*C-R HR*	*Laps Wkload*	*HR*	*BP*	*lb*	*BPs, Arrhythmias, Med. Changes, Symptoms, etc.*
WEEK 1	50	140/84	78	72	B-3, R-2 W-3, R-2 B-3, R-2 W-3, R-2	76–72 78–74 76–72 78–74	0.8 KP 3 Laps 0.8 KP 3 Laps	48	128/80	160	Pt. tolerance good No pain on bike, pain level 1 walking 7 min cool-down No arrhythmias BP 1st B—144/82 BP 2ndW—138/82 20′ Inter. CRE$_x$
WEEK 2	48	138/82	78	70	B-4, R-1 W-4, R-1 B-4, R-1 W-4, R-1 B-4, R-1	78 78 76 80 78	0.9 KP 5 Laps 0.9 KP 6 Laps 0.8 KP	68	118/78	159	Pt. tolerance good Pain level 1 walking 7 min cool-down BP 1stW—138/80 BP 3rd B—126/80 25′ Continuous CRE$_x$
WEEK 3	50	138/74	78–80	72	B-5 W-5 B-5 W-5 B-5	76 80 78 80 78	0.8 KP 6 Laps 0.8 KP 5 Laps 0.8 KP	70	126/70	158	Pt. tolerance good Pain level 1 to 2 walking 6 min cool-down No arrhythmias BP 2nd B—132/72 25′ Continuous CRE$_x$
WEEK 4	60	126/74	78–80	72	B-5 W-5 B-5 W-5 B-5	78 80 80 80 80	0.9 KP 6 Laps 1.0 KP 6 Laps 0.9 KP	60	126/70	158	Pt. tolerance good 6 min cool-down No arrhythmias BP only prn 25′ Continuous CRE$_x$

				Exercise	HR	Workload			Duration	Comments
WEEK 5	54	128/72	80 / 72	B-5 W-5 B-5 W-5	80 78 80 80	1.0 KP 6 Laps 1.0 KP 6 Laps	60 /	124/70	BP only prn	Pt. tolerance good 6 min cool-down
				B-5 W-5	80 80	0.9 KP 6 Laps	/		158.5	30' Continuous CRE$_x$	No arrhythmias
WEEK 6	72	160/90	76 / 72	B-5	74	0.7 KP	70 /	128/80	BP p̄ 2nd Bike—132/84	↓Target Hr. Pt. tired, worked overtime all week
				W-5	76	4 Laps				BP p̄ 2nd Walk—130/80	
				B-5	74	0.7 KP					
				W-5 B-5 W-5	76 74 74	5 Laps 0.7 KP 4 Laps	/		158	30' Continuous CRE$_x$	7 min cool-down
WEEK 7	54	120/70	80 / 72	B-5 W-5 B-5	78 80 78	1.0 KP 6 Laps 1.0 KP	62 /	118/70	BP only prn	Pt. tolerance good 6 min cool-down
				W-5 B-5 W-5	80 78 80	6 Laps 1.0 KP 6 Laps	/		157	35' Continuous CRE$_x$	No arrhythmias
WEEK 8	54	118/70	80 / 68	B-5 W-5 B-5 W-5	78 80 80 80	1.0 KP 6 Laps 1.1 KP 6 Laps	70 /	114/68	BP prn	Pt. tolerance good 6 min cool-down
				B-5 W-5 B-5 W-5	80 80 80 80	1.1 KP 6 Laps 1.1 KP 6 Laps	/		157	40' Continuous CRE$_x$	No arrhythmias

Continued

TABLE 12-6 Summary of a 12-Week Cardiac Exercise Program for Case Study 8, Chapter 9 (Continued)

Date	Rest HR	Rest BP	HR TARGET	HR W-UP	C-R Work Type-Min*	C-R HR	Laps Wkload	Cool-Down HR	Cool-Down BP	Wt. lb	Comments — BPs, Arrhythmias, Med. Changes, Symptoms, etc.
WEEK 9	50	118/70	80	72	B-10 W-5 B-10 W-5 B-10	80 80 80 80 80	1.1 KP 6–7 Laps 1.1 KP 7 Laps 1.1 KP	68	112/68	156	BP prn — Pt. tolerance good, 6 min cool-down 40' Continuous CRE$_x$ — No arrhythmias
WEEK 10	48	120/70	80	74	B-10 W-7 B-10 W-7 B-10	80 80 80 80 80	1.2 KP 10 Laps 1.2 KP 10 Laps 1.2 KP	64	114/68	156	BP prn — Pain Level 1 s/t cramping, 5 min cool-down 44' Continuous CRE$_x$ — No arrhythmias
WEEK 11	48	118/68	80	68	B-10 W-10 B-10 W-10	78 80 80 80	1.2–1.3 KP 13 Laps 1.3 KP 14 Laps	62	112/64	156	BP prn — Pt. tolerance good, Pain level 1, 5 min cool-down 45' Continuous CRE$_x$ — No arrhythmias
WEEK 12	46	118/70	80	72	B-10 W-10 B-10 W-10 B-5	80 80 80 80	1.3 KP 14–15 Laps 1.3 KP 14–15 Laps	64	110/60	156	BP prn — Pt. tolerance good, Pain level 1, 5 min cool-down 45' Continuous CRE$_x$ — No arrhythmias

*B = Bike; W = Walk; R = Rest.
Re-evaluation

ing or actual pain occurred and that he was breathing slowly and rhythmically and not holding his breath.

A muscular strength and endurance training program was not initially prescribed for this patient, but such a program was begun after week 7 of his CR training.

This patient was also referred for nutrition education regarding cardiovascular disease and a lipid-lowering diet regimen (see Chapter 13). He was within his ideal body weight range, and his percent body fat and body mass index (BMI) were also within acceptable limits.

A summary of this patient's course of exercise treatment is shown in Table 12–6. Note that, as physiologic responses to exercise training occurred, the THR remained relatively constant, but the workload was increased to compensate for the improvements in CR endurance and to maintain the HR on target.

As the patient's BP response to exercise improved, the need for BP measurement during exercise bouts declined. However, during week 6, when he worked overtime and his BP and HR were unusually high at rest, he was frequently monitored. Note also (see Table 12–6) that the unusually high resting HR and BP required an adjustment in the THR and the workload.

Keeping the THR low and increasing the length of the cool-down period during the 12 weeks of training enabled the patient to tolerate the CR exercise well and exhibit no arrhythmias. Gradual increases in the length of time he walked enabled him to exercise with manageable pain (less than level 2).

CASE STUDY 1, CHAPTER 10

This section describes the rehabilitative course for the patient in Case Study 1, Chapter 10. The initial exercise prescription is summarized in Table 12–7. The prescription is based on the results of a symptom-limited cycle ergometer test. (Table 10–3 gives the results of this exercise test.)

This patient's assessment was remarkable for her severe obstructive pulmonary disease, desaturation during exercise, and the recorded bronchospastic response to exercise. Reviewing Table 10–3, although the $\dot{V}E$max was predicted to be 23.8 liters per minute based on pre-exercise FEV_1 of 0.68 liters per minute ($FEV_1 \times 35 = \dot{V}E$max), the actual maximum voluntary ventilation (MVV) was only 17.8 liters per minute. This patient achieved a maximum minute ventilation ($\dot{V}E$max) of 16.8 during her exercise test. This calculates to $\dot{V}E$max/MVV ratio of 94 percent, showing she is quite close to her respiratory maximum. A general guideline is that if a patient comes to within 10 liters of his or her MVV, a pulmonary end point is considered. Symptoms of shortness of breath usually terminate the test before MVV equals $\dot{V}E$max.

This patient also revealed a significant bronchospastic response after exercise. Her FEV_1 value before exercise of 0.68 liters per second to her post exercise FEV_1 of 0.60 liters per second shows an 11.7 percent decrease. A drop of 10 percent or more is considered significant for exercise-induced bronchospasm.

Arterial blood gas values changed considerably during exercise as well. This patient became more hypoxemic. Clearly, some supplemental oxygen support was necessary for the exercise session. Although there was an increase in the car-

TABLE 12–7 Pulmonary Exercise Prescription for Case Study 1, Chapter 10

Exercise Rx

Name _____Case Study 1, Chapter 10_____ (F)   M   Age _61_   Date _____

Pack-years _45_   Ht. (in.) _65_   Wt. (lb) _124_

Dx: COPD, Asthma, Orthostatic hypotension, S/P Mastectomy

Meds: Tamoxatrin, imipramine, Ventolin MDI, Atrovent MDI, Slo-phyllin, Ativan

Comments: ECG normal before and after exercise. Quit smoking 8 years ago. Termination: Leg fatigue

GXT Data: Date Performed _4/5_   Where: _____Clinic X_____

Rest HR _108_   Protocol: _____Modified cycle_____

Max HR _123_   Max METs: _2.8_

Re-evaluation scheduled _7/12_

PFT Interpretation: Bronchospastic response to exercise moderately severe mechanical and diffusion limitations

C-R Rx:
   Functional Capacity (METs) = 40% to 85% of Max METs

$$= .40 \text{ to } .85 \times \underline{\quad 2.8 \quad}$$

$$= 1.1 \text{ to } 2.4 \text{ METs}$$

THRR (bpm) = (Max HR − Rest HR)(.40 to .85) + (Rest HR)

$$= 114–121 \text{ bpm}$$

RPE (10-point scale) = _4 to 5_

Type of Exercise _X_ Bike _____ Row _X_ Walk _____ Walk/Jog

_____ Stairs _X_ Arm ergometry

Circuit program: 10-min walk, 5-min bike (20 watts), 5 min arm ergometer, RPE not to exceed 5

Length of session: _____20 min_____   Frequency: _3 ×/wk_

Comments: Suggest Ventolin and Atrovent MDIs prior to ex. 16 stairs at home, work on pacing.

Flexibility Rx: General flexibility exercises with emphasis on head, neck, and shoulders.

Muscular strength and endurance Rx: Not applicable at this time. If METs increase, consider light weights later.

Monitoring and Oxygen Needs:

Telemetry _____   Oximetry _X_

Supplementary oxygen _3 liters_

Comments: Dropped PaO_2 during exercise. Oximetry evaluation with 3 liters of oxygen with exercise. Keep sats above 88%

bon dioxide level and she became somewhat more acidotic, the values were within the normal ranges.

Her ECG was normal throughout her exercise session, and her exercise termination was a result of leg fatigue.

Using the Karvonen formula, her THRR is calculated as follows:

$$(\text{Maximum HR} - \text{resting HR})(40\% \text{ to } 85\%) + \text{resting HR} = \text{THR}$$
$$(123 - 108)(40\% \text{ to } 85\%) + 108 = 114 \text{ to } 121 \text{ bpm}$$

Because this patient tested quite close to her respiratory maximum and has severe obstructive pulmonary disease with no compounding system disease, it was decided that she could exercise close to the maximum THRR. Using a THR of 80 percent of the HR reserve results in a THR of 120 bpm.

It was suggested that the patient use her metered dose inhaler (MDI) bronchodilators before the exercise session to help avoid the bronchospasm induced by exercise. Because she was always encouraged to use those drugs just before exercise, her resting heart rate was often elevated before the beginning of exercise. Therefore the THR was not strictly used; instead, symptoms and RPE dictated the exercise session.

The patient was placed (by the attending physician) on 3 liters per minute of nasal cannula oxygen during exercise sessions, which resulted in oxygen saturation of no less than 92 percent. Because of the initial need for oximetry monitoring, exercise was prescribed for the patient on stationary equipment: treadmill, cycle, and arm ergometer. Midway through the second week of exercise, oximetry readings were stable and oxygen saturation was checked only periodically. She was then free to ambulate out-of-doors on the track. Because the ability to walk out-of-doors was one of the goals she had set for the rehabilitation process, outdoor walking was strongly encouraged. Compliance with the rehabilitation program and with a home program is greater if the patient's goals are incorporated in the rehabilitation program.

This patient had a 15-minute warm-up session that included 10 minutes of general flexibility with special attention to the shoulders and neck. Care was taken to perform the exercises properly so that stretching was done on exhalation only to discourage the Valsalva maneuver. Rest periods between stretching exercises were given as needed. No pain should be experienced with the flexibility exercises. This patient was able to do the exercises on a mat on the floor. The remainder of the warm-up was done on a treadmill (5 minutes) at a perceived slow pace (RPE of 3). A cycle ergometer pedaled at 10 to 15 mph with no resistance could have been chosen as a warm-up as well. Her warm-up was maintained at 15 minutes throughout the rehabilitative process.

The CR endurance training began with ambulation, cycle ergometry, and arm ergometry. A circuit program allows for a variety of exercise modes to increase the specificity of training as well as to maintain interest in the activities. The patient accomplished three exercise sessions the first week with no symptoms of muscle soreness, fatigue, or joint pain. The program included 5 minutes of activity interspersed with rest periods. Exercise progression would be accomplished by increasing the amount of continuous activity until 30 minutes could be completed. Table 12–8 provides a weekly summary of the exercise performed. Exercise progression can be inferred from reviewing the chart.

TABLE 12–8 Summary of 8-Week Pulmonary Exercise Program for Case Study 1, Chapter 10

Date	Rest		HR		C-R Training						Cool-Down		O₂	Comments
	HR	BP	THRR THR	W-UP	C-R Work Type-Min*	HR	RPE	RR	%Sat	Distance Workload	HR	BP	Liters/Min	BPs, Arrhythmias, Med. Changes, Symptoms, etc.
WEEK 1	114	144/92	114–121	114	W-5 R-5 W-5 R-5 B-5 A-2 R-2 A-2	116 120 120	3–4 5	28 30 92		1400 ft 20 W 15 W	108	136/90	3L	Meds prior to exercise, 15-min warm-up % sats remain 90–93 range throughout program Spot check & paddles—NSR 10-min cool-down Patient seen 3×/wk
WEEK 2	108	130/84	114–121	120 112	W-5 R-2 W-5 B-5 R-3 A-3 R-2 A-3	120 120 120	4 4 5	30 92		1800 ft 20W 15 W	114	134/88	3L	Med before exercise, 15 min warm-up Sats on 3L remain good Oximeter spot check only Ambulated out-of-doors 10-min cool-down Oxygen delivered at home, portable pack filled Home exercise program of 10 to 15 min walking given Patient seen 3×/wk

											Comments
WEEK 3	114	114–121 120 114	140/80	W-10 R-2 W-10 A-3 R-2 A-3	120 120	24 30 30	4 5 5	1700 ft 1700 ft	108	15 W 144/86	3L	Med before exercise. 15 min warm-up Walk out-of-doors—enjoying being outside Walking intermittently 20 min per day 10-min cool-down Pacing taught 2 flights of stairs 2 stairs per exhalation Patient seen 3×/wk
WEEK 4	114	114–121 120	134/76	W-15 R-2 W-13 B-5 A-3 R-2 A-3	120 120	30	5	3200 ft 3000 ft 20 W	114	134/80	3L	Meds taken, 15-min warm-up 10-min cool-down Enjoys out-of-doors (hates arm ergometer) Continue pacing on stairs Home program: constant 20-min walk
WEEK 5	112	114–121 120 116	128/74	W-23½ A-4 R-2 A-4	123	28	5	4500 ft	120	126/78	3L	Meds before exercise,15-min warm-up, 10-min cool-down Diaphragmatic breathing after cool-down Patient decreased 2×/wk
WEEK 6	108	114–121 120 108	126/80	W-25 B-5 A-3½ R-2 A-4	120 123	30 28	4½	5000 ft 20 W	114	124/80	3L	Meds taken, 15-min warm-up Stairs: 3 flights, 2 stairs/breath pacing Home program increased to 25 min Walking 5 times a week 10-min cool-down Patient seen 2×/wk

Continued

TABLE 12–8 Summary of 8-Week Pulmonary Exercise Program for Case Study 1, Chapter 10 (*Continued*)

Date	Rest		HR		C-R Training					Cool-Down		O₂	Comments
	HR	*BP*	*THRR THR*	*W-UP*	*C-R Work Type-Min**	*HR*	*RPE*	*RR*	*%Sat*	*Distance Workload*	*HR*	*BP*	*Liters/ Min*	*BPs, Arrhythmias, Med. Changes, Symptoms, etc.*
	106		114–121		W-30	126		30		5000 ft	110			Meds taken, 15-min warm-up
			120	110	A-5	120	3	30		20W		140/84	3L	Stairs: 3 flights, 2:1 pacing
		134/80					4							Continuous down whole 3 flights
														10-min cool-down
														Home program—good compliance
WEEK 7														Seen 2×/wk
	108		114–121		W-30	126		30		5000 ft	112			Oximetry check on 2 liters during ex
			120	110	A-5	118	4			20 W		136/88	2–3	SaO₂ down to 86%
		134/90												Returned to 3 liters/min
														All goals met
														Discharged from rehab
WEEK 8														1 month follow-up

Cool-down was accomplished by ambulating again on the treadmill at an RPE of 3. Flexibility exercises were repeated, and the HR was taken. Occasionally, this patient had an elevated HR after her 10 minutes of cool-down. When that occurred, diaphragmatic breathing was practiced for 5 to 10 minutes with a continued decline in HR approaching resting. The patient was not dismissed from the rehabilitation session until her HR had returned to a reasonable resting level.

At week 2, pulsed portable home oxygen (demand oxygen delivery system) was supplied by a home care service company. A home exercise program was begun, and compliance was fair. The patient was hindered by the 16 stairs at home. Therefore, during week 3 of the rehabilitation program, stair climbing was substituted for biking.

During the final week of her pulmonary rehabilitation program, her physician asked her to perform exercise using a reduced amount of oxygen: 2 liters per minute. Oxygen saturation was found to decrease to 86 percent during exercise, and the patient showed changes in her exercise performance and RPE values. At that time, 3 liters per minute of oxygen delivered by nasal cannula was reinstituted.

By week 8 of pulmonary rehabilitation, all the patient's goals and the goals of the staff had been met. She was ambulating out of doors for 30 continuous minutes. She was able to climb two flights of stairs by using the pacing technique without becoming short of breath. She was able to descend two flights of stairs with no sensation of dyspnea. All formal lectures had been attended, and all informal teaching had been completed. The patient graduated from the program with a follow-up scheduled 1 month later.

CASE STUDY 3, CHAPTER 10

This section describes the course of rehabilitation for the patient in Case Study 3, Chapter 10. The initial exercise prescription written for this patient is given in Table 12–9. The prescription is based on the results of a physical assessment, including a symptom-limited graded exercise test. (Table 10–5 gives the results of the exercise test.)

Important considerations in the assessment of this patient are the moderately severe obstructive pulmonary disease, baseline ST-segment depression of 2 to 3 mm that does not change with exercise, an exercise test that did not reach anaerobic threshold, a disproportionately increased heart rate to workload ratio (a sign of cardiac limitation or deconditioning) and a $\dot{V}Emax/MVV$ ratio of 97%. The test was stopped because of fatigue and dyspnea.

Using the Karvonen formula, the patient's THRR was calculated as follows:

$$(\text{Maximum HR} - \text{resting HR})(40\% \text{ to } 85\%) + \text{resting HR} = \text{THRR}$$
$$(96 - 84)(40\% \text{ to } 85\%) + 84 = 88 \text{ to } 94 \text{ bpm}$$

Because the patient had signs of deconditioning and/or cardiac involvement and he stopped his exercise test for fatigue and dyspnea, the THR was set at the lowest end of THRR, or 88 bpm. This patient was monitored during exercise by both telemetry and oximetry, which necessitated walking on a treadmill and using a stationary bicycle for the exercise modes. Distance walked and bicycle

TABLE 12–9 Pulmonary Exercise Prescription for Case Study 3, Chapter 10

Exercise Rx

Name _____ Case Study 3, Chapter 10 _____ (F) M   Age _69_   Date _____

Pack-years _70_   Ht. (in.) _72.4_   Wt. (lb) _147_

Dx: COPD, Pneumoconiosis, HTN, CAD, S/P MI, L CVA, PVD, gout, ulcers

Meds: Lasix, ASA, Diltiazem, Alipurinol, digoxin, Lanoxin, NTG

Comments: ST-seg depression pre- and post-exercise. HR is disproportionately increased indicating cardiac limitation, smokefree 11 years. Termination: Dyspnea and fatigue.

GXT Data: Date Performed _5/11/_   Where: _____

Rest HR _84_   Protocol: _____ Modified treadmill _____

Max HR _96_   Max METs: _____ 3.1 _____

Re-evaluation scheduled _/ /_

PFT Interpretation: Moderately severe obstructive disease no change with exercise.

C-R Rx:
  Functional Capacity (METs) = 40% to 85% of Max METs

$$= .40 \text{ to } .85 \times \underline{\quad 3.1 \quad}$$

$$= \underline{1.2 \text{ to } 2.6 \text{ METs}}$$

THRR (bpm) = (Max HR − Rest HR)(.40 to .85) + (Rest HR)

$$= \underline{88-94} \text{ bpm}$$

RPE (10-point scale)   = _4_

Type of Exercise _X_ Bike _____ Row _X_ Walk _____ Walk/Jog

_____ Stairs _____ Arm ergometry

Cycle 50 rpm no resistance 2 sets of 3 min each with rests 1–2 min.

Walking 3–5 min with 1–2 min rests

Length of session: _12–15 min ex, 4–8 min rest_   Frequency: _5 ×/wk_

Comments: Intersperse rest periods as needed. No upper extremity work as yet. Progression: 15 min continuous exercise.

Flexibility Rx: General flexibility, special attention to L upper and lower extremity

Monitoring and Oxygen Needs:

Telemetry _X_   Oximetry _X_

Supplementary oxygen indicated during ex session

Comments: Decreased O_2 sats to 87% and increased heart rate with low-level exercise. Suggest telemetry and oximetry during exercise session.

workloads were recorded, as were physiologic parameters (subjective and objective) at those work levels. Functional gains were used to motivate the patient to continue with the exercise program. Upper extremity work was not begun until it was clear that the patient had developed some cardiopulmonary endurance. Education sessions, both group (formal) and individual (informal), began immediately.

At first, this patient required 15 minutes to get through the warm-up sessions. His warm-up included flexibility exercises modified so that he could do them in the sitting position in a chair. The therapist who demonstrated the exercises to the patient made it clear that the actual stretching motion of each exercise should be made during exhalation, thus avoiding the Valsalva maneuver, which has been known to increase blood pressure and close small airways impairing breathing. At first, it was continually necessary to remind the patient to continue to breathe throughout each exercise. Rest periods were needed to allow the patient to recover his breathing.

After stretching, the patient continued the warm-up session by performing, at a low effort level, the activity that he was to perform for the cardiopulmonary endurance exercise. In this case, the activity was treadmill walking, and the warm-up level was the perceived slow pace of 3 on the RPE scale. (An alternative warm-up and cardiopulmonary endurance exercise was pedaling on a stationary bicycle.)

The cardiorespiratory endurance training involved short bouts of aerobic activity interspersed with rest periods. The patient was initially able to perform 3 minutes of exercise with 2 minutes of rest. Oximetry showed a SaO_2 decrease from 96 to 86 percent. Telemetry revealed some HR irregularities, including occasional unifocal PVCs and three couplets. The ST segment did not change from baseline. A rhythm strip was recorded and sent to his physician for further evaluation. He did not achieve his THR of 88. However, because his resting HR was 12 bpm below his resting HR on the day of his test, and because he had increased his HR linearly with this workload while maintaining an appropriate RPE, the CR training session was felt to be adequate.

The CR endurance training activity was modified to promote cool-down and was completed in 10 minutes. This time, since the patient was already on the bicycle, cycling at 25 rpm, no resistance was added. Flexibility exercises followed the cool-down, again with emphasis on the need for a continuous breathing pattern during all phases of activity.

The patient returned to the program 2 days later with no symptoms of joint pain, muscle soreness, or fatigue. The program was then determined to be adequate for him. The physician ordered 1 liter of oxygen via nasal cannula during the exercise session. Exercise progression was undertaken, as tolerated, by increasing the amount of time within each activity until 15 to 30 minutes of continuous activity could be accomplished.

On the Sunday preceding the second week of pulmonary rehabilitation, the patient was seen in the emergency room (ER) for shortness of breath and headache. He was treated with bronchodilators and 3 liters of nasal cannula oxygen. His symptoms resolved, and he was released from the ER. There was no change in his medication schedule.

His second week of pulmonary rehabilitation began with an increase in his resting BP. Therefore, his BP was taken during the exercise session rather than only at rest and after cool-down. His BP was 182/94 mm Hg with an oxygen saturation of 84 percent during his second set of walking. A rhythm strip was taken; it showed one couplet and multifocal PVCs. The patient began the normal cool-down phase of the rehabilitation program, and his physician was called. The pa-

Text continued on page 372

TABLE 12–10 Summary of Pulmonary Exercise Program for Case Study 3, Chapter 10

Date	Rest		HR		C-R Training						Cool-Down		O₂	Comments
	HR	BP	THRR THR	W-UP	C-R Work Type-Min*	HR	RPE	RR	%Sat	Distance Workload	HR	BP	Liters/Min	BPs, Arrhythmias, Med. Changes, Symptoms, etc.
WEEK 1	72	162/74	88–96 / 88	82	W-3 / R-3 / W-3 / R-3 / B-3 / R-3 / B-3	78 / 78 / 86	5 / 4–6	30	24 / 30 / 86	800 ft / 50 rpm / No resistance	78	162/78	—	15-min warm-up; HR irregular—send strip; Good understanding of RPE scale; Oxygen sats down from 96 to 86; MD orders 1 liter/min oxygen exercise; 10-min cool-down; Seen 3 ×wk
WEEK 2	72	148/100	88–96 / 88	82	W-4 / R-3 / W-2	84 / 90	5–6	30	84	1200 ft	80	182/94	1 L/min	15-min warm-up; Patient to ER on Sunday for shortness of breath, headache; no change in med; BP up today; BP during 2nd set walking 182/94, HR 80, SaO₂ 84%, EKG showed occasional PVCs at ex and recovery, one coupling; Cool-down initiated (10 min); Session stopped, MD notified; Pt seen only once this week

WEEK 3	78	148/80	88–96	88	80	W-9 R-3 W-9 B-5 R-3 B-5	84	84–90	5	24 30 90	2400 ft 20 W	82 160/80	2 L/min	Exercise session now on 2 liters O_2 per MD order; O_2 set up at home for exercise and sleep; 15-min warm-up; Longer periods of exercise tolerated; Telemetry shows occasional PVCs, no couplets; 10-min cool-down; Pt seen 3 ×/wk
WEEK 4	72	164/80	88–96	88	80	W-12 R-2 W-10 R-2 B-5	78	84	5	30 90	2600 ft 20 W	78 150/74	2 L/min	15-min warm-up; 2 unifocal PVCs at max ex.; Began stairs with pacing; Begin spot check HR/remove telemetry; 10-min cool-down; Began home program of walking 10 min/rest/10 min; Pt see 3 ×/wk

Continued

TABLE 12-10 Summary of Pulmonary Exercise Program for Case Study 3, Chapter 10 (*Continued*)

Date	Rest HR	Rest BP	THRR/THR	W-UP HR	C-R Work Type-Min*	C-R HR	RPE	RR	%Sat	Distance Workload	Cool-Down HR	Cool-Down BP	O₂ Liters/Min	Comments: BPs, Arrhythmias, Med. Changes, Symptoms, etc.
WEEK 5	66	150/74	88–96 / 88	72	W-15 / R-3 / B-5 / A-3 / R-3 / A-3	84 / 78	5	24	90	2400 ft / 20 W	72	148/80	2	15-min warm-up; Discontinue oximetry; Normal sinus rhythm; Add arm ergometry; 10-min cool-down; Arm ergometry began at 15 watts
WEEK 6	72	166/82	88–96 / 88	74	W-15 / A-3 / R-3 / A-3	84 / 84	5	24 / 26		2400 ft / 15 W	76	164/86	2	15-min warm-up; Normal sinus rhythm; 10-min cool-down
WEEK 7	72	162/82	88–96 / 88	76	W-15 / R-3 / W-15 / B-5 / A-3 / R-3 / A-3	78 / 88	5	30		5000 ft / 25 W / 20 W	74	156/84	2	15-min warm-up; 13 stairs up & down, pacing; 10-min cool-down; Pt seen 3 ×/wk

	Resting HR	THR				BP (rest)	Activity		HR		Duration (min)			METs / Workload			HR	BP	RPE	Comments
WEEK 8	72	88–96			76	156/80	W-20 B-10 A-5	78 90		5	30		3800 ft 25 W 20 W		76	152/84	2				15-min warm-up Good control of respiration Pacing during ADLs reported Home program: 20 min continuous exercise 10-min cool-down Pt seen 2 ×/wk
WEEK 9	74	88–96	90		78	164/86	W-25 B-10 A-5	90 90 90		5	30 30		4000 ft 25 W 20 W		78	158/84	2				10-min warm-up Independent in warm-up & cool-down Increase THR to 90—with RPE at 5 Occasional PVCs at peak seen on scope 5-min cool-down Pt seen 1 ×/wk Good compliance with home program
FINAL SESSION	72	88–96	90		76	148/84	W-30 B-10 A-5	90 90 90		5	27 30 30		4800 ft 25 W 20 W		80	154/80	2				10-min warm-up Spot checks show occasional unifocal PVCs 5-min cool-down

tient was excluded from pulmonary rehabilitation until physician clearance to continue was obtained.

The patient returned for week 3 of rehabilitation with a change in oxygen dose only. During exercise, 2 liters per minute of oxygen were to be administered, and nocturnal oxygen was used at home. The patient continued in the exercise program with no further incidents. Telemetry was discontinued during week 4, although spot checking with paddles was continued for the duration of the exercise sessions. Oximetry was discontinued on week 5; the patient began ambulating on the outdoor track and arm ergometry was added. Progression of exercise is shown on the sample data sheets in Table 12–10.

By the end of his pulmonary rehabilitation program, this patient had achieved all the long-term goals established at the onset of his program. He had attended all of the formal lectures in the series and had completed all of the individual counseling sessions. He was independent in his exercise program, was able to accomplish 30 minutes of continuous exercise, and was successful in the use of the RPE scale. Because he made such significant gains in abilities, he was elected "valedictorian" of his graduating class. He was encouraged to continue his exercise regimen at home and was given the opportunity to join the open exercise program that meets every other week at the clinic. He became one of the most motivated and motivating participants in the open exercise program.

PATIENTS REQUIRING SPECIAL CONSIDERATION

At one time, the majority of patients referred for cardiac rehabilitation were those who were recovering from uncomplicated MIs. Currently, many patients who were once considered too unstable for cardiac rehabilitation are now being referred for cardiopulmonary rehabilitation services. Patients who are candidates for cardiopulmonary rehabilitation include those with angina pectoris, diabetes mellitus, peripheral vascular disease, restrictive pulmonary disease, pulmonary hypertension, exercise-induced bronchospasm, arthritis or other orthopedic limitations, heart transplantation, and compensated heart failure. Other candidates are elderly patients, those recovering from CABG, PTCA, or other revascularizations, and obese patients. In these and similar cases, the exercise prescription must be modified to enable the patient to adjust physiologically and psychologically to exercise therapy. This section briefly addresses guidelines for exercise therapy that are specific to patients that may need modification and/or special supervision during their exercise therapy sessions.

Angina Pectoris

Patients with stable angina are excellent candidates for exercise therapy. The object of the exercise therapy is to increase the functional capacity of the patient so that more physical exercise can be performed below the angina threshold. In this case, special consideration must be given to the ongoing evaluation of the angina, the extent of warm-up and cool-down periods, and the intensity of the cardiovascular endurance training period. Evaluation of the angina involves careful documentation of each episode as the patient describes it, according to the type of pain, the location of the pain, factors that may have precipitated an episode, and the methods used to relieve the pain. In addition, the clinician can usually observe and should record unique mannerisms or other subtle changes in coloring or demeanor exhibited by the patient during an episode. Ongoing evaluation of patients with stable angina is critical because any change in either the frequency or the intensity of the episodes warrants immediate medical investigation. Because of adverse hypotensive responses that may occur, careful observation is required of patients for whom prophylactic use of nitroglycerin or long-acting nitrates has been prescribed. During the exercise session, the patient's THR should remain approximately 10 to 15 beats below the anginal or ischemic threshold.[8,19,30]

Diabetes Mellitus

To prescribe exercise properly, the clinician must identify whether or not the patient has Type I (insulin-dependent) diabetes (IDDM) or Type II (non-insulin-dependent) diabetes (NIDDM). Type I diabetes is the result of a pancreatic deficiency in insulin production and the Type I diabetic must depend on regular administration of exogenous insulin. Type II diabetes is a complex disease characterized by increased insulin resistance and impaired insulin secretion. Type II diabetes affects nearly 20 percent of people 65 to 74 years of age and accounts for 90 to 95 percent of all cases of diabetes in the United States. Type II diabetes is usually diagnosed after age 40, is often associated with obesity, and is typically treated with dietary modification, exercise, oral hypoglycemic medication, and in some cases, exogenous insulin.[31–35]

Exercise programs are contraindicated for poorly controlled or uncontrolled diabetic patients, i.e., blood glucose values greater than 300 mg/dL.[32] The hypoglycemic effect of exercise is a major problem that exercising diabetics may encounter. This effect may occur as a result of the increased mobilization of depot insulin during exercise and may be exacerbated if the insulin injection site is in the exercising muscle. Because exercise creates an insulinlike effect, exercising diabetics may have to alter their insulin and carbohydrate (CHO) intake before exercise to avoid hypoglycemic events.[31] The risk of hypoglycemic events may be minimized if the following precautions are taken:

1. Blood glucose is monitored frequently if the patient is taking insulin or oral hypoglycemic agents.
2. The insulin dose is decreased (by 1 to 2 units as prescribed by the physician).
3. The diabetic patient exercises 1 to 2 hours following a meal.
4. When the blood glucose is below 100 mg/dL, the CHO intake should be increased approximately 30 grams (g) before exercising.
5. For each 30 to 60 minutes of moderate exercise the diabetic patient needs to ingest 10 to 15 g CHO as he or she exercises.
6. Insulin should be injected in an area such as the abdomen and not in actively exercising muscles.
7. The patient needs to be knowledgeable of the signs and symptoms of hypo- and hyperglycemia.
8. The diabetic patient needs to exercise with a partner.[31,32,36]

Generally, diabetic patients with cardiac disease can participate in the same modes of activity as nondiabetic patients with cardiac disease. However, special precautions must be taken when the patient is taking medications that potentiate exercise-induced hypoglycemia. For example, beta-blockers and other medications may reduce the patient's ability to perceive hypoglycemic symptoms.[31]

Type I diabetic patients should exercise daily, if possible, to assist in the maintenance of a regular pattern of diet and insulin dosage. Because the frequency of exercise is high, the duration may be decreased to 20 to 30 minutes. The intensity of the exercise session should be prescribed within the normal range (40 to 85 percent of functional capacity) and on the basis of HR. The diabetic patient with autonomic neuropathy, however, may demonstrate chronotropic insufficiency (altered HR response) during exercise. Such patients may also be unable to perceive angina or other symptoms of ischemia. Therefore, they must be carefully monitored, and the RPE methods (Chapter 11) may prove to be helpful in prescribing their exercise intensity.[37,38]

Type II diabetic patients should exercise 5 days per week, if possible, to enhance caloric expenditure. To assist in controlling body weight, the duration of exercise may be from 40 to 60 minutes. Because the frequency and duration of exercise for Type II patients are high, the intensity of the exercise should be maintained in lower to moderate end of the THR range.[32,37,38]

Diabetic patients should avoid exercising in excessive hot or cold environments. Patients with neuropathy have insensitive feet and should avoid exercises that involve running, a potentially traumatizing activity. Diabetic patients with active proliferative retinopathy, like all patients with cardiac disease, should avoid strenuous activities associated with Valsalva-like maneuvers. Proper footwear must be worn and the patient should be instructed to inspect his or her feet daily and after exercise.[32,37] Blood glucose levels should be monitored before exercise, during the first 30 minutes following exercise and may be necessary for 4 to 6 hours following the exercise.[38]

Peripheral Vascular Disease

Peripheral vascular disease (PVD) is an imprecise term indicating diseases of the arteries and veins of the extremities.[39] Other terms for various diseases of the extremities include peripheral arterial disease (PAD), arteriosclerosis obliterans (ASO), atherosclerosis obliterans, peripheral arterial occlusive disease, and similar diseases.[40] As used in this text, PVD is a generic term used to describe the muscle ischemia that results when a person with disease performs walking activities. The classic symptom of PVD is intermittent claudication, which presents as pain, cramping, or aching in the calf, thighs, and/or buttocks. Intermittent claudication is precipitated by walking and is relieved promptly by rest.[41,42]

The major goals of treatment include relieving the symptoms of intermittent claudication, improving functional capacity, and improvement in walking ability. Education for risk factor modification is especially important because cigarette smoking, diabetes mellitus, hyperlipidemia, and hypertension are major risk factors for PVD.[40-43] The subjective gradation of pain (Table 12–11) is a useful technique for evaluating the pain over a period of time and one method of measuring improvements in exercise tolerance. This technique also aids in writing the exercise prescription, when progressing the patient to higher work levels, and can be used as part of the outcome assessment for evaluating the efficacy of the cardiac rehabilitation program.

Patients with significant peripheral vascular disease are at a higher risk of having associated coronary and cerebral vascular disease than those without peripheral im-

TABLE 12-11 Subjective Gradation of Pain in Patients
with Peripheral Vascular Disease

Grade 1 Definite discomfort or pain but only of initial or modest level (established but minimal)
Grade 2 Moderate discomfort or pain from which the patient's attention can be diverted by a
         number of common stimuli (e.g., conversation)
Grade 3 Intense pain from which the patient's attention cannot be diverted (short of Grade 4)
Grade 4 Excruciating and unbearable pain

Source: From American College of Sports Medicine: ACSM's Guidelines for Exercise Testing and Prescription, ed 5. Williams & Wilkins, Baltimore, 1995, p 213, with permission.

pairment.[42] Therefore, an increase in resting systolic BP warrants significant reduction in the THR for the exercise session. Failure of BP to normalize justifies termination of an exercise therapy session. The patient with claudication may initially benefit from intermittent exercise but should be progressed to continuous low-level exercise as soon as it can be tolerated. Exercise therapy sessions should be increased in duration (to 60 minutes) at a low level before the intensity is increased. Initially, two exercise periods per day may be beneficial if each session is at least 20 minutes in length. Ideally, the mode of aerobic exercise should include as much walking as the patient can tolerate. Alternative activities suitable for the patient with intermittent claudication include cycling, rowing, and stair climbing.[8,40,42,44] A recent study has indicated that stair climbing may be safer than walking for claudication patients because similar levels of ischemia were found to occur at a lower cardiovascular demand.[44] More research into the long-term effects of this mode of activity on patients with PVD is needed.

Chronic Heart Failure

Chronic heart failure (CHF) is a complex syndrome of impaired ventricular function and restricted cardiac output that is characterized by an intolerance to low-level exercise which results in the clinical symptoms of fatigue and/or dyspnea. CHF is frequently a result of severe left ventricular dysfunction (LVD) and is often also referred to as congestive heart failure, although patients with stable chronic heart failure often do not show evidence of congestion in pulmonary or peripheral circulations.[45] Mortality from CHF increases with increasing age and it is estimated that 10 percent of the population over 75 years of age are afflicted with CHF.[45,46] Because of the high-risk status of LVD and CHF patients, at one time, they were excluded from cardiac rehabilitation programs. Recently, however, it has been determined that exercise training can have beneficial effects on patients with impaired ventricular function. As a result of cardiac rehabilitation, patients with CHF have been found to exhibit positive training effects including decreased resting heart rates, improved exercise performance, and an enhanced feeling of well-being.[45-48]

In addition to exercise training, the comprehensive rehabilitation program should include diet counseling, drug therapy, and frequent follow-up. Before exercise training, it is desirable for the patient with CHF to possess a functional capacity of at least 3 METs, and a left ventricular ejection fraction (LVEF) greater than 20 percent. If possible, the initial exercise evaluation should include direct measurement of $\dot{V}O_2$ since estimation of functional capacity from exercise time may be in error.[19,48]

Exercise training should be prescribed at the low end of the THRR or functional capacity (40 to 60 percent) and should begin with intermittent aerobic activity of 2 to 4 minutes of exercise followed by 1 to 2 minutes of rest. If tolerated, the initial cardiovascular exercise sessions should last for 10 to 15 minutes. According to patient response, the length of the exercise bouts can be gradually increased until a goal of 30 to 40 minutes of continuous exercise training can be tolerated.[19,48] Because HR response to exercise in the CHF patient may be impaired, frequent monitoring of BP and ECG combined with rating of perceived exertion (RPE) is important.[19,48] Depending on patient responses, frequency of training for the CHF patient should be 3 to 5 times per week. The CHF patient is likely to require at least 10 minutes of warm-up before each exercise session, and the duration of exercise should be increased before intensity.[48]

The clinician needs to be aware of signs and symptoms that indicate deterioration in cardiovascular status and worsening of CHF. These symptoms include a weight gain of 1 kg (~2 lb) or more within a 2-day period, increased heart rate and dyspnea, pulmonary edema as indicated by ascultation, and abnormal heart sounds (particularly S_3 gallop and regurgitant murmurs). If any of these symptoms occur, exercise should be terminated immediately and the patient should be referred for evaluation and treatment.[45] The patient with CHF is at risk for sudden death as a result of arrhythmias due primarily to ventricular tachycardia and ventricular fibrillation. Conditions that may precipitate these arrhythmias are hypokalemia, hypomagnesemia, and digoxin toxicity.[45]

Cardiac Transplantation

Five-year cardiac transplantation survival rates have been reported to be 72 percent.[49] In spite of the improved survival rates during the past few years, many patients with a heart transplant are not referred for cardiac rehabilitation because of potential limitations to exercise. These limitations include graft rejection, pulmonary hypertension, peripheral vascular and metabolic abnormalities, side effects of immunosuppressive drugs, and very low exercise tolerance following surgery.[50] However, patients who have engaged in cardiac rehabilitation programs have been shown to improve functional capacity, increase the duration of their ability to exercise, raise the anaerobic threshold, improve ventilatory responses to exercise, and increase peak heart rates.[46,50]

As a result of heart transplantation, the transplanted heart is no longer innervated by the autonomic system. Because the resting heart rate is no longer under vagal control, resting heart rates in patients with transplants are likely to be approximately 100 bpm. Humoral regulation becomes the primary physiologic mechanism for increasing the cardiac output which is necessary in response to exercise training.[19,49,50] The increase in cardiac output is a result of circulating catecholamines and the response to exercise in the patient with a transplant tends to be delayed and blunted. Because of higher resting heart rates and lower maximum heart rates, the heart rate range of the patient is approximately 40 to 50 bpm. Resting plasma lactate levels are higher and maximum lactate levels are lower in the transplanted patient compared with those observed in normal subjects. However, there seems to be an earlier onset of anaerobiosis in the patient with a transplant, and it is recommended that exercise therapy be prescribed at an intensity that does not cause significant elevations of blood lactate concentration.[49,50] Because heart rate responses during rest and exercise are atypical in the patient with a transplant, using an RPE of 12 to 14 and a MET level below the ventilatory threshold has been reported to be effective in establishing the initial exercise prescription intensity.[49-52] Duration of each exercise session depends on patient response, but can range between 30 and 60 minutes of intermittent or continuous aerobic activity performed 3 to 5 days per week. Modes chosen for the patient with a transplant are much the same as for other patients with cardiac conditions and include walking, cycling, rowing, stair-stepping, and perhaps walk-jogging.[8,50] Longer periods of warm-up and cool-down are also recommended.[19]

The clinician responsible for the rehabilitation of the patient with a heart transplant should be aware of, and monitor the side effects of, the immunosuppressive drug regimen that the patient with a transplant must follow. Cyclosporin causes hypertension and prednisone has a number of side effects, including sodium and fluid retention, loss of muscle mass, glucose intolerance, osteoporosis, redistribution of fat from extremities to torso, gastric irritation, increased appetite, ulcers, increased susceptibility to infection, and increased excretion of potassium. The clinician must also be alert to organ rejection (as indicated by biopsy scores) and terminate exercise sessions until the condition is reversed.[19]

Restrictive Pulmonary Disease

Restrictive disease creates an inability to adequately increase minute ventilation in response to increasing workload. The result is oxygen desaturation with exercise. This patient population should be referred for pulmonary rehabilitation. The benefits of a pulmonary rehabilitation program can be produced in such patients as well as in those with obstructive pulmonary disease. The use of oximetry can help ensure the safety of exercise intensity in patients with restrictive lung disease. The use of RPE also is important in this group of patients for monitoring exercise intensity.

PULMONARY HYPERTENSION

Patients who present with pulmonary hypertension often have a relatively fixed cardiac output. Therefore, with the onset of exercise, dyspnea, fatigue, and syncope can occur. Exercise must be tailored to low intensity levels and monitored by HR, BP, and oximetry. The benefits of exercise training in this population are, as yet, not encouraging, but judicious use of exercise in these patients is justified. Breathing retraining, energy-saving techniques, pacing, education, and group support are of undeniable benefit to this group.

EXERCISE-INDUCED BRONCHOSPASM

Exercise-induced bronchospasm (EIB) usually occurs 6 to 8 minutes after the onset of high levels of continuous exercise. The exercising environment is particularly important to patients with EIB. Cold air, low humidity, and pollutants can exacerbate their symptoms. By minimizing the potential hazards, exercise can be accomplished. The appropriate use of warm-up activities is necessary to decrease possible bronchospasm. Bronchodilators administered before exercise may help prevent exercise-induced bronchoconstriction. Swimming is the aerobic exercise of choice for patients with EIB because of its controlled environment, availability, and aerobic nature. (For more information on EIB, see Chapter 6.)

Osteoarthritis and Orthopedic Limitations

Osteoarthritis is a degenerative disease affecting the weight-bearing joints, especially the knee. It has been estimated that 33 percent of the adult population over the age of 63 have osteoarthritis of the knee, and the incidence of the disease is 3 times more prevalent in older women than in older men.[53,54] To date, there are no treatments that affect the underlying disease process and therapy usually includes medication and surgical procedures designed to relieve the pain. Recently, reports indicate that exercise training, which includes aerobic activity, muscular strength training, and flexibility exercises, can improve the pain and disability associated with osteoarthritis of the knee.[55] Exercise that produces excessive stress on osteoarthritic or injured joints should be avoided and the exercise prescription should emphasize exercises to increase range of joint motion, muscular strength, and functional capacity. Activities that place stress on weight-bearing joints during periods of inflammation are contraindicated. Initially, intermittent, low-intensity cardiovascular exercise characterized by short bouts of exercise and rest intervals appears to be tolerated better than continuous exercise in orthopedically limited patients. Nutrition counseling and education for weight management is also indicated for the patient with cardiac disease who is overweight.[56]

Obesity

Obesity is highly correlated with primary risk factors for disease, including hypertension, hyperlipidemia, diabetes mellitus, and CHD. Reductions in body fat have been shown to produce beneficial effects on risk factors for CHD, and the obese patient with cardiac disease should be counseled initially as to nutrition and weight management interventions and long-term follow-up for weight maintenance and lifestyle modification should be provided by the rehabilitation staff.[57,58] In most cases, because moderate exercise can be sustained for long periods of time, exercise therapy for the obese patient should be of long duration (maximum of 60 minutes) and low intensity to avoid stressing the weight-bearing joints.[31] Exercise intensity can be prescribed by THR, but a recent study has reported that, for the obese patient, the formula for predicting maximum heart rate should be as follows:[59]

$$\text{Predicted maximum heart rate} = 200 - 0.5 \times \text{Age}$$

Once the predicted maximum heart rate is calculated, it can be used in conventional methods to predict target heart rate range (see Chapter 11).

ENVIRONMENTAL CONSIDERATIONS

In addition to the exercise therapy session, selected patients should be encouraged to exercise at home, and once a patient has "graduated" from the formal exercise program, he or she is likely to continue the exercise regimens at home. As part of a comprehensive rehabilitation program, it is important to teach patients how to palpate their own pulses, to appropriately self-monitor their exercise, and to rate their perceived exertions. It is also important to educate the patient about the effects that various environmental factors may have on their ability to exercise. Major environmental concerns are extremes in temperature and humidity. Altitude and air pollution are major factors for patients with pulmonary disease and should be discussed with patients who exercise regularly in areas where the air quality is poor and/or the altitude is high.

Heat

When ambient temperatures range between 40° and 75°F and the humidity is 65 percent or below, conditions are generally recognized as favorable for exercise. In hot weather, however, the body temperature rises faster than usual during exercise and extra precautions must be observed. The harmful effect of higher temperatures is exacerbated by increases in relative humidity. In an environment of high heat and high humidity, the body struggles to dissipate heat and to cool itself. The natural cooling of the body through the evaporation of sweat is ineffective in an environment in which the humidity is high. As the core temperature rises the following increases are noted: heart rate, absolute stroke volume, blood flow to the skin, venous compliance, core temperature, body temperature, and sweating. Factors that decrease in response to increased heat and humidity are stroke volume, splanchnic blood flow, renal blood flow, urine production, central blood volume, plasma volume, and total body water.[60]

It has been estimated that the heart rate during exercise increases 1 to 1.5 bpm for every increase in temperature above 25°C (~75°F). In a hot and wet environment (high humidity), the increase is approximately 3.5 bpm. One advantage of using a THR to establish exercise intensity is that, during conditions of high heat and high humidity, the heart rate will increase because of the environmental conditions. To stay within the appropriate THRR, the exercising individual will have to decrease the intensity of the exercise.[60,61] For safety, it is important to teach patients to palpate their heart rates and to be competent in self-monitoring intensity of exercise. Patients should be instructed as to the best time of day to exercise, how to avoid excessive heat and humidity, the appropriate clothing to wear, and the signs and symptoms of heat intolerance (e.g., chills, lightheadedness, dizziness, nausea, and so forth).[61]

Cold

Exposure to cold temperatures results in peripheral vasoconstriction (increased peripheral resistance), which produces an increase in arterial BP. Because of the increased myocardial demand during exercise and the increased peripheral resistance caused by exposure to cold, the exercising patient with cardiac disease may reach ischemic threshold more rapidly and consequently may experience anginal pain. Activities performed in a cold environment that involve the upper body increase metabolic demand and are not recommended for the patient with CHD (e.g., shoveling snow). Because of the decrease in the angina threshold, patients should be instructed not to perform high-intensity activity in a cold environment.[62]

Cold also affects the pulmonary patient in the form of cold-induced bronchospasm. The cold air that reaches the tracheobronchial tree causes bronchoconstriction, which makes exercise difficult and unpleasant. Wearing a scarf around the nose and mouth provides a reservoir of warmed air. However, indoor exercise via stationary bicycle, treadmill, or ambulation in a mall may prove to be more advantageous for patients with cardiac and pulmonary disease.

Although ischemic responses are related to extremes in temperature and humidity, the same responses have been observed in cardiac patients at rest and when there were only moderate changes in temperature.[62,63] All patients should be educated as to the dangers associated with exposure to extremes in temperature. It should also be emphasized that, in addition to awareness of ambient temperature extremes during exercise, the effects of temperature extremes in all aspects of daily living should be buffered. This includes taking precautions when bathing and showering, going from air-conditioned buildings or cars into extreme heat (and vice versa), and drinking very cold or hot beverages. Patients should also be informed of the appropriate clothing to wear in cold weather.

MOTIVATION, COMPLIANCE, AND PSYCHOSOCIAL ISSUES

The goals of outpatient rehabilitation programs are to develop the best possible comprehensive prescribed therapeutic regimen for each patient and to enhance compliance with that regimen once the desired patient outcomes have been attained. For the rehabilitation program to be successful, patients must adhere to their programs for months and years following the termination of the formal program. All efforts must be made for follow-up and to have the patient understand the factors involved with compliant behavior, and plans must be made to incorporate successful strategies whenever and wherever possible.

Data concerning compliance to established exercise regimens are somewhat confusing. Some have reported that compliance to cardiac rehabilitation exercise programs is 80 percent for the first 3 months, approximately 60 percent at 12 months, and only about 50 percent for long-term treatment regimens.[46,64,65] Other data obtained from long-term follow-up of cardiac rehabilitation programs indicate that noncompliance may be as low as 20 percent over 5 years and as high as 90 percent with "heavy exercise" after 6 to 9 years.[66] Long-term compliance to the exercise component of the rehabilitation seems to be the result of educating patients as to why and how they should exercise and motivating them to adhere to the exercise regimen.[18] Most likely, the questions that remain regarding compliance and motivation will be answered through future research in this area.

Instructional Staff

The key to the success of any program is the competence of the instructional staff. The clinicians responsible for comprehensive rehabilitation programs must have a thorough and accurate knowledge of exercise physiology and the principles of assessment and exercise prescription. They must promote the educational components of rehabilitation and address the psychosocial status and needs of the patients. Many of the techniques used to motivate patients are simple and almost instinctive to individuals who are sincere in their desire to help others achieve outcomes to which they themselves are dedicated. The instructional staff must provide positive role models for the patients and must always maintain an enthusiastic attitude toward exercise and other lifestyle changes. This type of behavior reinforces patients' attitudes toward the rehabilitative process. They perceive that the changes they are making in their exercise and other habits can and must be a lifetime commitment.

Improving patient compliance involves breaking down barriers to compliance and motivating patient compliance by reinforcing, extrinsically and intrinsically, positive health behaviors. The methods used to achieve these goals are not only educational but also behavioral.

EDUCATIONAL TECHNIQUES

Education can be provided in a number of formal and informal situations. The types of educational experience provided by the rehabilitation program will be limited by the staff, facilities, and location of the program. The types of experience that might be provided include patient education manuals (written at the appropriate reading level), informal patient education sessions (discussions before, during, and after exercise therapy sessions, bulletin boards), and formal patient education (lectures and individual counseling sessions with or without spouse). Recommended lecture topics for the cardiac and/or pulmonary patient are given in Tables 12–12 and 12–13.

BEHAVIORAL TECHNIQUES

At one time, behavioral therapy focused on changing behavior and relied primarily on classical conditioning responses (Pavlovian) to elicit behavior change. Currently, models of behavior change, as used in health care, have also focused on the importance of social and cognitive factors. Social learning theory depicts human functioning related to behavioral, cognitive, and environmental factors.[67] To effect behavior change, social learning theory stresses the importance of self-efficacy or self-confidence because people are not likely to undertake behavior changes when they lack confidence that they will succeed. The following four factors have been found to influence self-efficacy:[67]

1. Information and persuasion. The role that health care professionals play in disseminating information and creating positive and realistic expectations as to the rate,

TABLE 12–12 Weekly Lecture Topics
for Cardiac Rehabilitation Programs

Risk Factors Associated with CHD
Anatomy and Physiology of the Heart: What Is a Heart
  Attack?
Angina: What Is Chest Pain?
Relation of Diet to Heart Disease
Human Sexuality and Heart Disease
Diet and Weight Management
Stress and Stress Management
Cigarette Smoking in Relation to Heart Disease
Medications Used in the Management of Heart Disease
  and Their Relationships to Exercise

Source: Adapted from the Cardiac Rehabilitation Program, Northeastern University, Boston, Mass.

**TABLE 12–13 Weekly Lecture Topics
for Pulmonary
Rehabilitation Programs**

Anatomy and Physiology of Respiratory Disease
Chronic Obstructive Pulmonary Disease (COPD)
Pulmonary Hygiene Techniques
Effects of Exercise
Nutrition and Pulmonary Disease
Energy-Saving Techniques
Stress Management and Relaxation
Smoking and Environmental Factors
Psychosocial Aspects of COPD
Diagnostic Techniques
General Management of COPD
Community Services
Film: *I Am Joe's Lung*
Signs and Symptoms of Pneumonia

Source: Adapted from the Pulmonary Rehabilitation Program
at Massachusetts Respiratory Hospital, Braintree, Mass.

magnitude, and effect of change is of paramount importance in behavior modification.

2. Observation of others. Lifestyle change is often a result of watching others, and rehabilitation staff members must be positive role models for their patients.

3. Successful performance of the behavior. Because patients are more likely to remember their failures, behavior modification programs often ask them to describe their previous attempts of changing a behavior (e.g., quitting smoking) to determine what they can do differently the next time.

4. Physiologic feedback. Daily documentation of patient exercise sessions can provide positive feedback to the patient because it is easy for the staff to point out increases in functional capacity, weight management, and other parameters included in each patient's exercise session. The post-GXT counseling and frequent follow-up can also have a strong influence on a patient's self-efficacy, behavior, and compliance with rehabilitation regimens.

PSYCHOSOCIAL VARIABLES, QUALITY-OF-LIFE ISSUES, AND OUTCOMES

Psychosocial variables have a great impact on patient compliance with the rehabilitation regimen and patient quality of life (QOL). The psychologic status and well-being of a patient include mood, anxiety, depression, and emotional well-being. Assessments of self-esteem, thoughts relating to the future, and feelings about personal relationships and critical life events can be used to indicate patient psychologic status and well-being.[68]

Social interactions and role functions indicate the patient's ability to assume person-to-person interactions basic to communal living. Assessments of patient interaction with family, friends, work associates, and the surrounding community are important in determining the social status of a patient.[68]

Ideally, assessment of psychosocial issues occurs during an acute cardiac illness so that patients at high risk for psychosocial complications can be given appropriate interventions. Identification of psychosocial difficulties (particularly adverse mood alterations) following the acute cardiac episode and/or delay in providing exercise rehabilitation has been associated with decreased benefits from exercise training.[69]

Assessing QOL includes not only psychosocial assessment but evaluations of physical functional status. QOL is a multidimensional concept that describes an individual's functional abilities, symptoms and their consequences, and the way in which a person feels and functions. Measurements of QOL are valuable for evaluating the effects or outcomes of cardiopulmonary rehabilitation programs.[70] Common outcomes following cardiac rehabilitation include survival, return to work, smoking cessation and other risk factor modifications, improvement in functional capacity, and improvement in QOL. Table 12–14 illustrates the health, clinical, and behavioral outcomes that may be assessed after cardiac rehabilitation intervention (see also Chapter 1). Several tools for assessing outcomes of cardiac rehabilitation programs are provided elsewhere,[68] and guidelines for rehabilitation staff members to construct their own questionnaires for assessing quality of life in cardiovascular disease are also available.[71]

It is obvious that the rehabilitation staff must carefully document patient status and progress in cardiopulmonary programs as a basis for outcomes assessment. All exercise therapy should be quantified in terms of work (e.g., METs, distance, speed), pa-

TABLE 12–14 Outcome Domains

Health	Clinical	Behavioral
I. Mortality	I. Physical	I. Medical regime
II. Morbidity	A. Weight	II. Diet
III. Quality of life	B. Blood pressure	III. Exercise
	C. Lipids	IV. Smoking cessation
	D. Oxygenation	V. Breathing retraining
	E. Functional capacity	VI. Relaxation skills
	F. Blood nicotine levels	VII. Social skills
	G. Blood medication levels	VIII. Recognition of impending
	1. Theophylline	complications
	2. Digoxin	
	H. Symptom management	
	1. Cough	
	2. Dyspnea	
	3. Angina	
	II. Psychosocial	
	A. Interpersonal function and dysfunction	
	B. Psychological status	
	C. Return to vocation and avocation independent living	
	III. Medical utilization	
	A. Medication usage	
	B. Hospitalization	
	C. Physician/emergency room visits	

Source: From American Association of Cardiovascular and Pulmonary Rehabilitation. Guidelines for Cardiac Rehabilitation Programs, ed 2. Human Kinetics, Champaign, 1995, p 74. Used by permission.

tient responses to exercise (e.g., heart rates, blood pressures, SAO_2), support measures (e.g., use of supplemental O_2, nitroglycerin), and adverse signs and symptoms (pain, arrhythmias). All communication with physicians, other health care professionals, and families that may affect patient outcomes should also be documented. Finally, a discharge summary should describe the course of treatment, the outcomes, and future plans for the patient.[68]

SUMMARY

Detailed case studies on two patients with cardiovascular disease and two patients with pulmonary disease have been presented to help the clinician better understand the principles relative to THR and RPE and the application of those principles to the daily cardiac and pulmonary exercise therapy session. Examples of readjustments in the exercise prescription based on feedback obtained from the exercise session (e.g., blood pressure, medication changes, oxygen saturation of the blood) have been included. These examples will alert the clinician to the necessity for periodic adjustments to the THR or RPE when individual physiologic measurements seem to be atypical. Additional modifications of the exercise prescription may be necessary for patients with cardiopulmonary disease who also have angina pectoris, diabetes mellitus, peripheral vascular disease, orthopedic limitations, and/or obesity. Guidelines for exercise prescription for patients with heart transplantation, left ventricular dysfunction, restrictive pulmonary disease, pulmonary hypertension, and exercise-induced bronchospasm are also included.

Initially, high-risk and selected intermediate-risk patients should be monitored continuously. Rhythm strips should be obtained during each exercise session for patients with cardiovascular complications. Continuous monitoring can be tapered to intermittent monitoring as the patient progresses. All patients should be instructed as to the effects of environmental extremes on HR and BP responses. They should be taught to palpate their own pulses and rate their perceived exertions so they can progress from Phase II to Phase III and then to home exercise safely. Suggestions for maintaining patient compliance with the established rehabilitation regimen include educational and behavioral techniques and the impact that psychosocial issues have on QOL, compliance and outcomes. Outcome measurement of rehabilitation intervention is important for the survival and future of cardiopulmonary rehabilitation.

REFERENCES

1. Hall, LK and Gettmen, LR: Policies and procedures in P&R programs. ACSM's Resource Manual for Guidelines for Exercise Testing and Prescription, ed 2. Lea & Febiger, Philadelphia, 1993, pp 562–569.
2. Wenger, NK et al: Cardiac Rehabilitation as Secondary Prevention. Clinical Practice Guideline. Quick Reference Guide for Clinicians, No. 17, Rockville, Md: U.S. Department of Health and Human Services, Public Health Service, Agency for Health Care Policy and Research and National Heart, Lung, and Blood Institute. AHCPR Pub. No. 96-0672. October, 1995.
3. Balady, GJ and Weiner, DA: Risk stratification in cardiac rehabilitation. J Cardpulm Rehabil 11(1):39–45, 1991.
4. American Association of Cardiovascular and Pulmonary Rehabilitation: Guidelines for Cardiac Rehabilitation Programs, ed 2. Human Kinetics, Champaign, 1995, pp 1–26.
5. Pashkow, FJ: Issues in contemporary cardiac rehabilitation: A historical perspective. J Am Coll Cardiol 21(3):822–834, 1993.
6. Leon, AS et al: Position paper of the American Association of Cardiovascular and Pulmonary Rehabilita-

tion. Scientific evidence of the value of cardiac rehabilitation services with emphasis on patients follow-ing myocardial infarction—Section I: Exercise conditioning component. J Cardpulm Rehabil 10(3): 79–87, 1990.

7. Hall, LK: Guidelines for cardiac rehabilitation: 1987 to 1990. J Cardpulm Rehabil 11(2):79–83, 1991.
8. Pollock, ML, Welsch, MA, and Graves, JE: Exercise prescription for cardiac rehabilitation. In: Pollock, ML and Schmidt, DH (eds): Heart Disease and Rehabilitation, ed 3. Human Kinetics, Champaign, 1995, pp 243–276.
9. Parmley, WW: Position report on cardiac rehabilitation: Recommendations of the American College of Cardiology. J Am Coll Cardiol 7(2):451–453, 1986.
10. American College of Sports Medicine: ACSM's Guidelines for Exercise Testing and Prescription, ed 5. Williams & Wilkins, Baltimore, 1995, pp 177–193.
11. American Association of Cardiovascular and Pulmonary Rehabilitation: op cit, p 94.
12. Herbert, WG and Herbert, DL. Legal considerations. In: Pollock, ML and Schmidt, DH (eds): Heart Disease and Rehabilitation, ed 3. Human Kinetics, Champaign, 1995, pp 433–439.
13. Herbert, DL and Herbert, WG. Medicolegal aspects of rehabilitation of the coronary patient. In: Wenger, NK and Hellerstein, HK (eds): Rehabilitation of the Coronary Patient, ed 3. Churchill Livingstone, New York, 1992, pp 566–580.
14. American Thoracic Society: Definitions, epidemiology, pathology, diagnosis, and staging. Am J Respir Crit Care Med 152:S78–S110, 1995.
15. American Thoracic Society: Evaluation of impairment/disability secondary to pulmonary disorders. American Review of Respiratory Diseases 133:1205–1209, 1986.
16. Reis, A: Position paper of the American Association of Cardiovascular and Pulmonary Rehabilitation. J Cardpulm Rehabil 10:418–441, 1990.
17. Berra, K: Cardiac and pulmonary rehabilitation: Historic and future needs. J Cardpulm Rehabil 11:8–15, 1991.
18. Franklin, BA et al: Hospital and home-based cardiac rehabilitation outpatient programs. In: Pollock, ML and Schmidt, DH (eds): Rehabilitation of the Coronary Patient, ed 3. Churchill Livingstone, New York, 1995, pp 209–227.
19. American College of Sports Medicine: Guidelines for Exercise Testing and Prescription, ed 4. Lea & Febiger, Philadelphia, 1991, pp 121–159.
20. Stamford, B: A stretching Primer. The Physician and Sportsmedicine 22(9):85–86, 1994.
21. Stamford, B. How to warm up and cool down your workout. The Physician and Sportsmedicine 23(9): 97–98, 1995.
22. American College of Sports Medicine: ACSM's Guidelines for Exercise Testing and Prescription, ed 5. Williams & Wilkins, Baltimore, 1995, pp 153–176.
23. Franklin, BA et al: Exercise and cardiac complications. The Physician and Sportsmedicine 22(2):56–68, 1994.
24. Franklin, BA et al: Resistance training in cardiac rehabilitation. J Cardpulm Rehabil 11(2):75–77, 1991.
25. Stralow, CR, Ball, TE, and Looney, M: Acute cardiovascular responses of patients with coronary disease to dynamic variable resistance exercise of different intensities. J Cardpulm Rehabil 13(4):255–263, 1993.
26. American Association of Cardiovascular and Pulmonary Rehabilitation: op cit, pp 27–56.
27. Squires, RW et al: Cardiovascular rehabilitation: Status, 1990. Mayo Clin Proc 65:731–755, 1990.
28. Temes, WC: Cardiac rehabilitation. In: Hillegass, EA and Sadowsky, HS (eds): Essentials of Cardiopul-monary Physical Therapy. Saunders, Philadelphia, 1994, pp 633–675.
29. Karvonen, M, Kentala, K, and Mustala, O. The effects of training on heart rate: A longitudinal study. An-nales Medicinae Experimentalis et Biologiae Fenniae 35:307, 1957.
30. American Association of Cardiovascular and Pulmonary Rehabilitation: op cit, pp 103–109.
31. American College of Sports Medicine: op cit, pp 206–219.
32. Gordon, NF: Exercise guidelines for patients with non-insulin dependent diabetes mellitus: An update. J Cardpulm Rehabil 14(4):217–220, 1994.
33. Helmrich, SP, Ragland, DR, and Paffenbarger, RS: Prevention of non-insulin dependent diabetes mellitus with physical activity. Med Sci Sports Exerc 26(7):824–930, 1994.
34. Kriska, AM, Blair, SN, and Pereira, MA: The potential role of physical activity in the prevention of non-insulin dependent diabetes mellitus: The epidemiological evidence. In: Holloszy, JO (eds): Exercise and Sport Sciences Reviews, Vol 22. Williams & Wilkins, Baltimore, 1994, pp 121–143.
35. Maki, KC, Abraira, C, and Cooper, RS: Arguments in favor of screening for diabetes in cardiac rehabilita-tion. J Cardpulm Rehabil 15(2):97–102, 1995.
36. Potera, C. When to eat. The Physician and Sportsmedicine 21(11):87–91, 1993.
37. American College of Sports Medicine: Guidelines for Exercise Testing and Prescription, ed 4. Lea & Febiger, Philadelphia, 1991, pp 161–186.
38. Hanson, P: Diabetic patients. In: Pollock, ML and Schmidt, DH (eds): Heart Disease and Rehabilitation, ed 3. Human Kinetics, Champaign, 1995, pp 357–365.
39. Thomas, CL (ed): Taber's Cyclopedic Medical Dictionary, ed 17. FA Davis, Philadelphia, 1993.
40. Hirsch, AT and Munnings, F: Intermittent claudication. The Physician and Sportsmedicine 21(6): 125–138, 1993.

41. Allen, RC and Smith, RB: Diseases of the peripheral arteries and veins. In: Schlant, RC and Alexander, RW (eds): Hurst's The Heart, ed 8. McGraw-Hill, New York, 1995, pp 381–388.
42. Regensteiner, JG, and Hiatt, WR: Exercise rehabilitation for patients with peripheral arterial disease. In: Holloszy, JO (ed): Exercise and Sport Sciences Reviews, Volume 23, Williams & Wilkins, Baltimore, 1995, pp 1–24.
43. Williams, LR et al: Vascular rehabilitation: Benefits of a structured exercise/risk modification program. J Vasc Surg 14:320–326, 1991.
44. Gardner, AW et al: Stair climbing elicits a lower cardiovascular demand than walking in claudication patients. J Cardpulm Rehabil 15(2):134–142, 1995.
45. Hanson, P: Exercise testing and training in patients with chronic heart failure. Med Sci Sports Exerc 26(5):527–537, 1994.
46. Balady, GJ et al: AHA medical/scientific position statement: Cardiac rehabilitation programs. Circulation 90(3):1602–1610, 1994.
47. Kavanaugh, T: Cardiac rehabilitation. In: Goldberg, L and Elliot, DL (eds): Exercise for Prevention and Treatment of Disease. FA Davis, Philadelphia, 1994, pp 48–75.
48. Normandin, EA et al: A comparison or conventional versus anaerobic threshold exercise prescription methods in subjects with left ventricular dysfunction. J Cardpulm Rehabil 13(2):110–116, 1993.
49. Brubaker, PH et al: Relationship of lactate and ventilatory thresholds in cardiac transplant patients. Med Sci Sports Exerc 25(2):191–196, 1993.
50. Badenhop, DT: Therapeutic role of exercise in patients with orthotopic heart transplant. Med Sci Sports Exerc 27(7):975–985, 1995.
51. Ehrman, J et al: Ventilatory threshold after exercise training in orthotopic heart transplant recipients. J Cardpulm Rehabil 12(2):126–130, 1992.
52. Shephard, RJ et al: Kinetics of the transplanted heart. J Cardpulm Rehabil 15(4):288–296, 1995.
53. Messier, SP: Osteoarthritis of the knee: an interdisciplinary perspective. Med Sci Sports Exerc 26(12):1427–1428, 1994.
54. Martin, DF: Pathomechanics of knee osteoarthritis. Med Sci Sports Exerc 26(12):1429–1434, 1994.
55. Ettinger, WH and Afable, RF: Physical disability from knee osteoarthritis: The role of exercise as an intervention. Med Sci Sports Exerc 26(12):1435–1440, 1994.
56. Messier, SP: Osteoarthritis of the knee and asociated factors of age and obesity: Effects on gait. Med Sci Sports Exerc 26(12):1446–1452, 1994.
57. Ballor, DL, Harvey-Berino, J, and Ades, PA: A healthy lifestyle is the treatment of choice for obesity in coronary patients. J Cardpulm Rahabil 15(1):14–18, 1995.
58. Perri, MG: Confronting the maintenance problem in the treatment of obesity. J Cardpulm Rehabil 13(3):164–266, 1993.
59. Miller, WC, Wallace, JP, and Eggert, KE. Predicting max HR and the HR-VO relationship for exercise prescription in obesity. Med Sci Sports Exerc 25(9):1077–1081, 1993.
60. Folinsbee, LJ: Heat and air pollution. In: Pollock, ML and Schmidt, DH (eds): Heart Disease and Rehabilitation, ed 3. Human Kinetics, Champaign, 1995, pp 327–342.
61. American College of Sports Medicine: ACSM's Guidelines for Exercise Testing and Prescription, ed 5. Williams & Wilkins, Baltimore, 1995, pp 288–296.
62. Pandolf, KB and Young, AJ: Altitude and cold. In: Pollock, ML and Schmidt, DH (eds): Heart Disease and Rehabilitation, ed 3. Human Kinetics, Champaign, 1995, pp 309–326.
63. Emmett, JD: A review of heart rate and blood pressure responses in the cold in healthy subjects and coronary artery disease patients. J Cardpulm Rehabil 15(1):19–24, 1995.
64. Burkett, PA: Practical issues for increasing exercise adherence. J Cardpulm Rehabil 12(1):18–19, 1992.
65. Vidmar, PM and Rubinson, L: The relationship between self-efficacy and exercise compliance in a cardiac population. J Cardpulm Rehabil 14(4):246–254, 1994.
66. Oldridge, NB: Patient compliance. In: Pollock, ML and Schmidt, DH (eds): Heart Disease and Rehabilitation, ed 3. Human Kinetics, Champaign, 1995, pp 393–404.
67. Miller, NH and Taylor, CB: Behavior modification for cardiovascular risk factor reduction. In: Pollock, ML and Schmidt, DH (eds): Heart Disease and Rehabilitation, ed 3. Human Kinetics, Champaign, 1995, pp 161–168.
68. American Association of Cardiovascular and Pulmonary Rehabilitation: op cit, pp 57–102.
69. Wenger, NK: Future directions in cardiac rehabilitation. In: Pollock, ML and Schmidt, DH (eds): Heart Disease and Rehabilitation, ed 3. Human Kinetics, Champaign, 1995, pp 447–453.
70. Loose, MS and Fernhall, B: Differences in quality of life among male and female cardiac rehabilitation participants. J Cardpulm Rehabil 15(3):225–231, 1995.
71. Guyatt, G et al: Assessing quality of life in cardiovascular disease: A general approach and an example in patients with myocardial infarction. Quality of Life in Cardiovascular Care 83:304–318, 1986.

CHAPTER 13

Risk Factor Modification

Although the rate of deaths from coronary heart disease (CHD) has decreased during the past 30 years, CHD remains the leading cause of premature death and disability in the United States and coronary artery disease (CAD) is the major factor in deaths caused by CHD.[1,2] High-technology care has increased the survival rates of patients with acute cardiac disease, but it has also increased the costs of medical care.[3] In an effort to reduce health care costs, more emphasis is being placed on primary and secondary prevention of CHD.[3,4] Primary and secondary prevention programs for CHD emphasize modification of cardiovascular disease risk factors through positive lifestyle changes. Current research indicates that positive lifestyle changes that modify the risk for CHD have reduced the rates of mortality and morbidity and are important behavioral approaches to the primary and secondary prevention of CHD.[5-23]

The American Heart Association (AHA) has identified risk factors that are believed to be directly associated with atherogenesis or to bring about a cardiovascular event. These major risk factors include heredity, age, male gender, smoking, hypertension, elevated blood cholesterol, and physical inactivity. Heredity, age, and male gender are classified as nonmodifiable risk factors, and smoking, hypertension, elevated blood cholesterol, and physical inactivity are considered to be modifiable risk factors. Factors that are believed to contribute to the risk of CHD are diabetes mellitus (Chapter 12), obesity (Chapter 12), and excess emotional stress.[23,24] In some cases these have been classified as major risk factors rather than factors contributing to risk.[25,26] It is not the purpose of this chapter to establish whether a risk factor directly or indirectly influences risk, but to discuss the factors that have been established as major risks. Increasing evidence supports the concept that cessation of smoking, control of blood pressure, decreases in plasma lipids, and regular physical activity are not only important factors in primary and secondary prevention but are also useful interventions and may promote the regression of CHD and prolong life.[8,13,16,20,22,27-36] Consequently, the purpose of the chapter is to discuss the major modifiable risk factors as determined by the AHA, as they are the factors that must be modified if CHD patients are to function as optimally as possible and reduce their risk of recurrent cardiovascular events.

CIGARETTE SMOKING

In the United States, cigarette smoking has been identified as the number one cause of preventable death and accounts for more than one in every six deaths, or over 400,000 deaths annually.[1] Over 115,000 of these deaths are caused by smoking-related CHDs and 27,500 are caused by cerebrovascular disease.[37,38] Smoking is also responsible for over 130,000 deaths related to cancer.[38] In adult men, smoking accounts for approximately 90 percent of all deaths from cancer of the lung, trachea, and bronchus. Smoking also accounts for approximately 60,000 deaths annually from chronic obstructive pulmonary disease (COPD), chronic bronchitis, and emphysema[38] (Chapter 14).

In a recent study to assess mortality from chronic disease in the United States, nine risk factors were examined singularly for their contribution to deaths from nine different diseases. Of all excess deaths, 33 percent were attributable to cigarette smoking.[39] The numbers and proportions of deaths attributable to risk factors for various chronic diseases are presented in Table 13–1.

People who smoke one pack or more of cigarettes a day have twice the number of heart attacks as nonsmokers. They also experience a 70 percent greater level of CHD risk and three times the rate of sudden death. People who smoke two or more packs of cigarettes a day have four times the number of coronary events as nonsmokers and a CAD mortality twice as high.[1,40] Although more research is needed, people exposed to passive smoking (sidestream or involuntary smoking) have also been shown to have higher rates of death due to CAD.[1] Passive smoking accounts for an estimated 3800 nonsmoker deaths from lung cancer each year.[38]

Although the prevalence of smoking has declined considerably in the United States in the past 25 years, the decline has been less pronounced in women than in men.[41,42] Women are also more likely than men to smoke the "low-yield" brands of cigarettes because they believe them to be safer than other kinds of cigarettes, but studies indicate that women who smoke low-yield cigarettes have virtually the same risk of myocardial infection (MI) as women who smoke the higher-yield brands.[41] Despite the recent decreases in the number of smokers, nearly one-third of all adults in the United States continue to smoke.[42] Cigarette smoking is currently more common among blacks and people of low socioeconomic status.[37,38,42]

Pathophysiologic Effects

Approximately 4000 compounds have been identified in cigarette smoke, including some that are pharmacologically active, toxic, carcinogenic, or antigenic.[1] The inhalation of cigarette smoke produces a number of cardiovascular responses in healthy subjects such as increases in both systolic and diastolic blood pressure, heart rate, and vasoconstriction of peripheral vessels. Nicotine appears to be the agent producing these responses through stimulation of the sympathetic nervous system, which in turn results in local and systemic catecholamine release.[43] These cardiovascular responses cause increases in myocardial oxygen demand that may exacerbate angina pectoris, induce ventricular ectopy, and evoke sudden death.[1,43]

The carbon monoxide in cigarette smoke has also been found to be a major contributor to CAD. Carbon monoxide bonds to hemoproteins such as hemoglobin, myoglobin, and cytochrome oxidase. On the average, the cigarette smoker has a fivefold increase in the carboxyhemoglobin level as compared with the nonsmoker. Carboxyhemoglobin is

TABLE 13-1 Numbers of Deaths and Proportions of Deaths (%) Attributable to Risk Factors for Nine Chronic Diseases*

Risk Factor	Coronary Heart Disease	Stroke	Obstructive Pulmonary Disease	Lung Cancer	Cervical Cancer	Breast Cancer	Colorectal Cancer	Cirrhosis	Diabetes	Total
Total no. deaths	593,111	149,204	71,099	125,511	4,543	40,534	55,811	26,151	37,178	1,103,142
Current/former smoking, %	148,879 (25.1)	35,931 (25.1)	57,791 (81.3)	108,164 (86.2)	1,443 (31.8)				9,703 (26.1)	361,911 (32.8)
Cholesterol level ≥5.20 mmol/L, %	253,194 (42.7)									253,194 (23.0)
Hypertension (systolic blood pressure ≥140 mm Hg), %	171,121 (28.9)	47,431 (31.8)							7,409 (19.9)	225,962 (20.5)
Obesity (≤110/130% of desirable weight), %	190,456 (32.1)	68,483 (45.9)							3,049 (8.2)	261,988 (23.7)
No regular exercise, %	205,254 (34.6)	43,063 (28.9)					8,369 (15.0)			256,686 (23.3)
Alcohol (≥1 oz of ethanol/day)								8,385 (32.1)		8,385 (0.7)
Diabetes, %	77,709 (13.1)	6,993 (4.7)								84,701 (7.7)
Never use mammography, %						7,823 (19.3)				7,823 (0.7)
Never use Papanicolaou screening, %					1,658 (36.5)					1,658 (0.2)

*Deaths attributed to risk factors are additive by row (i.e., risk factors), but not by column (i.e., disease).
Source: Adapted from Hahn,[39] JAMA 264:2654, 1990, with permission.

an inactive form of hemoglobin that has no oxygen-carrying capacity. With increases in the carboxyhemoglobin level, there is a shift in the hemoglobin dissociation curve resulting in a shift to the left and a reduction in the ability of hemoglobin to deliver oxygen to the tissues (Chapter 10). In compensation for the decreased oxygen delivery capacity, smokers maintain a higher mean hemoglobin level than nonsmokers. Women smokers have a significantly higher mean hemoglobin level than women who have stopped smoking or have never smoked.[44] Mean hemoglobin and carboxyhemoglobin levels have been reported to increase progressively with the number of cigarettes consumed per day. This effect of smoking may mask the detection of anemia.[44] Venous carboxyhemoglobin levels have been reported to have a positive relationship to onset of angina pectoris, MI, and intermittent claudication.[1]

The combined effects of nicotine and carbon monoxide have been shown to reduce plasma high-density lipoprotein (HDL) levels, to increase platelet aggregation, and to increase the levels of plasma fibrinogen, all of which increase the tendency for thrombosis development. Cigarette smoking increases automaticity and decreases the ventricular threshold, which results in increased frequency of arrhythmias and sudden death.[1]

When CAD is present, cigarette smoking can cause an imbalance between myocardial oxygen supply and demand, primarily through the impairment of oxygen transport and utilization. Pulmonary dysfunction associated with smoking can also produce a tissue hypoxia and possible decrease in coronary blood flow (Chapter 14).

Clinical Assessment of Smoking Behavior

Clinicians in cardiopulmonary rehabilitation have the opportunity and means to modify smoking behavior in their patients. For patients who quit smoking after MI, there is a reduction of reinfarction, sudden cardiac death, and total mortality when these patients are compared with patients who continue to smoke.[24,41,45] A detailed history of the patient's use of all types of tobacco should be assessed at the time of entry into the rehabilitation program and reviewed every 3 to 6 months. Through self-reporting and clinician-taken medical history, most patients are honest about their habits and readily admit the deleterious effects of smoking

An assessment of pulmonary function (Chapter 10) that includes measurement of vital capacity and forced expiratory volume in 1 second (FEV_1) should be taken early in life for heavy smokers (2 or more packs per day). Routine annual chest x-rays are also recommended for heavy smokers.[46]

Cessation of smoking is the single most effective way to reduce the risk of CHD and other atherosclerotic diseases.[47] The risk of cancer and heart disease also decreases rapidly after a patient quits smoking. After 2½ years of not smoking, the risk of lung cancer decreases by 50 percent. The risk of a heart attack is the same as that of a nonsmoker within 3 to 5 years of smoking cessation, and within 5 to 10 years, the risk of major health problems deceases to a level just slightly above the risk of people who have never smoked.[48]

Smoking cessation and maintenance of cessation appear to be complicated phenomena characterized by physiologic and psychologic dependence. Nicotine is highly addictive and has both stimulating and tranquilizing effects, depending on the dosage.[8] There is some evidence to suggest that nicotine may increase the production of endorphins, which may explain why nicotine can reduce the perception of pain and increase the feeling of well-being.[48] The psychologic effects of smoking are related to many situations and emotional aspects of a person's life that can "trigger" the need for a cigarette. Examples of such situations include the consumption of coffee or alcohol, the end of a meal, or instances of anger, boredom, and the like.[8,48]

To help the patient stop smoking, several approaches may be taken, including pharmacologic intervention, behavioral interventions, and other techniques including acupuncture and hypnosis.

PHARMACOLOGIC AGENTS

The parmacologic agents that appear to be the most successful in smoking cessation are nicotine polacrilex (Nicorette) and the transdermal nicotine patch (Habitrol, Nicoderm, Nicotrol, and Prostep). These agents provide partial replacement for the nicotine previously obtained from cigarettes and make the withdrawal symptoms in the initial phase of smoking cessation less severe. When Nicorette (nicotine gum) is chewed, the nicotine is released from the medication and absorbed through the mucous membranes.[48] Nicorette is available without a prescription and instructions for its use should be accompanied by a program of behavioral modification.

The transdermal nicotine patch is available in several strengths and is ideal for use in nicotine tapering. Six-month abstinence rates for people receiving the nicotine patch were 26 percent compared with 12 percent for those receiving a placebo.[49] Use of the transdermal nicotine patch decreases the intensity of withdrawal symptoms, but its use should also be accompanied by a program of behavioral intervention.

Two newer methods for delivery of nicotine to the patient who is attempting to quit smoking include a nicotine spray and a nicotine inhaler.[50] Data as to the effectiveness of the nicotine spray and/or inhaler as an aid to smoking cessation are not yet available.

BEHAVIORAL INTERVENTIONS

Clinical trials have demonstrated the effectiveness of patient counseling and smoking cessation techniques involving various combinations of counseling, distribution of literature, and nicotine replacement therapy.[37,38] Smoking cessation counseling should be offered on a frequent basis to all patients who smoke cigarettes, cigars, or pipes, and to those who use smokeless tobacco. The effectiveness of behavioral interventions varies with age, level of education, years of negative behaviors, and the nature of the intervention.[42,51,52]

One intervention that has been found effective in smoking cessation programs is rapid smoking. This method is characterized by having the patient inhale smoke from his or her cigarette every 6 seconds until the patient no longer desires to take another puff. This intervention creates an aversion to smoking, but should be used only with guidance from a trained health care professional.[48]

Once a patient has quit smoking, a behavioral technique used to assist in maintaining smoking cessation is that of relapse prevention. This technique teaches patients to anticipate situations in which they will be tempted to smoke and to devise strategies to avoid relapse (smoking) in those situations.[48]

ADDITIONAL TECHNIQUES

Smokers (and people who want to lose weight) try to find easy methods to modify their behaviors and change their negative habits. Some are attracted to hypnosis, acupuncture, drugs, lotteries, relaxation training, and other techniques in hopes of finding an easy way to quit smoking.

The health care professional who is assisting patients in smoking cessation may find the following guidelines useful:[48]

1. Advise the smoker to quit.
2. Work with the patient to develop a specific plan and date for cessation of smoking.
3. Encourage the patient's efforts to quit smoking and provide support during difficult times.
4. Respond to concern about weight gain and suggest that the patient increase physical activity and eat low-fat foods and low-calorie snacks.

The major conclusions of a recent report on smoking cessation techniques revealed the following:[38,45]

1. Most smokers quit on their own.
2. Interventions using multiple and frequent reinforcements are more successful than those relying on a single intervention technique.
3. The greatest problem in cessation programs is relapse, and preparation for it should be included in the overall smoking cessation strategy.
4. When coupled with other interventions, nicotine replacement may facilitate cessation rates.
5. Health care professionals should facilitate multicomponent strategies that incorporate the use of behavioral techniques and scheduled reinforcement.

Assisting the patient with cardiopulmonary disease with smoking cessation should be a high priority for the rehabilitation staff. The patient should be informed in lay terms about the adverse effects of smoking. The information can be contained in a patient education manual or provided as supplemental material for distribution during individual or group counseling. Formal group therapy is not always required to help a patient stop smoking. Many cardiopulmonary patients will have stopped smoking on the advice of their physicians before entering a formal exercise rehabilitation program. Therefore, the role of the rehabilitation staff becomes primarily one of reinforcing the patient's compliance with his or her self-motivated behavioral change. Compliance with positive behavior change may be reinforced by reminding the patient of the reason(s) that motivated him or her to stop smoking. The most common reasons are as follows:

1. Concern over effects on health (particularly fear of recurring coronary events)
2. Desire to set an example for others
3. Recognition of the unpleasant aspects of smoking, i.e., nicotine stains, foul-smelling clothing, expense
4. Desire to exercise self-control

Because smoking is one of the most serious of the risk factors associated with CHD, the rehabilitation staff must make a concentrated effort to motivate patients to stop smoking and to educate and encourage patients who have stopped so that the chances of their resuming the habit are significantly reduced (see Chapter 14).

Measurement of Smoking Outcomes

Smoking cessation and relapse prevention can be measured through self-reporting and use of biochemical measures. A major disadvantage of using self-reporting (questionnaires, interviews, daily logs) is that patients may not accurately report their smoking behaviors. Physiologic measures that indicate smoking status include serum thiocyanate, expired carbon monoxide, or levels of cotinine in the saliva, urine, or plasma. Cotinine is a metabolite of nictoine and has a half-life of 16 to 20 hours; thiocyanate, a metabolite of hydrogen cyanide, remains in the plasma for up to 14 days. In cases in which biochemical data are not available, confirmation of smoking status by a spouse or family member may be helpful.[53]

HYPERTENSION

Hypertension, defined as a systolic blood pressure (SBP) equal to or greater than 140 mm Hg and/or a diastolic blood pressure (DBP) equal to or greater than 90 mm Hg, or individuals already taking anti-hypertensive medications, occurs in approximately 50 million Americans.[54] Although the number of people with hypertension has decreased in the past few years, hypertension remains the most common cardiovascular disease and afflicts approximately 20 percent of the population. However, in the black population, the prevalence of hypertension is 25 to 30 percent.[55]

Hypertension is well established as a primary risk factor for CHD, cerebrovascular disease, congestive heart failure, and renal disease.[56] It increases with age, and mortality from all causes increases progressively with higher levels of both SBP and DBP. Higher levels of SBP, DBP, or both are associated with increased risks of morbidity, mortality, and disability.[54] Hypertension is also more prevalent in the presence of other well-identified risk factors including excessive dietary fat intake, obesity, elevated lipids, smoking, diabetes mellitus, excessive alcohol intake, and sedentary lifestyle.[45,54]

The Joint National Committee on Detection, Evaluation, and Treatment of High Blood Pressure revised the classification and standards for blood pressures in 1993.[54] The new classification describes the stages of hypertension as determined by two or more measurements on two or more visits. All stages of hypertension are associated with greater risk of nonfatal and fatal cerebrovascular disease (CVD) and renal disease (Table 13–2). When systolic and diastolic blood pressures fall into different classifications, the higher category should be selected to classify the individual's blood pressure (BP) status. For example, if a patient's blood pressure were 160/94 mm Hg, the individual should be classified as stage 2. If the blood pressure were 180/120, the individual would be classified as stage 4 (Table 13–2).[54] Isolated systolic hypertension (ISH) is defined as a SBP measurement equal to or greater than 140 mm Hg, and a DBP of less than 90 mm Hg. A person with a blood pressure measurement of 170/85 mm Hg would be classified as stage 2 ISH. Ideally, the SBP should be 120 mm Hg or less, and the DBP should be 80 mm Hg or less.[54,57]

Clinically, hypertension is classified as either primary or secondary. Primary hypertension is also known as essential hypertension and accounts for approxi-

TABLE 13–2 Classification of
Blood Pressure for Adults Aged 18
Years and Older

Category	Systolic, mm Hg	Diastolic, mm Hg
Normal	<130	<85
High normal	130–139	85–90
Hypertension*		
Stage 1 (Mild)	140–159	90–99
Stage 2 (Moderate)	160–179	100–109
Stage 3 (Severe)	180–209	110–119
Stage 4 (Very severe)	≥210	≥120

*Average of two or more measurements on two or more visits.

Source: From The Fifth Report of the Joint National Committee on Detection, Evaluation, and Treatment of High Blood Pressure. US Department of Health and Human Services, National Heart, Lung, and Blood Institute, Bethesda. Publication No. 95-1088, 1995, p. 4.

mately 95 percent of patients with sustained high BP. The causes of primary hypertension are not well understood, but several regulatory mechanisms are known to contribute to the development of primary hypertension. Among these factors are abnormal sympathetic control of cardiac output and peripheral resistance, abnormal renal and metabolic control of vascular volume, and abnormal control of endothelial-mediated vasodilation.[55,58] The combination of neurohumoral and metabolic abnormalities contributes to gradual increases in vascular resistance, which may result from activation of the sympathetic nervous system and pressor hormones such as angiotensin. Increases in circulating catecholamines, hyperinsulinemia, alterations in renin levels, and an imbalance in calcium and sodium concentrations in vascular smooth muscle have been identified as contributing factors to the development of essential hypertension.[55,58]

Secondary hypertension accounts for approximately 5 percent of patients with sustained hypertension. The major causes of secondary hypertension include renal, endocrine, and vascular impairment. Renal vascular disease causes an increased release of renin, which stimulates the conversion of plasma angiotensinogen to angiotensin-II, a powerful vasoconstrictor that stimulates the release of aldosterone and causes renal retention of sodium and water. Tumors of the adrenal medulla and adrenal cortex, although not usually encountered, also cause secondary hypertension.[55,58]

Regardless of cause, hypertension has been shown to be a powerful risk factor for CHD. A recent Framingham Study update emphasized that the risk of sudden death more than doubled when blood pressure was mildly elevated.[59] More important was the discovery that isolated systolic hypertension was a prognostic factor for major cardiovascular events. Isolated systolic hypertension was reported to be the most common form of hypertension and accounted for 57.4 percent of all hypertensive conditions in men 65 or older and for 65.1 percent in women 65 or older.[59]

Evaluation of Hypertension

Errors in measurement of blood pressure can result from equipment, observer, and/or patient factors. The American Heart Association (AHA) recommends that baseline blood pressure not be measured immediately after a taxing or stressful situation. Patients should have refrained from smoking, eating, and ingestion of caffeine for at least 30 minutes. The average should be taken of two or more measurements with the patient seated comfortably with the arm bared, supported, and at heart level. If the first two measurements differ by more than 5 mm Hg, additional readings should be obtained. Hypertension should be confirmed on more than one reading at each of three separate visits.[54,60]

Lifestyle Modification for Treatment of Hypertension

The goal of treating patients with hypertension is to present morbidity and mortality and to control blood pressure by the least invasive procedure possible.[54] Once hypertension has been confirmed, a comprehensive history, physical examination, and pathologic assessment should be administered. Because of the possible adverse side effects, cost, and mortality associated with the pharmacologic treatment of hypertension, there is an increasing interest in treating patients with mild, moderate, and severe hypertension by lifestyle modification (previously termed nonpharmacologic treatment). Several lifestyle interventions merit review for their contribution to the primary and secondary prevention of CHD through blood pressure control.[61,62] The initial lifestyle interventions include reduction of sodium intake, reduction of body weight in overweight people, moderation of alcohol intake, and initiation of a regular program of aerobic exercise. Although not directly related to hypertension, cigarette smoking is a major risk factor for CVD, and hypertensive patients should be encouraged not to smoke. The lifestyle interventions should be tried for 3 to 6 months before pharmacologic therapy is considered.[54,57]

SODIUM REDUCTION

A blood-pressure-lowering effect from restriction of sodium has been recognized for some time. The Intersalt Study examined the relation of electrolyte excretion to blood pressure in over 10,000 people throughout the world. Data from this multicenter epidemiologic study revealed a significant correlation between sodium intake and blood pressure. Sodium and the sodium/potassium ratio were significantly related to the blood pressure of the subjects independent of other factors. A reduction in daily sodium intake of 100 mg was associated with a decrease in systolic pressure of 3.5 mm Hg. Other results revealed that, after adjusting for confounding variables, both body mass index and alcohol consumption were positively, significantly, and independently associated with blood pressure.[63,64]

In recent years there has been a re-evaluation of the role of sodium in human blood pressures because of two observations. First, not all individuals respond to an excessive sodium intake with an increase in blood pressure. Second, not all individuals show a decrease in blood pressure as a result of a reduction in sodium and/or extracellular fluid volume by dietary sodium restriction or diuretic administration.[65] New observations suggest that sodium sensitivity or resistance of blood pressure may be the result of genetics or acquired abnormalities and require further investigation.

The average American diet contains about 5 to 10 grams of sodium per day, which is approximately two to three times the recommended amount of 1100 to 3300 mg. Approximately 30 to 50 percent of dietary sodium is in the form of salt added in food preparation or at the table. The remainder of dietary sodium is in the food itself or in added preservatives or chemicals. It would appear prudent for all individuals, even those who are apparently healthy, those with a family history of hypertension, and especially those with documented CHD, to moderate sodium intake in order to reduce the development of hypertension. The reduction of discretionary and nondiscretionary salt and a decrease in sodium-rich foods appears advisable for most patients. Limitations of intake to 1.5 to 2.5 g of sodium (approximately 4 to 6 g of salt) per day is not known to produce serious adverse consequences.[66] Blood pressure may be controlled by this degree of sodium restriction in some patients with stage 1 hypertension and may reduce the medication requirements in some patients on pharmacologic therapy.[54] Make cardiac patients aware of the sodium content of frequently used prepared food items by analyzing their eating patterns and instructing the patients as to the types and amounts of low-sodium foods that should be part of a healthy diet.

WEIGHT REDUCTION

Because obesity and hypertension are closely associated, weight reduction is an important lifestyle intervention.[54,67,68] In 40 to 80 percent of obese patients with hypertension, even modest weight reduction was found to result in sustained decrease in blood pressure to or toward normal levels.[67] The deposition of excess fat in the abdominal (truncal) area, with an increased waist-to-hip-ratio above 0.85 in women and 0.95 in men, is positively correlated not only with hypertension but also with dyslipidemia, diabetes, and increased mortality from CHD[1,69-72] (see Chapters 9 and 12).

The mechanisms for a decrease in blood pressure associated with weight loss are not fully understood and the impact of long-term weight reduction on the incidence of cardiovascular complications in overweight patients with hypertension has not been fully assessed. Weight reduction using a diet low in saturated fat and cholesterol lowers the risk by decreasing important atherogenic risk factors. In an effort to control hypertension in overweight patients with stage I hypertension, a weight loss program, combined with other lifestyle modifications, should be tried for a minimum of 3 to 6 months before initiating pharmacologic therapy.[54]

ALCOHOL REDUCTION

Elevated blood pressure has been associated with increased alcohol intake and can cause antihypertensive therapy to be less effective.[73] Alcohol intake can also cause an increase in body weight, triglyceride levels, and uric acid levels and may impair ventricular function and induce atrial and ventricular arrhythmias.

Complications imposed by medications and their side effects make abstinence from alcohol the prudent choice for most cardiac patients. Patients should be informed about the dangers associated with alcohol consumption and the decision as to whether a patient is permitted to consume alcohol is one that must be made in conjunction with the primary physician. Hypertensive patients who drink alcoholic beverages should limit their daily intake to 1 ounce, or the amount of ethanol contained in 2 ounces of a 100 proof beverage, 8 ounces of wine, or 24 ounces of beer.[54]

PHYSICAL CONDITIONING AND HYPERTENSION

Although some controversy exists, mounting evidence indicates that regular aerobic exercise can be beneficial in the prevention and treatment of hypertension.[54,55,58,74-76] The recommended mode, intensity, frequency, and duration of activity are generally the same as for apparently healthy individuals. The exercise intensity should be low to moderate (40 to 60 percent of $\dot{V}O_2$max) at a duration of 30 to 60 minutes for 3 to 5 days per week. High-intensity aerobic activity and isometric activities are not recommended.[54,77]

ADDITIONAL CONCERNS

Although an AHA Task Force has reported that stress can elevate blood pressure, it has not been proven to lead to sustained hypertension.[78] At the present time, there is minimal evidence to support the theory that relaxation techniques or biofeedback, in and of themselves, can serve as effective means of treatment of mild, moderate, or severe hypertension.[62]

Recent research has examined the actions of such intracellular ionic abnormalities as elevated levels of cytosolic free calcium in hypertension.[78] High levels of free calcium have been reported to correlate with elevated blood pressure, which suggests that hypertension may be a condition of excess cytosolic free calcium. Conversely, other studies report that there is an inverse relationship between dietary calcium and blood pressure.[79] Observations of higher levels of free magnesium have been reported to coincide with lower systolic and diastolic blood pressures.[78] Current studies are examining the roles that magnesium, calcium, sodium, and pH, or free hydrogen ions, play in hypertension and other metabolic syndromes.[78] Although controversy exists, there is agreement that control of hypertension should involve the safest means possible for the CHD patient by using a combination of the nonpharmacologic interventions described above.[54]

Pharmacologic Treatment of Hypertension

Pharmacologic treatment of hypertension centers around several available drugs. Diuretics, beta-blockers, calcium antagonists, and angiotensin-converting enzyme (ACE) inhibitors are widely used to treat hypertension. The choice of drug is often related to the severity of hypertension, presence of target organ damage (TOD), presence of diabetes mellitus, or other major risk factors for CHD and stroke.[54,57,80,81] The primary goal of pharmacologic treatment is to maximize blood pressure control to normal, or near normal, levels with minimal side effects.

The Fifth Report of the Joint National Committee (JNC V) on Detection, Evaluation, and Treatment of High Blood Pressure has revised its standards for pharmacologic treatment of high blood pressure. Figure 13–1 shows the treatment algorithm for hypertension.[54] If, after 3 to 6 months of appropriate lifestyle modifications, the blood pressure remains at or above 140/90 mm Hg, it is recommended that pharmacologic treatment be initiated. For patients with stage 1 and stage 2 hypertension, initial drug therapy of a single drug is recommended. The JNC V has reported that the two classes of drugs preferred for initial drug therapy are diuretics and beta-blockers. Although the "alternative" drugs (calcium antagonists, ACE inhibitors, alpha-receptor blockers, and the alpha-beta blocker) have been shown to be effective in lowering blood pres-

TREATMENT ALGORITHM

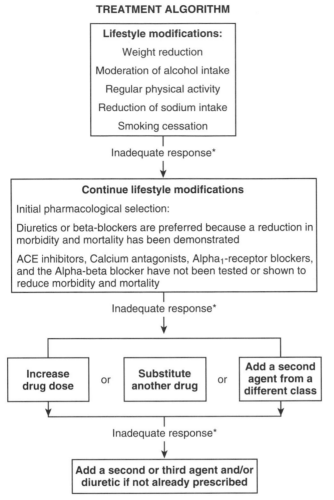

FIGURE 13-1. Treatment Algorithm for Hypertension. From The US Department of Health and Human Services. The Fifth Report of the Joint National Committee on Detection, Evaluation, and Treatment of High Blood Pressure. NIH Publication No. 95-1088, Bethesda, MD, 1995, p. 16.

sure, they have not been as well studied as diuretics and beta-blockers and are recommended when the latter two have not been effective.[54]

Patients with stage 3 and 4 hypertension may not respond to pharmacologic monotherapy (one drug), and it may be necessary to add a second or third antihypertensive medication for control of hypertension. The JNC V has recommended similar procedures for pharmacologic therapy for stages 3 and 4 hypertensives as was described for stages 1 and 2.[54]

There is some reason to be cautious in the use of the JNC V recommendation that diuretics and beta-blockers be the drugs of choice in the initial treatment of hypertension. Thiazide diuretics and beta-blockers may have adverse metabolic effects on blood lipid levels, glucose, and uric acid; these factors should be taken into consideration before recommendations for drug therapy are implemented. Thiazide diuretics produce a pattern of elevating total cholesterol, triglycerides, low-density lipoprotein (LDL) cholesterol, and very-low-density lipoprotein (VLDL) cholesterol. Other adverse effects are hypokalemia and increased arrhythmias. Careful dietary counseling and supplemental potassium may be required, as well as frequent evaluation of serum potassium levels. Diuretics are often the first-line agents for many hypertensive patients, but they may not be the best choice for patients who are exercising.[82,83]

The effects of selective and nonselective beta-blockers in the treatment of hypertension have been well documented. As with thiazide diuretics, beta-blockers, both selective and nonselective, can adversely affect triglycerides and HDL.[82,83]

Calcium channel blockers and ACE inhibitors do not appear to have the adverse effects on lipid metabolism that the diuretics and beta-blockers have. In addition, in post-MI patients with left ventricular dysfunction or chronic heart failure, ACE inhibitors have been found to enhance the life-lengthening effects of beta-blockers.[57,82–84] It is obvious that more research is needed to determine the medications of choice for hypertensive therapy. Table 13–3 gives a summary of the hypertensive agents recommended by the JNC V.

In summary, cardiopulmonary rehabilitation programs provide an opportunity for continued monitoring of blood pressure and supervision of adherence to medications. Hypertension is a major indication for pharmacologic therapy in primary and secondary prevention of hypertension if such lifestyle modifications as regular endurance training, sodium restriction, moderate use of alcohol, smoking cessation, and weight reduction (in overweight individuals) are not adequate to control blood pressure.

Measurement of Outcomes in Hypertension

The effect of various lifestyle interventions and/or pharmacologic therapy on systolic and diastolic blood pressures are measured by taking the blood pressure after 5 minutes of rest while the patient is seated[53] (see earlier section of this chapter on evaluation of blood pressure). The cardiac rehabilitation staff have an excellent opportunity to monitor blood pressures and to note if lifestyle interventions and/or medications are effectively controlling hypertension and to recommend adjustments in treatment as indicated.

PLASMA CHOLESTEROL, LIPOPROTEINS, AND TRIGLYCERIDES

There is no longer any doubt about the causative relationship linking elevated cholesterol levels to increased rates of premature CHD and to the progression of disease among those with established atherosclerosis.[1,25,56,85–88] Desirable blood cholesterol levels are those below 200 mg/dL. Blood cholesterol levels of 200 to 239 mg/dL are classified as borderline high and those above 240 mg/dL are considered high.[25] Clinical trials have demonstrated that lowering levels of serum cholesterol reduces morbidity and mortality both in persons with established CHD and those without CHD. Hence, cholesterol-lowering regimens that include education, dietary modification, physical activity, and risk factor reduction are recommended for primary and secondary prevention of CHD.[25]

Text continued on page 404

TABLE 13–3 Antihypertensive Agents

Type of Drug	Usual Dosage Range (Total mg/day)*	Frequency (Once/day unless otherwise noted)	Mechanisms	Comments
INITIAL ANTIHYPERTENSIVE AGENTS				
Diuretics				• For thiazide and loop diuretics, lower doses and dietary counseling should be used to avoid metabolic changes.
Thiazides and related agents:			Decreased plasma volume and decreased extracellular fluid volume, and decreased cardiac output initially, followed by decreased total peripheral resistance with normalization of cardiac output. Chronic effects include a slight decrease in extracellular fluid volume.	• More effective antihypertensive than loop diuretics except in patients with serum creatinine ≥221 µmol/L (2.5 mg/dL).
Bendroflumethiazide	2.5–5			
Benzthiazide	12.5–50			
Chlorothiazide	125–500	twice		• Hydrochlorothiazide or chlorthalidone is generally preferred; were used in most clinical trials.
Chlorthalidone	12.5–50			
Cyclothiazide	1.0–2			
Hydrochlorothiazide	12.5–50			
Hydroflumethiazide	12.5–50			
Indapamide	2.5–5			
Methyclothiazide	2.5–5			
Metolazone	0.5–5			
Polythiazide	1.0–4			
Quinethazone	25.0–100			
Trichlormethiazide	1.0–4			
Loop diuretics:			See thiazides.	• Higher doses of loop diuretics may be needed for patients with renal impairment or congestive heart failure.
Bumetanide	0.5–5	twice		
Ethacrynic acid	25.0–100	twice		• Ethacrynic acid is the only alternative for patients with allergy to thiazide and sulfur-containing diuretics.
Furosemide	20.0–320	twice		

Drug	Dose range	Frequency	Mechanism	Comments
Potassium sparing:				• Weak diuretics.
Amiloride	5–10	once or twice	Increased potassium reabsorption.	• Used mainly in combination with other diuretics to avoid or reverse hypokalemia from other diuretics.
Spironolactone	25–100	twice or thrice	Aldosterone antagonist.	• Avoid when serum creatinine ≥221 μmol/L (2.5 mg/dL).
Triamterene	50–150	once or twice		• May cause hyperkalemia, and this may be exaggerated when combined with ACE inhibitors or potassium supplements.
Adrenergic inhibitors				
Beta-blockers:			Decreased cardiac output and increased total peripheral resistance. Decreased plasma renin activity. Atenolol, betaxolol, bisoprolol, and metoprolol are cardioselective.	• Selective agents will also inhibit beta$_2$-receptors in higher doses, e.g., all may aggravate asthma.
Atenolol	25–100†			
Betaxolol	5–40			
Bisoprolol	5–20			
Metoprolol	50–200	once or twice		
Metoprolol (extended release)				
Nadolol	50–200			
Propranolol	20–240†	twice		
Propranolol (long acting)	40–240			
Timolol	20–40	twice		
Beta-blockers with intrinsic sympathomimetic activity (ISA):			Acebutolol is cardioselective.	• No clear advantage for agents with ISA except in those with bradycardia who must receive a beta-blocker; they produce fewer or no metabolic side effects.
Acebutolol	200–1200†	twice		
Carteolol	2.5–10†			
Penbutolol	20–80†			
Pindolol	10–60†	twice		
Alpha-beta blocker:			Same as beta-blockers plus alpha$_1$-blockade	• Possibly more effective in blacks than other beta-blockers.
Labetalol	200–1200	twice		• May cause postural effects, and titration should be based on standing blood pressure.
Alpha1-receptor blockers:			Block postsynaptic alpha$_1$-receptors and cause vasodilation.	• All may cause postural effects, and titration should be based on standing blood pressure.
Doxazosin	1.0–16			
Prazosin	1.0–20	twice or thrice		
Terazosin	1.0–20			

Continued

401

TABLE 13-3 Antihypertensive Agents (*Continued*)

Type of Drug	Usual Dosage Range (*Total mg/day*)*	Frequency (*Once/day unless otherwise noted*)	Mechanisms	Comments
ACE inhibitors			Block formation of angiotensin II, promoting vasodilation and decreased aldosterone. Also increased bradykinin and vasodilatory prostaglandins.	• Diuretic doses should be reduced or discontinued prior to starting ACE inhibitors whenever possible to prevent excessive hypotension.
Benazepril	10.0–40†	once or twice		
Captopril	12.5–150†	twice		• Reduced dose of those drugs marked "†" in patients with serum creatinine ≥221 μmol/L (2.5 mg/dL).
Cilazapril	2.5–5.0	once or twice		
Enalapril	2.5–40†	once or twice		
Fosinopril	10.0–40	once or twice		
Lisinopril	5.0–40†	once or twice		• May cause hyperkalemia in patients with renal impairment or in those receiving potassium-sparing agents.
Perindopril	1.0–16†	once or twice		• Can cause acute renal failure in patients with severe bilateral renal artery stenosis or severe stenosis in an artery to a solitary kidney.
Quinapril	5.0–80†	once or twice		
Ramipril	1.25–20†	once or twice		
Spirapril	12.5–50	once or twice		
Calcium antagonists			Block the inward movement of calcium ion across cell membranes and cause smooth muscle relaxation.	• These agents also block the slow channels in the heart and may reduce sinus rate and produce heart block.
Diltiazem	90–360	thrice		
Diltiazem (sustained release)	120–360	twice		
Diltiazem (extended release)	180–360			
Verapamil	80–480	twice		
Verapamil (long acting)	120–480	once or twice		
Dihydropyridines				• Dihydropyridines are more potent peripheral vasodilators than diltiazem and verapamil and may
Amlodipine	2.5–10			
Felodipine	5–20			
Isradipine	2.5–10	twice		

Drug	Dosage range	Frequency	Mechanism	Comments
Nicardipine	60–120	thrice		• cause more dizziness, headache, flushing, peripheral edema, and tachycardia.
Nifedipine	30–120	thrice		
Nifedipine (GITS)	30–90			

SUPPLEMENTAL ANTIHYPERTENSIVE AGENTS

Centrally acting alpha$_2$-agonists

Drug	Dosage range	Frequency	Mechanism	Comments
Clonidine	0.1–1.2	twice	Stimulate central alpha$_2$-receptors that inhibit efferent sympathetic activity.	• Clonidine patch is replaced once a week. • None of these agents should be withdrawn abruptly. Avoid in nonadherent patients.
Clonidine TTS (patch)**	0.1–0.3	once weekly		
Guanbenz	4–64	twice		
Guanfacine	1–3			
Methyldopa	250–2000	twice		

Peripheral acting adrenergic antagonists

Drug	Dosage range	Frequency	Mechanism	Comments
Guanadrel	10–75	twice	Inhibits catecholamine release from neuronal storage sites.	• May cause serious orthostatic and exercise-induced hypotension.
Guanethidine	10–100			

Rauwolfia alkaloids:

Drug	Dosage range	Frequency	Mechanism	Comments
Rauwolfia root	50–200	twice	Depletion of tissue stores of catecholamines	
Reserpine	0.05§–0.25	once or twice		

Direct vasodilators

Drug	Dosage range	Frequency	Mechanism	Comments
Hydralazine	50–300	twice to four times	Direct smooth muscle vasodilation (primarily arteriolar)	• Hydralazine is subject to phenotypically determined metabolism (acetylation). • For both agents: should treat concomitantly with a diuretic and a beta-blocker due to fluid retention and reflex tachycardia
Minoxidil	2.5–80	once or twice		

*The lower dose indicated is the preferred initial dose, and the higher dose is the maximum daily dose. Most agents require 2 to 4 weeks for complete efficacy, and more frequent dosage adjustments are not advised except for severe hypertension. The dosage range may differ slightly from the recommended dosage in the "Physicians' Desk Reference" or package insert.

†Indicates drugs that are excreted by the kidney and require dosage reduction in the presence of renal impairment (serum creatinine ≥221 μmol/L [2.5 mg/dL]).

**Weekly patch is 1, 2, 3 equivalent to 0.1–0.3 mg per day.

§0.1 mg dose may be given every other day to achieve this dosage.

Source: From The Fifth Report of the Joint National Committee on Detection, Evaluation, and Treatment of High Blood Pressure. National Heart Lung and Blood Institute Publication No. 95-1088, Bethesda, 1995, pp 18–20.

The association between elevated serum cholesterol levels and an increased risk of CHD is directly related to the low-density lipoprotein (LDL) fraction of total cholesterol and inversely proportional to high-density lipoprotein (HDL) levels.[87]

Cholesterol and Lipoproteins

Cholesterol is a fatlike substance (lipid) found in cell membranes and is necessary for normal bodily functions, including the transport and storage of body energy and the production of steroid hormones and bile acids. Cholesterol is circulated in the blood in particles containing both lipid and proteins (lipoproteins). Plasma lipoproteins are a major constituent in a complex transport system that allows exogenous and endogenous lipid to be transported between the liver, intestine, and peripheral tissues. Because lipoproteins are not water soluble, they must combine with other substances (apolipoproteins) to be transported in the circulatory system. The major classes of lipoproteins are chylomicrons, LDL, HDL, and very-low-density lipoproteins (VLDL).[25,89]

CHYLOMICRONS

Chylomicrons are derived from dietary fat and cholesterol and synthesized in the intestinal mucosa. Triglycerides constitute approximately 85 percent of their lipid component (triglyceride-rich chylomicrons). When newly ingested triglycerides enter the intestine through the diet, they are hydrolyzed to fatty acids and monoglycerides by pancreatic lipase. Chylomicrons rapidly transport the converted dietary lipids into the circulatory system and throughout the body. They deliver most of their fatty acids to the peripheral cells within a few minutes and reach their highest concentration in plasma 2 to 4 hours following a meal. The chylomicron remnants are cleared from the bloodstream by the liver within 10 to 12 hours after ingestion. Thus, a 14-hour fasting blood sample is recommended to obtain a reliable triglyceride measurement.[89,90]

LOW-DENSITY LIPOPROTEINS

Low-density lipoproteins are the major carriers of cholesterol in plasma, and approximately 60 to 75 percent of the total plasma cholesterol is found in LDL. Consequently, increases in the level of total blood cholesterol are usually the result of increases in LDL cholesterol. The LDL core consists almost entirely of cholesterol esters. Approximately 75 percent of the serum LDL is cleared by the liver and the remainder is cleared by the extrahepatic tissues.[91] LDL originates from catabolism of triglyceride-rich lipoproteins, VLDL, and VLDL remnants. Approximately 30 to 40 percent of the VLDL and VLDL remnants are converted to LDL. The rest are removed by the hepatic LDL receptors. Low-density lipoprotein delivers cholesterol to tissues via a specific, high-affinity LDL receptor, which controls the uptake of cholesterol by cells as well as intracellular cholesterol synthesis. Low-density lipoprotein-receptor activity appears to be a key regulator of LDL-cholesterol concentrations.[89] The LDL molecule is small in size and has been shown to pass through the intima to initiate and sustain the process of atherosclerosis. It has been suggested that modified or oxidized LDL is taken up by endothelial cells and smooth muscle cells 3 to 10 times more rapidly than native LDL and can therefore accelerate endothelial injury and progression of lesions.[92,93] Three basic abnormalities appear to contribute to the development of high serum cholesterol levels, and the major component of each is LDL. The first cause of elevated LDL is a decrease in LDL-receptor activity, which leads to a delayed clearance of LDL and VLDL remnants. This delay in clearance can result in a greater conversion of VLDL remnants to LDL. The second abnormality is an overproduction of LDL caused by an overproduction of apolipoprotein B by the liver (see the section in this chapter on apolipoproteins) and the decreased uptake of VLDL or VLDL remnants. The final mechanism of hypercholesterolemia is the overloading of LDL molecules with cholesterol esters.[91,94]

Accurate quantification of LDL cholesterol in the clinical laboratory is difficult. Because all cholesterol in plasma is present on lipoproteins, the concentration of LDL cholesterol in fasting plasma can be estimated from measurements of total cholesterol, total triglycerides, and HDL cholesterol. If the triglyceride value is below 400 mg/dL (4.5 mmol/L), one can divide the triglyceride value by five to estimate the VLDL-cholesterol level. Because the total serum cholesterol is the sum of LDL cholesterol, HDL cholesterol, and VLDL cholesterol, the LDL cholesterol level can be estimated by the following equation:[25]

$$\text{LDL-cholesterol} = \text{total cholesterol} - \text{HDL-cholesterol} - \frac{\text{Triglycerides}}{5}$$

If the triglyceride level is greater than 400 mg per dL, LDL cholesterol should not be estimated, but ultracentrifugation of the serum in a specialized laboratory would provide a more accurate LDL-cholesterol level.[25] Plasma LDL-cholesterol levels should be determined after 9 to 12 hours of fasting. The desirable level of LDL for the person without CHD or other atherosclerotic disease is less than 130 mg/dL. Borderline-high-risk LDL cholesterol occurs when a person has 130 to 159 mg/dL and two or more risk factors. High-risk LDL cholesterol occurs when the LDL level is 160 mg/dL or greater. For patients with CHD or other atherosclerotic disease, the optimal LDL cholesterol is 100 mg/dL or less. In primary prevention of CHD, patients who are borderline and high-risk should be referred for diet and exercise therapy. Drug therapy may be initiated in these patients if diet and exercise interventions are not effective and the LDL cholesterol is equal to, or exceeds, 190 mg/dL in patients without two additional risk factors, or 160 mg/dL in patients with two or more CHD risk factors.[25]

In the patient with known CHD or other atherosclerotic disease and a higher than optimal LDL cholesterol level (greater than 100 mg/dL), pharmacologic intervention may be necessary. In CHD patients with LDL cholesterol 100 mg/dL or lower, secondary prevention via diet and exercise therapy is recommended.[25]

The evidence that elevated LDL cholesterol is a cause of CHD has been well established from epidemiologic, genetic, and animal investigations.[70,95] Clinical trials have demonstrated that lowering the LDL cholesterol by dietary and/or drug interventions can reduce the incidence of CHD.[1,25,89] Although more research is needed in this area, regular physical activity has been shown to positively alter the composition of the LDL particle.[96]

HIGH-DENSITY LIPOPROTEINS

HDLs are the smallest particles in the major classes of lipoproteins, and they have the highest density. They are composed of approximately 50 percent proteins, 18 percent cholesterol, and very little triglyceride. HDL is synthesized in both the liver and small intestine and plays an important role in lipid metabolism by transporting cholesterol from the cells back to the liver, where they are metabolized into bile or bile salts and used in further digestion or excreted from the body via the intestines. This reverse cholesterol transport may be the method whereby HDL protects the body from developing atherosclerosis.[89] HDL cholesterol consists of two major subfractions: HDL_2 and HDL_3. It is thought that HDL_3 is the likely precursor to HDL_2, and HDL_2 is the final acceptor of cholesterol in the reverse cholesterol transport process.[89,90]

A reduced level of HDL is associated with an increased risk for CHD and is considered to be a major risk factor for CHD. Conversely, higher levels of HDL have been found to reduce the incidence of CHD.[25,89,97–100] Although controversial, the plasma levels of both HDL_2 and HDL_3 appear to be cardioprotective.[101]

HDL cholesterold levels below 35 mg/dL are considered to be low. Modifications in behavior including weight reduction in the obese patient, smoking cessation, and increased aerobic exercise, have been shown to raise levels of HDL-cholesterol.[25,97,100,102] Caution should be used with a patient taking medications that lower HDL levels, e.g., beta-adrenergic blockers, and alternate agents may need to be prescribed.

VERY-LOW-DENSITY LIPOPROTEINS

Very-low-density lipoproteins (VLDL) are triglyceride-rich lipoproteins that are manufactured in the liver and transported to adipose tissue or muscle for storage or use. The lipid component of VLDLs is approximately 50 percent triglyceride and 22 percent cholesterol. VLDL breakdown occurs in a series of steps during which triglycerides are removed progressively by tissue lipoprotein lipase. Once the triglycerides are hydrolyzed, the VLDL remnant can follow one of two pathways. VLDL remnants can be taken up directly by the liver or they can be converted into LDLs. Usually, about 60 to 70 percent of the VLDL remnants are removed by the liver and the remainder are converted to LDL. Thus, VLDL is a precursor of LDL. The mechanism whereby some VLDL remnants are converted to LDL, or the precise contribution of VLDL to atherogenesis or CHD risk, remains unknown.[25,89,97,102,103]

APOLIPOPROTEINS

Apolipoproteins are the protein subcomponents on the surface of lipoproteins that help deliver the lipoproteins to their sites of metabolism and degradation. They play an important role in maintaining the structural integrity of lipoproteins and in the regulation of metabolic enzymes. Fourteen apolipoproteins have been identified, and much remains to be learned about the biologic functions of the various apolipoproteins.[89,97]

Quantitative analysis and the role of apolipoproteins in identifying individuals at risk for CHD have received considerable attention. The most promising research has focused on two apolipoproteins that have been related to risk for developing CAD: apolipoprotein A–I (apo A–I) and apolipoprotein B (apo B). Apo A–I is the major protein component of the HDL group and apo B is the principal LDL protein moiety. Individuals with elevated concentrations of A–I have been found to have lower incidence of CAD; apo B has been correlated with increased risk for CAD.[89,97] Recent evidence has suggested that measurements of apo A–I and apo B may provide a stronger indication of CHD risk than concentrations of plasma lipids or HDL or LDL cholesterol.[1,89,104] Although currently the measurement of apolipoproteins is not practical, in some lipid disorders the measurements can aid in detection of the underlying cause as well as the effects of various interventions. Evidence as to the effects of diet and regular physical activity on the concentrations of apo-I and apo B provide inconclusive results, and more research in this area is likely to be done.[1,89,97,105]

Triglycerides

Triglycerides are combinations of glycerol and fatty acids. Because these lipids are insoluble in water, triglycerides are transported in the circulation in combination with protein (lipoproteins). Triglycerides are produced in the liver from carbohydrate food sources and are also found in ingested food. Increased levels of triglycerides in the blood can result from heritable defects or may be secondary to various endocrine and metabolic disorders (e.g., diabetes). The relation between serum triglyceride levels and cardiovascular disease is controversial. In most population studies, serum triglyceride levels were not independently predictive of CHD after being statistically corrected for such associated risk factors as total serum cholesterol, low HDL cholesterol, cigarette smoking, insulin, age, fasting blood glucose, physical inactivity, and alcohol intake.[1,25,106] Rather than being a direct cause of atherogenesis, elevated triglyceride levels are usually present with other atherogenic lipoprotein abnormalities that are more directly associated with CHD, such as small, dense LDL particles and low levels of HDL cholesterol.[107] Some patients with borderline or high triglyceride levels and a strong family history of premature cardiovascular disease may have familial combined hyperlipidemia, which also increases the risk of CHD. The most common lipoprotein abnormalities produced by hypertriglyceridemia are increased levels of chylomicron remnants and VLDL remnants as well as decreased levels of HDL cholesterol.[25]

Classification according to triglyceride levels in the blood are as follows:[25]

Category	Serum Triglyceride Levels
Normal triglycerides	Less than 200 mg/dL
Borderline high triglycerides	200 to 400 mg/dL
High triglycerides	400 to 1000 mg/dL
Very high triglycerides	Greater than 1000 mg/dL

Modifications in lifestyle are the recommended principal therapies for abnormal blood lipid levels in which elevated triglycerides are a component. Recommended modifications include normalizing body weight, regular aerobic exercise, smoking cessation, restriction of alcohol use, and consumption of a diet low in saturated fat and cholesterol. Lipid-lowering drug therapy may also be considered according to individual patient circumstances.[25]

Severe Forms of Hypercholesterolemia

FAMILIAL HYPERCHOLESTEROLEMIA

Familial hypercholesterolemia (FH) is an autosomal-dominant disorder characterized by a defect in the gene encoding for the LDL receptor, which is either absent or nonfunctional. The gene for the LDL receptor is normally inherited from both parents. In very rare incidences, individuals inherit two abnormal genes for LDL receptors and intracellular cholesterol production is out of control. This causes serum cholesterol levels to be in the range of 600 to 1000 mg per dL. The disorder occurs in one in a million people and leads to atherosclerosis by the age of 10 years with rare survival past 20 years.[94] The heterozygous form of FH occurs in 1 in 500 people in whom an abnormal gene for the LDL receptor is inherited from only one parent. The affected individual has only one-half of the number of LDL receptors, and serum cholesterol levels are in the 350 to 450 mg per dL range. Patients with heterozygous FH are prone to premature CHD, usually do not respond adequately to dietary therapy alone, and often require a combination of lipid-lowering medications to bring LDL cholesterol under control.[25]

FAMILIAL COMBINED HYPERLIPIDEMIA

Familial combined hyperlipidemia (FCHL) is another autosomal-dominant disorder characterized by multiple patterns of hyperlipidemia phenotypes occurring in a single family. Approximately 1 to 2 percent of the American population appear to have FCHL, with about one-third of the affected patients having elevated VLDL cholesterol, one-third having increases in LDL cholesterol alone, and the remainder having either elevated VLDL and LDL or elevated VLDL and chylomicrons. The primary defect appears to be overproduction of VLDL by the liver, and patients also exhibit high levels of apolipoprotein B (apo B). Approximately 10 to 15 percent of patients with MI before 60 years of age have FCHL.[25,94] Treatment of FCHL includes weight reduction, control of diabetes (if present), and restriction of dietary saturated fat and cholesterol. When lifestyle changes are ineffective, pharmacologic therapy may have to be initiated.[25]

SEVERE PRIMARY HYPERCHOLESTEROLEMIA

Severe primary hypercholesterolemia is often called polygenic because a definite monogenic inheritance of elevated LDL cholesterol (greater than 220 mg/dL) cannot be demonstrated. The word "polygenic" can be considered to mean that several different defects might cause a monogenic form of moderate hypercholesterolemia. Several metabolic abnormalities, such as mild defects in LDL-receptor function, overproduction of apolipoprotein B-100, and an increased cholesterol absorption, have been identified and are thought to be responsible for polygenic hypercholesterolemia. Patients in this category often do not respond to dietary treatment and require pharmacologic intervention to lower LDL cholesterol.[25,94]

FAMILIAL DYSBETALIPOPROTEINEMIA

Familial dysbetalipoproteinemia (type 3 hyperlipoproteinemia) is relatively uncommon and occurs in about 1 in every 5000 people in the United States. An abnormal apolipoprotein E interferes with the normal metabolism of VLDL and chylomicrons which leads to their accumulation as well as to elevated levels of cholesterol and triglycerides. Cholesterol levels usually range from 300 to 600 mg/dL and triglycerides range from 400 to 800 mg/dL or higher. Patients with this hyperlipidemia are characterized by the physical findings of palmar tuberous xanthomas, premature CHD, and peripheral vascular disease. Frequently these patients are obese, glucose-intolerant, and hyperuricemic. Treatment of this condition includes a diet low in saturated fat and cholesterol and a program to control body weight. Pharmacologic interventions may be necessary to reduce circulating VLDL and chylomicron remnants.[25]

EVALUATION OF PATIENT RISK-FACTOR MODIFICATION

Regular evaluation of patient compliance with risk-factor modification is a standard procedure while the patient is participating in the formal supervised program. However, once the patient leaves the supervised program and is continuing with his or her program in a community-based facility or at home, compliance with the prescribed plan for risk-factor modification, exercise, and psychosocial issues can be assessed through regularly scheduled conferences and evaluations. These follow-up evalutions (either in person or by phone) should be scheduled at intervals as determined by the medical status of the patient. It is recommended that the patient receive nutrition counseling quarterly during the first year of follow-up and annually (or more often if necessary) thereafter.[25]

Rehabilitation staff members should note that in the initial stages of rehabilitation, too much change will defeat the purpose of behavior modification. Patients must not be overwhelmed by the changes they are asked to make in their lifestyles. To ensure success in modifying behavior, care must be taken to apply developmental principles to the establishment of goals.

Dietary Intervention

Generally, the goals of dietary intervention are to decrease the levels of serum cholesterol, especially LDL cholesterol, because evidence indicates that lowering of LDL cholesterol decreases the incidence of CHD. Three major factors appear to contribute to high levels of serum cholesterol:

1. A high intake of dietary cholesterol
2. A high intake of saturated fat
3. An imbalance between caloric intake and energy expenditure leading to overweight and obesity

The first approach to treatment of high blood cholesterol include dietary modification, weight control, and increased physical activity.[1,25,108–116]

Dietary Recommendations

The most widely recommended diet modifications to manage serum cholesterol levels are referred to as the Step I and Step II Diets. Both are designed to reduce the intake of saturated fatty acids and cholesterol and to eliminate intake of excess calories. When diet therapy is indicated, the therapy usually begins with the Step I Diet (Table 13–4), which recommends a daily fat intake of 30 percent or less of total calories, less than 10 percent of total intake in saturated fatty acids, and less than 300 mg per day of cholesterol. The patient usually remains on this regimen for 3 months. If, at the end of that time, the cholesterol levels remain high, the patient is progressed to the Step II

TABLE 13-4 Dietary Therapy for High Blood Cholesterol

Nutrient*	Recommended Intake		
	Step I Diet		Step II Diet
Total Fat		30% or less of total calories	
Saturated fatty acids	8–10% of total calories		Less than 7% of total calories
Polyunsaturated fatty acids		Up to 10% of total calories	
Monounsaturated fatty acids		Up to 15% of total calories	
Carbohydrates		55% or more of total calories	
Protein		Approximately 15% of total calories	
Cholesterol	Less than 300 mg/day		Less than 200 mg/day
Total calories		To achieve and maintain desirable weight	

*Calories from alcohol not included.
Source: From U.S. Department of Health and Human Services. The Second Report of the Expert Panel on Detection, Evaluation, and Treatment of High Blood Cholesterol in Adults. National Heart, Lung, and Blood Institute, Bethesda. Publication No. 93-3095, 1993, p II-2.

Diet. The Step II Diet further reduces the saturated fatty acid intake to less than 7 percent of total calories and cholesterol to less than 200 mg per day. Patients usually remain on diet therapy (combined with exercise) for at least 6 months, after which, if cholesterol levels remain high, drug therapy may be considered.[25] Table 13–5 gives examples of foods to choose or decrease for the Step I and Step II Diets.

Additional dietary regimens have been used to treat various types of hyperlipidemic disorders. One of the earliest dietary regimens for treatment of CHD was the Pritikin Diet.[115] This diet is characterized by a reduction in daily cholesterol and total dietary fat, allows no meat consumption except small amounts of fish or chicken, and recommends that 75 to 80 percent of daily caloric intake come from primarily complex carbohydrates. Some of the guidelines for the Pritikin Diet are as follows:[115]

Reduction of daily cholesterol to 100 mg or less
Dietary fat should be 10% or less of total calories
With the exception of small amounts of fish or fowl, meat consumption is not recommended
Protein should be limited to 10 to 15% of daily calories and be derived primarily from vegetable sources
Caffeine or alcohol ingestion is not recommended
Ingestion of fiber should equal 35 or more g per day
Sodium intake should be restricted to 1600 mg per day

Another regimen, the Ornish Diet,[111] is characterized by grouping foods into 5 categories, with Group 1 being the most healthful and Group 5 being the least healthful. Ornish's "reversal" diet is characterized as follows:

It is a vegetarian diet
Less than 10% of daily caloric consumption should be from fat

TABLE 13–5 Examples of Foods to Choose or Decrease for the Step I and Step II Diets*

Food Group	Choose	Decrease
Lean meat, poultry and fish ≤5–6 oz. per day	Beef, pork, lamb—lean cuts well trimmed before cooking Poultry without skin Fish, shellfish Processed meat—prepared from lean meat, e.g., lean ham, lean frankfurters, lean meat with soy protein or carrageenan	Beef, pork, lamb—regular ground beef, fatty cuts, spare ribs, organ meats Poultry with skin, fried chicken Fried fish, fried shellfish Regular luncheon meat, e. g., bologna, salami, sausage, frankfurters
Eggs ≤4 yolks per week, Step I ≤2 yolks per week, Step II	Egg whites (two whites can be substituted for one whole egg in recipes), cholesterol-free egg substitute	Egg yolks (if more than four per week on Step I or if more than two per week on Step II); includes eggs used in cooking and baking
Low-fat dairy products 2–3 servings per day	Milk—skim, ½%, or 1% fat (fluid, powdered, evaporated), buttermilk Yogurt—nonfat or low-fat yogurt or yogurt beverages Cheese—low-fat natural or processed cheese Low-fat or nonfat varieties, e.g., cottage cheese—low fat, nonfat, or dry curd (0 to 2% fat) Frozen dairy dessert—ice milk, frozen yogurt (low fat or nonfat) Low-fat coffee creamer Low-fat or nonfat sour cream	Whole milk (fluid, evaporated, condensed), 2% fat milk (lowfat milk), imitation milk Whole milk yogurt, whole milk yogurt beverages Regular cheeses (American, blue, Brie, cheddar, Colby, Edam, Monterey Jack, whole-milk mozzarella, Parmesan, Swiss), cream cheese, Neufchatel cheese Cottage cheese (4% fat) Ice cream Cream, half & half, whipping cream, nondairy creamer, whipped topping, sour cream Coconut oil, palm kernel oil, palm oil
Fats and oils ≤6–8 teaspoons per day	Unsaturated oils—safflower, sunflower, corn, soybean, cottonseed, canola, olive, peanut Margarine—made from unsaturated oils listed above, light or diet margarine, especially soft or liquid forms Salad dressings—made with unsaturated oils listed above, low-fat or fat free Seeds and nuts—peanut butter, other nut butters Cocoa powder	Butter, lard, shortening, bacon fat, hard margarine Dressings made with egg yolk, cheese, sour cream, whole milk Coconut Milk chocolate

Continued

411

TABLE 13–5 Examples of Foods to Choose or Decrease for the Step I and Step II Diets* (*Continued*)

Food Group	Choose	Decrease
Breads and cereals 6 or more servings per day	Breads—whole-grain bread, English muffins, bagels, buns, corn or flour tortilla Cereals—oat, wheat, corn, multigrain Pasta Rice Dry beans and peas Crackers, low-fat—animal-type, graham, soda crackers, breadsticks, melba toast Homemade baked goods using unsaturated oil, skim or 1% milk, and egg substitute—quick breads, biscuits, cornbread muffins, bran muffins, pancakes, waffles	Bread in which eggs, fat, and/or butter are a major ingredient; croissants Most granolas High-fat crackers Commercial baked pastries, muffins, biscuits
Soups	Reduced- or low-fat and reduced-sodium varieties, e.g., chicken or beef noodle, minestrone, tomato, vegetable, potato, reduced-fat soups made with skim milk	Soup containing whole milk, cream, meat fat, poultry fat, or poultry skin
Vegetables 3–5 servings per day	Fresh, frozen, or canned, without added fat or sauce	Vegetables fried or prepared with butter, cheese, or cream sauce
Fruits 2–4 servings per day	Fruit—fresh, frozen, canned, or dried Fruit juice—fresh, frozen, or canned	Fried fruit or fruit served with butter or cream sauce
Sweets and modified fat desserts	Beverages—fruit-flavored drinks, lemonade, fruit punch Sweets—sugar, syrup, honey, jam, preserves, candy made without fat (candy corn, gumdrops, hard candy), fruit-flavored gelatin Frozen desserts—low-fat and nonfat yogurt, ice milk, sherbert, sorbet, fruit ice, popsicles Cookies, cake, pie, pudding—prepared with egg whites, egg substitute, skim milk or 1% milk, and unsaturated oil or margarine; ginger snaps; fig and other fruit bar cookies, fat-free cookies; angel food cake	Candy made with milk chocolate, coconut oil, palm kernel oil, palm oil Ice cream and frozen treats made with ice cream Commercial baked pies, cakes, doughnuts, high-fat cookies, cream pies

*Careful selection of processed foods is necessary to stay within the sodium <2400 mg guideline.
Source: From U.S. Department of Health and Human Services. The Second Report of the Expert Panel on Detection, Evaluation, and Treatment of High Blood Cholesterol in Adults. National Heart, Lung, and Blood Institute, Bethesda. Publication No. 93-3095, 1993, pp II-11-13.

Cholesterol intake should be no more than 5 mg per day

With the exception of nonfat dairy products and egg whites, no animal products are recommended

Ingestion of no more than one tablespoon of oil per day is recommended

A major characteristic of diet modification for primary and secondary prevention of CHD is the reduction of fat content in the daily diet. Table 13–6 gives a summary of low-fat diet objectives. The staff dietitian or nutritionist and the referring physician play the major roles in determining each patient's dietary regimen. However, every rehabilitation staff person shares responsibility for keeping abreast of current trends and research in dietary management of CHD patients.

Pharmacologic Therapy

Patients whose LDL cholesterol remains elevated following at least 6 months of diet and exercise therapy should probably be recommended for drug treatment. Candidates for drug therapy in primary prevention of CHD include those whose LDL cholesterol remains equal to or greater than 190 mg/dL, who have no CHD, and who have no more than one additional risk factor; and those whose LDL cholesterol remains equal to or greater than 160 mg d/L, have no CHD, but have two or more additional risk factors.[25]

Patients with CHD whose serum LDL cholesterol levels are 130 mg/dL or greater should probably be referred for pharmacologic intervention. The goal for the CHD patient is to decrease the LDL cholesterol to 100 mg/dL or lower. In most patients, drug therapy with a single drug in combination with diet therapy should be effective. If the goal of pharmacologic therapy (100 mg/dL) is not reached within 3 months with a single medication, it may be appropriate to add a second agent.[25]

TABLE 13–6 Summary of Low-Fat Objectives

1. Reduce the consumption of beef, pork, and lamb.
2. Substitute poultry, fish, and meat substitutes for beef, lamb, and, pork.
3. Prepare poultry and seafood without added fat.
4. Increase consumption of meatless meals.
5. Prepare rice, macaroni, and other grains without added fat.
6. Prepare vegetables without added fat.
7. Reduce the consumption of margarine and peanut butter as spreads for breads and rolls.
8. Eliminate butter totally.
9. Use only fat-free salad dressings.
10. Use only low-fat breads and cereals.
11. Use only skim and low-fat dairy products.
12. Avoid egg yolks.
13. Avoid commercial baked goods (cakes, pies, cookies).
14. Avoid foods high in sodium, and do not add salt at the table.
15. Limit the use of sugar in coffee and tea and on cereal.
16. Substitute fruit toppings for jams, preserves, jellies, honey, syrup, and molasses.
17. Use only recommended dessert recipes.
18. Drink decaffeinated coffee and caffeine-free herb teas.
19. Limit alcoholic beverages.

Source: From Frye, N, et al. A Comprehensive Guide to Cardiac Rehabilitation. The Methodist Hospital, Houston, TX, 1982, with permission.

Three major classes of blood lipid medications are available for lipid management: bile acid sequestrants, nicotinic acid, and HMG CoA reductase inhibitors.

BILE ACID SEQUESTRANTS

The available bile acid sequestrants are cholestyramine and colestipol. These sequestrants have been shown to effectively reduce LDL cholesterol and CHD risk, and their long-term use appears to be safe. Because the sequestrants are not absorbed from the gastrointestinal tract, they do not cause systemic toxicity. The bile acid sequestrants are the drugs of first choice when drug therapy is warranted for men under 45 years of age and for women under 55 years who have isolated elevations of LDL cholesterol in the range of 160 to 220 mg/dL. Because, in some patients, the sequestrants may increase serum triglycerides, they are not recommended as a single-drug therapy in patients with high triglycerides (triglycerides greater than 500 mg/dL). They have also been found to be effective in patients with borderline high-risk LDL-cholesterol levels who have multiple risk factors or established CHD. In combination with the statins (see subsequent section on HMG CoA reductase inhibitors) they have also been found to be effective in patients with severe hypercholesterolemia.[25] Table 13–7 gives a summary of the bile acid sequestrants.

NICOTINIC ACID

Nicotinic acid, or niacin, is a water-soluble B vitamin. It has been found to positively affect all lipids and lipoproteins when given in doses well above the daily vita-

TABLE 13–7 Summary of Bile Acid Sequestrants

Available drugs	Cholestyramine, colestipol
Lipid/lipoprotein effects	LDL-cholesterol — ↓ 15–30%
	HDL-cholesterol — ↑ 3–5%
	Triglycerides — No effect or increase
Major use	To lower LDL-cholesterol
Contraindications	
Absolute	Familial dysbetalipoproteinemia
	Triglycerides >500 mg/dL
Relative	Triglycerides >200 mg/dL
Reduce CHD risk	Yes
Long-term safety	Yes
Major side/adverse effects	Upper and lower gastrointestinal complaints
	Decrease absorption of other drugs
Usual daily dose	Cholestyramine — 4–16 g
	Colestipol — 5–20 g
Maximum daily dose	Cholestyramine — 24 g
	Colestipol — 30 g
Available preparations	
Cholestyramine	9 g packets (4 g drug)
	378 g bulk
Cholestyramine "light"	5 g packets (4 g drug)
	210 g bulk
Colestipol	5 g packets (5 g drug)
	500 g bulk

Source: From The Second Report of the Expert Panel on Detection, Evaluation, and Treatment of High Blood Cholesterol in Adults. National Heart, Lung, and Blood Institute, Bethesda. Publication No. 93-3095, 1993, p III-4.

min requirement. Nicotinic acid has been found to lower serum total cholesterol, LDL cholesterol, and triglyceride levels and also raises the levels of HDL cholesterol. It has also been shown to reduce the risk of recurrent MI and to reduce total mortality in patients with coronary disease.[25] Nicotinic acid has been found to be especially useful in patients with moderately elevated LDL cholesterol who also have increased triglycerides and low HDL cholesterol. There are four major side effects from nicotinic acid therapy: gastrointestinal symptoms including nausea, vomiting, and peptic ulcers; hepatotoxicity; hyperuricemia and gout; and hyperglycemia. Nicotinic acid should be used cautiously in a noninsulin-dependent diabetic, and all patients taking nicotinic acid should be monitored on a regular basis by a health professional. Crystalline nicotinic acid is the preferred form of nicotinic acid administration because sustained-release preparations have been reported to increase hepatotoxicity and are recommended only under special circumstances.[25] Table 13–8 gives a summary of nicotinic acid.

HMG CoA REDUCTASE INHIBITORS

The HMG CoA reductase inhibitors are also referred to as the "statins," namely, lovastatin, pravastatin, and simvastatin. The HMG CoA reductase inhibitors inhibit a rate-limiting enzyme in cholesterol synthesis and reduce the biosynthesis of cholesterol. Because of this inhibition, the hepatocytes increase the release of LDL receptors, which enhances the clearance of LDL from the plasma. The statins have been found to lower LDL cholesterol, decrease triglycerides and VLDL cholesterol, and in some cases increase the HDL cholesterol. The statins are usually prescribed to reduce LDL choles-

TABLE 13–8 Summary of Nicotinic Acid

Available drugs	Crystalline nicotinic acid
	Sustained-release (or slow release) nicotinic acid (not FDA approved)
Lipid/lipoprotein effects	LDL-cholesterol - ↓ 10–25%
	HDL-cholesterol - ↑ 15–35%
	Triglycerides - ↓ 20–50%
Major use	Useful in most lipid and lipoprotein abnormalities
Contraindications	
Absolute	Chronic liver disease
Relative	Non–insulin-dependent diabetes mellitus (NIDDM), severe gout, or hyperuricemia
Reduce CHD risk	Yes
Long-term safety	Yes for crystalline form; uncertain for sustained-release form
Major side/adverse effects	Flushing, hepatotoxicity, hyperglycemia, hyperuricemia or gout, and upper gastrointestinal complaints; hepatotoxicity especially for sustained-release form
Usual daily dose	Crystalline nicotinic acid -1.5–3 g
	Sustained-release nicotinic acid -1–2 g
Maximum daily dose	Crystalline nicotinic acid -6 g
	Sustained-release nicotinic acid -2 g
Available preparations	Many preparations by various manufacturers for both crystalline and sustained-release nicotinic acid

Source: From The Second Report of the Expert Panel on Detection, Evaluation, and Treatment of High Blood Cholesterol in Adults. National Heart, Lung, and Blood Institute, Bethesda. Publication No. 93-3095, 1993, p III-6.

TABLE 13-9 Summary of HMG CoA Reductase Inhibitors

Available drugs	Lovastatin, pravastatin, simvastatin
Lipid/lipoprotein effects	LDL-cholesterol - ↓ 20–40%
	HDL-cholesterol - ↑ 5–15%
	Triglycerides - ↓ 10–20%
Major use	To lower LDL-cholesterol
Contraindications	
Absolute	Active or chronic liver disease
Relative	Concomitant use of cyclosporine, gemfibrozil, or niacin
Reduce CHD risk	Yes*
Long-term safety	Extensive clinical use and 1- and 2-year safety data in controlled trials, 5-year data are available only from uncontrolled trials
Usual daily dose	Lovastatin–10–40 mg
	Pravastatin–10–40 mg
	Simastatin–5–20 mg
Maximum daily dose	Lovastatin–80 mg
	Pravastatin–40 mg
	Simvastatin–40 mg
Available preparations	
Lovastatin	10, 20, 40 mg tablets
Pravastatin	10, 20, 40 mg tablets
Simvastatin	5, 10, 20, 40 mg tablets

*Angiographic trials employing combination therapy of a statin with a resin and/or nicotinic acid showed reduced progression and increased regression of coronary artery lesions.

Source: From The Second Report of the Expert Panel on Detection, Evaluation, and Treatment of High Blood Cholesterol in Adults. National Heart, Lung, and Blood Institute, Bethesda. Publication No. 93-3095, 1993, p. III-8.

terol in patients with severe forms of hypercholesterolemia or established CHD. Because data on long-term safety are limited, and unless hypercholesteremia is severe, the sequestrants, rather than the statins, are usually the drugs of first choice in young adults. Gastrointestinal disturbances are the most common side effects, although they have been known to cause elevated hepatic transaminases and myopathy (muscle aches and weakness with concomitant use of cyclosporine, gemfibrozil, or niacin) and to increase creatine kinase values more than 10 times the upper limit of normal. Statins are not recommended for patients with myopathy or active liver disease.[25] Table 13–9 summarizes the HMG CoA reductase inhibitors.

ADDITIONAL PHARMACOLOGIC INTERVENTIONS

Several medications are available for treatment of blood lipid levels, but their effectiveness and safety have not been well established. The fibric acid derivatives, gemfibrozil and clofibrate, are primarily effective in lowering triglyceride levels and may increase HDL cholesterol levels in some patients. Clofibrate is recommended for patients with very high triglycerides who are at risk for pancreatitis. Gemfibrozil is used in the treatment of patients with very high triglycerides and for primary prevention of CHD in patients with combined elevated LDL cholesterol, high triglycerides, and low HDL cholesterol who have no known CHD. The fibric acid derivatives are not routinely used to lower cholesterol levels and reduce the risk of CHD. To determine the effectiveness and safety of the fibric acid derivatives, more research is needed and is likely to be forthcoming, as there is much interest in pharmacologic treatment of high serum cholesterol.[25]

Probucol is an antioxidant that is thought to retard the oxidative modification of LDL particles and prevent the formation of foam cells, an important component of atherosclerotic lesions. Probucol is generally used to treat patients who have not been treated successfully with other cholesterol-lowering medications. It has been found to lower serum LDL cholesterol in some patients, but in most patients, it has also been found to lower HDL cholesterol. Currently, there is no defined use for Probucol, and more research into its effectiveness and safety is needed.[25]

Estrogen replacement has been found, in uncontrolled studies, to reduce the rates of CHD in women. Estrogen has also been reported to have positive effects on osteoporosis. However, the potential carcinogenic effects of estrogen replacement in primary and secondary prevention of CHD have not been well established, and women taking estrogen replacement therapy should be monitored for development of uterine and breast cancer.[25]

Many new cholesterol-lowering drugs are currently in various phases of development and testing. The research regarding vigorous lifestyle modification to include diets low in fat (particularly saturated fat), regular aerobic exercise, reduction in body weight (if needed), smoking cessation, relaxation techniques, and pharmacologic intervention (if necessary), have reported positive results in primary and secondary prevention of CHD. The rehabilitation team of professionals in medicine, clinical exercise physiology, nursing, physical therapy, psychosocial, and behavior fields and nutrition have excellent opportunities to assist patients in achieving their individual goals in the retardation, stabilization, and reversal of their disease processes.[117,118]

Measurement of Lipid Outcomes

A complete fasting lipid profile is recommended before and after cardiac rehabilitation intervention. The profile should include blood levels of total cholesterol, triglycerides, HDL cholesterol, and LDL cholesterol.[53] Caution should be taken in interpreting blood lipid results obtained too soon (within 8 weeks) after AMI, CABG, or infection because the event can cause errors in lipid values.[119] Regular follow-up of each patient is also recommended in accordance with individual circumstances.

PHYSICAL INACTIVITY

The American Heart Association has recently classified inactivity as a major risk for CHD.[23] The first Surgeon General's report on activity and health[120] is explicit in stating that a substantial improvement in health and quality of life can be achieved by including moderate amounts of physical activity in daily routines. The report also states that regular physical activity reduces the risk of premature mortality, coronary heart disease, hypertension, colon cancer, and diabetes mellitus. Regular physical activity has also been reported to improve mental health and is important for the health of muscles, bones, and joints.[120] The physiologic adaptations of the body to aerobic exercise, the methods for patient assessment, guidelines for exercise prescription, and exercise therapy have been thoroughly discussed in other chapters of this text and will not be duplicated here. The reader is referred to Chapters 4, 9, 10, 11, and 12 for specific information about exercise therapy.

SUMMARY

The primary modifiable risk factors associated with increased incidence of CHD have been identified. They include cigarette smoking, hypertension, high serum cholesterol levels (particularly LDL cholesterol), and physical inactivity. They have been discussed in regard to their primary physiologic effects and current trends in the detection, management, and treatment of these factors. In most cases, treatment involves not only medical management but also lifestyle modifications that include exercise, normalizing body weight, dietary changes, and perhaps relaxation techniques. Increasing evidence supports the continuing need for quality cardiac rehabilitation programs that use a multidisciplinary approach as an adjunct to the medical and surgical management of the patient with CHD.

REFERENCES

1. Leon, AS: Scientific rational for preventive practices in atherosclerotic and hypertensive cardiovascular disease. In: Pollock, ML and Schmidt, DH (eds): Heart Disease and Rehabilitation, ed 3. Human Kinetics, Champaign, 1995, pp 115–146.
2. Agency for Health Care Policy and Research: Ischemic heart disease PORT publishes latest findings. Research Activities No. 183:1, Mar/April, 1995.
3. American Association of Cardiovascular and Pulmonary Rehabilitation: Secondary prevention of cardiovascular and pulmonary diseases under health care reform. In: News & Views, 9(3):3, summer, 1995.
4. American Association of Cardiovascular and Pulmonary Rehabilitation: Health care reform in the 1990s. J Cardpulm Rehabil 14(1):11–12, 1994.
5. American Association of Cardiovascular and Pulmonary Rehabilitation. Guidelines for Cardiac Rehabilitation Programs, ed 2. Human Kinetics, Champaign, 1995, pp 57–85.
6. Burnett, RE and Blumenthal, JA: Biobehavioral aspects of coronary artery disease: Considerations for prognosis and treatment. In: Pollock, ML and Schmidt, DH (eds): Heart Disease and Rehabilitation, ed 3. Human Kinetics, Champaign, 1995, pp 41–55.
7. Eaton, CB et al: Physical activity and coronary heart disease risk factors. Med Sci Sports Exerc 27(3):340–346, 1995.
8. Foster, C, Schrager, M, and Cohen, J: The value of cardiac rehabilitation: Secondary prevention. In: Pollock, ML and Schmidt, DH (eds). Heart Disease and Rehabilitation, ed 3. Human Kinetics, Champaign, 1995, pp 177–183.
9. Frasure-Smith, N: The Montreal heart attack readjustment trial. J Cardpulm Rehabil 15(2):103–106, 1995.
10. Frasure-Smith, N, Lesperance, F, and Talajic, M: Depression after myocardial infarction. Circulation 91:999–1005, 1995.
11. Hare, DL et al: Cardiac rehabilitation based on group light exercise and discussion. J Cardpulm Rehabil 15(3):186–192, 1995.
12. Kannel, WB: Epidemiologic insights into atherosclerotic cardiovascular disease—from the Framingham study. In: Pollock, ML and Schmidt, DH (eds): Heart Disease and Rehabilitation, ed 3. Human Kinetics, Champaign, 1995, pp 3–16.
13. LaFontaine, T: The role of lipid management by diet and exercise in the progression, stabilization, and regression of coronary artery atherosclerosis. J Cardpulm Rehabil 15(4):262–268, 1995.
14. DeBusk, RF et al: A case-management system for coronary risk factor modification after acute myocardial infarction. Ann Intern Med 120:721–729, 1994.
15. Nelson, DV et al: Six-month follow-up of stress management training versus cardiac education during hospitalization for acute myocardial infarction. J Cardpulm Rehabil 14(6):384–390, 1994.
16. Niebauer, J et al: Five years of physical exercise and low fat diet: Effects on progression of coronary artery disease. J Cardpulm Rehabil 15(1)L47–64. 1995.
17. Powell, KE and Blair, SN: The public health burdens of sedentary living habits: Theoretical but realistic estimates. Med Sci Sports Exerc 26(7):851–856, 1994.

18. Taylor, CB and Berra, K. Assessing depression. J Cardpulm Rehabil 14(6):376–377, 1994.
19. Joreteg, T et al: Evaluation of outcomes in patients post cardiac event following participation in cardiac rehabilitation or conventional medical management. J Cardpulm Rehabil 15(5):366, 1995.
20. Rosenson, RS: Reversing coronary artery disease. Phys Sports Med 22(11):59–64, 1994.
21. American Association of Cardiovascular and Pulmonary Rehabilitation: Round table: The primary prevention of coronary artery disease. J Cardpulm Rehabil 14(2):79–86, 1994.
22. Friedman, DB: Exercise and the Heart. U of Texas, Southwestern Medical Center, Dec 9, 1993.
23. American Heart Association: 1993 Heart Facts. American Heart Association Publication No. 550362, Dallas, 1993.
24. American College of Sports Medicine Position Stand: Exercise for patients with coronary artery disease. Med Sci Sports Exerc 26(3):i–iv, 1994.
25. US Department of Health and Human Services: National Cholesterol Education Program. Second Report of the Expert Panel on Detection, Evaluation, and Treatment of High Blood Cholesterol in Adults (Adult Treatment Panel II). National Institutes of Health, Bethesda. NIH Publication No. 93–3095, 1993.
26. American College of Sports Medicine: ACSM's Guidelines for Exercise Testing and Prescription, ed 5. Williams & Wilkins, Baltimore, 1995, pp 12–26.
27. American Heart Association. Position statement: Cardiac rehabilitation programs. Circulation 90(3):1602–1610, 1994.
28. Froelicher, VF et al: Exercise and the Heart. Mosby-Year Book, St. Louis, 1993, pp 347–377.
29. Hambrecht, R et al: Various intensities of leisure time physical activity in patients with coronary artery disease: Effects of cardiorespiratory fitness and progression of coronary atherosclerotic lesions. J Am Coll Cardiol 22:468–477, 1993.
30. Ornish, D et al: Can lifestyle changes reverse coronary heart disease? Lancet 336(8708):129–133, 1990.
31. Paffenbarger, RS and Blair, SN: Exercise in the primary prevention of coronary artery disease. In: Pollock, ML and Schmidt, DH (eds): Heart Disease and Rehabilitation, ed 3. Human Kinetics, Champaign, 1995, pp 169–176.
32. Paffenbarger, RS et al: Changes in physical activity and other lifeway patterns influencing longevity. Med Sci Sports Exerc 26(7):857–865, 1994.
33. Paffenbarger, RS et al: The association of changes in physical-activity level and other lifestyle characteristics with mortality among men. N Engl J Med 328:538–545, 1993.
34. Sherman C: Reversing heart disease: Are lifestyle changes enough? The Physician and Sportsmedicine 22(1):91–95, 1994.
35. Schuler, G et al: Regular physical exercise and low-fat diet: Effects on progression of coronary artery disease. Circulation 86:1–11, 1992.
36. Hurst, JW: Coronary heart disease: The overview of a clinician. In: Wenger, NK and Hellerstein, HK (eds): Rehabilitation of the Coronary Patient, ed 3. Churchill Livingstone, New York, 1992, p 14.
37. US Department of Health and Human Services: Reducing the health consequences of smoking: 25 years of progress. A report of the Surgeon General. Publication No. DHHS PHS 89–8411, Rockville, MD, 1989.
38. US Preventive Services Task Force: Counseling to prevent tobacco use. In: Guide to Clinical Preventive Services: An Assessment of the Effectiveness of 169 Interventions Report of the US Preventive Services Task Force. Williams & Wilkins, Baltimore, 1989, p 289.
39. Hahn, RA et al: Excess deaths from nine chronic diseases in the United States, 1986. JAMA 264:2654, 1990.
40. Caspersen, CJ and Heath, GW: The risk factor concept of coronary heart disease. In: ACSM's Resource Manual for Guidelines for Exercise Testing and Prescription, ed 2. Lea & Febiger, Philadelphia, 1993, pp 151–167.
41. Rosenberg, L, Palmer, JR, and Shapiro, S: Decline in the risk of myocardial infarction among women who stop smoking. N Engl J Med 322:213, 1990.
42. Fiore, MC et al: Trends in cigarette smoking in the United States: The changing influence of gender and race. JAMA 261:249, 1989.
43. American College of Sports Medicine: Guidelines for Exercise Testing and Prescription, ed 4. Lea & Febiger, Philadelphia, 1991, pp 121–159.
44. Nordenberg, D, Yip, R, and Binkin, NJ: The effects of cigarette smoking on hemoglobin levels and anemia screening. JAMA 264:1556, 1990.
45. Miller, HN et al: Position paper of the American Association of Cardiovascular and Pulmonary Rehabilitation: The efficacy of risk factor intervention and psychosocial aspects of cardiac rehabilitation. J Cardpulm Rehabil 10(6):198–209, 1990.
46. Grundy, SM et al: Cardiovascular and risk factor evaluation of healthy American adults: A statement for physicians by an ad hoc committee appointed by the steering committee. American Heart Association. Circulation 75:1340A, 1987.
47. LaCroix, AX et al: Smoking and mortality among older men and women in three communities. N Engl J Med 324:1619–1625, 1991.
48. Gottlieb, AM, Sachs, DP, and Newman, BR: Smoking Cessation. In: ACSM's Resource Manual for Guidelines for Exercise Testing and Prescription, ed 2. Lea & Febiger, Philadelphia, 1993, pp 483–488.

49. Transdermal Nicotine Study Group: Transdermal nicotine for smoking cessation: Six-month results from two multicenter controlled clinical trials. JAMA 266:3133, 1991.
50. Silagy, C et al: Meta-analysis on efficacy of nicotine replacement therapies in smoking cessation. Lancet 343(8890):139–142, 1994.
51. US Department of Health and Human Services: The health benefits of smoking cessation: A report of the Surgeon General. Public Health Service, Rockville, Publication No. DHHS 90–8416, 1990.
52. Morbidity and mortality weekly report 39:653, 1990. Smokers' belief about the health benefits of smoking cessation, US Committee, 1989. JAMA 264:1933, 1990.
53. Pashkow, P et al: Outcome Measurement in Cardiac and Pulmonary Rehabilitation: by the AACVPR Outcomes Committee. J Cardpulm Rehabil 15(6):394–405, 1995.
54. US Department of Health and Human Services: The Fifth Report of the Joint National Committee on Detection, Evaluation, and Treatment of High Blood Pressure. National Institutes of Health, Bethesda, NIH Publication No. 95–1008, 1995.
55. Hanson, P: Pathophysiology of chronic diseases and exercise training. In: ACSM's Resource Manual for Guidelines for Exercise Testing and Prescription, ed 2. Lea & Febiger, Philadelphia, 1993, pp 187–196.
56. Goldberg, L and Eliott, DL: Exercise as treatment for essential hypertension. In: Goldberg, L and Eliott, DL (eds): Exercise for Prevention and Treatment of Illness, FA Davis, Philadelphia, 1994, pp 27–47.
57. Roffman, DS: JNC V: Implications for management of hypertension. J Cardpulm Rehabil 14(1):21–24, 1994.
58. Hanson, P and Rueckert, P: Hypertension. In: Pollock, ML and Schmidt, DH (eds). Heart Disease and Rehabilitation, ed 3. Human Kinetics, Champaign, 1995, pp 343–356.
59. Kannel, WB: CHD risk factors: A Framingham Study update. Hosp Pract (Off Ed) 25:122, 1990.
60. Frohlich, ED et al: Recommendations for human blood pressure determination by sphygmomanometers. Report of a special task force appointed by the Steering Committee, American Heart Association. Hypertension 11:209A–222A, 1988.
61. Treatment of Mild Hypertension Research Group: The treatment of mild hypertension study: A randomized, placebo-controlled trial of a nutritional-hygienic regimen along with various drug monotherapies. Arch Intern Med 151:1413–1423, 1991.
62. Trials of Hypertension Prevention Collaborative Research Group: The effects of nonpharmacologic interventions on blood pressure of persons with high normal levels: Results of the Trials of Hypertension Prevention, Phase I. JAMA 267:1213–1220, 1992.
63. Stamler, J et al: INTERSALT study findings: Public health and medical care implications. Hypertension 14:570, 1989.
64. Sanders, E (ed): Lifestyle factors may affect hypertension, data shows. National Medical Association News, July/Aug:1, 1990.
65. Weinberger, MH: Salt intake and blood pressure in humans. Contemporary Nutrition 13:1, 1988.
66. Melby, CL, Lyle, RM, and Hyner, GC: Beyond blood pressure screening: A rationale for promoting the primary prevention of hypertension. American Journal of Health Promotion 3:5, 1988.
67. Alexander, JK: Obesity and the cardiovascular system. Hypertension 16:43, 1990.
68. Alexander, JK: The heart and obesity. In: Hearst, JW (ed): The Heart, ed 7. McGraw-Hill, New York, 1990.
69. Verrill, D, et al: Recommended guidelines for body composition assessment in cardiac rehabilitation. J Cardpulm Rehabil 14(2):104–121, 1994.
70. Ades, PA, Ross, SJ, and Poehlman, ET: Body composition-coronary risk factor interactions in older female coronary patients. J Cardpulm Rehabil 15(5):352, 1995.
71. Alexander, JK: Obesity and the cardiovascular system. In: Schlant, RC and Alexander, RW (eds): Hurst's The Heart, ed 8. McGraw-Hill, New York, 1995, pp 297–300.
72. Smith, CR: Fat distribution linked to mortality risk. The Physician and Sportsmedicine 21(5):40, 1993.
73. World Hypertension League: Alcohol and hypertension—implications for management: A consensus statement by the World Hypertension League. J Hum Hypertens 5:1854–1856, 1991.
74. Martin, JE, Dubbert, PM, and Cushman, WC: Controlled trial of aerobic exercise in hypertension. Circulation 81:1560–1567, 1990.
75. Kelemen, MH et al: Exercise training combined with antihypertensive drug therapy. Effects on lipids, blood pressure, and left ventricular mass. JAMA 263:2766–2771, 1990.
76. World Hypertension League: Physical exercise in the management of hypertension: A consensus statement by the World Hypertension League. J Hypertens 9:283–287, 1991.
77. American College of Sports Medicine: ACSM's Guidelines for Exercise Testing and Prescription, ed 5. Williams & Wilkins, Baltimore, 1995, pp 206–219.
78. Resnick, LM: Ionic hypothesis: The link between hypertension, obesity, insulin resistance, and left ventricular hypertrophy. Practical Cardiology 16(1):36, 1990.
79. Hamet, P et al: Interactions among calcium, sodium, and alcohol intake as determinants of blood pressure. Hypertension 17(Suppl I):I-150–I-154, 1991.
80. Ames, RP: Antihypertensive therapy and risk factors for coronary heart disease. Pract Cardiol 15(10):49, 1989.

81. Tanji, JL: Hypertension. Part 2. The role of medication. The Physician and Sportsmedicine 18(8):87, 1990.
82. Ames, RP: op cit.
83. Tanki, JL, and Batt, ME: Management of Hypertension. The Physician and Sportsmedicine 23(2):47–55, 1995.
84. Roffman, DS: Angiotensin converting enzyme inhibitors in cardiovascular disease, part two. J Cardpulm Rehabil 13(2):83–86, 1993.
85. Fletcher, BJ, et al: Dietary intake and blood cholesterol in an active elderly population. J Cardpulm Rehabil 13(2):80–82, 1993.
86. Johnson, CL et al: Declining serum total cholesterol levels among US adults: The national health and nutrition examination surveys. JAMA 269(23):3002–3008, 1993.
87. Kannel, WB: Epidemiologic insights into atherosclerotic cardiovascular disease—from the Framingham Study. In: Pollock, ML and Schmidt, DH (eds): Heart Disease and Rehabilitation, ed 3. Human Kinetics, Champaign, 1995, pp 3–16.
88. Rifkind, BM and Rossouw, JE: Lowering cholesterol. J Cardpulm Rehabil 12(2):87–91, 1992.
89. Durstine, LJ and Haskell, WL. Effects of exercise training on plasma lipids and lipoproteins. In: Holloszy, JO (ed): Exercise and Sport Sciences Reviews, Vol 22. Williams & Wilkins, Baltimore, 1994, pp 477–521.
90. Grundy, SM: Metabolism of triglyceride-rich lipoproteins. In: Cholesterol and Coronary Disease: Reducing the Risk. Science and Medicine, New York, 1988, p 4.
91. Grundy, SM and Vega, GL: Causes of high blood cholesterol. Circulation 81:412, 1990.
92. Steinberg, D and Witztom, JL: Lipoproteins and atherogenesis: Current concepts. JAMA 264:3047, 1990.
93. Steinberg, D et al: Beyond cholesterol: Modifications of low-density lipoprotein that increases its atherogenicity. N Engl J Med 320:915, 1989.
94. Grundy, SM: Classification of Lipid Disorders. Gower Medical Publishing, New York, 1990, pp 2–3.
95. American Heart Association Task Force on Cholesterol Issues: The cholesterol facts: A summary of the evidence relating to dietary fats, serum cholesterol, and coronary heart disease. A joint statement by the American Heart Association and the National Heart, Lung, and Blood Institute. Circulation 81:1721, 1990.
96. Houmard, JA et al: Effects of exercise training on the chemical composition of plasma LDL. Arterioscler Thromb Vasc Biol 14:325–330, 1994.
97. Goldberg, L and Elliot, DL: The use of exercise to improve lipid and lipoprotein levels. In: Exercise for Prevention and Treatment of Illness. FA Davis, Philadelphia, 1994, pp 189–209.
98. Rifkind, BM: High-density lipoprotein cholesterol and coronary artery disease: Survey of the evidence. Am J Cardiol 66:3A–6A, 1990.
99. Friedman, DB: Exercise and the Heart. Southwestern Medical Center, University of Texas, December, 1993, pp 6–7.
100. Lavie, CJ, Milani, RV, and Boykin, C: High-density lipoprotein cholesterol is the strongest lipid risk factor in elderly coronary patients. J Cardpulm Rehabil 13(5):334, 1993.
101. Stampfer, MJ et al: A prospective study of cholesterol, apolipoproteins, and the risk of myocardial infarction. N Engl J Med 323:373–381, 1991.
102. Spate, TL and Keyser, RE: Effects of exercise intensity on HDL profile. J Cardpulm Rehabil 13(5):340, 1993.
103. Havel, RJ: Role of triglyceride-rich lipoproteins in progression of atherogenesis. Circulation 81:694, 1990.
104. Scanu, AM and Fless, GM: Lipoprotein (a): Heterogeneity and biological relevance. J Clin Invest 85:1709, 1990.
105. Rauramaa, R et al: Inverse relation of physical activity and apolipoprotein AI to blood pressure in elderly women. Med Sci Sports Exerc 27(2):164–169, 1995.
106. American College of Sports Medicine. ACSM's Guidelines for Exercise Testing and Prescription, ed 5. Williams & Wilkins, Baltimore, 1995, pp 29–48.
107. Grundy, SM: Cholesterol and coronary heart disease: Future directions. JAMA 264:3053, 1990.
108. American Heart Association: The American Heart Association Diet. American Heart Association, Dallas, 1991.
109. Barnard, ND, Scherwitz, LW, and Ornish, D: Adherence and acceptability of a low-fat, vegetarian diet among patients with cardiac disease. J Cardpulm Rehabil 12(6):423–431, 1992.
110. Hiser, E: The Mediterranean diet and cardiovascular disease. J Cardpulm Rehabil 15(3):179–182, 1995.
111. Ornish, D: Eat More, Weigh Less. HarperCollins, New York, 1993.
112. Pritikin, R: The New Pritikin Program. Simon & Schuster, New York, 1990.
113. Rosati, KG and Spencer, M: Implementing progressive "reversal" cardiac diets in a hospital setting. J Cardpulm Rehabil 12(1):13–20, 1994.
114. U.S. Department of Health and Human Services. Step by Step: Eating to Lower Your High Blood Cholesterol. National Institutes of Health, Bethesda. NIH Publication No. 94–2920, 1994.
115. Pritikin, N: The Pritikin Program for Diet and Exercise. Bantam Books, New York, 1979.

116. Dattilo, AM: Reinforcing the Step II Diet in patients with coronary heart disease. J Cardpulm Rehabil 14(2):97–101, 1994.
117. Haskell, WL et al: Effects of intensive multiple risk factor reduction on coronary atherosclerosis and clinical events in men and women with coronary artery disease: The Stanford Coronary Risk Intervention Project (SCRIP). Circulation 89:975–990, 1994.
118. LaFontaine, T: loc cit.
119. Snyder, P: Cholesterol measurement following a cardiac event. J Cardpulm Rehabil 14(6):371–372, 1994.
120. Physical Activity and Health. A Report of the Surgeon General (Executive Summary). U.S. Department of Health and Human Services, National Institutes of Health, Bethesda, Md, 1996.

CHAPTER 14

Additional Components of Pulmonary Rehabilitation

Although aerobic exercise training is an integral part of pulmonary rehabilitation, the pulmonary patient requires additional information to optimize his or her exercise capabilities and to improve the quality of life. The topics presented below are often termed "adjuncts" to pulmonary rehabilitation, but the inference that they are somehow of secondary importance is inaccurate. The following discussion covers the essential elements of a pulmonary rehabilitation program: secretion removal techniques, ventilatory muscle training and breathing re-education, energy-saving techniques, and smoking cessation.

SECRETION-REMOVAL TECHNIQUES

Secretion retention can occur when there is an increase in the amount of secretions produced by the goblet cells and mucous glands that line the tracheobronchial tree (as in bronchiectasis, chronic bronchitis, and asthma), a change in the composition of the secretions (as in cystic fibrosis), or a decrease in the action of the cilia within the tracheobronchial tree (caused by immotile cilia or smoking). In any case, the resultant increase in secretions can interfere with ventilation and the diffusion of oxygen and carbon dioxide. An assessment of the pulmonary system will identify the areas of secretion retention (Chapter 10). An individualized program of secretion removal techniques directed to the areas of involvement can optimize a patient's ventilation and improve gas exchange capabilities.

Patients with secretion retention may improve their performance of an exercise regimen if the proper secretion removal techniques are provided before the exercise session. The following discussion includes the techniques of postural drainage, percussion, shaking, vibration, self-care techniques, and airway clearance as they pertain to the patient population who might participate in an outpatient pulmonary rehabilitation program. There is no intent to cover all patients who are acutely ill with pulmonary dysfunctions.

423

Postural Drainage

Positioning a patient in such a way that the bronchus of the involved lung segment is perpendicular to the ground is the basis for postural drainage. By using gravity, the positioning assists the mucociliary transport system in removing excessive secretions from the tracheobronchial tree. Lorin and Denning[1] found that secretion clearance improved in patients with cystic fibrosis when postural drainage coupled with coughing was compared with coughing alone. Postural drainage can be used by itself as a treatment program. Each appropriate postural drainage position is maintained for at least 5 minutes and may last up to 20 minutes if large amounts of secretions are present. An appropriate method of airway clearance (e.g., coughing) should be encouraged during and after each postural drainage position. Postural drainage can also be used in conjunction with other manual techniques (described in this chapter) as part of a treatment program.

Standard postural drainage positions are pictured in Figure 14–1. Although they are the optimal positions for gravity drainage of specific lung segments, they may not be realistic for some patients. The standard position for postural drainage could make a patient's respiratory status, or a concomitant problem, worse. Modification of the standard positions may prevent any untoward effects and still enhance secretion removal. The following list of precautions should be considered before instituting postural drainage with patients enrolled in an outpatient pulmonary rehabilitation program. They are relative precautions rather than absolute contraindications.

A. Precautions for the use of the Trendelenberg position (bed in a tipped, head-down position)
   1. Circulatory problems: such as pulmonary edema, congestive heart failure, hypertension
   2. Abdominal problems: such as obesity, abdominal distention, hiatal hernia, nausea, recent food consumption
   3. Shortness of breath made worse with the Trendelenberg position
B. Precautions for the use of the sidelying position
   1. Vascular problems: such as axillofemoral bypass graft
   2. Musculoskeletal problems: such as arthritis, recent rib fracture, shoulder bursitis, tendonitis, making positioning uncomfortable

This list is not meant to be all-inclusive, but it does provide the reader with a range of dysfunction that should be considered before instituting postural drainage.

Percussion

Percussion (or clapping) is a force rhythmically applied with the therapist's cupped hands to the patient's chest wall (Fig. 14–2). The percussion technique is applied to a specific area on the thorax that corresponds to an underlying involved lung segment. The appropriate site for the application of the percussion technique is shown in Figure 14–1. The technique is typically administered from 2 to 5 minutes (or to patient tolerance) to each involved lung segment, although there have been reports in the literature of 30 seconds to 20 minutes of percussion.[2,3] Percussion is thought to release the pulmonary secretions from the wall of the airways and into the lumen of the air-

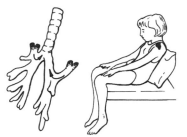

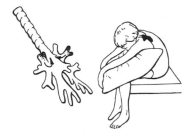

UPPER LOBES Apical Segments

Bed or drainage table flat.

Patient leans back on pillow at 30° angle against therapist.

Therapist claps with markedly cupped hand over area between clavicle and top of scapula on each side.

UPPER LOBES Posterior Segments

Bed or drainage table flat.

Patient leans over folder pillow at 30° angle.

Therapist stands behind and claps over upper back on both sides.

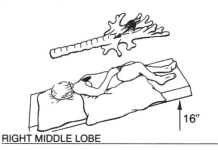

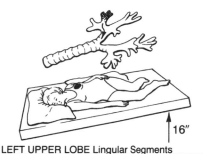

RIGHT MIDDLE LOBE

Foot of table or bed elevated 16 inches.

Patient lies head down on left side and rotates ¼ turn backward. Pillow may be placed behind from shoulder to hip. Knees should be flexed.

Therapist claps over right nipple area. In females with breast development or tenderness, use cupped hand with heel of hand under armpit and fingers extending forward beneath the breast.

LEFT UPPER LOBE Lingular Segments

Foot of table or bed elevated 16 inches.

Patient lies head down on right side and rotates ¼ turn backward. Pillow may be placed behind from shoulder to hip. Knees should be flexed.

Therapist claps with moderately cupped hand over left nipple area. In females with breast development or tenderness, use cupped hand with heel of hand under armpit and fingers extending forward beneath the breast.

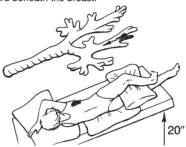

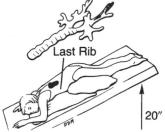

LOWER LOBES Lateral Basal Segments

Foot of table or bed elevated 20 inches.

Patient lies on abdomen, head down, then rotates ¼ turn upward. Upper leg is flexed over a pillow for support.

Therapist claps over uppermost portion of lower ribs. (Position shown is for drainage of right lateral basal segment. To drain the left lateral basal segment, patient should lie on his or her right side in the same posture).

LOWER LOBES Posterior Basal Segments

Foot of table or bed elevated 20 inches.

Patient lies on abdomen, head down, with pillow under hips. Therapist claps over lower ribs close to spine on each side.

FIGURE 14–1. Postural drainage.

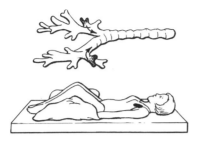

UPPER LOBES Anterior Segments

Bed or drainage table flat.

Patient lies on back with pillow under knees.

Therapist claps between clavicle and
nipple on each side.

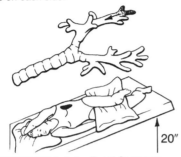

LOWER LOBES Anterior Basal Segments

Foot of table or bed elevated 20 inches.

Patient lies on side, head down, pillow under knees.

Therapist claps with slightly cupped hand over lower
ribs. (Position shown is for drainage of <u>left</u> anterior
basal segment. To drain the right anterior basal
segment, patient should lie on his or her left side in
same posture).

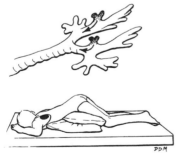

LOWER LOBES Superior Segments

Bed or table flat.

Patient lies on abdomen with two pillows under hips.

Therapist claps over middle of back at tip of scapula
on either side of spine.

FIGURE 14–1. *Continued.* (From Rothstein, JM,
Roy, SH, and Wolf, SL: The Rehabilitation Specialist's Handbook, ed. 2. FA Davis, Philadelphia,
1998, pp. 534–535, with permission.)

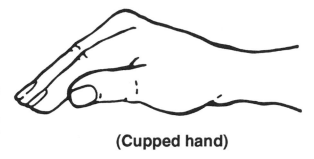

FIGURE 14–2. Cupped hand for the percussion technique. (From the National Cystic Fibrosis Foundation, Courtesy of Bettina C. Hilman, MD, with permission.)

(Cupped hand)

way.[4] Unfortunately, this process seems to be nondirectional; that is, the secretions may be moved closer to the glottis or deeper into the pulmonary parenchyma. When percussion is coupled with the appropriate postural drainage position for a specific lung segment, the probability of secretion removal is enhanced.[5-7] Because percussion is a force directed to the thorax, there are conditions that must be evaluated before its use.

A. Precautions for the use of percussion
   1. Circulatory: such as hemoptysis, coagulation disorders (increased partial thromboplastin time (PTT) or prothrombin time (PT), decreased platelet count below 50,000, and medications that interfere with coagulation)
   2. Musculoskeletal: such as fractured ribs, flail chest, degenerative bone disease

Again, the list is by no means all-inclusive. It does provide some general guidelines that deserve consideration when percussion is part of the therapeutic regimen. It should also be noted that some modification of this technique to enhance patient tolerance can occur.

Shaking

Shaking is used to hasten the removal of secretions via the mucociliary transport system. Following a deep inhalation, a bouncing maneuver is applied to the rib cage throughout the expiratory phase of breathing. The shaking maneuver is applied to a specific area on the thorax that corresponds to the underlying involved lung segment (Fig. 14–3). It is commonly used following percussion in the appropriate postural drainage position.[8,9] Five to seven deep inhalations, each followed by shaking on exhalation, are adequate to promote secretion clearance without risking possible hyperventilation. Because the technique is a force applied to the thorax, the same precautions as noted in the application of percussion are needed.

Vibration

The sustained co-contraction of the therapist's upper extremities produces a vibration that is transmitted from the therapist's hands to the patient's thorax during the expiratory phase of respiration. Vibration can also be produced by a mechanical device

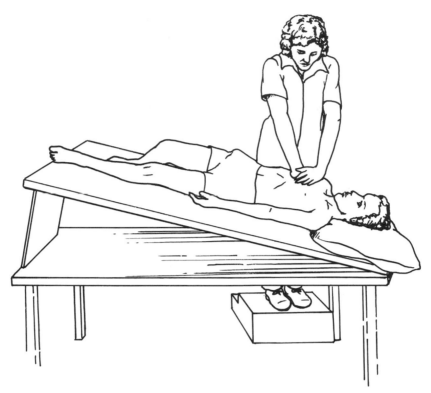

FIGURE 14–3. Shaking being performed over the involved right anterior segment, upper lobe. (From the National Cystic Fibrosis Foundation, Courtesy of Bettina C. Hilman, MD, with permission.)

and transmitted to the patient's chest wall. Again, it is applied to a specific area on the thorax that corresponds to an underlying involved lung segment. Vibration is used to enhance the mucociliary transport system. Because little or no pressure is placed on the thorax during the vibration technique, there are no contraindications to its use. Vibration is often used when percussion and shaking are contraindicated. Postural drainage positions, if appropriate, can be coupled with vibration to optimize effectiveness.

Airway Clearance

Once the secretions have been mobilized with postural drainage, percussion, and shaking or vibration, removing them from the airways is necessary. Coughing is the most common and easiest means of clearing the airway. There are many variations of the cough maneuver. For the patient enrolled in a pulmonary rehabilitation program, the cough, huff, and forced expiratory technique (FET) are most often used.

COUGH

A cough is the simplest way in which to clear secretions from the upper airways. It is produced by a coordinated effort made up of the following steps: inhale deeply, close the glottis, create an increased intrathoracic pressure by contracting the abdominal muscles ("bearing down"), and then release the glottis and expel the air while continually contracting the abdominal muscles.[10] Expiratory flow rates during a cough can be as high as 70 mph. The upright sitting position has been found to produce the highest expiratory flow rates and is therefore thought to be the most effective position for coughing.[11]

HUFF

A huff uses many of the same coordinated steps as the cough with the omission of a closed glottis. The patient is asked to take a deep inhalation and rapidly contract the abdominal muscles for a series of forced expirations through an "open" airway. It is as if the patient were saying "Ha, ha, ha." High intrathoracic pressure generated during the compression phase of coughing can close off small airways in some patients with chronic obstructive pulmonary disease (COPD). If the air is trapped behind the closed airway, the cough becomes ineffective. A huff has been shown to stabilize collapsible airway walls, making expiration and secretion removal more effective in this patient population.[12]

FORCED EXPIRATORY TECHNIQUE

The performance of the forced expiratory technique (FET), also called active cycle of breathing technique (ACBT), is characterized by breathing control and huffing from mid to low lung volumes. The patient is first taught breathing from the lower chest (diaphragmatic breathing). He or she is then asked to inhale a medium-sized breath of air and, from that point, to contract the abdominal muscles to produce a huff.[13]

The sequence of performing this technique is summarized as follows:[14]

1. Breathing control
2. Thoracic expansion exercises (with or without percussion and shaking)
3. Breathing control
4. One or two huffs from mid to low lung volumes
5. Breathing control

As secretions accumulate in the more central airways, one or two huffs or coughs from high lung volumes can be used to clear the secretions.

FET is thought to milk the more peripheral airways of their secretions and make overall lung clearance more effective.[15] This technique has been used alone and in conjunction with other secretion removal techniques with various outcomes. It has been effective in patients with COPD, asthma, and cystic fibrosis and is currently the treatment of choice in many cystic fibrosis centers in England.[16]

Self-Administered Secretion-Removal Techniques

A variety of new devices and techniques have been developed in hopes of allowing the patient more independence in the clearing of excessive secretions from the airways of the lungs. The best use of these new techniques (i.e., appropriate patient population, severity of disease state) is currently under investigation.

The flutter VRP1 is a pipelike device with a steel ball-bearing inside. Exhalation through the apparatus results in the ball bearing within the pipe to be quickly and repeatedly raised and dropped creating a fluttering or oscillation that is transmitted back to the airway. This vibration may aid in patients' abilities to independently eliminate excessive mucus from their airways. Studies to date on the efficacy of secretion removal with the flutter device have not been conclusive.[17–19] Further study regarding short- and long-term outcomes and the appropriate patient populations are needed.

Positive expiratory pressure (PEP) masks are tight-fitting facial masks that provide expiratory resistance to the patient, usually in the range of 15 to 20 mm Hg. The positive pressure is used to maintain open airways and allow better secretion removal. Some investigators use cycles of controlled breathing with the mask in place (8 to 10 breaths),[20] followed by an airway clearance technique such as a cough or huff, while others use the mask for a number of minutes with no interruption.[21] There does not yet seem to be consensus on how to apply this technique nor which patient populations might best benefit from it.

Autogenic drainage involves three stages of breathing maneuvers:

Stage 1: A series of breaths thought to be used to unstick secretions from the airways. Stage one requires breathing at low lung volumes, from the middle tidal volume into expiratory reserve volume.

Stage 2: A series of breaths thought to help collect mucus in the middle airways. This stage is performed by breathing at high lung volumes, from low inspiratory reserve volume down to the expiratory reserve volume.

Stage 3: A final series of breaths used to remove secretions from the central airways. This is done by breathing in high lung volumes (upper inspiratory reserve volume) and, with small bouts of coughing, reduce the amount of air in the lungs to end tidal volume.

Each stage has a controlled inspiration, a short stop where the inspiratory level is maintained, followed by expiration. In stages 1 and 2, the expiration is rapid but controlled, avoiding high flow rates that might result in airway collapse. Stage 3 allows for coughing.[22]

Various studies have compared autogenic drainage with other forms of secretion removal techniques, with differing outcomes.[23–25] The major consideration in the use of autogenic drainage is the amount of training needed before independence and the concentration required during the performance of the treatment.[24]

Self-management is a major goal in pulmonary rehabilitation. Research in the next few years may assist the pulmonary rehabilitation team in determining the applicability of these devices to their patient populations, allowing independence and self-care.

In summary, the combination of postural drainage, percussion, shaking, vibration, self-care techniques, and airway clearance directed to specific areas of secretion retention can remove excessive pulmonary secretions, improve ventilation, and subsequently improve gas exchange. Patients with secretion retention who participate in a pulmonary rehabilitation program might benefit from a session of secretion-removal techniques before the exercise session.

VENTILATORY MUSCLE TRAINING AND BREATHING RE-EDUCATION

The inability to increase ventilation sufficiently is often the limiting factor in activities and exercise tolerance of patients with pulmonary dysfunction. Optimizing the ventilatory function may improve exercise tolerance and the ability to perform work. Ventilatory muscle training has been used to improve the strength and endurance of the muscles of ventilation, which may increase the ability to exercise. Breathing re-education teaches a more efficient pattern of ventilation, which in some patients may decrease the work of breathing and the feeling of breathlessness.

Ventilatory Muscle Training

The ventilatory muscles can be physiologically trained in a manner similar to the training of other skeletal muscles. Traditionally, skeletal muscles are trained by either loading them against a high resistance for strengthening or by high-frequency repetition for enhancing endurance. In general, skeletal muscles, particularly ventilatory muscles, have the capacity for specificity of training. Whereas general aerobic exercise alone may improve the strength and endurance of the ventilatory muscles,[26] specific training regimens for those muscles have been suggested.[27] Leith and Bradley[28] report a 55 percent increase in the strength and a 19 percent increase in the endurance of the ventilatory muscles following a 5-week training program.

There are specific devices, inspiratory muscle trainers (IMTs), that load the inspiratory muscles via graded apertures. The patient breathes in through the narrowed opening, which loads the inspiratory muscles and thereby trains the muscles of inspiration.[29] Exhalation is unresisted in most IMT devices. Exercise programs that provide both strength and endurance training of the inspiratory muscles can be formulated. Training sessions are recommended at a frequency of one to two times per day and a duration of 15 to 30 minutes.[29,30] By changing the size of the opening, the intensity of training can be modulated.

An appropriate exercise intensity can be determined in either of two ways. First, the maximum static inspiratory mouth pressure (MSIP) from functional residual capacity is determined. Inspiratory muscle strengthening programs then begin by using an opening that provides a resistance between 15 and 30 percent of MSIP working up to higher percentages as the training progresses.[31-33] Some studies have used as much as 80 percent of MSIP for training.[34] A second way to determine exercise intensity is to select the smallest aperture (opening) the patient can tolerate for a 10-minute exercise period.[29] Endurance training would use a lower percent of MSIP, or the opening that would allow a longer exercise duration.

As with any exercise regimen for the musculoskeletal system, the exercise must be done properly to achieve the desired results. Patients can develop alternative breathing patterns that lessen the resistance placed on the ventilatory system by the inspiratory muscle trainer, usually a slower, deeper breath. A controlled pattern of breathing must be sustained to maintain an appropriate inspiratory load (intensity) throughout the program.

The objective of this type of training is to decrease the oxygen consumption of the inspiratory muscles during ventilation, and thereby improve exercise capacity.[35] By training the inspiratory muscles, patients may be able to decrease the work of breathing, inspiratory time[36] (which allows for a longer expiratory time), increase ability to perform activities of daily living,[37] and the sensation of dyspnea.[38] Inspiratory muscle training in conjunction with lower extremity exercise or generalize exercise training may enhance the ability to increase exercise tolerance.[32,39] Patients may also be more able to resist ventilatory muscle fatigue. This is advantageous during exercise sessions as well as during exacerbations of the respiratory disease.

Breathing Re-education

DIAPHRAGMATIC BREATHING

Teaching diaphragmatic breathing, although not a physiologic training technique, has been shown to lower the respiratory rate, increase the tidal volume per breath and decrease the sensation of dyspnea in some patients. Instructing a patient in diaphragmatic breathing exercises begins by placing him or her in the comfortable semi-Fowler's (reclined sitting) position. The patient's own hand is placed over the costochondral angle. "Sniffing" is then used to facilitate the contraction of the diaphragm, allowing the patient to palpate the muscle and ensuring proper hand placement. Allowing the hand to rise during inspiration and fall during expiration encourages a relaxed and efficient pattern of ventilation. It is most desirable to inspire nasally, thus ensuring a slow, even inspiration. Oral exhalation provides for the least resistance to air flow.

Decreasing the use of accessory muscles also decreases the work of breathing. Biofeedback can emphasize the proper use of the diaphragm and inhibit the use of accessory muscles during the ventilatory cycle.

Even though a good breathing pattern is often taught in a semi-recumbent, comfortable position, a progression must be established.[31] The continued use of that same breathing pattern during sitting, standing, walking, and stair climbing is necessary to make breathing re-education useful in the overall rehabilitation of the patient with pulmonary disease.

Not all patients seem to benefit from the use of diaphragmatic breathing.[40] As the patient learns the technique, the instructor must watch for paradoxic movement (or an increase in an existing paradoxic movement) of the thorax. If no benefit is noted by the patient or the therapist after a trial of diaphragmatic breathing, then the natural breathing pattern of the patient may be the more efficient method.

PURSED-LIPS BREATHING

The pursed-lips breathing technique is performed by inhaling through the nose and exhaling through pursed lips (as though the patient were about to whistle). The abdominal muscles may or may not be used for exhalation. Many patients have "found" this technique without any instruction. The therapist can ensure that pursed-lips breathing is done correctly and that it is maintained during exercise and any other activity that may result in shortness of breath.

Pursed-lips breathing, when used by patients with COPD, has been shown to decrease respiratory rates, increase tidal volumes,[35] and decrease the sensation of dyspnea.[41] Some authors have demonstrated an improvement in arterial oxygenation.[42] It may delay or prevent airway collapse and allow better gas exchange.[43]

Both techniques of ventilatory muscle training and breathing re-education strive to decrease the work of breathing. When they are incorporated in the exercise session, a more effective exercise program may be performed.

ENERGY-SAVING TECHNIQUES

Patients with pulmonary dysfunction may become dyspneic while performing varying levels of activities of daily living (ADLs). The activities that produce dyspnea are thereafter often avoided. The result may be a dependence on others, with both physical and emotional consequences. During the initial evaluation, the therapist must determine which ADLs are problematic. The individual's goals for the rehabilitation program should reflect the difficulties and offer resolution of the problems. Instruction in the use of energy-saving techniques (ESTs) should be part of the patient's treatment plan. Regaining the ADLs can renew a patient's independence and sense of well-being.

ESTs should be used when the usual performance of an activity would precipitate dyspnea. An EST combines the techniques of assistive and adaptive equipment, activity planning and preparation, pacing, and efficient breathing patterns. Together, the techniques lower the energy expenditure and the oxygen consumption of an activity.

Assistive and Adaptive Equipment

The use of assistive and adaptive equipment *alone* can allow a patient to perform an activity. A patient with pulmonary disease who has moderate obesity over the abdomen may become dyspneic while putting on shoes and socks. The task can be accomplished without dyspnea by using a stocking aid and long-handled shoehorn. A patient with moderate to severe dyspnea often finds it very difficult to shower, because the activity requires long periods of standing, bending, upper extremity work, and frequency of breath holding. The patient may be able to shower by using a shower bench, soap on a rope, a hand-held shower nozzle, a long-handled brush, and a terry cloth bathrobe. Assistive equipment may include even a microwave oven, because it requires less cooking time and little attention during cooking and may allow a patient to better prepare more nutritious meals more frequently with decreased levels of dyspnea. These are only a few examples of how assistive and adaptive equipment can be used in pulmonary rehabilitation.

Activity Planning and Preparation

Activity planning and preparation is another key component of energy-saving techniques. The scheduling, organizing, and prioritizing of tasks can make a difference in the functional abilities of patients with pulmonary disease.[44] Many bouts of dyspnea can be avoided by efficient scheduling of activities. Activities that most significantly increase the demands on the cardiopulmonary system should be spaced throughout the day, week, and month to allow maximum rest and recovery time between activities. They should also be scheduled around availability of friends and relatives to assist in the more demanding work. Many patients with pulmonary disease find the mornings most difficult. Performing as many activities as possible the evening before and organizing the tasks ahead can make the mornings less demanding. Meal preparation is another important activity that often is not performed adequately because of dyspnea. Even when the meal is prepared, the patient may have become too fatigued to eat. Proper organization from the start of meal preparation can minimize the demands of the activity. Proper planning ensures that only one trip to the refrigerator or cupboard is necessary. Commonly used meal ingredients and utensils should be very accessible to the preparation site. Meals can be prepared while seated instead of standing. With careful planning and preparation for an activity, it can be completed without dyspnea or fatigue. Activities such as cooking should be performed in areas with good ventilation and oxygen precautions when applicable.

Pacing

Pacing is another integral component of ESTs and pulmonary rehabilitation. It is so simple in nature that the patient is somehow expected to know and use the concept intuitively. This is often not the case, however, and pacing has to be taught. Pacing can be defined as the performance of an activity within the limits or boundaries of the patient's breathing capacity. Often that means the activity must be divided into components so that it is performed at a tempo that does not exceed the patient's breathing limitations. For example, stair climbing is performed only on exhalation and by taking one or two steps at a time. The patient is asked to remain on that step until there is full recovery of his or her breathing. The next two or three steps are ascended, again on exhalation, followed by a rest period for breathing recovery. The sequence is continued until the full flight of stairs is accomplished without dyspnea. (Pursed-lip breathing and recovery breathing should also be used with pacing when necessary.)

Often a patient may complain that an activity took too long to perform or that he or she felt foolish walking that way. To the patient, pacing is viewed as slowing down. It is often helpful to prove to the patient that the pacing technique may actually save time. First, ask the patient to climb a flight of stairs his or her own way. A person with COPD typically climbs the stairs in the following manner: an upward look at the awesome task ahead, ascent of the first few steps, some shortness of breath, and then an increase in the speed of ascent to ensure that the top will be reached. By the time the patient reaches the top, he or she is visibly dyspneic, and it may take several minutes to regain control of respirations. Time the activity from the onset of stair climbing until breathing is recovered at the top of the stairs. Now repeat the task with pacing. With pacing, the task will undoubtedly take less time and the patient will remain comfortable throughout. As to looking foolish, how foolish did the patient appear to be at the top of the stairs in the first climb while gasping for air? The patient should also expect that the activity will look much more coordinated with practice.

The goal of pacing is to complete an activity safely and without dyspnea. Pacing can and should be part of every activity that would otherwise cause dyspnea. By dividing activities into component parts and interspersing rest periods between components, the total activity can be completed without dyspnea or fatigue.

Pacing should be used in such tasks as ADLs, ambulating, stair climbing, and lifting. It is not a technique to be used during the aerobic portion of a pulmonary rehabilitation program. During exercise, some shortness of breath should, and will, occur.

SMOKING CESSATION

Smoking is the primary cause of COPD[45] as well as a contributing cause of many other disease processes.[46] Therefore a special focus on smoking cessation should be included in all pulmonary rehabilitation programs. The benefits of being smoke-free have long been assumed. Participants in the Lung Health Study, patients with mild to moderate air flow obstruction who quit smoking, showed an age-related decline in FEV_1 that was less dramatic than that of the group of continued smokers.[47] In other words, lung function will be better over time when patients quit smoking than it will be if they continue to smoke. Although only mild to moderate airflow obstruction was studied, this conclusion seems to encourage smoking cessation for all patients with lung disease.

TABLE 14–1 Types of Smoking-Cessation Techniques

Propaganda	Therapy programs
Mass media messages	Smoking-cessation clinics
Posters	Group therapy
Brochures	Individual counseling
	Psychotherapy
Drugs	Hypnosis
Lobeline	
Dextroamphetamine	Behavior modification
Imipramine	Self-monitoring
Nicotine gum	Stimulus control
	Contingency management
Aversion–satiation	Self-management
Rapid smoke	Desensitization
Imagination	Role-playing
Smoky air in face or mouth	Self-punishment
Electric shock	Values clarification
	Sensory deprivation
Cognitive approach	Gradual reduction
Information	Problem solving
Books	
Articles	Other
Physician's order	Prayer
	Meditation
Affective approach	Relaxation
Fear	Exercise
	Acupuncture

Source: From Peters, J and Lim, V: Smoking cessation techniques. In Hodgkin, J et al. (eds): Pulmonary Rehabilitation: Guidelines to Success. Butterworth Publishers, Boston, 1984, p. 94. Used by permission of J. Hodgkin, MD.

Patients are classified into four categories according to smoking habits: those who never smoked, those who used to smoke, those who are currently smoking but would like to quit, and finally, those who are currently smoking and wish to continue smoking. For the two groups of nonsmokers, the hazards of primary smoke and passive ambient smoke need to be emphasized. The effects of smoking and the benefits of being smokeless must be reinforced.[48]

The currently smoking patient demands careful consideration. A patient who has the desire to quit smoking, regardless of personal success, needs assistance to break the behavior pattern most effectively. There are many smoking cessation techniques; examples are cold turkey, behavior modification,[49] rapid smoking,[50] cognitive approach,[51] and nicotine replacement regimens[52,53] (Table 14–1; also see Chapter 13). No single method has a higher long-term success rate than another. A comprehensive treatment approach incorporating many different smoking cessation strategies has a higher abstention rate than any single specific technique.[54–57] It is well known that persons in smoking cessation programs have a low percentage of abstinence after 5 years (22 percent in the Lung Health Study).[47] Often, patients need to quit multiple times before they become successful nonsmokers.

It is the role of the clinician to guide the patient toward smoking cessation, not necessarily to provide the service. The American Lung Association and the American Cancer Society are good sources of available smoking cessation centers. It is very important that the clinician be a sympathetic and encouraging professional during the process of smoking cessation.

A patient who has no intention of quitting smoking may need to be dealt with quite differently. The patient must fully understand the consequences of smoking and how the habit is altering the degree of illness. If the patient still plans to smoke, the benefits of continuing in a pulmonary rehabilitation program are questionable. There may be little or no motivation for being well, for being responsible for one's own care, or for complying with the demands of pulmonary rehabilitation.

NUTRITION

Patients with COPD have a 15 percent increase in energy expenditure at rest resulting from the increase in the work of breathing.[45] These patients therefore require more calories per day than their peers who do not have lung disease. Patients with cystic fibrosis, with their combined problems of malabsorption and increased work of breathing, may require up to 50 percent more calories per day than the average person.[58] However, eating certain foods and large meals is difficult for many patients with pulmonary disease. The preparation of food, the need to hold the breath during swallowing, the side effects of medication regimens, and the limitations of diaphragmatic excursion as a result of a full stomach can make eating uncomfortable and unpleasant. As a result, patients may lose their appetites and lose weight; they could become malnourished. Muscle strength, endurance, and the ability to ward off infection are affected. Small, more frequent meals and readily available snacks may provide better nutrition, patient comfort, and compliance. The usefulness of altering the fats to carbohydrates ratio in a patient's diet have not yet been shown to be beneficial. Nutritional counseling to identify individual dietary needs is often important for overall wellness.

SUMMARY

In summary, pulmonary rehabilitation is more than an exercise therapy session. A comprehensive care plan that will "return the patient to the highest possible functional capacity allowed by his pulmonary handicap and overall life situation"[59] is the goal of pulmonary rehabilitation. Additional components of the exercise sessions, secretion removal techniques, ventilatory muscle training and breathing re-education, energy-saving techniques, smoking cessation, and nutritional requirements are imperative to meet that goal, and they have been presented in this discussion.

REFERENCES

1. Lorin, M and Denning, C: Evaluation of postural drainage for measurement of sputum volume and consistency. Am J Phys Med 50(5):215–219, 1971.
2. Murphy, M, Concannon, D, and Fitzgerald, M: Chest percussion: Help or hindrance to postural drainage? Ir Med J 76:189–190, 1983.

3. Zidulka, A et al: Clapping or percussion causes atelectasis in dogs and influences gas exchange. J Appl Physiol 66(6):2833–2838, 1989.
4. Kigin, C: Advances in chest physical therapy. In: Current Advances in Respiratory Care. American College of Chest Physician, Park Ridge, 1984.
5. Chopra, S et al: Effects of hydration and physical therapy on tracheal transport velocity. American Review of Respiratory Diseases 115:1009–1014, 1977.
6. Denton, P: Bronchial secretions in cystic fibrosis. Am Rev Respir Dis 86:41–46, 1962.
7. Mazzocco, M et al: Physiologic effects of chest percussion and postural drainage in patients with bronchiectasis. Chest 88:360–363, 1985.
8. Frownfelter, D: Chest Physical Therapy and Pulmonary Rehabilitation: An Interdisciplinary Approach, ed 2. Year Book Medical Publishers, Chicago, 1987.
9. Zack, M and Oberwaldner, B: Chest physiotherapy: The mechanical approach to antiinfective therapy in cystic fibrosis. Infection 15(5):381–384, 1987.
10. Starr, J: Lesson 8, In Touch Series. American Physical Therapy Association, Alexandria, Va, 1990.
11. Starr, J: The effect of position and trial on the effectiveness of cough in the postoperative patient. Boston University, 1980. Unpublished thesis.
12. Hietpas, B, Roth, R, and Jensen, W: Huff coughing and airway patency. Respiratory Care 24(8):710–713, 1979.
13. Partridge, C, Pryor J, and Webber, B: Characteristics of the forced expiration technique. Physiotherapy 75:193–194, 1989.
14. Pryor, JA: Respiratory Care. Churchill Livingstone, New York, 1991, pp 80–82.
15. Sutton, P et al: Assessment of the forced expiratory technique: Postural drainage and directed coughing in chest physiotherapy. European Journal of Respiratory Disease 64:62–68, 1983.
16. Prasad, S: Current concepts in physiotherapy. J R Soc Med 86 (suppl 20): 23–29, 1993.
17. Konstan, M, Stern, R, and Doershuk, C: Efficacy of the flutter device for airway mucus clearance in patients with cystic fibrosis. J Pediatr 124:689–693, 1994.
18. Pryor J et al: The flutter VRP1 as an adjunct to chest physiotherapy in cystic fibrosis. Respir Med 88: 677–681, 1994.
19. Swift G et al: Use of flutter VRP1 in the management of patients with steroid dependent asthma. Respiration 61:126–129, 1994.
20. Pfleger A, et al: Self administered chest physiotherapy in cystic fibrosis: A comparative study of high pressure PEP and autogenic drainage. Lung 170:323–330, 1992.
21. Larsen K et al: Mask physiotherapy in patients after heart surgery: A controlled study. Intensive Care Med 21:469–474, 1995.
22. Schoni, M: Autogenic drainage: A modern approach to physiotherapy in cystic fibrosis: J R Soc Med 82 (suppl 16): 32–37, 1989.
23. Giles D et al: Short term effects of postural drainage on oxygen saturation and sputum recovery in patients with cystic fibrosis. Chest 108(4):952–954, 1995.
24. Miller S et al: Chest physiotherapy in cystic fibrosis: A comparative study of autogenic drainage and the active cycle of breathing techniques with postural drainage. Thorax 50:165–169, 1995.
25. Thomas, J, Cook, D, and Brooks, D: Chest physical therapy management of patients with cystic fibrosis: A meta-analysis. American Review of Respiratory Diseases 151:846–850, 1995.
26 Keens, T et al: Ventilatory muscle endurance training in normal subjects and patients with cystic fibrosis. American Review of Respiratory Diseases 116:853–860, 1977.
27. Kim, M: Respiratory muscle training: Implications for patient care. Heart lung 13:333–340, 1984.
28. Leith, D and Bradley, M: Ventilatory muscle strength and endurance training. J Appl Physiol 41:508–516, 1976.
29. Sonne, L and David, J: Increased exercise performance in patients with severe COPD following inspiratory resistive training. Chest 81:436–439, 1982.
30. Chen, H, Dukes, R, and Martin, B: Inspiratory muscle training in patients with chronic obstructive pulmonary disease. American Review of Respiratory Diseases 131:251–255, 1985.
31. Darbee, J and Cerney, F (eds.): Exercise testing and exercise conditioning for children with lung dysfunction. In: Irwin, S and Tecklin J: Cardiopulmonary Physical Therapy, ed 2. Mosby, Philadelphia, 1990, pp 469–470.
32. Weiner, D, Azgad, Y, and Ganam R: Inspiratory muscle training combined with general exercise reconditioning in patients with COPD. Chest 102:1351–1356, 1992.
33. Weiner, P et al: Inspiratory muscle training in patients with bronchial asthma. Chest 102:357–361, 1992.
34. Berry, M et al: Inspiratory muscle training and whole body reconditioning in chronic obstructive pulmonary disease: A controlled randomized trial. Am J Respir Crit Care Med 153:1812–1816, 1996.
35. Belman, M and Mittman, C: Ventilatory muscle training improves exercise capacity in chronic obstructive pulmonary disease patients. American Review of Respiratory Diseases 121:273–280, 1980.
36. Flynn, M et al: Threshold pressure training, breathing pattern and exercise performance in chronic airflow obstruction. Chest 95:535–540, 1989.
37. Dekhurzen, P, Folgering, H, and van Herwaarden, C: Target flow inspiration muscle training during pulmonary rehabilitation in patients with COPD. Chest 99:128–133, 1991.
38. Harver, A, Mahler, D, and Daubenspeck J: Targeted inspiratory muscle training improves respiratory

muscle function and reduces dyspnea in patients with chronic obstructive disease. Ann Intern Med 111:117–124, 1989.

39. Wanke, T et al: Effects of combined inspiratory muscle and cycle ergometer training on exercise performance in patients with COPD. Eur Respir J 7:2205–2211, 1994.

40. Sachner, M et al: Effects of abdominal and thoracic breathing on breathing pattern components in normal subjects and in patients with chronic obstructive pulmonary disease. American Review of Respiratory Diseases 130:584–587, 1984.

41. Mueller, T, Petty, T, and Filley, G: Ventilation and arterial blood gas changes induced by pursed lips breathing. J Appl Physiol 28:784–789, 1970.

42. Tiep, B et al: Pursed lips breathing training using ear oximetry. Chest 90:218–221, 1986.

43. Adkins, H: Improvement of breathing ability in children with respiratory muscle paralysis. Phys Ther 48:577–581, 1968.

44. Thoman, R, Stoker, G, and Ross, J: The efficacy of pursed-lips breathing in patients with chronic obstructive pulmonary disease. American Review of Respiratory Diseases 93:100–106, 1966.

45. American Thoracic Society: Standards for the diagnosis and care of patients with chronic obstructive pulmonary disease. Am J Respir Crit Care Med 152:S78–S121, 1995.

46. Kigin, C: Breathing exercises for the medical patient: The art and the science. Phys Ther 70(11):700–706, 1990.

47. Anthonisen, N et al: Effects of smoking intervention and the use of an inhaled anticholinergic bronchodilator on the rate of decline of FEV_1: The lung health study. JAMA 272(19):1497–1505, 1994.

48. Burki, N: Pulmonary Diseases. Medical Examination Publishing, Garden City, NY, 1982, p 271.

49. American Thoracic Society: Standards for the diagnosis and care of patients with chronic obstructive pulmonary disease (COPD) and asthma. American Review of Respiratory Diseases 136(1):225–244, 1987.

50. Relinger, J et al: Utilization of adverse rapid smoking in groups: Efficacy of treatment and maintenance procedures. J Consult Clin Psychol 45(2):245–249, 1977.

51. Peters, J and Lim, V: Smoking cessation techniques. In: Hodgkin, J, Zorn, E, and Connors, G (eds): Pulmonary Rehabilitation: Guidelines to Success. Butterworth Publishers, Boston, 1984, pp 91–120.

52. Tang, J, Law, M, and Wald, N: How effective is nicotine replacement therapy in helping people to stop smoking? BMJ 308:21–26, 1994.

53. Fiore, M et al: Tobacco dependence and the nicotine patch: Clinical guidelines for effective use. JAMA 268:2687–2694, 1992.

54. Fielding, J: Smoking effects and control: Part I. N Engl J Med 313(8):491–498, 1985.

55. Harris, M and Rothberg, C: A self-control approach to reducing smoking. Psychol Rep 31:165–166, 1972.

56. Russell, M, Raw, M, and Jarvis, M: Clinical use of nicotine chewing gum. BMJ 280(6231):1599–1602, 1980.

57. Horn, D and Waingrow, S: Some dimensions of a model for smoking behavior change. Am J Public Health (Supp 56)12:21–26, 1966.

58. Tecklin, J: Pediatric Physical Therapy. Lippincott, Philadelphia, 1989, p 165.

59. American Thoracic Society: Pulmonary Rehabilitation. American Review of Respiratory Diseases 124:663–666, 1981.

APPENDIX A

Patient Program Application Forms*

Dear

Enclosed are the preliminary application forms that we discussed via telephone. Please complete the enclosed forms as indicated (x).

_____ Medical and Personal History Form
_____ Dietary Profile Form
_____ Insurance Information Form
_____ Medical Release Authorization Form

These forms must be completed by you and returned to _____ before your therapy can be initiated. Referral forms will be forwarded to your personal physician, cardiologist, and/or other medical specialist for specific medical information that we require.

Upon receiving your forms and the physician referral forms, we will contact you to schedule an orientation/observation session. Instructions for the session are enclosed in this mailing. When you are contacted to schedule your orientation/observation session, record the date and time of your appointment on this form.

_____ offers complete rehabilitative services. Whether you are a patient (cardiac, diabetic, arthritic, postsurgical, etc.) requiring a prescribed rehabilitation program, or a person seeking help in beginning an exercise and/or weight-control program, the staff works as a team to design and supervise an individualized program for you. Our staff of physicians, exercise and medical physiologists, registered nurses, physical therapists, nutritionists, and other health professionals work together to promote health through lifestyle modification and applied education.

The specific needs of each individual are considered; therefore, the appropriate treatment, as well as the cost of treatment will vary among patients. Your medical/health insurance will pay for the major portion of your treatment; however,

---

*Courtesy of Bio-Energetiks Rehabilitation, Prospect, Pa.

the percentage of reimbursement is dependent upon individual insurance policies. Transportation costs incurred during treatment are also tax-deductible.

Please do not hesitate to contact me if you have any questions regarding our services or the completion of the enclosed forms.

Sincerely,

Director

PLEASE COMPLETE AND RETURN TO:

Medical and Personal History Forms: PLEASE PRINT

NAME: _____ AGE ____ SEX ____ BIRTHDATE ____/____/____

I. Conditions which you have had/or currently have:

	Yes	No	Unknown	Date Occurred
Allergies	___	___	_____	_____
Specify			_____	
Congenital heart defect	___	___	_____	_____
Rheumatic fever	___	___	_____	_____
Heart murmur	___	___	_____	_____
Vascular diseases:	___	___	_____	_____
Coronary artery disease	___	___	_____	_____
Artery diseases, other	___	___	_____	_____
Varicose veins	___	___	_____	_____
Leg cramps (claudication)	___	___	_____	_____
Phlebitis	___	___	_____	_____
Heart attack(s)	___	___	_____	_____
High blood pressure	___	___	_____	_____
Hyperlipidemia (elevated cholesterol, triglycerides)	___	___	_____	_____
Obesity (more than 20 lb above ideal weight)	___	___	_____	_____
Diabetes	___	___	_____	_____
Gout	___	___	_____	_____
Hernia(s)	___	___	_____	_____
Epilepsy	___	___	_____	_____
Arthritis	___	___	_____	_____
Specify (knees, elbows, spine, etc.)			_____	
Injuries to:				
Back	___	___	_____	_____
Muscles	___	___	_____	_____
Bones	___	___	_____	_____
Joints	___	___	_____	_____
Lung disease	___	___	_____	_____
Kidney disease	___	___	_____	_____
Liver disease	___	___	_____	_____
Psychological/emotional problems	___	___	_____	

II. Operations: Date Occurred

1. _____ _____
2. _____ _____
3. _____ _____
4. _____ _____
5. _____ _____

III. Other medical problems:

_____

_____

_____

IV. Current medications & dosages:
          MEDICATIONS   DOSAGES

_____   _____
_____   _____
_____   _____
_____   _____
_____   _____
_____   _____

V. Risk Factors:
   A. <u>Family History</u>: Have any of your relatives had?

                              Yes   No   Unknown
      Heart attacks   ___   ___   _____
         Specify relative   _____
      High blood pressure   ___   ___   _____
         Specify relative   _____
      Hyperlipidemia   ___   ___   _____
         Specify relative   _____
      Heart operations   ___   ___   _____
         Specify relative   _____
      Diabetes   ___   ___   _____
         Specify relative   _____
      Other diseases   _____

   B. <u>Smoking</u>: Did you smoke in the past? _____ Age when you started smoking
      _____ Do you smoke now? _____ If you have stopped smoking, when
      did you and why? _____
      _____
      Currently smoking: cigarettes   cigars   pipe   (please circle)
      Number per day? _____ .

   C. <u>Diet</u>: Present weight _____ lb   Weight 1 year ago _____ lb
      Weight at age 21 _____ lb
      Are you dieting presently? _____ Why? _____
      What type of diet? _____

   D. <u>Employment/Occupation</u>:
      Current employment status:
      Full time _____   Retired _____   Unemployed _____
      Part time _____   Disabled _____
      Occupation _____ Number of years _____
      Employer _____
      Do you plan to return to this job or continue in the occupation? _____
      Physical activity required in occupation:

                              Almost All   (½)+   (½)   −(½)   Almost None
      Time spent sitting   _____   ___   ___   ___   _____
      Time spent walking   _____   ___   ___   ___   _____
      Time spent standing   _____   ___   ___   ___   _____
      Time spent standing/sitting
         with arm work   _____   ___   ___   ___   _____
      Lifting or carrying heavy objects: Seldom   Sometimes   Often
                                        (please circle one)
                              Approximate weight range ____ to ____ lb

Transportation to and from work: (please circle one of the following)
   car   bus   railroad   ferry   subway   walking
If walking to work: (please circle one)
   Less than 1 block   1–2 blocks   3–4 blocks   5–9 blocks
   10–19 blocks   1 mile   2 miles+
Working hours per week: (please circle one)
Less than 25   25–35   36–40   41–50   51+

E. <u>Physical Activity</u>:
In addition to your occupation, do you exercise on a regular basis? _____
If so, list your activities:

ACTIVITY	NUMBER OF TIMES PER WEEK
_____	_____
_____	_____
	_____

Have you previously participated in an exercise class or program? _____
If so, describe the activities you performed: _____
_____

F. <u>Stress</u>:

Are you:	Yes	No
Frustrated when waiting in line, <u>often</u> in a hurry to complete work or keep appointments, <u>easily</u> angered, irritable?	____	____
Impatient when waiting, <u>occasionally</u> hurried, or <u>occasionally</u> moody?	____	____
Comfortable when waiting, <u>seldom</u> rushed, and easygoing?	____	____

PLEASE COMPLETE AND RETURN TO:

Name _____

Dietary Information Form

1. Are you on a specialized diet at this time? _____ yes _____ no
2. If so, what type of diet? (e.g., low salt, low fat, number of calories, etc.)
   _____
3. Who recommended this diet? _____
4. Have you recently gained or lost weight? _____ yes _____ no
5. If yes, how much gained? _____ lost? _____
6. Describe your use of salt. _____
7. Check all of the following commercially prepared foods which you use:
   _____ Canned, dehydrated, or frozen soups or stews
   _____ Canned or frozen casseroles
   _____ Frozen dinners
   _____ Pretzels, chips, or snack crackers
   _____ Fast-food chain foods
8. Do you eat meals out frequently (3 times per week or more)? _____
9. Name any foods you *cannot* eat. _____
10. What foods would be particularly hard for you to give up? _____
    _____

Daily Dietary Habits

List foods and beverages commonly consumed. Include alcohol, sugar, milk, or cream
used in beverages, butter or margarine used, and dressing used on salads.

Breakfast:

Lunch:

Dinner:

Snacks:

Food Preference: <u>Check</u> the foods that you eat almost every day. <u>Circle</u> the foods that
                 you eat at least once a week.

Milk and Dairy Products:
___ whole milk   ___ 2% milk   ___ skim milk   ___ buttermilk
___ evap. milk   ___ cream   ___ cheese   ___ prc. cheese and spreads
___ cottage cheese   ___ yogurt   ___ ice cream   ___ low-fat cottage cheese

Vegetables/Legumes:
___ green and yellow beans   ___ carrots   ___ lettuce and salad greens
___ beets   ___ corn   ___ broccoli, brussel sprouts
___ sweet potatoes   ___ peas   ___ lima beans
___ squash   ___ potatoes   ___ cabbage
___ tomatoes   ___ baked beans   ___ dried beans

Fruits and Juices:
___ citrus fruits   ___ citrus juice   ___ pineapple   ___ pineapple juice
___ apples   ___ peaches   ___ bananas   ___ apple juice
___ grapes   ___ grape juice   ___ cherries
___ berries   ___ prune juice   ___ plums

Breads/Cereals/Pasta:
___ cereal, dry, unsweet.   ___ cereal, dry, sweet.   ___ cereal, cooked
___ muffins   ___ bread   ___ rice
___ biscuits   ___ crackers   ___ rolls
___ macaroni   ___ spaghetti   ___ noodles

Meat/Fish/Poultry/Eggs:
___ eggs   ___ beef   ___ bacon   ___ shellfish
___ liver   ___ pork   ___ frankfurters
___ cold cuts   ___ poultry   ___ fish

Fats/Oils/Snacks:
___ salad dressing   ___ pastries   ___ peanuts and other nuts
___ margarine   ___ cookies   ___ potato chips and other chips
___ butter   ___ candy   ___ popcorn
___ oil   ___ pie   ___ cake
___ peanut butter

PLEASE COMPLETE AND RETURN TO:

Insurance Information Form

Patient's Name _____ Date ____/____/____
        (Last, First, MI)
Address _____ Phone: Home _____
_____   Work _____
                        Zip Code
Patient's Date of Birth _____
Insurance Company _____
Address _____
Telephone Number _____
Insured's Name _____ Insured's Date of Birth _____
        Last, First, MI   SS# ____-____-____
Insured's Employer _____ Occupation _____
Insured's relationship to patient ____ self ____ spouse ____ child ____ other
Insurance ID Number _____
Group Name or Number _____
Are you covered by any other plans which provide medical benefits or services?
____ yes ____ no
If "yes," list all other insurance companies or service plans providing coverage:
Company Name _____ Insured's Name _____
Company Address _____ ID Number _____
_____ Group Name or Number _____
                        Zip Code
Referring Physician: _____
Most recent diagnosis/symptoms   Date illness/injury
1. _____   _____
2. _____   _____
3. _____   _____
4. _____   _____
Date of first treatment _____
I certify that the above information is correct to the best of my knowledge.
_____
                        SIGNATURE

PLEASE COMPLETE AND RETURN TO:

Medical Records Release Authorization

TO: _____

_____
(Physician's Address)

I HEREBY AUTHORIZE AND REQUEST YOU TO RELEASE TO:

Records and/or pertinent information in your possession concerning my
illness/treatment.

Name _____ Date ___/___/___

Address _____

Signature: _____
(If relative, state relationship)

Witness: _____

Instructions for Orientation/Observation Sessions

Name _____

Appointment _____ _____ _____
                        Month   Date   Time

Clothing

Bring soft-soled shoes, e.g., tennis or walking shoes, socks, cotton shorts and a cotton shirt; and wear no unnecessary jewelry. (If you are more comfortable in slacks, feel free to wear them).

DO NOT WEAR A NYLON SHIRT.

Day of the Orientation/Observation Session:
1. Do not eat for at least 2 hours preceding the session.
2. Do not vary your medications (regular).
3. Do not ingest coffee, tea, coke, or other stimulants.
4. Do not engage in excessive physical activity.
5. Do not ingest alcohol or other depressants.
6. Do not smoke for at least 2 hours preceding the session.

The procedures will take approximately 1 hour and are not particularly stressful or uncomfortable to most people. You should try to remain as relaxed as possible during all of the procedures.

Referring Physician Forms*

To _____ M.D.

We have been contacted by _____
concerning participation in one of our rehabilitation programs.

The enclosed form must be completed and returned to us prior to the initiation of therapy. Your recommendations concerning your patient's participation in the program will be adhered to completely. Please do not hesitate to contact us should you have any questions regarding your patient's therapy.

Thank you for your time and consideration.

_____

*Courtesy of Bio-Energetiks Rehabilitation, Prospect, Pa.

PLEASE COMPLETE AND RETURN TO:

Referring Physician Form

Patient's Name _____ Age _____
Etiology: _____
Diagnosis(es): ____ _____
Medications: _____
Blood Analysis: Date _____ CBC: Hgb __ HCT __ WBC __ Diff __
                      Lipids: Trig __ Chol __ HDL __ LDL __ HDL/Chol __
Urinalysis: Date _____ _   Alb _____   Glucose _____   Micro _____ _
Other Tests (please attach findings): ____ _____
Treadmill Report (if applicable):
     Date of test   ____/____/____   Protocol ____ _____
     Resting heart rate _____   Resting BP _____/_____
     MAX heart rate _____ bpm   MAX BP _____/_____
     Maximum METs _____
12-Lead ECG Interpretation/Comments (Rhythm/abnormalities): _____
_____
_____

STAT and PRN Orders
     1. Nitroglycerin 1/150 gr. SL PRN for chest pain.
     2. Lidocaine 50 mg. bolus IVP for PVCs 6–7/min. or V-bigeminy or V-tachycardia.
     3. Atropine 0.6 mg. IVP q 2–3 hrs. PRN for heart rate 40/min.
     4. Oxygen Intranasal 2–6 liters/min. PRN.
     5. Hang 250 D_5W and run at KVO rate.
     6. Defibrillate for ventricular fibrillation:
        Start at: 200–300 joules delivered energy; if no results 360 joules delivered
          energy.
     7. Additional (specify): _____
_____
_____
_____

                                   _____, M.D.
                                       Signature
                    Date ____/____/____

Physician Re-Referral Form

Patient's Name _____ Date ____/____/____
Address _____ Telephone _____
Date of conducted laboratory evaluation or exercise session episode _____
_____
_____
_____

YOU RECOMMEND:
_____ 1. Discontinue participation in the cardiac rehabilitation program.
_____ 2. Temporarily discontinue participation in the cardiac rehabilitation program
         while further investigation procedures are conducted. Probable date of renewed
         participation _____ .
_____ 3. Continue participation in the cardiac rehabilitation program while further
         investigative procedures are conducted. Probable date of completion of investi-
         gative procedures _____ .
_____ 4. Continue participation in the cardiac rehabilitation program. No further
         investigative procedures to be conducted.

Physician's Name _____ Date ____/____/____

Physician's Signature _____

Informed Consent Forms*

Graded Exercise Tolerance Test Informed Consent

I, the undersigned, authorize the _____ Diagnostic Laboratory to administer and conduct the Exercise Tolerance Test. This test is designed to measure my fitness for work and/or sport; to determine the presence or absence of clinically significant heart disease; and/or to evaluate the effectiveness of my current therapy.

I understand that the test will require that I either walk on a motor-driven treadmill or pedal a bicycle ergometer. During the performance of physical activity, my electrocardiogram will be monitored and my blood pressure will be measured at periodic intervals and recorded. Exercise will be progressively increased until I attain a predetermined endpoint corresponding to a moderate work level, or become distressed in any way, or develop an abnormal response the administrator of the test considers significant, whichever of the above occurs first.

Every effort will be made to conduct the test in such a way as to minimize discomfort and risk. However, I understand that in performing diagnostic tests on individuals with pre-existing medical problems (diagnosed or undiagnosed) that there are potential risks associated with such tests. In particular, an exercise tolerance test may elicit episodes of transient light-headedness, fainting, chest discomfort, or leg cramps, and very rarely heart attack or death may occur. I further understand that emergency equipment, drugs, and trained personnel are available to provide usual and customary care in unusual situations that may arise including: basic and advanced life support and transportation of a patient by ambulance to the nearest hospital.

Questions: _____

_____

Reply: _____

_____

_____   ___/___/___   _____   ___/___/___
       Witness   Date   Signature of Patient   Date

_____

*Courtesy of Bio-Energetiks Rehabilitation, Prospect, Pa.

452

Informed Consent/Release

1. Explanation of Program

You will be participating in a rehabilitation program that will include physical exercise, nutritional counseling, and patient education and may include stress management/relaxation therapy. The intensity and type of exercise you will perform will be based on your cardiovascular response to an initial graded exercise tolerance test that will be performed at the _____ clinic or by your personal physician within 1 month prior to beginning your exercise therapy. You may also be given other tests as needed to estimate body composition, desirable weight, lung function, various physiological parameters, personality traits, and stress levels. You will be given instructions regarding the amount and kind of regular exercise you should do. Exercise treatment visits will be available on a regularly scheduled basis. Your exercise prescription may be adjusted by the staff depending on your progress. You will be given the opportunity for re-evaluation at regularly scheduled intervals after beginning the rehabilitation program. Other re-evaluations may be recommended as needed. Progress reports will be sent to your personal physician on a regular basis.

2. Monitoring

Your blood pressure will be monitored regularly as part of your program. You will be taught to monitor your own pulse rate before, during, and after each exercise session. In addition, ECG monitoring will be performed as a routine part of your program and according to individual needs.

3. Risks and Discomforts

In rehabilitating individuals with pre-existing medical problems (diagnosed or undiagnosed), there exists the possibility of certain physiological changes occurring during the exercise treatment visits. These changes include abnormal blood pressures, fainting, and irregular heart beats, and in rare instances a heart attack or death may occur. We emphasize that every effort will be made to minimize the danger associated with the aforementioned changes by review of referring physician information, preliminary examination, and through observations of your exercise sessions. Emergency equipment, drugs, and trained personnel are available to provide basic life support at times when unusual situations arise. A registered nurse, physician, or emergency medical technician are available to provide advanced life support within a reasonable period of time. If required, patients may be transported by ambulance to the nearest hospital.

4. Benefits to be Expected

Participation in the rehabilitation program may not benefit you directly in any way. The results obtained may help in evaluating the types of activities in which you might engage safely in your daily life. No assurance can be given that the rehabilitation program will increase your functional capacity, although widespread research and experience indicates that improvement is usually achieved.

5. Responsibility of the Participant

To gain expected benefits you must give priority to <u>regular attendance and adherence to prescribed amounts of intensity, duration, frequency, and type of activity.</u>
To assure the safest exercise environment:

DO NOT: A. Withhold any information pertinent to symptoms from the professional staff.

            B. Exceed target heart rate.

            C. Exercise when you do not feel well.

            D. Exercise within 2 hours after eating.

            E. Exercise after drinking alcoholic beverages.

            F. Expose yourself to extremes in temperature; e.g., hot shower after exercising, saunas, steam baths, and similar extreme temperatures, as well as iced or hot drinks.

            G. Undertake isometric or straining exercise.

DO: A. Report any unusual symptom you experience before, during, or after exercise.

            B. Before leaving the site, check out with a member of the staff.

6. Use of Medical Records

The information obtained during evaluation performed at the clinic and/or while I am a participant in the rehabilitation program will be treated as privileged and confidential. It is not to be released or revealed to any person except my referring physician without my written consent. The information obtained, however, may be used for statistical analysis or scientific purpose with my right to privacy retained.

7. Inquiries

Any questions about the rehabilitation program are welcome. If you have doubts or questions, please ask us for further explanation.

8. Freedom of Consent

Your permission to engage in this rehabilitation program is voluntary. You are free to deny consent if you so desire, both now and at any point in the program.

I acknowledge that I have read this form in its entirety or it has been read to me and that I understand the rehabilitation program in which I will be engaged. I accept the rules and regulations set forth. I consent to participate in the _____ rehabilitation program.

Questions: _____

Response: _____

9. Release

I have read the foregoing and I understand it. Any questions that have occurred to me have been answered to my satisfaction. Therefore, for guidance and supervision in exercise therapy, life-style change counseling, and/or diet therapy, I hereby for myself, my heirs, Executors and Administrators, waive and release any and all rights and claims for damages I may now and hereafter have against the staff of the _____ Rehabilitation Program, its Agents, Representatives or Assigns and Consultants.

_____	_____	_____
Signature of Patient	Signature of Director	Signature of Witness
Date _____	Date _____	Date _____

APPENDIX D

Emergency Procedures, Medications, and Basic Emergency Equipment*

Standing Emergency Orders

The following emergency procedures have been adapted to make these procedures more practical to the real environment of the prehospital setting and are presented as guidelines only. Keep in mind that the prehospital setting is very different from the hospital setting in terms of the advanced surgical procedures used in care of cardiac and other trauma patients. Also, it should be noted that there is more than one acceptable way to manage most situations. Clinicians must seek advice from the medical director as to how emergency situations might best be handled in specific areas of the country.

General Procedures

The following orders delegate authority to the nurse to initiate emergency and resuscitative treatment in the absence of a physician. All patients participating in rehabilitation programs provided by _____ shall be covered under these orders—with or without a written order by the physician.

The following is the basic outline for all procedures and medications covered by this policy:

A. Initial response to emergency
   1. Evacuation of the exercise area. When an emergency situation arises, the staff shall immediately order evacuation of the exercise area. Patients should exit to the hallway area and proceed to cool-down. Patients should remain outside the exercise area until the compromised patient has been safely transported out of the building.
   2. Notify the _____ ambulance authority. Use the emergency message posted by the phone.
   3. Notify the physician in charge.

---

*Courtesy of Bio-Energetiks Rehabilitation, Prospect, Pa.

B. Initiate CPR, if indicated, until a monitor/defibrillator is available. All nursing personnel must be certified in basic life support (BLS) as described by the AHA or Red Cross. Certification must be current and evidence of certification must be on file at each clinic.

C. Defibrillation: Only for pulseless ventricular tachycardia (VT) or ventricular fibrillation (VF):
Start at 200 joules; if no change, 200 to 300 joules; if no change, 360 joules, maximal output. Do not perform CPR between shocks. Quickly assess cardiac rhythm on the monitor between each defibrillation to assess for further need for defibrillation.

D. Initiating IV therapy: All patients in a life-threatening situation must have a route whereby IV therapy can be administered if necessary. The nurse may start an IV of 0.9 normal saline solution (NSS).

E. ECG: In an emergency or unstable situation, for example, patient experiencing persistent chest pain, obtain a 12-lead ECG and monitor cardiac rhythm continuously PRN.

F. Oxygen: Give intranasal O_2, PRN 2 L/min rate. To increase flow rate, notify physician.

Procedures for Specific Situations Including Administration of Medications

A. Hypotension: Systolic BP <90 mm Hg
                    Symptomatic HR >60 bpm
  1. Elevate feet
  2. Notify physician
  3. Obtain ECG

B. Fainting
  1. Lay patient in lateral recumbent position
  2. Use ammonia ampules
  3. Give O_2 PRN
  4. Notify physician
  5. Obtain ECG

C. Symptomatic Bradyarrhythmias: Ventricular rate <60 bpm
                    Signs (low BP, shock, pulmonary congestion, CHF, acute MI)
                    Symptoms (chest pain, SOB, decreased consciousness)
  1. Notify ambulance and physician
  2. Assure adequate airway and ventilation; O_2 PRN
  3. IV therapy
  4. If HR <60 bpm, give atropine: 0.5 to 1.0 mg IV bolus up to 0.04 mg/kg. Transcutaneous pacing (TCP) is class I, if available.
  5. Obtain ECG
     If circulatory collapse and loss of consciousness occur, proceed to BLS measures appropriate to shock and/or other arrhythmia.

D. Asystole: Carotid pulse = Absent
                    Confirm asystole in more than one lead as the rhythm may be VF in another lead; in which case the patient should be promptly defibrillated.
  1. Begin BLS, notify ambulance and physician
  2. Obtain ECG and give O_2
  3. Immediate consideration of TCP

4. If no response:
   a. IV therapy
   b. Intubate
   c. Give epinephrine: 1 mg IV push, may repeat every 3 to 5 min.
   d. Give atropine: 1 mg IV, repeat every 3 to 5 min up to 0.04 mg/kg
   e. Sodium bicarbonate: 1 mEq/kg is class I if patient has known preexisting hyperkalemia.
5. If a change in cardiac rhythm occurs, proceed to appropriate cardiac arrhythmia protocol.
6. Continue the following sequence if asystole persists:
   a. Epinephrine: 0.5 mg (5 mL) q 5 min IV bolus
   b. Atropine: 0.5 mg IV bolus q 5 min to maximum 2 mg
7. If a change in rhythm occurs, proceed to appropriate arrhythmia protocol
8. Obtain ECG

E. Symptomatic PVCs: New onset of PVCs, PVCs >6/min, R on T phenomenon, change in mental status with symptomatic PVCs, salvos
1. Notify physician
2. Assure adequate airway and ventilation, O_2 PRN
3. IV therapy
4. Obtain ECG strips, 12-lead if possible
5. Give lidocaine: 50 to 100 mg IV bolus: dose (1 mg/kg)
6. Begin lidocaine drip, premixed 2 g/500 mL D5/W at 2 to 3 mg/min (30 to 45 mL/hr) (30 to 45 mcg tts/min)
7. Additional 50 mg bolus (0.5 mg/kg) may be given q 5 min if necessary to total of 225 mg
8. Increase infusion by 1 mg/min with additional bolus to a maximum of 4 mg/min (60 mL/hr) (60 mcg tts/min)
9. Watch for signs of toxicity—slurred speech, altered consciousness, muscle twitches, seizures
10. If change in rhythm occurs, follow appropriate cardiac rhythm sequence

F. PVCs due to bradycardia: Ventricular rate <60 bpm
                            Patient symptomatic
                            Systolic BP <90 mm Hg
1. Notify physician and ambulance
2. Assure adequate airway and ventilation
3. Give atropine: 0.5 mg IV bolus, repeat q 5 min to total dosage of 2 mg
4. If ineffective in increasing HR to >60 bpm and overriding PVCs, start isuprel drip. Mix 1 mg in 250 mL D5/W (4 mcg/mL): titrate between 2 to 20 mcg/min to maintain HR 60–100 bpm and override PVCs. Isuprel is Class IIb or Class III at higher doses and is a last choice treatment due to tendency to cause myocardial ischemia.

G. Ventricular Tachycardia: Patient conscious and symptomatic
1. Notify ambulance and physician
2. Provide adequate airway and ventilation and give O_2 PRN
3. IV therapy
4. Obtain ECG strips and 12 lead if possible
5. If HR >150 bpm with compromised BP Cardiovert 50 joules
6. Give lidocaine: 50 to 100 mg IV bolus; dose (1 mg/kg)
7. Begin lidocaine drip premixed 2 g/500 mL D5/W (Start at 2 mg/min, 30 mL/hr)

8. Additional 50 mg bolus (0.5 mg/kg) may be given q 5 min if necessary to a total of 225 mg
9. Increase infusion by 1 mg/min with additional bolus to a maximum of 4 mg/min
10. Watch for CNS signs of possible lidocaine toxicity—slurred speech, altered consciousness, muscle twitching, seizures
11. If change in rhythm occurs, follow appropriate cardiac rhythm sequence

H. Ventricular Tachycardia/Ventricular Fibrillation: Patient unconscious
   1. Notify ambulance and physician
   2. Obtain ECG strips
   3. Witnessed and monitored: defibrillate 200 joules; if no response, 200 to 300 joules; if no response, 360 joules
   4. Initiate CPR; intubate; obtain IV access
   5. Give epinephrine: 1 mg IV push, may repeat every 3 to 5 min
   6. Perform CPR for 30 to 60 seconds
   7. Defibrillate 360 joules
   8. Administer class IIa medications if persistent VT
   9. Defibrillate 360 joules after each dose of medication (drug-shock, drug-shock)

I. Supraventricular Tachycardia: Patient symptomatic, for example, change in mental status, systolic BP <90 mm Hg
   1. Notify physician
   2. Assure adequate airway, ventilation and O_2 PRN
   3. Obtain ECG
   4. Attempt to convert rhythm by instructing patient to perform Valsalva maneuver
   5. Perform carotid massage (under direct physician supervision only)
   6. IV therapy

Medications

1. Atroprine sulfate: 0.1 mg/mL in 10-mL syringe
   Dosage: 0.5 mg–1.0 mg = 5 to 10 mL
   Repeat at 5-min intervals to achieve desired HR generally, do not exceed 2 mg
2. Dopamine: 200 mg in 5-mL ampule
   Dosage: 200 mg in 250 mL D5/W = 800 mcg/mL
   Infusion: 2 to 10 mcg/kg/min
3. Epinephrine: 1:10,000 solution, 0.1 mg/mL in 10-mL syringe
   Dosage: 0.5 mg to 1.0 mg = 5 to 10 mL IV
        Repeat dose q 5 min PRN in cardiac arrest
   Infusion: 1 mg in D5/W (4 mcg/mL in 250 mL; 2 mcg/mL in 500 mL)
        Rate: 1 mcg/min for maintenance of BP
4. Isoproterenol (Isuprel): 0.2 mg/mL in 5-mL ampule
   Dosage: 1 mg in D5/W (4 mcg/mL in 250 mL; 2 mcg/mL in 500 mL)
   Infusion: 2–20 mcg/min; titrate; beware of PVCs
5. Lidocaine: 1% (10 mg/mL; 100 mg/10 mL) and 2% (20 mg/mL; 100 mg/5 mL)
        for IV bolus
        for infusion after bolus: 4% (40 mg/mL; 1 g/25 mL)
   Infusion: 1 to 4 mg/min

For breakthrough ventricular ectopy, additional 50 mg bolus q 5 min to suppress ectopy—total 225 mg; increase drip: 4 mg/min

6. Procainamide: 100 mg/mL in 10 mL ampule for IV bolus
                  500 mg/mL in 2 mL ampules for infusion p bolus

Dosage: 20 mg/min until:
   a. Dysrhythmia suppressed
   b. Hypotension ensues
   c. QRS widens by 50%
   d. Total of 1 g given

All Orders and Medication Instructions Approved

_____ M.D _____

Medical Director   Date

_____

Clinic

Basic Emergency Equipment

Portable cart
Automatic external defibrillator (AED)
IV lines, needles, syringes
Ambu bags
Airways and O_2 tank
ECG equipment
Stethoscope
Sphygmomanometer
Pulse oximeter

APPENDIX E

Flexibility Exercises*

Stretching I

Discontinue any exercise that causes you pain or discomfort.
Do not hold your breath—breathe slowly and deeply.
Stretch slowly and gently—no bouncing.
Try not to strain. Relax while you stretch.

1. Wall Stretch

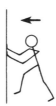

Stand facing wall with feet a shoulder-width apart. Take one step forward with right leg, bending knee. Keep back heel on floor. Place hands a shoulder-width apart on the wall for support. Hold. Repeat with other leg.

2. Stand and Reach

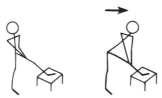

Using a bench or stool, place one foot up on bench, keeping leg straight. Slowly extend arms down leg. Hold. Repeat with other leg.

*Courtesy of Bio-Energetiks Rehabilitation, Prospect, Pa.

3. Standing Foot Hold

Stand with left hand on chair or wall for support. Bend right leg and grasp foot with right hand. Gently pull foot toward body. Repeat with other leg.

4. Groin Stretch

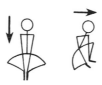

Sit on mat with feet together. Place hands on ankles. Gently pull them in close to hips. Slowly bend forward, keeping back straight. Relax. Repeat.

5. Straddle

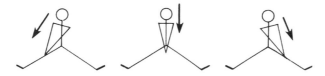

Sit on mat with legs apart extended straight out. Extend arms out, reaching toward right foot. Return to center. Reach toward left foot. Return to center and reach forward. Relax. Keep back straight.

6. Spinal Twist

Sitting on mat, extend right leg to front, and place left foot on mat on other side of right knee. Reach over left leg with right arm. Use left hand behind you for balance. Turn upper body to left, looking over left shoulder. Repeat to other side.

7. Curl Stretch

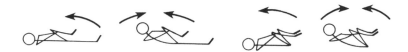

Lie on back on mat with legs extended. Bring right knee up to chest. Hold hands just below knee. As you stretch slowly, bring head up toward knee. Relax. Repeat with other knee. Relax. Bring both knees up and slowly curl head up. Relax.

8. Neck Limber

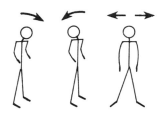

Seated or standing, pull head down toward chest and hold for 10 seconds. Return to starting position and then pull head back and hold for 10 seconds. Repeat for left and right side and as many angles in between as you wish.

9. Arm Circle

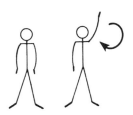

Seated or standing, begin with right arm, depressing shoulder down toward floor with arm extended. Continue to raise arm slowly up toward ceiling and around toward back. Keep arm extended and stretch throughout movement. Repeat with other arm.

Flexibility and Muscular Strength and Endurance Data Sheet

Name _____

Kinetic Activities

| | Flexibility Exercises | | | | | | Muscular Strength and Endurance | | | | | | |
Date	Calf	Hamstring	Quads	Groin	Trunk	Shoulder	Neck	1	2	3	4	5	6	BP

Index